Dr. N. M. Foley
Dept. of Respiratory Medicine
Royal United Hospital
Bath
BA1 3NG

Noninvasive Ventilation
Second Edition

European Respiratory Monograph 41
November 2008

Editor in Chief
K. Larsson

This book is one in a series of European Respiratory Monographs. Each individual issue provides a comprehensive overview of one specific clinical area of respiratory health, communicating information about the most advanced techniques and systems needed to investigate it. It provides factual and useful scientific detail, drawing on specific case studies and looking into the diagnosis and management of individual patients. Previously published titles in this series are listed at the back of this book with details of how they can be purchased.

Noninvasive Ventilation
Second Edition

Edited by
J-F. Muir, N. Ambrosino and A.K. Simonds

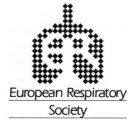

European Respiratory
Society

Published by European Respiratory Society Journals Ltd ©2008
November 2008
Hardback ISBN: 978-1-904097-61-7
Paperback ISBN: 978-1-904097-62-4
ISSN: 1025-448x
Printed by Latimer Trend & Co. Ltd, Plymouth, UK

Business matters (enquiries, advertisement bookings) should be addressed to: European Respiratory
Society Journals Ltd, Publications Office, 442 Glossop Road, Sheffield, S10 2PX, UK.
Tel: 44 114 2672860; Fax: 44 114 2665064; E-mail: Monograph@ersj.org.uk

The European Respiratory Monograph

Number 41

November 2008

CONTENTS

The Guest Editors

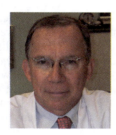 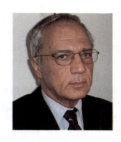 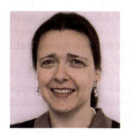

J-F. Muir N. Ambrosino A.K. Simonds

The Guest Editors

J-F. Muir is a Professor of Pulmonology and Head of both the Respiratory Diseases Dept and Respiratory Intensive Care unit at the Rouen University Hospital, France. He has a special interest in acute and chronic mechanical ventilation and sleep studies.

N. Ambrosino's research activity has been devoted to: chronic obstructive pulmonary disease, respiratory critical care, pulmonary rehabilitation and home respiratory care. He has also contributed to the development of the use of noninvasive mechanical ventilation techniques in acute and chronic respiratory failure with several clinical trials and original experimental studies. He was the former head of the Pulmonary Rehabilitation Working Group of the European Respiratory Society, and he currently sits on the editorial boards of several international journals.

A.K. Simonds is a Consultant in Respiratory Medicine at Royal Brompton Hospital, London. She runs the Home Ventilation service for adults and children and has a long term clinical and research interest in acute and chronic: noninvasive ventilation, new ventilatory modes, neuromuscular disorders, sleep disordered breathing, endstage lung disease, palliative care and ethics.

Preface

The view on treatment of patients with severe respiratory disorders in general, and of patients with severe chronic obstructive pulmonary disease in particular, has changed during the past decades. The former, often nihilistic, approach has changed into an attitude towards more active engagement in, and treatment of, severely ill patients. In this context, noninvasive ventilation (NIV) has been brought into focus as a valuable alternative treatment, both in acute respiratory failure and chronic respiratory diseases. The growing interest in NIV has been reflected in the *European Respiratory Monograph* (*ERM*) through the years and the present issue on NIV is a comprehensive review of the field. It updates areas that were covered in the previous 2001 *ERM* edition and adds a number of new aspects on how NIV may be an option in the treatment of patients with primary respiratory and nonrespiratory disorders. In the current issue there are new chapters on treatment of acute and chronic respiratory failure in obese patients. Acute respiratory failure in immunocompromised patients has been given its own chapter and there are specific chapters on the use of NIV in pre-hospital patients and in palliative care. Furthermore, treatment of cardiogenic pulmonary oedema with NIV has a devoted chapter.

The present updated and extended *ERM* on NIV, written and edited by the most appreciated experts in the field, is a must for every clinician who makes contact with patients who suffer from acute or chronic respiratory failure, in whom NIV may be considered. This issue will certainly constitute a highly appreciated source of information and knowledge, both for clinicians and scientists.

K. Larsson
Editor in Chief

INTRODUCTION

J-F. Muir*, N. Ambrosino[#,¶], A.K. Simonds[+]

*Pneumology and Respiratory Intensive Care Unit, Rouen University Hospital, Rouen, France, [#]Pulmonary Diseases and Respiratory Intensive Care Unit, Cardio-Thoracic Dept, University Hospital Pisa, Pisa, and [¶]Weaning and Pulmonary Rehabilitation Unit, Auxilium Vitae, Volterra, Italy, and [+]Academic Unit of Sleep and Breathing, Royal Brompton Hospital, London, UK.

Correspondence: J-F. Muir, Service de Pneumologie et Unité de Soins Intensifs Respiratoires, Hôpital de Bois-Guillaume, CHU de Rouen, 76031 Rouen, France. Fax: 33 232889000; E-mail: jean-francois. muir@chu-rouen.fr

In August 2001, the first edition of a *European Respiratory Monograph* (*ERM*) devoted to noninvasive mechanical ventilation (NIV) was published [1]. Now is a good time for a second edition, in order to take into account and consolidate views on the numerous developments that have occurred on a variety fronts.

NIV is not a recent concept, having been developed in the 19th century. Subsequent milestones date from the 1950s, with the iron lung in the polio era; the 1960s, with the first attempts at mask ventilation; the 1970s, when mouth ventilation was used increasingly; and the 1980s, when nasal interfaces improved and pressure support ventilation emerged. The 1990s and the first decade of the 21st century have highlighted the importance of pressure support ventilation and of sleep investigation in respiratory medicine, and have demonstrated the changing profile of the underlying causes of chronic and acute respiratory failure, the disease of this century, in particular the growing burden of morbid obesity.

The current *ERM* has been thoroughly renewed and rewritten. We hope that it will afford medical teams daily confronted with acute and chronic respiratory failure a substantial overview of the new aspects of NIV, including pathophysiological indications, technology and monitoring. It is essential that these developments are understood if, over time, we want to improve survival and also optimise ventilator–patient interaction and health-related quality of life.

We would like to warmly thank all the contributors for their enthusiasm and hard work and, in addition, acknowledge K. Larsson (Editor in Chief) and the European Respiratory Society Publications Dept for their excellent technical help.

References

1.   Muir JF, Ambrosino N, Simonds AK, eds. Noninvasive Mechanical Ventilation. *Eur Respir Mon* 2001; 16.

Eur Respir Mon, 2008, 41, ix. Printed in UK - all rights reserved. Copyright ERS Journals Ltd 2008; European Respiratory Monograph; ISSN 1025-448x.

Part I

Acute respiratory failure
and NIV

Physiological rationale of noninvasive mechanical ventilation use in acute respiratory failure

G. Prinianakis, M. Klimathianaki, D. Georgopoulos

Intensive Care Medicine Dept, University Hospital of Heraklion, University of Crete, Heraklion, Greece.

Correspondence: D. Georgopoulos, Dept of Intensive Care, University Hospital of Heraklion, University of Crete, Heraklion, Crete 71110, Greece. Fax: 30 2810392636; E-mail: georgop@med.uch.gr

Introduction

The present article will begin with a general presentation of the effects of noninvasive mechanical ventilation (NIMV) on the respiratory and cardiovascular systems. It is important to note that these are the physiological effects of NIMV and that they are applicable during both normal conditions and various disease states. Depending on the pathophysiology of respiratory failure of any given disease state, the various physiological effects of NIMV may have relatively greater or lesser importance or may even be undesirable. Consequently, knowing the underlying pathophysiology is fundamental for adapting NIMV mode and parameters to the specific disease state in order to maximise benefits and minimise any adverse effects. A short review of major pathophysiological patterns in relation to NIMV physiology is included.

Effect of NIMV on respiratory mechanics

Equation of motion

The simplified equation of motion:
$$P_{tot(t)} = P_{res(t)} + P_{el(t)} \tag{1}$$
describes the relationship between any driving pressure ($P_{tot(t)}$) applied to the respiratory system (RS) at any time (t), and the opposing resistive ($P_{res(t)}$) and elastic ($P_{el(t)}$) pressures of the RS (inertia is considered to be negligible).

$P_{res(t)}$ is the pressure dissipated to overcome resistance to flow:
$$P_{res(t)} = V'_{(t)} \cdot R_{rs} \tag{2}$$
where $V'_{(t)}$ is instantaneous gas flow and R_{rs} is the resistance of the RS.

$P_{el(t)}$ is the elastic recoil pressure exerted by the RS when volume increases above passive functional residual capacity (FRC),
$$P_{el(t)} = V_{(t)} \cdot E_{rs} \tag{3}$$
where $V_{(t)}$ is instantaneous volume relative to passive FRC, and E_{rs} is the elastance of the RS. Note that tidal volume (V_T) is not always equal to volume above passive FRC. When dynamic hyperinflation (DH) exists, at end-expiration the RS has not reached passive FRC and the trapped volume exerts additional outward elastic recoil pressure, which is called "intrinsic positive end-expiratory pressure" (PEEPi). When the next

Eur Respir Mon, 2008, 41, 3–23. Printed in UK - all rights reserved. Copyright ERS Journals Ltd 2008; European Respiratory Monograph; ISSN 1025-448x.

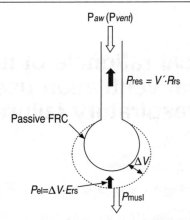

Fig. 1. – Schematic representation of pressures acting on the respiratory system during assisted mechanical ventilation. Pressure generated by inspiratory muscles (P_{mus}I) and ventilator (P_{aw}) drive inspiratory flow (V') into the lungs (open arrows), which is opposed by resistive (P_{res}) and elastic (P_{el}) pressures (closed arrows). R_{rs}: resistance of respiratory system; FRC: functional residual capacity; ΔV: change in volume; E_{rs}: elastance of the respiratory system.

inspiration starts, P_{tot} must first overcome the elastic threshold of PEEPi before any flow is produced and V_T enters the RS. Thus, equation 3 may be rewritten as:

$$P_{el(t)} = V_{T(t)} \cdot E_{rs} + PEEPi \qquad (4)$$

where $V_{T(t)}$ is the instantaneous V_T.

The equation of motion is always applicable to the RS at any phase of the respiratory cycle (*i.e.* during inspiration or expiration) and regardless of the ventilation mode (*i.e.* spontaneous breathing, invasive or noninvasive mechanical ventilation (MV), assisted or controlled MV, pressure or volume targeted *etc.*).

During spontaneous breathing, the only P_{tot} applied to the RS is that generated by the respiratory muscles $P_{mus(t)}$, while during MV (invasive or non-invasive), the inspiratory pressure provided by the ventilator $P_{aw(t)}$ is also incorporated into the equation (fig. 1), which can then be expressed as follows:

$$P_{tot(t)} = P_{mus(t)} + P_{aw(t)} = V'_{(t)} \cdot R_{rs} + V_{T(t)} \cdot E_{rs} + PEEPi \qquad (5)$$

Effect of continuous positive airway pressure/PEEP

During continuous positive airway pressure (CPAP)/PEEP, a constant positive pressure is applied to the RS throughout the respiratory cycle (*i.e.* during both inspiration and expiration), while the patient breathes spontaneously. Since this pressure is constant, it does not generate flow and it does not increase V_T [1, 2] and it can not be considered to be a form of noninvasive ventilation in a strict sense; yet, it exerts important effects to respiratory system mechanics.

FRC increase. When CPAP/PEEP is applied, passive FRC is increased by a volume ΔV that depends on the E_{rs} and can be calculated from:

$$CPAP = \Delta V \cdot E_{rs} \qquad (6)$$

or

$$\Delta V = CPAP / E_{rs} \qquad (7)$$

In other words, CPAP supplies the P_{tot} to overcome the additional P_{el} imposed by the additional volume (ΔV) above passive FRC. The effect of this increase might be beneficial or detrimental, depending on the underlying pathophysiology.

This increase in FRC might prevent or reverse atelectasis, and thus improve shunt and ventilation/perfusion (V'/Q') relationships and gas exchange. Alternatively, when excessive, it might cause hyperinflation and increase of functional dead space volume (V_D), therefore worsening V'/Q' relationships. Excessive FRC increase will also pose a mechanical disadvantage to the inspiratory muscles, because it shortens their length and according to their length–strength relationship, their capacity to produce pressure will be reduced. This is very important for the diaphragm, which becomes increasingly flattened when FRC increases. The disadvantaged inspiratory muscles will also have to work on a less steep portion of the RS pressure–volume curve (*i.e.* E_{rs} increases). All these physiological effects of CPAP should be appreciated when choosing the appropriate CPAP/PEEP level for a given patient.

Decrease of elastic workload due to DH. When DH is present, the disadvantaged inspiratory muscles have to overcome the additional elastic threshold of PEEPi before generating inspiratory flow [3]. This additional elastic workload may be significant. When CPAP/PEEP is applied externally, it supplies all or part of the driving pressure required to overcome PEEPi, and equation 5 can be expressed as:

$$P_{tot(t)} = P_{mus(t)} = V'(t) \cdot R_{rs} + V_{T(t)} \cdot E_{rs} + (PEEPi - CPAP) \tag{8}$$

for spontaneous breathing with CPAP. It is obvious that pressure generated by inspiratory muscles is not wasted to overcome PEEPi and thus is available for generating inspiratory flow and pull air into the lungs. Thus, CPAP may indirectly increase V_T by unloading the inspiratory muscles.

For NIMV with assisted inspiration, equation (5) becomes:

$$P_{tot(t)} = P_{mus(t)} + P_{aw(t)} = V'(t) \cdot R_{rs} + V_{T(t)} \cdot E_{rs} + (PEEPi - PEEP) \tag{9}$$

Again PEEP applied externally unloads the inspiratory muscles in exactly the same manner presented for CPAP [1]. Additionally, it permits faster and easier triggering of the assisted inspiration, thus improving patient–ventilator synchrony.

This effect of CPAP/PEEP is of major importance in clinical situations where DH is significant (*i.e.* disease states with obstructive pathophysiology pattern like chronic obstructive pulmonary disease (COPD) or asthma).

Effect of positive inspiratory pressure

During NIMV with assisted inspiration, PEEP is combined with positive inspiratory pressure. The delivery of positive inspiratory pressure is triggered by the patient's inspiratory effort, and usually titrated to produce either constant volume (assist volume control; AVC) or constant pressure (pressure-support ventilation; PSV). In both modes, equation 9 is applicable. It is evident, from equation 9, that $P_{aw(t)}$ delivered by the ventilator is meant to act as an "additional inspiratory muscle"; this is true for PSV but not for AVC.

AVC. In this mode, inspiratory pressure delivered by the ventilator is titrated in order to achieve a preset constant volume target. This ensures that the preset volume will be delivered, despite any changes in the mechanical properties of the RS and in the magnitude of the patient's inspiratory effort. The minimum inspiratory effort required by the patient is to trigger the ventilator. Alternatively, when the patient increases their inspiratory effort, due to increased ventilatory needs, the inspiratory pressure delivered by the ventilator will decrease in order to keep the constant volume target [4]. The greater the patient's inspiratory effort, the lesser the ventilator's assistance. The ventilator might even deliver negative inspiratory pressure (*i.e.* pull air back), when the patient makes an adequately strong inspiratory effort, in order not to exceed the preset volume target (fig. 2e and f). Thus, in AVC the ventilator antagonizes, rather than assists, the patient. Additionally, it has been shown that some home ventilators are inaccurate in delivering the preset V_T, especially when faced with deteriorating mechanical properties of the RS [5]. For this reason, AVC has been disfavored for use as NIMV in the acute setting [6] and, currently, is used merely for home NIMV for patients with chronic respiratory failure due to neuromuscular disease [7, 8]. Therefore, this mode of ventilation will not be focused on any further.

Pressure support. In this mode, inspiratory pressure delivered by the ventilator is constant to the preset pressure level, regardless of the magnitude of the patient's inspiratory effort (fig. 2c and d). In this mode, the ventilator truly acts as an "additional inspiratory muscle", increasing $P_{tot(t)}$ and thus increasing V_T and minute ventilation (V'_E) [2]. It also unloads the fatigued inspiratory muscles [2] by decreasing their inspiratory work of breathing and oxygen consumption. For these reasons, it has gained widespread acceptance as a mode of delivering NIMV in both the acute and chronic setting [6–8]. However, caution is needed because, despite the perceived simplicity in its settings, inspiratory and expiratory synchronisation with patient's respiratory effort is not always optimal (see section on patient–ventilator interaction). Patient–ventilator dys-synchrony is very common with PSV, and its effects may diminish or even totally cancel out the beneficial role of PSV [9].

With PSV, breath-by-breath delivered V_T will depend on not only the pressure-support level, but also on the patient's inspiratory effort and the mechanical properties of the RS (*i.e.* R_{rs}, E_{rs}, presence of DH). When the patient increases their inspiratory effort, they are able to partially increase the delivered V_T (within the limits of patient–ventilator interaction) while the ventilator's assistance remains constant [4]. Thus, in PSV, the ventilator assists the patient with constant pressure support and certainly does not antagonise; however, it does not follow up and does not adapt according to the patient's ventilatory needs (fig 2c and d). The only assist mode capable of adapting to the patient's breathing pattern and ventilatory needs is proportional assist ventilation (PAV).

Ventilators with mixed volume and pressure-targeted modes. In an effort to combine the advantages of pressure- and volume-targeted modes into one ventilation mode, new hybrid modes such as average volume-assured pressure support [10] and adaptive servoventilation [11] have recently been introduced in the NIMV setting.

PAV

With PAV, inspiratory pressure delivered by the ventilator is instantaneously adapted to keep up with the patient's instantaneous inspiratory effort. When the patient increases their inspiratory effort due to increased ventilatory needs, the ventilator proportionally increases the delivered P_{aw} [4]. When the patient terminates their inspiratory effort, it is immediately sensed by the ventilator, which promptly terminates the delivered P_{aw} and thus patient–ventilator synchrony is optimised.

In contrast to the previously mentioned assist modes, a preset target level of volume, pressure or flow does not exist. What is preset is only the proportionality between the patient's inspiratory effort and the ventilator's assistance.

The principle underlying PAV is that any changes in instantaneous flow represent changes in patient's inspiratory effort. Again, equation 9 is applicable.

Flow and volume leaving the ventilator are continuously measured. When the patient increases $P_{mus(t)}$, alveolar pressure will decrease and this will cause additional instantaneous flow (and volume) to leave the ventilator. This is sensed by the ventilator

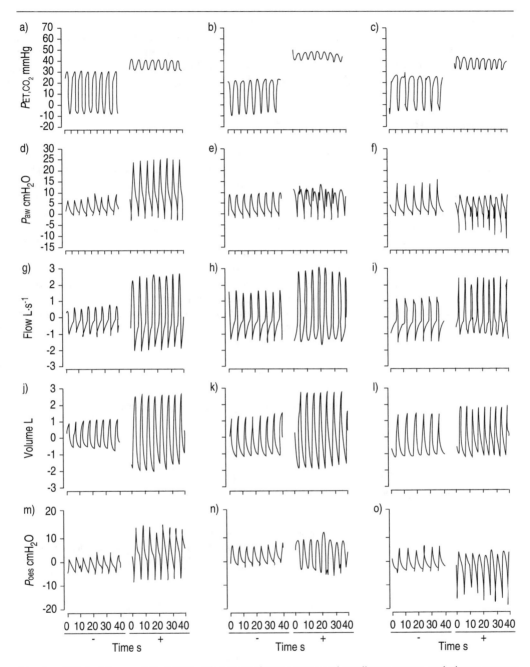

Fig. 2. – Effect of increased inspiratory drive on respiratory motor and ventilatory output, and airway pressure during different modes of noninvasive assisted mechanical ventilation. End-tidal carbon dioxide tension (P_{ET,CO_2}), airway pressure (P_{aw}), flow (inspiration up), volume (inspiration up), and oesophageal (P_{oes}) pressure in a representative subject during a, d, g, j, m) proportional assist ventilation, b, e, h, k, n) pressure support and c, f, i, l, o) assist-volume control without (-) and with (+) CO_2 challenge. Of note is the different response in P_{aw} after CO_2 challenge between the different modes of support. 1 mmHg = 0.133 kPa. Reproduced from [4].

which responds by instantaneously increasing $P_{aw(t)}$ proportionally to the sensed increase in instantaneous flow (and volume). Further details on PAV design and application [12] are beyond the scope of this article. What is important for NIMV physiology is the improved patient–ventilator synchrony and the breath-by-breath adaptability of the delivered assist according to the patient's ventilatory needs (fig 2a and b).

Cardiovascular effects of NIMV

The cardiovascular effects of (both invasive and noninvasive) MV are complex and mediated through different mechanisms, often interdependent or counteracting (fig. 3) [14].

The most important cardiovascular effects of NIMV are: decreased venous return (VR); decreased left ventricle (LV) afterload; decreased work of breathing (WOB) and oxygen consumption; and effect on pulmonary vascular resistance (RV afterload).

Any change in pleural pressure during the respiratory cycle will be transmitted to the heart; therefore, the pressure gradients for both systemic VR (preload to RV and LV) and systemic arterial outflow (LV afterload) will also change [15].

Spontaneous inspiratory efforts decrease pleural pressure, which can become extremely negative during acute or chronic respiratory failure, when respiratory system mechanics and when lung gas exchange properties are altered [16–18]. When positive inspiratory pressure is applied and the respiratory muscles are unloaded, these negative pleural pressure swings during inspiration will be decreased or even abolished. Furthermore, PEEP/CPAP increases pleural pressure during expiration [18, 19].

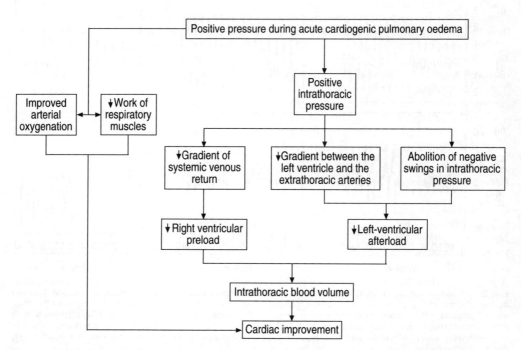

Fig. 3. – Schematic physiological effects of positive-pressure ventilation in a case of acute cardiogenic pulmonary oedema. Reproduced from [13] with permission from the publisher.

Decreased VR (RV and LV preload)

Any NIMV-induced increase in pleural pressure will increase right atrial pressure and consequently decrease the pressure gradient for systemic VR, which will decrease. This will lead to a decrease of both Rv and LV preload. The consequences will depend on the underlying cardiovascular status [20]. If the patient is relatively hypovolaemic, or has pre-existing Rv failure, then NIMV may severely impede VR, leading to a decreased Cardiac output (CO), decreased mixed venous oxygen saturatution (Sv,O_2) and paradoxical worsening of arterial oxygen saturation (Sa,O_2), or even cardiovascular collapse [21]. Conversely, in hypervolaemic congestive heart failure, this NIMV-induced decrease in VR is much less, yet beneficial [22, 23].

Decreased LV afterload

The exaggerated negative pleural pressure swings during laboured spontaneous breathing increase LV afterload, while NIMV-induced increase in pleural pressure will decrease it. For the normal heart, cardiac function is mostly preload rather than afterload dependent [19], so the effects of pleural pressure on LV afterload have limited clinical significance. Conversely, when LV is dilated, with impaired contractility, cardiac function heavily depends on afterload. For such patients the beneficial effects of NIMV on LV afterload reduction are of major clinical importance [19, 20, 22, 23] .

Decreased WOB and oxygen consumption by respiratory muscles

During lung disease states the respiratory WOB and consequently oxygen consumption by respiratory muscles is severely increased. This causes a shift of blood flow to the respiratory muscles, so that for the same CO blood flow and oxygen delivery to other organs will be decreased, leading to peripheral tissue hypoperfusion, lactic acidosis and decreased Sv,O_2 (due to a greater oxygen extraction ratio by the hypoxic tissues). As a consequence, Sa,O_2 will also decrease, even without any other change in lung gas exchange properties. These effects are greater in patients with a limited cardiovascular reserve, who are unable to increase CO in response to the increased demand. Even NIMV may unload the respiratory muscles and decrease their oxygen consumption [18], thus increasing oxygen delivery to other organs, increasing Sv,O_2 and Sa,O_2 and decreasing lactic acidosis [14].

Effect on pulmonary vascular resistance (RV afterload)

Pulmonary capillaries are situated within the alveolar septa, therefore they are subject to compression by adjacent alveolar pressure. They are also subject to hypoxic pulmonary vasoconstriction (HPV) when adjacent alveolar oxygen partial pressure PA,O_2 falls below 7.98 kPa (60 mmHg). NIMV (mainly CPAP/PEEP application) may reverse HPV by inducing recruitment of atelectatic regions, thus reducing PVR. Adversely, when NIMV induces hyperinflation (excess PEEP) rather than recruitment, pulmonary capillaries are compressed and PVR is increased. This increase in Rv afterload, if severe, may precipitate acute Rv failure, again also depending on the previous cardiovascular status of the patient.

For interpreting and anticipating the cardiovascular effects of NIMV, apart from knowledge of the aforementioned mechanisms, the physician should also be aware of three important points as follows. First, the importance of underlying cardiovascular status (including intravascular volume, ventricular pump function and myocardial reserve), as it was presented above. Furthermore, the cardiovascular response to NIMV-induced increase in pleural pressure may be used as a clue to the underlying haemodynamic status of the patient. Secondly, P_{aw} is variably transmitted to the pleural space; positive airway pressures (inspiratory pressure and CPAP/PEEP) delivered by the ventilator are variably transmitted to the pleural space ($P_{pleural}$) depending on the RS mechanical properties, particularly on the compliance of the lungs (CL) *versus* the compliance of the chest wall (CCW). When CL is low, pressure is mostly dissipated to inflate the stiff lungs (high transpulmonary pressure required). Conversely, when CL is high, little pressure is dissipated to inflate the compliant lungs (low transpulmonary pressure required) and, thus, pressure is mostly transmitted to the pleural place. This effect is exaggerated when CCW is low, which means that a high $P_{pleural}$ is dissipated to inflate the stiff chest wall (high distending pressure required across the chest wall). Therefore, pressure transmitted to the pleural space and thus affecting cardiovascular structures depends on not only the magnitude of P_{aw}/PEEP delivered by the ventilator but also the RS mechanical properties. Finally, Withdrawal of MV is accompanied by the opposite cardiovascular effects. Withdrawal of NIMV in patients with limited cardiovascular status may precipitate myocardial ischaemia and heart failure, which might manifest as overt acute cardiogenic pulmonary oedema (ACPO) or as otherwise unexplained weaning failure.

Patient–ventilator interaction during NIMV

During assisted modes of mechanical ventilation, including noninvasive ventilation, the synchrony between patient and ventilator is fundamental for successful patient outcome. Synchrony is defined as the condition when the ventilator fully meets the patient's ventilation demands. In other words, the patient's neural timing and flow demand coincide with ventilator timing and flow supply, a condition which rarely occurs in daily clinical practice. During NIMV, dys-synchrony is even worse because of the presence of air leaks and the alert status of the patients. These factors make the problem of patient–ventilator synchrony during NIMV more complex than that described for invasive mechanical ventilation.

The dys-synchrony between patient and ventilator depends on factors related both to the ventilator and the patient [24, 25]. The ventilator-related factors include the triggering variable, the variable that controls gas delivery, and the cycling off criterion. Patient-related factors include the respiratory system mechanics and the P_{mus} characteristics.

The trigger variable

Commonly used trigger variables during NIMV are flow or pressure trigger. With these variables, the patient effort must generate a preset decrease in airway pressure or in ventilator bias flow in order to trigger the assisted breath. NAVA *et al.* [26] found that in both normal and COPD patients, flow triggering is better than pressure triggering in terms of patient inspiratory effort and triggering delay.

Under certain conditions, however, the inspiratory muscle contraction does not trigger the ventilator, a dys-synchrony phenomenon called "missing" or "ineffective" effort occurs [27, 28]. Ineffective efforts are common in patients who exhibit DH, due to excessive level of mechanical support and altered mechanical properties. Indeed, excessive support results in high V_T, which, in combination with a long time constant, may force the mechanical inspiration to invade into the patient's neural expiration. Consequently, the following inspiratory effort is likely to begin at end expiratory lung volume above passive FRC, which may lead to ineffective effort.

Recently, a new microprocessor-controlled positive pressure ventilatory assist system has been introduced (BiPAP Vision; Respironics, Pittsburg, PA, USA), which has new algorithms to trigger the ventilator. These are designed to improve patient–ventilator interaction, with the flow waveform mainly used to trigger the ventilator. This method of triggering is referred to as the "shape signal method". It is based on the generation of a new flow signal (flow-shape signal) by offsetting the signal from the actual flow by 0.25 L·s^{-1} and delaying it for 300 ms. This intentional delay causes the flow shape signal to be slightly behind the patient's actual flow rate. As a result, a sudden decrease in expiratory flow, due to an inspiratory effort will cross the shape signal and this creates a signal for ventilator triggering (fig. 4). This triggering method was found to be more sensitive to patient effort than the flow triggering, with less ineffective patient efforts [29]. Similarly, the flow-shape signal can be used to terminate the mechanical breath.

A new ventilation mode called neurally adjusted ventilatory assist (NAVA) has recently been developed, in which the ventilator supports the patient effort according to the diaphragm electrical activity [30]. With this mode, synchrony between neural and mechanical timing should be guaranteed at any phase of respiration despite PEEPi or altered respiratory mechanics. Indeed, animal studies have shown that NAVA can be effective in delivering noninvasive ventilation, even when the interface is excessively leaky, and can unload the respiratory muscles while maintaining synchrony with the subject's demand [30]. Improved patient–ventilator interactions have been shown in humans, during helmet NIMV using NAVA *versus* conventional triggering methods [31].

Interfaces choice is also important to improve patient–ventilator synchrony. NAVALESI *et al.* [32] have demonstrated, in COPD patients, that the helmet significantly worsens patient–ventilator synchrony when compared with the facemask; indicated by longer delays between inspiratory muscle effort and support delivery, both at the onset and at the end of inspiration, and by the occurrence of wasted efforts.

NIMV use may improve the respiratory system mechanics and decrease DH. DIAZ *et al.* [33] showed that when NIMV is applied to severe stable hypercapnic COPD patients, it significantly decreases pulmonary hyperinflation and inspiratory loads, due to the adoption of a slow deep-breathing pattern by the patients.

In everyday clinical practice, a more-sensitive trigger threshold is set, in order to reduce the number of ineffective efforts; however, this strategy in not always advantageous. By setting a more sensitive threshold in the presence of air leaks, water in the ventilator circuit or large heart stroke volume may lead to a mechanical breath that is not patient triggered. This dys-synchrony phenomenon is called autotriggering [25]. Therefore, when ventilator trigger level is set, the lowest possible threshold, that does not result in autotriggering, should be chosen.

The variable that controls gas delivery

During NIMV, either AVC or PSV can be used as ventilation mode. Generally, it is accepted that patients with poor respiratory drive are the appropriate candidates to receive AVC. GIRAULT *et al.* [34] studied the physiological effects of the two modes, in patients suffering from acute respiratory failure. Briefly, they found that both modes of gas delivery are efficient in improving breathing pattern and gas exchange. These physiological effects though are achieved with a lower inspiratory workload but at the expense of a higher respiratory discomfort with AVC compared with PSV mode [34].

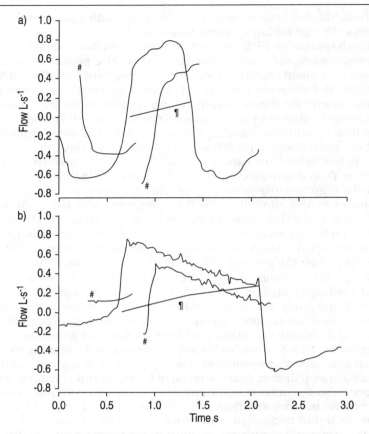

Fig. 4. – Flow–time waveform in two patients ventilated with a Vision ventilator on pressure support mode. Inspiration is down and expiration is up. The flow shape signal, generated by offsetting (0.25 L·s⁻¹;) and delaying (300 ms) the actual flow during inspiration and expiration (#) and the electronic signal rising in proportion to actual inspiratory flow in each breath (¶) are shown. a) Mechanical breath was triggered and terminated by the shape method. During expiration the actual flow decreased abruptly (due to the onset of inspiratory effort), crossed the flow shape signal and triggered the ventilator. Reproduced from [29] with permission from the publisher.

Usually, assist level is set according to clinical and/or physiological variables. VITACCA *et al.* [35] demonstrated that when using clinical variables to set pressure support, almost half of their home ventilated patients showed ineffective efforts. Even by using more invasive techniques, such as gastric and oesophageal balloons, they did not totally avoid patient–ventilator dys-synchrony [35].

PAV is a ventilatory mode in which the ventilator follows the patient's neural output (see preceding section on PAV), so, in theory, it achieves perfect patient–ventilator interaction. Generally, using PAV noninvasively may improve gas exchange and dyspnoea [36, 37], but no difference was found in terms of patient–ventilator synchrony when compared with PSV in stable COPD patients [38]. Furthermore, these studies have demonstrated no differences in clinical endpoints, such as mortality, number of endotracheal intubations and length of hospital stay [36, 37].

PAV is underused in everyday clinical practice because setting the ventilator parameters is complex. In fact, the ventilator settings must be adjusted every time the patient's mechanical proprieties change. "PAV+", a new sophisticated option of PAV, which semicontinuously estimates patient's mechanical properties noninvasively, may simplify PAV application in clinical practice [39].

Recently, the effects of varying pressurisation rate, the incremental increase in P_{aw} per time unit, have been assessed in 15 COPD patients on NIMV. No significant differences were found in breathing pattern and gas exchange between four different pressurisation rates. The fastest rate seemed to reduce the pressure–time product, an estimate of oxygen consumption of diaphragm; however, this resulted in increased air leaking and worse patient tolerance, as measured with a visual scale. Patient–ventilator synchrony was assessed by calculating the ratio between the neural and mechanical inspiratory time. With the fastest pressurisation rate, this ratio was shorter, indicating that the mechanical inspiration invaded into the patient neural expiration. Two factors seemed to determine NIMV tolerance: the presence of high air leaks and the dys-synchrony between neural and mechanical inspiratory time [40].

During noninvasive ventilation, setting pressure-support level is difficult because of the presence of mask air leaks. SCHETTINO *et al.* [41] have shown that the leaks increase in proportion to the pressure delivered into the mask. Although modern ventilators compensate for mask leaking, still any pressure support increase may lead to decreased V_T because of leaks [41].

The cycling-off criterion

Ventilators permit transition from inspiration to expiration according to a predetermined cycling-off criterion. The most commonly used criterion is the decrease of inspiratory flow to a predetermined percentage of peak inspiratory flow.

During noninvasive ventilation, the presence of leaks may lead to a prolonged mechanical inspiration because inspiratory flow does not reach the cycling-off criterion. Consequently, the machine's inspiration invades into the patient's expiratory phase, a phenomenon known as delayed cycling-off. CALDERINI *et al.* [42] have compared time cycling with flow cycling and they found that using time-cycling criterion essentially reduced the inspiratory effort and WOB, and improved expiratory synchronisation (fig. 5).

Every effort should be made to minimise mask air leaks. However, excessive tightness of the mask may lead to patient discomfort and NIMV intolerance. It should be noted that high pressurisation rate increases air leakage despite sufficient mask fitting, which may provoke delayed cycling off (fig. 6) [40].

COPD: physiological role of NIMV

The cardinal feature of COPD pathophysiology is DH. DH is the result of expiratory flow limitation (EFL), due to the increased R_{rs} and compliance of the respiratory system (C_{rs}) which prolong the time constant ($\tau = R_{rs} \times C_{rs}$) for lung emptying and increase the end-expiratory lung volume above passive FRC. DH poses important mechanical disadvantages for the inspiratory muscles, which have to overcome additional elastic load (PEEPi) to initiate inspiratory flow (or trigger the ventilator during MV [43] and must also operate on the flat part of the C_{rs} curve (fig. 7). Conversely, the pressure generating capacity of the shortened inspiratory muscles is additionally limited by DH (fig. 8). These pathophysiological mechanisms apply to stable COPD, but are further exaggerated during exacerbations [44].

NIMV is capable of partly reversing this pathophysiology and thus unloading the respiratory muscles (fig. 8). PEEP/CPAP decreases the elastic workload due to DH, because it supplies all or part of the P_{tot} required to overcome PEEPi and initiate

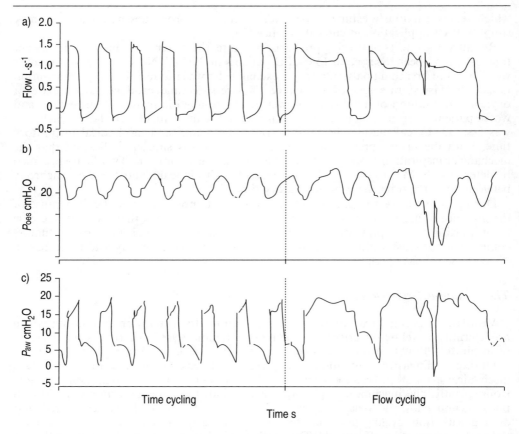

Fig. 5. – A representative experimental record of a) flow, b) oesophageal pressure (Poes) and c) airway pressure (Paw) in a patient treated with noninvasive mechanical ventilation using time and conventional flow percentage as cycling-off criteria. The perfect synchronisation between patient and machine during time cycling off criterion. With flow cycling off criterion, the prolonged mechanical assist into the neural expiratory time results into wasted next inspiratory effort, as evident by the following negative deflections on the Poes curve. Reproduced from [42] with permission from the publisher.

inspiratory flow (or trigger the ventilator). The addition of positive inspiratory pressure further unloads the inspiratory muscles and increases VT, V'E and improves gas exchange [1, 46]. NIMV has been used with favorable physiological and clinical outcomes for both stable COPD (PSV and AVC) [1] and for exacerbations (mostly PSV [46] and recently PAV), as well as to facilitate weaning from invasive MV.

In a principal study of NIMV during COPD exacerbation, APPENDINI *et al.* [46] showed that PEEP/CPAP set between 80% and 90% of dynamic PEEPi decreased the diaphragmatic pressure-time product (PTPdi), and additional PSV further decreased PTPdi, increased VT and V'E and improved gas exchange.

During stable COPD, long term NIMV has been shown to decrease inspiratory muscle workload due to dynamic PEEPi [35]. The beneficial effects of long-term NIMV seem to persist also during the period of daytime spontaneous breathing. WINDISCH *et al.* [47] showed that controlled nocturnal NIMV therapy is capable of increasing VT and V'E during the three subsequent hours of daytime spontaneous breathing and of sustaining increased diurnal VT and V'E. It has also been shown that PSV induces a decrease of daytime lung hyperinflation, as quantified by the decreased total lung

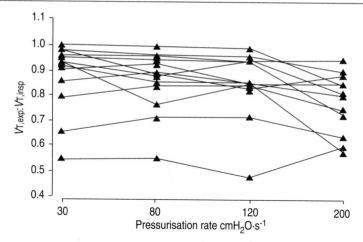

Fig. 6. – Amount of air leaks through the mask, as assessed by the ratio between expiratory ($V_{T,exp}$) and inspiratory tidal volume ($V_{T,insp}$) in the different values of pressurisation rate for each patient. The amount of leak was bigger at highest (200 cmH$_2$O·s^{-1}) pressurisation rate. Reproduced from [40] with permission from the publisher.

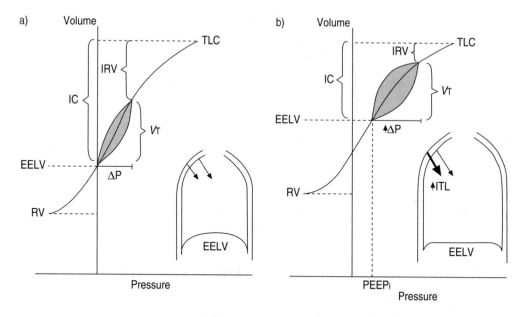

Fig. 7. – Schematic representation of mechanical effects of chronic obstructive pulmonary disease (COPD) exacerbation. Representative pressure–volume plots during a) stable COPD and b) COPD exacerbation. During exacerbation, worsening expiratory flow limitation results in dynamic hyperinflation with increased end-expiratory lung volume (EELV) and residual volume (RV). Corresponding reductions occur in inspiratory capacity (IC) and inspiratory reserve volume (IRV). Total lung capacity (TLC) is unchanged. As a result, tidal breathing becomes shifted rightward on the pressure–volume curve, closer to TLC. Mechanically, increased pressures must be generated to maintain tidal volume (V_T). At EELV during exacerbation, intrapulmonary pressures do not return to zero, representing the development of intrinsic positive end-expiratory pressure (PEEPi), which imposes increased inspiratory threshold loading (ITL) on the inspiratory muscles; during the subsequent respiratory cycle, PEEPi must first be overcome in order to generate inspiratory flow. From [44] with permission.

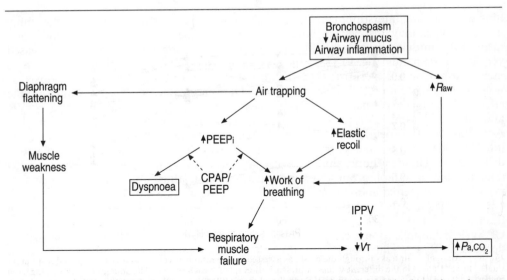

Fig. 8. – Schematic physiological effects of noninvasive mechanical ventilation in chronic obstructive pulmonary disease. Continuos positive airway pressure (CPAP)/ positive end-expiratory pressure (PEEP) decreases the elastic work of breathing because it supplies all or part of the driving pressure required to overcome intrinsic PEEP (PEEPi) and initiate inspiratory flow. The addition of inspiratory positive pressure ventilation (IPPV) further unloads the inspiratory muscles and increases tidal volume (VT) and decreases arterial carbon dioxide tension (Pa,CO_2). Raw: airway resistance. Published from [45] with permission from the publisher.

capacity (~10%), FRC (~25%) and residual volume (~35%), and the increased VT (~180 mL) [33]. Mouth occlusion pressure (P0.1), a measure of inspiratory drive, also decreases, while 6 min walking distance increases [48]. NIMV (PSV plus PEEP) has also been reported to exert positive cardiovascular effects in stable COPD patients, including improved heart rate variability, decreased circulating natriuretic peptide levels and enhanced functional performance [49]. There is no consensus regarding the titration to optimal level of PSV [35, 50, 51] . Noninvasive PAV has also been studied for stable COPD, and was comparable to PSV in increasing VT and V'E, and in unloading inspiratory muscles [38].

Recently, a method to noninvasively detect expiratory flow limitation by the difference between mean inspiratory and expiratory reactance, measured with a forced-oscillation technique has been proposed for titration of CPAP/PEEP level in stable COPD patients, so that increase of operating lung volumes, by PEEP/CPAP, above the levels imposed by EFL and concomitant disadvantageous effects may be avoided [52].

Congestive heart failure: physiological role of NIMV

NIMV in the setting of congestive heart function (CHF) has three major goals: to improve cardiac function; to unload the respiratory muscles; and to improve gas exchange. It is mainly used for management of ACPO, but it has also been studied in chronic stable CHF.

ACPO

ACPO represents a vicious cycle of progressive LV (systolic and/or diastolic) failure, which results in a progressive decrease in systemic CO as well as increase in extravascular lung water in lung interstitium and alveoli. The interstitial oedema, apart from worsening gas exchange, may also cause lung resistance and elastance to increase; therefore, inspiratory muscles must generate greater pressure swings to sustain the increased ventilatory demands (fig. 9) [18, 19]. Oxygen consumption by respiratory muscles is increased but cannot be satisfied by the already limited CO, thus metabolic acidosis, as well as progressive muscle fatigue, may occur. Of even greater clinical importance are the effects of the increased negative intra-thoracic pressure swings on the failing heart; VR and thus RV (and LV) preload increases, while LV afterload also increases [19]. Additionally, the overloaded RV may become dilated and, through ventricular interdependence (*i.e.* interventricular septum shift), may further impose LV diastolic dysfunction. These pathophysiological mechanisms not only increase myocardial oxygen demand but also compromise oxygen delivery and, thus, may further precipitate myocardial ischaemia and worsen heart failure.

NIMV has mostly been studied in LV systolic failure (*i.e.* with a decreased ejection fraction (EF)), and has consistently been shown to break this vicious cycle (fig. 3). CPAP/PEEP application increases expiratory pleural pressure [18, 19], and consequently decreases VR, RV and LV preload, RV dilatation, and improves LV diastolic function [53]. It additionally decreases LV afterload by decreasing LV transmural pressure during systole [18, 19] and, thus, also improves LV systolic function, decreases LV stroke work and decreases myocardial oxygen consumption [54]. It has also been shown to unload the inspiratory muscles [18, 19]. End-expiratory lung volume increases [55], thus improving lung gas-exchange properties and respiratory mechanics [18, 56–58].

The addition of positive inspiratory pressure (mainly studied is PSV), and recently PAV may further unload the inspiratory muscles [59, 60], decrease or even totally

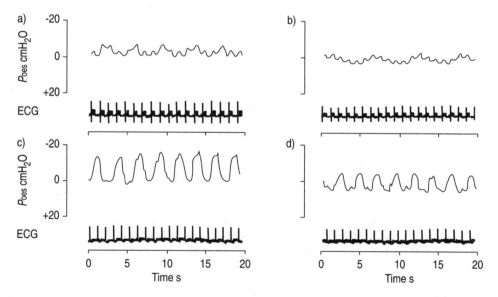

Fig. 9. – Oesophageal pressure (*P*oes) and electrocardiogram recordings from a healthy subject (a and b) and a patient with congestive heart failure (CHF; c and d) at baseline (a and c) and on 10 cmH$_2$O of continuous positive airway pressure (CPAP; b and d). Note that in the healthy subject, CPAP caused both end-expiratory *P*oes and peak inspiratory *P*oes to become more positive but caused no change in the amplitude of the inspiratory *P*oes swing. Respiratory rate also decreased. In the patient with CHF, the *P*oes amplitude at baseline was greater than in the healthy subject. On CPAP, end-expiratory *P*oes becomes more positive and *P*oes amplitude is reduced, such that peak inspiratory *P*oes becomes more positive. Respiratory rate did not change. Reproduced from [19], with permission from the publisher.

abolish the detrimental negative inthrathoracic pressure swings, and may also decrease inspiratory muscle work of breathing and oxygen consumption.

It is important to note that these direct effects of NIMV take advantage of the heart–lung interactions and occur above and beyond any change in gas exchange. Gas exchange is also greatly improved, both by the improved gas exchange properties of the lung and by the indirect effect of increased cardiac output and decreased oxygen consumption by the inspiratory muscles [18].

NIMV has also been studied in LV diastolic failure (*i.e.* with a preserved EF > 45%), and is also associated with clinical improvement [61], although debate exists about its exact pathophysiological effects in this setting [62]. The NIMV-induced decrease in cardiac preload and LV end-diastolic volume (LVEDV) may be detrimental and actually decrease stroke volume in patients with impaired diastolic filling, which displays a steep curve for LV diastolic pressure in relation to volume. Indeed, BENDJELID *et al.* [61] showed that, in a small group of patients presenting with ACPO with preserved systolic function, CPAP decreased LVEDV, albeit to a lesser degree compared with patients with systolic dysfunction, and does not increase LV EF. Yet, CPAP was associated with consistent clinical improvement even in the diastolic dysfunction group [61]. A possible explanation of these findings might be that patients with diastolic dysfunction who present with ACPO, in contrast to stable diastolic HF, might already be excessively volume overloaded, so that any decrease in preload and LVEDV has beneficial rather than detrimental effects, setting LV in a more favorable position on its compliance curve. In addition, noncardiac-function beneficial effects of NIMV (*i.e.* decreased work and oxygen cost of breathing, improved gas exchange and lung mechanical properties) may contribute to the clinical benefit. Nevertheless, treating physicians should be aware of a possible detrimental effect of NIMV-induced preload decrease in patients with LV diastolic failure, depending on their underlying RV and LV function and hydration status.

Chronic CHF

NIMV in chronic CHF exerts similar effects to those presented above for ACPO, since pathophysiology is similar, and many of the studies presented previously were performed on stable rather than acutely decompensated CHF patients [19, 53, 54]. Additionally, it has been shown that CPAP may increase the low heart rate variability these patients exhibit and is recognised as a poor prognostic factor [55].

Nocturnal long-term NIMV (mainly CPAP but also adaptive servoventilation) has been used for the management of central sleep apnoea and Cheyne–Stokes respiration (CSA-CSR), which is a cardinal feature of chronic CHF [11, 63–66]. CPAP improves cardiac function, as evidenced by the increased LV ejection, decreased mitral regurgitation and decreased plasma atrial natriuretic and norepinephrine levels [58, 63, 64]. Similar effects have been shown when pressure support is added (BiPAP) [65]. Exercise capacity also improved [57, 63]. Although, the clinical significance of long-term NIMV in CHF with CSA-CSR is doubtful, especially in the face of potent pharmacological treatments like β-blockers that have been introduced in the management of stable CHF [63, 66].

It should be noted that CPAP has been successfully used in the management of obstructive sleep apnoea (OSA) which is a major comorbidity in many patients with CHF [66, 67]. Although beyond of the scope of this discussion about the physiological basis of NIMV in CHF, again the beneficial effect of CPAP on cardiac function is mainly mediated by keeping the obstructed upper airway open and thus abolishing the detrimental large negative inspiratory intrathoracic pressure swings [68].

NIMV during weaning

Reverse pathophysiological mechanisms are expected to occur during abrupt withdrawal of NIMV and shift from positive to negative intrathoracic pressures, culminating in: a) increased VR and cardiac preload; b) increased LV afterload; c) decreased LV diastolic compliance due to myocardial ischaemia and/or biventricular interdependence; and d) increased WOB and increased myocardial oxygen consumption [67]. These mechanisms may precipitate ACPO and myocardial ischaemia. Although these effects have mainly been studied during withdrawal from invasive MV [69], they are also applicable in the NIMV setting and treating physicians should be aware of and expect possible worsening of cardiac function during weaning from NIMV.

NIMV has been proposed as a tool for weaning from invasive MV, in patients who failed a spontaneous breathing trial. VITACCA *et al.* [70] showed that in patients affected by chronic respiratory disorders who failed to sustain spontaneous breathing, postextubation PSV delivered non-invasively was equally effective in reducing work of breathing and dyspnoea level, and in improving arterial blood gases compared with pre-extubation, invasively delivered PSV.

Conclusion

Thorough understanding of the physiological effects of noninvasive mechanical ventilation on respiratory system mechanics and heart–lung interactions, as well as the principles of patient–ventilator interaction are fundamental for rational noninvasive mechanical ventilation application in the clinical setting. Noninvasive mechanical ventilation effects should be interpreted in the context of the pathophysiology of the underlying disease and the cardiovascular status of the patient. Pathophysiological rationale for the two most common acute noninvasive mechanical ventilation applications, in chronic obstructive pulmonary disease exacerbations and acute cardiogenic pulmonary oedema, were presented as an example.

Summary

Noninvasive mechanical ventilation (NIMV) exerts multiple effects on respiratory (functional residual capacity increase, elastic workload decrease due to dynamic hyperinflation and decrease of inspiratory muscle workload) and cardiovascular systems (left ventricle afterload decrease, venous return and right ventricle preload decrease and O_2 consumption decrease). The relative importance of these effects depends on the underlying pathophysiology. Chronic obstructive pulmonary disease and acute cardiogenic pulmonary oedema are two of the most common NIMV indications and are used in the present chapter as an example of rational physiological application of NIMV.

For optimal performance of NIMV, attention must be paid to patient–ventilator interaction during NIMV, by tailoring mode (assist volume control, pressure-support ventilation or proportional assist ventilation) and trigger and cycling-off parameters to the specific patient needs.

In conclusion, when NIMV is rationally applied to carefully chosen patients with the appropriate indication, it has physiological effects similar to those of invasive mechanical ventilation, with fewer complications.

Keywords: Acute cardiogenic pulmonary oedema, cardiovascular effects, COPD, noninvasive mechanical ventilation, patient–ventilator interaction, respiratory effects.

References

1. Vanpee D, El Khawand C, Rousseau L, Jamart J, Delaunois L. Effects of nasal pressure support on ventilation and inspiratory work in normocapnic and hypercapnic patients with stable COPD. *Chest* 2002; 122: 75–83.

2. L'Her E, Deye N, Lellouche F, *et al.* Physiologic effects of noninvasive ventilation during acute lung injury. *Am J Respir Crit Care Med* 2005; 172: 1112–1118.

3. Yan S, Kayser B. Differential inspiratory muscle pressure contributions to breathing during dynamic hyperinflation. *Am J Respir Crit Care Med* 1997; 156: 497–503.

4. Mitrouska J, Xirouchaki N, Patakas D, Siafakas N, Georgopoulos D. Effects of chemical feedback on respiratory motor and ventilatory output during different modes of assisted mechanical ventilation. *Eur Respir J* 1999; 13: 873–882.

5. Lofaso F, Fodil R, Lorino H, *et al.* Inaccuracy of tidal volume delivered by home mechanical ventilators. *Eur Respir J* 2000; 15: 338–341.

6. Schönhofer B, Sortor-Leger S. Equipment needs for noninvasive mechanical ventilation. *Eur Respir J* 2002; 20: 1029–1036.

7. Lloyd-Owen SJ, Donaldson GC, Ambrosino N, *et al.* Patterns of home mechanical ventilation use in Europe: results from the Eurovent survey. *Eur Respir J* 2005; 25: 1025–1031.

8. Janssens JP, Derivaz S, Breitenstein E, *et al.* Changing patterns in long-term noninvasive ventilation: a 7-year prospective study in the Geneva Lake area. *Chest* 2003; 123: 67–79.

9. Nava S, Bruschi C, Fracchia C, Braschi A, Rubini F. Patient-ventilator interaction and inspiratory effort during pressure support ventilation in patients with different pathologies. *Eur Respir J* 1997; 10: 177–183.

10. Storre JH, Seuthe B, Fiechter R, *et al.* Average volume-assured pressure support in obesity hypoventilation: a randomized crossover trial. *Chest* 2006; 130: 815–821.

11. Philippe C, Stoïca-Herman M, Drouot X, *et al.* Compliance with and effectiveness of adaptive servoventilation versus continuous positive airway pressure in the treatment of Cheyne-Stokes respiration in heart failure over a six month period. *Heart* 2006; 92: 337–342.

12. Younes M. : Proportional-Assist Ventilation. *In*: Martin T, Ed. Principles and Practice of Mechanical Ventilation. McGraw-Hill, 2006; pp. 335–364.

13. Monnet X, Teboul JL, Richard C. Cardiopulmonary interactions in patients with heart failure. *Curr Op Crit Care* 2007; 13: 6–11.

14. Pinsky MR. Cardiovascular issues in respiratory. *Chest* 2005; 128: Suppl. 2, 592S–597S.

15. Bradley TD, Hall MJ, Ando S, Floras JS. Hemodynamic effects of simulated obstructive apneas in humans with and without heart failure. *Chest* 2001; 119: 1827–1835.

16. Noble WH, Kay JC, Obdrzalek J. Lung mechanics in hypervolemic pulmonary edema. *J Appl Physiol* 1975; 38: 681–687.

17. Naughton MT, Rahman MA, Hara K, Floras JS, Bradley TD. Effect of continuous positive airway pressure on intrathoracic and left ventricular transmural pressures in patients with congestive heart failure. *Circulation* 1995; 91: 1725–1731.

18. Lenique F, Habis M, Lofaso F, Dubois-Randé JL, Harf A, Brochard L. Ventilatory and hemodynamic effects of continuous positive airway pressure in left heart failure. *Am J Respir Crit Care Med* 1997; 155: 500–505.

19. Naughton M, *et al.* Effect of CPAP on respiratory mechanics in heart failure. *Am J Respir Crit Care Med* 1995; 151 (A706).

20. De Hoyos A, Liu PP, Benard DC, Bradley TD. Haemodynamic effects of continuous positive airway pressure in humans with normal and impaired left ventricular function. *Clin Sci (Lond)* 1995; 88: 173–178.

21. Ambrosino N, Nava S, Torbicki A, *et al.* Haemodynamic effects of pressure support and PEEP ventilation by nasal route in patients with stable chronic obstructive pulmonary disease. *Thorax* 1993; 48: 523–528.

22. Baratz DM, Westbrook PR, Shah PK, Mohsenifar Z. Effect of nasal continuous positive airway pressure on cardiac output and oxygen delivery in patients with congestive heart failure. *Chest* 1992; 102: 1397–1401.

23. Bradley TD, Holloway RM, McLaughlin PR, Ross BL, Walters J, Liu PP. Cardiac output response to continuous positive airway pressure in congestive heart failure. *Am Rev Respir Dis* 1992; 145: 377–382.

24. Slutsky AS. Mechanical ventilation. American College of Chest Physicians' Consensus Conference. *Chest* 1993; 104: 1833–1859.

25. Kondili E, Prinianakis G, Georgopoulos D. Patient–ventilator interaction. *Br J Anaesth* 2003; 91: 106–119.

26. Nava S, Ambrosino N, Bruschi C, Confalonieri M, Rampulla C. Physiological effects of flow and pressure triggering during non-invasive mechanical ventilation in patients with chronic obstructive pulmonary disease. *Thorax* 1997; 52: 249–254.

27. Georgopoulos DB, Anastasaki M, Katsanoulas K. Effects of mechanical ventilation on control of breathing. *Monaldi Arch Chest Dis* 1997; 52: 253–262.

28. Tobin MJ, Jubran A, Laghi F. Patient–ventilator interaction. *Am J Respir Crit Care Med* 2001; 163: 1059–1063.

29. Prinianakis G, Kondili E, Georgopoulos D. Effects of the flow waveform method of triggering and cycling on patient–ventilator interaction during pressure support. *Intensive Care Med* 2003; 29: 1950–1959.

30. Sinderby C, Navalesi P, Beck J, *et al.* Neural control of mechanical ventilation in respiratory failure. *Nat Med* 1999; 5: 1433–1436.

31. Beck J, Brander L, Slutsky AS, Reilly MC, Dunn MS, Sinderby C. Non-invasive neurally adjusted ventilatory assist in rabbits with acute lung injury. *Intensive Care Med* 2008; 34: 316–323.

32. Navalesi P, Costa R, Ceriana P, *et al.* Non-invasive ventilation in chronic obstructive pulmonary disease patients: helmet *versus* facial mask. *Intensive Care Med* 2007; 33: 74–81.

33. Díaz O, Bégin P, Torrealba B, Jover E, Lisboa C. Effects of noninvasive ventilation on lung hyperinflation in stable hypercapnic COPD. *Eur Respir J* 2002; 20: 1490–1498.

34. Girault C, Richard JC, Chevron V, *et al.* Comparative physiologic effects of noninvasive assist-control and pressure support ventilation in acute hypercapnic respiratory failure. *Chest* 1997; 111: 1639–1648.

35. Vitacca M, Nava S, Confalonieri M, *et al.* The appropriate setting of noninvasive pressure support ventilation in stable COPD patients. *Chest* 2000; 118: 1286–1293.

36. Gay PC, Hess DR, Hill NS. Noninvasive proportional assist ventilation for acute respiratory insufficiency. Comparison with pressure support ventilation. *Am J Respir Crit Care Med* 2001; 164: 1606–11.

37. Wysocki M, Richard JC, Meshaka P. Noninvasive proportional assist ventilation compared with noninvasive pressure support ventilation in hypercapnic acute respiratory failure. *Crit Care Med* 2002; 30: 323–329.

38. Porta R, Appendini L, Vitacca M, *et al.* Mask proportional assist *vs* pressure support ventilation in patients in clinically stable condition with chronic ventilatory failure. *Chest* 2002; 122: 479–488.

39. Kondili E, Prinianakis G, Alexopoulou C, Vakouti E, Klimathianaki M, Georgopoulos D. Respiratory load compensation during mechanical ventilation – proportional assist ventilation with load-adjustable gain factors *versus* pressure support. *Intensive Care Med* 2006; 32: 692–699.

40. Prinianakis G, Delmastro M, Carlucci A, Ceriana P, Nava S. Effect of varying the pressurisation rate during noninvasive pressure support ventilation. *Eur Respir J* 2004; 23: 314–320.

41. Schettino GP, Tucci MR, Sousa R, Valente Barbas CS, Passos Amato MB, Carvalho CR. Mask mechanics and leak dynamics during noninvasive pressure support ventilation: a bench study. *Intensive Care Med* 2001; 27: 1887–1891.

42. Calderini E, Confalonieri M, Puccio PG, Francavilla N, Stella L, Gregoretti C. Patient–ventilator asynchrony during noninvasive ventilation: the role of expiratory trigger. *Intensive Care Med* 1999; 25: 662–667.

43. Elliott MW, Mulvey DA, Moxham J, Green M, Branthwaite MA. Inspiratory muscle effort during nasal intermittent positive pressure ventilation in patients with chronic obstructive airways disease. *Anaesthesia* 1993; 48: 8–13.

44. O'Donnell DE, Parker CM. COPD exacerbations. 3: Pathophysiology. *Thorax* 2006; 61: 354–361.

45. Organized jointly by the American Thoracic Society, the European Respiratory Society, the European Society of Intensive Care Medicine, and the Société de Réanimation de Langue Française, and approved by ATS Board of Directors, December. International consensus conferences in intensive care medicine: noninvasive positive pressure ventilation in acute respiratory failure. *Am J Respir Crit Care Med 2001* 2000; 163: 283–291.

46. Appendini L, Patessio A, Zanaboni S, *et al.* Physiologic effects of positive end-expiratory pressure and mask pressure support during exacerbations of chronic obstructive pulmonary disease. *Am J Respir Crit Care Med* 1994; 149: 1069–1076.

47. Windisch W, Dreher M, Storre JH, Sorichter S. Nocturnal non-invasive positive pressure ventilation: physiological effects on spontaneous breathing. *Respir Physiol Neurobiol* 2006; 150: 251–160.

48. Díaz O, Bégin P, Andresen M, *et al.* Physiological and clinical effects of diurnal noninvasive ventilation in hypercapnic COPD. *Eur Respir J* 2005; 26: 1016–1023.

49. Sin DD, Wong E, Mayers I, *et al.* Effects of nocturnal noninvasive mechanical ventilation on heart rate variability of patients with advanced COPD. *Chest* 2007; 131: 156–163.

50. Köhnlein T, Welte T. Noninvasive ventilation in stable chronic obstructive pulmonary disease. *Eur Respir J* 2003; 21: 558.

51. Windisch W, Kostić S, Dreher M, Virchow JC Jr, Sorichter S. Outcome of patients with stable COPD receiving controlled noninvasive positive pressure ventilation aimed at a maximal reduction of Pa,CO_2. *Chest* 2005; 128: 657–662.

52. Dellacà RL, Rotger M, Aliverti A, Navajas D, Pedotti A, Farré R. Noninvasive detection of expiratory flow limitation in COPD patients during nasal CPAP. *Eur Respir J* 2006; 27: 983–991.

53. Mehta S, Liu PP, Fitzgerald FS, Allidina YK, Douglas Bradley T. Effects of continuous positive airway pressure on cardiac volumes in patients with ischemic and dilated cardiomyopathy. *Am J Respir Crit Care Med* 2000; 161: 128–134.

54. Kaye DM, Mansfield D, Naughton MT. Continuous positive airway pressure decreases myocardial oxygen consumption in heart failure. *Clin Scie (Lond)* 2004; 106: 599–603.

55. Butler GC, Naughton MT, Rahman MA, Bradley TD, Floras JS. Continuous positive airway pressure increases heart rate variability in congestive heart failure. *J Am Coll Cardiol* 1995; 25: 672–679.

56. Lin M, Chiang HT. The efficacy of early continuous positive airway pressure therapy in patients with acute cardiogenic pulmonary edema. *J Formos Med Assoc* 1991; 90: 736–743.

57. Wittmer VL, Simoes GM, Sogame LC, Vasquez EC. Effects of continuous positive airway pressure on pulmonary function and exercise tolerance in patients with congestive heart failure. *Chest* 2006; 130: 157–163.

58. Naughton MT, Liu PP, Bernard DC, Goldstein RS, Bradley TD. Treatment of congestive heart failure and Cheyne-Stokes respiration during sleep by continuous positive airway pressure. *Am J Respir Crit Care Med* 1995; 151: 92–97.

59. Chadda K, Annane D, Hart N, Gajdos P, Raphaël JC, Lofaso F. Cardiac and respiratory effects of continuous positive airway pressure and noninvasive ventilation in acute cardiac pulmonary edema. *Crit Care Med* 2002; 30: 2457–2461.

60. Rusterholtz T, Bollaert PE, Feissel M, *et al.*, Continuous positive airway pressure vs. proportional assist ventilation for noninvasive ventilation in acute cardiogenic pulmonary edema. *Intensive Care Med* 2008; 34: 840–846.

61. Bendjelid K, Schütz N, Suter PM, *et al.* Does continuous positive airway pressure by face mask improve patients with acute cardiogenic pulmonary edema due to left ventricular diastolic dysfunction? *Chest* 2005; 127: 1053–1058.

62. Agarwal R, Gupta D. Is the decrease in lvedv the mechanism of action of continuous positive airway pressure in diastolic heart failure? *Chest* 2005; 128: 1891–1892.

63. Bradley TD, Logan AG, Kimoff RJ, *et al.* Continuous positive airway pressure for central sleep apnea and heart failure. *N Engl J Med* 2005; 353: 2025–2033.

64. Tkacova R, Liu PP, Naughton MT, Bradley TD. Effect of continuous positive airway pressure on mitral regurgitant fraction and atrial natriuretic peptide in patients with heart failure. *J Am Coll Cardiol* 1997; 30: 739–745.

65. Noda A, Izawa H, Asano H, *et al.* Beneficial effect of bilevel positive airway pressure on left ventricular function in ambulatory patients with idiopathic dilated cardiomyopathy and central sleep apnea-hypopnea: a preliminary study. *Chest* 2007; 131: 1694–1701.

66. Arzt M, Bradley TD. Treatment of sleep apnea in heart failure. *Am J Respir Crit Care Med* 2006; 173: 1300–1308.

67. Yoshinaga K, Burwash IG, Leech JA, *et al.* The effects of continuous positive airway pressure on myocardial energetics in patients with heart failure and obstructive sleep apnea. *J Am Coll Cardiol* 2007; 49: 450–458.

68. Tkacova R, Rankin F, Fitzgerald FS, Floras JS, Bradley TD. Effects of continuous positive airway pressure on obstructive sleep apnea and left ventricular afterload in patients with heart failure. *Circulation* 1998; 98: 2269–2275.

69. Lamia B, Monnet X, Teboul J. Weaning-induced cardiac dysfunction. *In:* V. JL ed. Yearbook of intensive care and emergency medicine. Berlin, Heidelberg, New York, Springer, 2005; pp. 239–245.

70. Vitacca M, Ambrosino N, Clini E, *et al.* Physiological response to pressure support ventilation delivered before and after extubation in patients not capable of totally spontaneous autonomous breathing. *Am J Respir Crit Care Med* 2001; 164: 638–641.

NIV: indication in case of acute respiratory failure in obstructive pulmonary diseases

N. Ambrosino*,#, A. Corrado¶

*Pulmonary Diseases and Respiratory Intensive Care Unit, Cardio-Thoracic Dept, University Hospital Pisa, Pisa, #Weaning and Pulmonary Rehabilitation Unit, Auxilium Vitae, Volterra and ¶Pulmonary Intensive Care Unit, Respiratory Sleep Disorders Diagnosis and Treatment Centre, Regional Reference Centre for Diagnosis and Treatment of Respiratory Insufficiency, University Hospital, Careggi, Florence, Italy.

Correspondence: N. Ambrosino, U.O. Pneumologia, Dipartimento Cardio-Toracico, Azienda Ospedaliero-Universitaria Pisana, Via Paradisa 2, Cisanello, 56124 Pisa, Italy. Fax: 39 050996779; E-mail: n.ambrosino@ao-pisa.toscana.it

The acute exacerbation of chronic obstructive pulmonary disease

The most severe patients with chronic obstructive pulmonary disease (COPD) are likely to undergo severe exacerbations of their disease often needing hospital admission [1]. Acute exacerbations of COPD (AECOPD) are important events in the natural course of disease [2] leading to worsening in lung function and in health-related quality of life [3, 4] and, when associated with acute respiratory failure (ARF), to severe short- and long-term prognosis [5, 6]. Although the relationship between AECOPD frequency and severity of airflow obstruction is not particularly close, prevalence of AECOPD increases with disease severity [7], and new evidence indicates a possible role for extrapulmonary factors in their genesis [8].

The pharmacological management of AECOPD is outside the scope of this chapter and can be found elsewhere [9]. A stepwise drug therapy is recommended for both home and hospital management. Hospital management includes proper assessment of severity, diagnosis of the cause, controlled oxygen therapy and/or mechanical ventilation with an early noninvasive approach as the first line of intervention [10, 11]. A very severe life-threatening episode requires direct admission into the intensive care unit (ICU). When the cause of acute-on-chronic respiratory failure due to AECOPD is reversible, medical treatment works to maximise lung function and reverse the precipitating cause, whereas ventilatory support aims to gain time by unloading respiratory muscles, increasing ventilation (thus reducing dyspnoea and respiratory rate) and improving arterial oxygenation and eventually hypercapnia and related respiratory acidosis [12].

Most of the complications of invasive mechanical ventilation (table 1) are related to the endotracheal intubation (ETI) or to the placement of a tracheostomy tube, to baro- or volu-trauma and to the loss of airway defence mechanisms; some others may follow the extubation or complicate long-term tracheostomy [13]. Different modalities of noninvasive mechanical ventilation may avoid most of these complications, ensuring at the same time a similar degree of efficacy [14]. Ventilation-acquired pneumonia (VAP) and other nosocomial infections are reduced by noninvasive ventilation, because the airway defence mechanisms are preserved and there is less requirement for invasive monitoring [15, 16]. These modalities enhance the patient's comfort by allowing for eating, drinking, coughing and communication, and avoiding the need for sedation, without an increase in costs and nurse workload compared with invasive mechanical

Eur Respir Mon, 2008, 41, 24–36. Printed in UK - all rights reserved. Copyright ERS Journals Ltd 2008; European Respiratory Monograph; ISSN 1025-448x.

Table 1. – Complications of invasive mechanical ventilation

Related to tube insertion
  Aspiration of gastric contents
  Trauma of teeth, pharynx, oesophagus, larynx and trachea
  Sinusitis (nasotracheal intubation)
  Need for sedation
Related to mechanical ventilation
  Arrhythmias and hypotension
  Barotrauma
Related to tracheostomy
  Haemorrhage
  Trauma of trachea and oesophagus
  False lumen intubation
  Stomal infections and mediastinitis
  Tracheomalacia, tracheal stenoses and granulation tissue formation
  Tracheo-oesophageal or tracheoarterial fistulas
Caused by loss of airway defence mechanisms
  Airway colonisation with Gram-negative bacteria
  Pneumonia
Occurring after removal of the endotracheal tube
  Hoarseness, sore throat, cough and sputum
  Haemoptysis
  Vocal cord dysfunction and laryngeal swelling

Reproduced from AMBROSINO and VAGHEGGINI [10].

ventilation [17]. Many devices have been used in the past to deliver noninvasive mechanical ventilation, including both noninvasive positive pressure ventilation (NPPV) and intermittent negative pressure ventilation (INPV), but in recent years there has been prevalent use of NPPV [18].

Noninvasive positive pressure ventilation

Although continuous positive airway pressure (CPAP) is not considered a form of ventilation since no inspiratory aid is applied, according to the International Consensus Conference in 2001 [19], NPPV is defined as any form of ventilatory support applied without ETI, and is considered to include: CPAP, with or without inspiratory pressure support; volume- and pressure-cycled systems; proportional assist ventilation; and the use of helium–oxygen (heliox) gas mixtures [20]. NPPV is one of the most important developments in pulmonology over the past 15 yrs [21]. Indeed, a study in 349 ICUs in 23 countries describing current mechanical ventilation practices and assessing the influence of interval randomised trials, when compared with findings from a 1998 cohort, found that, in 2004, the use of NPPV increased (11.1 versus 4.4%) [22].

Different conditions leading to acute or acute-on-chronic respiratory failure have been treated with NPPV, but only a few are supported by strong evidence. NPPV leads to prevention of ETI in patients with AECOPD (the topic of this chapter) or acute cardiogenic pulmonary oedema, in immunocompromised patients, and is also a means of weaning from invasive mechanical ventilation in patients with AECOPD who undergo ETI. Weaker evidence supports the use of NPPV for patients with post-operative or post-extubation ARF, patients with ARF due to asthma exacerbations, pneumonia, acute lung injury or acute respiratory distress syndrome, during bronchoscopy, or as a means of pre-oxygenation before ETI in critically ill patients with severe hypoxaemia [10, 11].

The goals of NPPV may be different according to the underlying pathologies. During AECOPD or acute asthma, the goal of NPPV is to reduce hypercapnia by unloading the respiratory muscles and increasing alveolar ventilation, thereby reducing hypercapnia, improving respiratory acidosis until the underlying problem can be reversed [18]. Several prospective, randomised, controlled studies [23–30], systematic reviews and meta-analyses [31–33] show a good level of evidence for clinical efficacy of NPPV in the treatment of ARF due to AECOPD. Compared with standard medical therapy alone, NPPV improved survival, reduced the need for ETI and the rate of complications, and shortened the hospital and ICU length of stay. Based on these observations, NPPV has been proposed as the first-line ventilatory strategy in this condition with different timing and location according to the level of ARF severity [10, 11, 34, 35].

Severity of ARF

In patients with "mild" AECOPD, without respiratory acidosis (pH >7.35), NPPV did not prove to be more effective than standard medical therapy in preventing ARF or in improving mortality and length of hospitalisation, whereas >50% of the patients did not tolerate NPPV [24, 36]. In patients with mild to moderate ARF, as assessed by pH levels between 7.30 and 7.35, NPPV was successfully administered to prevent ETI in different settings, including the ward [29]. In even more severely ill patients (pH <7.25), the rate of NPPV failure was inversely related to the severity of respiratory acidosis, rising to 52–62% [26, 28]. The use of NPPV as an alternative to the ETI did not affect the mortality rate or the duration of ventilatory support, but the patients treated with NPPV underwent a lower rate of complications (*e.g.* VAP or difficult weaning) [30].

Severe encephalopathy was considered a contraindication to NPPV due to the concern that a depressed sensorium would predispose the patient to aspiration [15]. More recent observations of NPPV use in patients with altered levels of consciousness due to hypercapnic ARF have been reported [37, 38]. In a prospective case–control multicentre study of patients with AECOPD and moderate to severe hypercapnic encephalopathy, the use of NPPV *versus* conventional (invasive) mechanical ventilation (CMV) was associated with similar short- and long-term survivals, fewer nosocomial infections and shorter durations of mechanical ventilation and hospitalisation in the subgroup of patients treated successfully with NPPV [39]. SCALA *et al.* [39] suggest an initial cautious NPPV trial in patients with AECOPD and hypercapnic encephalopathy, as long as there are no other contraindications and the technique is administered by an experienced team in a closely monitored setting where ETI is always readily available (table 2).

Asthma

In contrast with AECOPD, the use of NPPV in severe exacerbation of asthma leading to ARF is supported by less evidence. MEDURI *et al.* [40] reported successful use of

Table 2. – Reported contraindications for noninvasive positive pressure ventilation

Cardiac or respiratory arrest
Severe encephalopathy
Severe gastrointestinal bleeding
Severe haemodynamic instability with or without unstable cardiac angina
Facial surgery or trauma
Upper airway obstruction
Inability to protect the airway and/or high risk of aspiration
Inability to clear secretions

NPPV in 17 episodes of status asthmaticus and severe ARF, as assessed by a mean pH of 7.25. NPPV resulted in a rapid improvement in physiological variables; only two patients required ETI. A retrospective, noncontrolled study reported favourable outcomes in 22 patients with status asthmaticus treated with NPPV because of persistent hypercapnia [41]. Other studies also report favourable outcomes [42]. Nevertheless, two more recent controlled trials reported inconclusive results [43, 44]. Owing to the small sample size of these studies, a recent Cochrane analysis concluded that evidence for use of NPPV in acute asthma was "promising" but "controversial" [45] and the British Thoracic Society Standards of Care Committee stated that NPPV "should not be used routinely in acute asthma", but that a trial might be considered in patients not promptly responding to standard treatments [46].

Successful NPPV

Successful use of NPPV in ARF due to AECOPD depends on the following several factors.

Clinical conditions. Selection of appropriate patients is crucial to the success of NPPV in AECOPD. Success of NPPV is not proven in conditions listed in table 2, which have been considered as exclusion criteria in randomised controlled trials [47]. Clinical judgment is important in taking decisions on NPPV and can be helped by predictive factors in the choice of this modality. An improvement in arterial blood gases and in sensorium, as assessed by means of the score described by KELLY and MATTHAY [48], or the response to NPPV of a combination of several clinical and physiological parameters after the first hour or two of treatment, are used as predictors of success or failure in COPD patients [49–51]. Airway colonisation by nonfermenting Gram-negative bacilli is strongly associated with NPPV failure [52]. Although these predictive factors must be kept in mind for successful NPPV, there is a caveat that, despite an initial brief improvement with NPPV, some COPD patients with severe ARF, particularly those with more severe functional impairment during the stable state, may have a late worsening (after >48 h), often requiring ETI [53].

Trained team. As with other therapies, NPPV application also follows a learning curve. With time, caregivers become more and more confident with NPPV, with success rates remaining stable or even improving despite increasing severity of treated patients [54]. A retrospective cohort study in French medical ICUs found that training in NPPV implementation may be an important factor in improving survival and reducing nosocomial infections in critical patients with AECOPD [55]. In this regard, JOLLIET et al. [56] reported that NPPV was not as time-consuming as they reported 10 yrs before [57].

Monitoring and location. Close clinical and functional monitoring is crucial, especially during the initial period of NPPV. The main concepts for adequate monitoring of NPPV can be summarised as follows: strict nurse supervision of respiratory and neurological conditions of patient; noninvasive monitoring; and preference for ventilators with availability of airway pressure, expired volume and airflow monitoring. The problem of monitoring is strictly related to the location for NPPV, which can actually determine NPPV outcome. Treating a severe hypoxaemia with or without hypercapnia might be dangerous in a general ward, whereas it is safer in a monitored high-technology setting like an ICU. In other words, selection of patients must take into account the location available to perform NPPV (fig. 1) [59]. Several studies support the effectiveness of

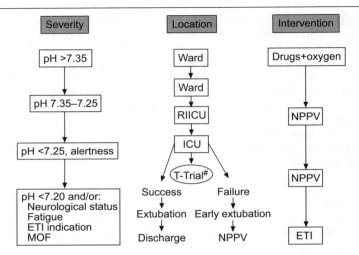

Fig. 1. – Flow chart of the application of noninvasive positive pressure ventilation (NPPV) in acute exacerbations of chronic obstructive pulmonary disease, according to the severity of acute respiratory failure. RIICU: respiratory intermediate intensive care unit; ICU: intensive care unit; ETI: endotracheal intubation; MOF: multiple organ failure. [#]: as described in [58]. Reproduced from AMBROSINO and VAGHEGGINI [10].

NPPV in the ICU, the respiratory intermediate ICUs, the general ward and the emergency departments [60]. Despite the demonstrated success of NPPV at least in some clinical conditions, the utilisation rates for NPPV vary enormously among different acute care hospitals within the same region [61]. In a survey of practice of NPPV in Ontario, Canada, the two most common indications for NPPV use were COPD and congestive heart failure [62]. Physician characteristics, such as awareness of the literature, were predictive of NPPV use for AECOPD, whereas perceived NPPV efficacy was predictive of use for many indications, including congestive heart failure. Recently, case series have also reported effectiveness of NPPV treatment in patients with moderate-to-severe ARF (pH <7.25) and AECOPD in general ward settings [63]. Given the prevalence of patients presenting with severe respiratory acidosis, further studies are needed to better outline the role of NPPV in non-ICU settings.

What's new?

The use of a heliox mixture seems very promising during NPPV in AECOPD in further reducing dyspnoea, work of breathing and length of hospital stay, but not in improving the success rate [64–67]. The use of heliox is difficult because of the lack of availability of approved heliox delivery systems, and appropriately designed randomised controlled trials are necessary in order to define the role for heliox mixtures during NPPV in AECOPD patients [68].

Despite the advantages of NPPV in ARF, a large number of failures are due to patient refusal to continue the often uncomfortable sessions. Therefore, sedation might have a role in success of this procedure. A cross-sectional web-based survey showed that most physicians infrequently use sedation and analgesic therapy for NPPV to treat ARF, but practices vary widely within and between specialties and geographic regions [69]. A recent pilot study showed that remifentanil-based sedation is safe and effective in the treatment of NPPV failure due to low tolerance [70].

Negative pressure ventilation

With negative-pressure ventilators the chest wall is exposed to subatmospheric pressure during inspiration, resulting in airflow into the lungs through the mouth and nose. When the pressure around the chest wall returns to atmospheric, expiration occurs passively owing to the elastic recoil of the lungs and chest wall [71].

All negative pressure devices have two major components: an applicator where a negative (subatmospheric) pressure is generated at the surface of the body during inspiration and a pump that effects pressure changes [71]. The cuirass (or shell) covers the anterior surface of the chest and upper abdomen. It is connected to the negative pressure pump through a tube and hose inlet on the centre. Standard sizes are available for commercial devices, whereas it is possible to tailor custom-made shells to patients with thoracic deformities [72]. All body suits, like the "pneumowrap" or "ponchowrap" applicators, are fitted over a rigid grid including the patient's ribcage and upper abdomen. The grid is anchored posteriorly with a backplate. The pneumowrap is attached to the negative pressure pump in a way similar to the cuirass.

The modern "iron lung" or a "tank ventilator" is made of aluminium and plastic. All the patient's body rests on a thin mattress except his/her head, which protrudes through a porthole at one end of the ventilator. In most designs, the head and the neck may rest to ensure comfort and to prevent upper airway collapse. Most tank ventilators have windows, allowing patient observation, and portholes through which catheters and monitor leads can be passed and which allow access to the patient for procedures. In some models, the patient's head can be raised so that aspiration may be prevented. Negative pressure is generated by bellows pumps incorporated into the structure of the ventilator or by separate rotary pumps. Most of the pumps used are pressure cycled, *i.e.* the ventilator will continue to develop a subatmospheric pressure until a set level is reached. With this modality the set pressure is the independent variable, whereas the tidal volume depends on the mechanical characteristics of the patient (besides the amount of leaks). With most tank ventilators the caregiver can set the pressure to be delivered during inspiration and expiration independently, and also set inspiratory and expiratory times [71]. Volume-cycled pumps have also been used; however, these devices cannot compensate for variable air leaks from the applicator and their use is limited. At the present time, there are five modes for delivering negative pressure ventilation: INPV, negative/positive pressure, continuous negative pressure (CNEP), negative pressure/CNEP and external high frequency oscillation [71].

INPV is the most commonly used mode. When operating in this mode, the respirator generates a set negative pressure around the body to initiate (or assist) inspiration. Expiration is passive and expiratory pressure at the anterior thoracic surface is atmospheric. During CNEP, subatmospheric pressure surrounds the patient throughout the respiratory cycle, the patient can breathe spontaneously or the respirator can be set to superimpose cycles of increased negative pressure. The clinical effect of CNEP is somewhat similar to that associated with positive end-expiratory pressure, but its cardiovascular effects differ [73]. All negative-pressure ventilators provide a control mode; additionally, some devices provide a "trigger" whereby patient-generated negative pressure at the nares or tracheotomy stoma initiates a machine breath. Other devices use a thermistor at the nares to trigger a breath. Nevertheless, up to now these modalities are still experimental.

Clinical studies

Early anecdotal reports [74–77] indicated a positive effect of INPV in ARF. Nevertheless, starting from the 1960s, COPD patients were generally treated with positive pressure ventilation through an endotracheal tube. More recently, there has been a renewed interest in INPV. Iron lung, cuirass and ponchowrap ventilators have been successfully used in AECOPD [78–81]. INPV was associated with good short- and long-term prognosis when used as first-line treatment in severe COPD patients with ARF [82, 83]. In a case–control study of very severe patients (pH 7.24, Acute Physiology and Chronic Health Evaluation II score 25), INPV was as effective as invasive mechanical ventilation and resulted in a similar length of hospital stay for the treatment of acute-on-chronic respiratory failure, but it was associated with a shorter duration of ventilation [84]. If NPPV is more successful with early application and lower severity of respiratory acidosis [49], the results of the study by CORRADO et al. [84] seem to indicate that INPV may be effective in a later stage of disease, similar to that requiring ETI. A possible explanation for the favourable effects of INPV in these studies [83, 84] may be a more beneficial effect on cardiopulmonary haemodynamics than seen with positive pressure ventilation [85]. Nevertheless, direct comparisons of INPV *versus* NPPV are not available. More recently, it has been reported that with sequential combination of INPV and NPPV, ETI was avoided in most unselected patients with acute-on-chronic respiratory failure needing ventilatory support [86, 87]. In recent years, the effectiveness of INPV for the treatment of acute-on-chronic respiratory failure in COPD patients has been confirmed in two case–control studies and in one randomised prospective control study [88, 89].

The studies suggest the following conclusions. 1) Physiological studies suggest that INPV is able to improve breathing pattern and arterial blood gases and to unload the respiratory muscles, thus fulfilling the aims of mechanical ventilation [71]. 2) Whereas prospective, randomised, controlled studies of INPV *versus* standard medical therapy are lacking, studies show that INPV, compared with CMV, had a similar degree of efficacy and was associated with a lower number of complications [83, 84]. 3) The most recent and "positive" reports come from one Italian centre only, and these results might also have been influenced by the specific expertise of that team. This clearly limits the potential widespread usefulness of the technique [82–84, 86, 88, 89]. 4) Uncontrolled but historically controlled retrospective and controlled but not randomised clinical studies show that INPV (by iron lung) is able to reduce the need for ETI and related complications even in patients with severe respiratory acidosis [71]. 5) Although the most recent reports are rather convincing on the usefulness of INPV in the treatment of acute or chronic respiratory failure, there are some difficulties in trying to introduce this modality in the vast majority of ICUs where NPPV is preferred as a noninvasive modality of mechanical ventilation [90]. The reason for this choice may be more due to the fact that iron lungs are more cumbersome and expensive than ventilators designed for NPPV, than due to the side-effects reported with those devices.

Advantages, contraindications and side-effects

Like NPPV, the major advantage of INPV is the avoidance of ETI and its related complications, while preserving physiological functions, such as speech, cough, swallowing and feeding. As with NPPV, bronchoscopic manoeuvres are allowed during INPV, which additionally may help techniques like laser therapy [91, 92]. Nevertheless, when treating patients with INPV several limitations should be considered. 1) The lack of upper airway protection, especially in unconscious and/or neurological patients, may result in aspiration, given the reported effect on the lower oesophageal sphincter, an effect to be prevented by pre-medication with metoclopramide [93]. 2) Upper airway obstruction may occur [94] or be enhanced in unconscious patients, in patients with neurological disorders with bulbar dysfunction and in those with sleep apnoeas syndrome.

Nevertheless, it has been reported that in unconscious patients with normal bulbar function, the placement of a nasogastric tube and the positioning of an oropharyngeal airway can minimise the risk of aspiration and/or airway collapsibility [78].

Conclusions

Noninvasive mechanical ventilation has assumed an important role in managing patients with acute respiratory failure due to acute exacerbations of chronic obstructive pulmonary disease. Even in conditions in which noninvasive positive pressure ventilation or intermittent negative pressure ventilation have strong evidence of success, patients should be monitored closely for signs of treatment failure and promptly intubated before a crisis develops. The application of either modality by a trained and experienced team, with careful patient selection and appropriate location and setting, should optimise patient outcomes. It must be clear that noninvasive mechanical ventilation is not a panacea, nor the "poor men's" technique of mechanical ventilation. Conversely, it cannot replace endotracheal intubation in all circumstances. With limited intermittent negative pressure ventilation facilities and expertise in most countries, it seems that noninvasive positive pressure ventilation will remain the most widely applied noninvasive ventilatory method, with intermittent negative pressure ventilation continuing as a viable option in some centres.

Summary

Noninvasive positive pressure ventilation (NPPV) and intermittent negative pressure ventilation (INPV) are techniques for delivering mechanical ventilation avoiding the complications of endotracheal intubation (ETI). We review the evidence supporting the use of noninvasive ventilation in acute respiratory failure (ARF) due to chronic obstructive pulmonary disease (COPD).
Strong evidence supports the use of NPPV for ARF to prevent ETI in patients with acute exacerbations of COPD. There is increasing evidence that in ARF due to COPD, INPV is as effective as NPPV and invasive mechanical ventilation and that a combination strategy of INPV and NPPV reduces the need for ETI. Noninvasive ventilation should be applied under close clinical and physiological monitoring for signs of treatment failure, and ETI should be promptly available in such cases. A trained team, careful patient selection and optimal choice of devices can optimise outcome.
Noninvasive mechanical ventilation is increasingly used in the management of ARF due to acute exacerbation of COPD. With limited INPV facilities and expertise in most countries, it seems that NPPV will remain the most widely applied noninvasive ventilatory method, with INPV continuing as a viable option in some centres.

Keywords: Acute respiratory failure, chronic obstructive pulmonary disease, endotracheal intubation, mechanical ventilation, noninvasive ventilation.

References

1.   Garcia-Aymerich J, Monsó E, Marrades RM, *et al.* Risk factors for hospitalization for a chronic obstructive pulmonary disease exacerbation. EFRAM study. *Am J Respir Crit Care Med* 2001; 164: 1002–1007.

2.   Celli BR, Barnes PJ. Exacerbations of chronic obstructive pulmonary disease. *Eur Respir J* 2007; 29: 1224–1238.

3.   Donaldson GC, Seemungal TA, Bhowmik A, Wedzicha JA. Relationship between exacerbation frequency and lung function decline in chronic obstructive pulmonary disease. *Thorax* 2002; 57: 847–852.

4.   Seemungal TA, Donaldson GC, Paul EA, Bestall JC, Jeffries DJ, Wedzicha JA. Effect of exacerbation on quality of life in patients with chronic obstructive pulmonary disease. *Am J Respir Crit Care Med* 1998; 157: 1418–1422.

5.   Connors AF Jr, Dawson NV, Thomas C, *et al.* Outcomes following acute exacerbation of severe chronic obstructive lung disease. The SUPPORT investigators (Study to Understand Prognoses and Preferences for Outcomes and Risks of Treatments). *Am J Respir Crit Care Med* 1996; 154: 959–967.

6.   Soler-Cataluña JJ, Martínez-García MA, Román Sánchez P, Salcedo E, Navarro M, Ochando R. Severe acute exacerbations and mortality in patients with chronic obstructive pulmonary disease. *Thorax* 2005; 60: 925–931.

7.   Dewan NA, Rafique S, Kanwar B, *et al.* Acute exacerbation of COPD: factors associated with poor treatment outcome. *Chest* 2000; 117: 662–671.

8.   Fabbri LM, Luppi F, Beghé B, Rabe KF. Complex chronic comorbidities of COPD. *Eur Respir J* 2008; 31: 204–212.

9.   Albert P, Calverley PM. Drugs (including oxygen) in severe COPD. *Eur Respir J* 2008; 31: 1114–1124.

10. Ambrosino N, Vagheggini G. Noninvasive positive pressure ventilation in the acute care setting: where are we? *Eur Respir J* 2008; 31: 874–886.

11. Hill NS, Brennan J, Garpestad E, Nava S. Noninvasive ventilation in acute respiratory failure. *Crit Care Med* 2007; 35: 2402–2407.

12. Laghi F, Tobin MJ. Indications for mechanical ventilation. *In*: Tobin MJ, ed. Principles and Practice of Mechanical Ventilation. 2nd Edn. New York, McGraw-Hill, 2006; pp. 129–162.

13. Epstein SK. Complications associated with mechanical ventilation. *In*: Tobin MJ, ed. Principles and Practice of Mechanical Ventilation. 2nd Edn. New York, McGraw-Hill, 2006; pp. 877–902.

14. Hill NS. Noninvasive positive-pressure ventilation. *In*: Tobin MJ, ed. Principles and Practice of Mechanical Ventilation. 2nd Edn. New York, McGraw-Hill, 2006; pp. 433–471.

15. Girou E, Schortgen F, Delclaux C, *et al.* Association of noninvasive ventilation with nosocomial infections and survival in critically ill patients. *JAMA* 2000; 284: 2361–2367.

16. Hess DR. Noninvasive positive-pressure ventilation and ventilator-associated pneumonia. *Respir Care* 2005; 50: 924–929.

17. Nava S, Evangelisti I, Rampulla C, Compagnoni ML, Fracchia C, Rubini F. Human and financial costs of noninvasive mechanical ventilation in patients affected by COPD and acute respiratory failure. *Chest* 1997; 111: 1631–1638.

18. Mehta S, Hill NS. Noninvasive ventilation. *Am J Respir Crit Care Med* 2001; 163: 540–577.

19. American Thoracic Society, European Respiratory Society, European Society of Intensive Care Medicine, Société de Réanimation de Langue Française. International Consensus Conferences in Intensive Care Medicine: noninvasive positive pressure ventilation in acute respiratory failure. *Am J Respir Crit Care Med* 2001; 163: 283–291.

20. MacIntyre NR. Principles of positive pressure mechanical ventilatory support. *In*: Ambrosino N, Goldstein RS, eds. Ventilatory Support for Chronic Respiratory Failure. New York, Informa Healthcare, 2008; pp. 13–27.

21. Garpestad E, Brennan J, Hill NS. Noninvasive ventilation for critical care. *Chest* 2007; 132: 711–720.

22. Esteban A, Ferguson ND, Meade MO, *et al.* Evolution of mechanical ventilation in response to clinical research. *Am J Respir Crit Care Med* 2008; 177: 170–177.
23. Bott J, Carroll MP, Conway JH, *et al.* Randomised controlled trial of nasal ventilation in acute ventilatory failure due to chronic obstructive airways disease. *Lancet* 1993; 341: 1555–1557.
24. Barbé F, Togores B, Rubí M, Pons S, Maimó A, Agustí AG. Noninvasive ventilatory support does not facilitate recovery from acute respiratory failure in chronic obstructive pulmonary disease. *Eur Respir J* 1996; 9: 1240–1245.
25. Celikel T, Sungur M, Ceyhan B, Karakurt S. Comparison of noninvasive positive pressure ventilation with standard medical therapy in hypercapnic acute respiratory failure. *Chest* 1998; 114: 1636–1642.
26. Conti G, Antonelli M, Navalesi P, *et al.* Noninvasive *versus* conventional mechanical ventilation in patients with chronic obstructive pulmonary disease after failure of medical treatment in the ward: a randomized trial. *Intensive Care Med* 2002; 28: 1701–1707.
27. Kramer N, Meyer TJ, Meharg J, Cece RD, Hill NS. Randomized, prospective trial of noninvasive positive pressure ventilation in acute respiratory failure. *Am J Respir Crit Care Med* 1995; 151: 1799–1806.
28. Brochard L, Mancebo J, Wysocki M, *et al.* Noninvasive ventilation for acute exacerbations of chronic obstructive pulmonary disease. *N Engl J Med* 1995; 333: 817–822.
29. Plant PK, Owen JL, Elliott MW. Early use of non-invasive ventilation for acute exacerbations of chronic obstructive pulmonary disease on general respiratory wards: a multicentre randomised controlled trial. *Lancet* 2000; 355: 1931–1935.
30. Squadrone E, Frigerio P, Fogliati C, *et al.* Noninvasive *versus* invasive ventilation in COPD patients with severe acute respiratory failure deemed to require ventilatory assistance. *Intensive Care Med* 2004; 30: 1303–1310.
31. Ram FS, Picot J, Lightowler J, Wedzicha JA. Non-invasive positive pressure ventilation for treatment of respiratory failure due to exacerbations of chronic obstructive pulmonary disease. *Cochrane Database Syst Rev* 2004; 3: CD004104.
32. Keenan SP, Sinuff T, Cook DJ, Hill NS. Which patients with acute exacerbation of chronic obstructive pulmonary disease benefit from noninvasive positive-pressure ventilation? A systematic review of the literature. *Ann Intern Med* 2003; 138: 861–870.
33. Lightowler JV, Wedzicha JA, Elliott MW, Ram FS. Non-invasive positive pressure ventilation to treat respiratory failure resulting from exacerbations of chronic obstructive pulmonary disease: Cochrane systematic review and meta-analysis. *BMJ* 2003; 326: 185–189.
34. Nava S, Navalesi P, Conti G. Time of non-invasive ventilation. *Intensive Care Med* 2006; 32: 361–370.
35. Elliott MW. Non-invasive ventilation in acute exacerbations of chronic obstructive pulmonary disease: a new gold standard? *Intensive Care Med* 2002; 28: 1691–1694.
36. Keenan SP, Powers CE, McCormack DG. Noninvasive positive-pressure ventilation in patients with milder chronic obstructive pulmonary disease exacerbations: a randomized controlled trial. *Respir Care* 2005; 50: 610–616.
37. Díaz GG, Alcaraz AC, Talavera JC, *et al.* Noninvasive positive-pressure ventilation to treat hypercapnic coma secondary to respiratory failure. *Chest* 2005; 127: 952–960.
38. Scala R, Naldi M, Archinucci I, Coniglio G, Nava S. Noninvasive positive pressure ventilation in patients with acute exacerbations of COPD and varying levels of consciousness. *Chest* 2005; 128: 1657–1666.
39. Scala R, Nava S, Conti G, *et al.* Noninvasive *versus* conventional ventilation to treat hypercapnic encephalopathy in chronic obstructive pulmonary disease. *Intensive Care Med* 2007; 33: 2101–2108.
40. Meduri GU, Cook TR, Turner RE, Cohen M, Leeper KV. Noninvasive positive pressure ventilation in status asthmaticus. *Chest* 1996; 110: 767–774.
41. Fernández MM, Villagrá A, Blanch L, Fernández R. Non-invasive mechanical ventilation in status asthmaticus. *Intensive Care Med* 2001; 27: 486–492.
42. Soma T, Hino M, Kida K, Kudoh S. A prospective and randomized study for improvement of acute asthma by non-invasive positive pressure ventilation (NPPV). *Intern Med* 2008; 47: 493–501.

43. Holley MT, Morrissey TK, Seaberg DC, Afessa B, Wears RL. Ethical dilemmas in a randomized trial of asthma treatment: can Bayesian statistical analysis explain the results? *Acad Emerg Med* 2001; 8: 1128–1135.

44. Soroksky A, Stav D, Shpirer I. A pilot, prospective, randomized, placebo-controlled trial of bilevel positive airway pressure in acute asthmatic attack. *Chest* 2003; 123: 1018–1025.

45. Ram FS, Wellington S, Rowe BH, Wedzicha JA. Non-invasive positive pressure ventilation for treatment of respiratory failure due to severe acute exacerbations of asthma. *Cochrane Database Syst Rev* 2005; 1: CD004360.

46. British Thoracic Society Standards of Care Committee. Non-invasive ventilation in acute respiratory failure. *Thorax* 2002; 57: 192–211.

47. Elliott MW. Non-invasive ventilation for acute respiratory disease. *Br Med Bull* 2005; 72: 83–97.

48. Kelly BJ, Matthay MA. Prevalence and severity of neurologic dysfunction in critically ill patients. Influence on need for continued mechanical ventilation. *Chest* 1993; 104: 1818–1824.

49. Ambrosino N, Foglio K, Rubini F, Clini E, Nava S, Vitacca M. Non-invasive mechanical ventilation in acute respiratory failure due to chronic obstructive pulmonary disease: correlates for success. *Thorax* 1995; 50: 755–757.

50. Confalonieri M, Garuti G, Cattaruzza MS, *et al.* A chart of failure risk for noninvasive ventilation in patients with COPD exacerbation. *Eur Respir J* 2005; 25: 348–355.

51. Nava S, Ceriana P. Causes of failure of noninvasive mechanical ventilation. *Respir Care* 2004; 49: 295–303.

52. Ferrer M, Ioanas M, Arancibia F, Marco MA, de la Bellacasa JP, Torres A. Microbial airway colonization is associated with noninvasive ventilation failure in exacerbation of chronic obstructive pulmonary disease. *Crit Care Med* 2005; 33: 2003–2009.

53. Moretti M, Cilione C, Tampieri A, Fracchia C, Marchioni A, Nava S. Incidence and causes of non-invasive mechanical ventilation failure after initial success. *Thorax* 2000; 55: 819–825.

54. Carlucci A, Delmastro M, Rubini F, Fracchia C, Nava S. Changes in the practice of non-invasive ventilation in treating COPD patients over 8 years. *Intensive Care Med* 2003; 29: 419–425.

55. Girou E, Brun-Buisson C, Taillé S, Lemaire F, Brochard L. Secular trends in nosocomial infections and mortality associated with noninvasive ventilation in patients with exacerbation of COPD and pulmonary edema. *JAMA* 2003; 290: 2985–2991.

56. Jolliet P, Abajo B, Pasquina P, Chevrolet JC. Non-invasive pressure support ventilation in severe community-acquired pneumonia. *Intensive Care Med* 2001; 27: 812–821.

57. Chevrolet JC, Jolliet P, Abajo B, Toussi A, Louis M. Nasal positive pressure ventilation in patients with acute respiratory failure. Difficult and time-consuming procedure for nurses. *Chest* 1991; 100: 775–782.

58. Ferrer M, Esquinas A, Arancibia F, *et al.* Noninvasive ventilation during persistent weaning failure: a randomized controlled trial. *Am J Respir Crit Care Med* 2003; 168: 70–76.

59. Ambrosino N, Corrado A. Obstructive pulmonary disease with acute respiratory failure. *In*: Muir JF, Ambrosino N, Simonds AK, eds. Noninvasive Mechanical Ventilation. *Eur Respir Mon* 2001; 16: 11–32.

60. Corrado A, Roussos C, Ambrosino N, *et al.* Respiratory intermediate care units: a European survey. *Eur Respir J* 2002; 20: 1343–1350.

61. Maheshwari V, Paioli D, Rothaar R, Hill NS. Utilization of noninvasive ventilation in acute care hospitals: a regional survey. *Chest* 2006; 129: 1226–1233.

62. Burns KE, Sinuff T, Adhikari NK, *et al.* Bilevel noninvasive positive pressure ventilation for acute respiratory failure: survey of Ontario practice. *Crit Care Med* 2005; 33: 1477–1483.

63. Crummy F, Buchan C, Miller B, Toghill J, Naughton MT. The use of noninvasive mechanical ventilation in COPD with severe hypercapnic acidosis. *Respir Med* 2007; 101: 53–61.

64. Jaber S, Fodil R, Carlucci A, *et al.* Noninvasive ventilation with helium-oxygen in acute exacerbations of chronic obstructive pulmonary disease. *Am J Respir Crit Care Med* 2000; 161: 1191–1200.

65. Jolliet P, Tassaux D, Roeseler J, *et al.* Helium-oxygen *versus* air-oxygen noninvasive pressure support in decompensated chronic obstructive disease: a prospective, multicenter study. *Crit Care Med* 2003; 31: 878–884.

66. Gainnier M, Forel JM. Clinical review: use of helium-oxygen in critically ill patients. *Crit Care* 2006; 10: 241.

67. Tassaux D, Gainnier M, Battisti A, Jolliet P. Helium-oxygen decreases inspiratory effort and work of breathing during pressure support in intubated patients with chronic obstructive pulmonary disease. *Intensive Care Med* 2005; 31: 1501–1507.

68. Hess DR. Heliox and noninvasive positive-pressure ventilation: a role for heliox in exacerbations of chronic obstructive pulmonary disease? *Respir Care* 2006; 51: 640–650.

69. Devlin JW, Nava S, Fong JJ, Bahhady I, Hill NS. Survey of sedation practices during noninvasive positive-pressure ventilation to treat acute respiratory failure. *Crit Care Med* 2007; 35: 2298–2302.

70. Constantin JM, Schneider E, Cayot-Constantin S, *et al.* Remifentanil-based sedation to treat noninvasive ventilation failure: a preliminary study. *Intensive Care Med* 2007; 33: 82–87.

71. Corrado A, Gorini M. Negative-pressure ventilation. *In*: Tobin MJ, ed. Principles and Practice of Mechanical Ventilation. 2nd Edn. New York, McGraw-Hill, 2006; pp. 403–419.

72. Newman JH, Wilkins JK. Fabrication of a customized cuirass for patients with severe thoracic asymmetry. *Am Rev Respir Dis* 1988; 137: 202–203.

73. Lockhat D, Langleben D, Zidulka A. Hemodynamic differences between continual positive and two types of negative pressure ventilation. *Am Rev Respir Dis* 1992; 146: 677–680.

74. Boutourline-Young HJ, Whittenberger JL. The use of artificial respiration in pulmonary emphysema accompanied by high carbon dioxide levels. *J Clin Invest* 1951; 30: 838–847.

75. Stone DJ, Schwartz A, Newman W, Feltman JA, Lovelock FJ. Precipitation by pulmonary infection of acute anoxia, cardiac failure and respiratory acidosis in chronic pulmonary disease; pathogenesis and treatment. *Am J Med* 1953; 14: 14–22.

76. Lovejoy FW Jr, Yu PN, Nye RE Jr, Joos HA, Simpson JH. Pulmonary hypertension. III. Physiologic studies in three cases of carbon dioxide narcosis treated by artificial respiration. *Am J Med* 1954; 16: 4–11.

77. Marks A, Bocles J, Morganti L. A new ventilatory assister for patients with respiratory acidosis. *N Engl J Med* 1963; 268: 61–67.

78. Corrado A, Gorini M, Villella G, De Paola E. Negative pressure ventilation in the treatment of acute respiratory failure: an old noninvasive technique reconsidered. *Eur Respir J* 1996; 9: 1531–1544.

79. Corrado A, Bruscoli G, Messori A, *et al.* Iron lung treatment of subjects with COPD in acute respiratory failure. Evaluation of short- and long-term prognosis. *Chest* 1992; 101: 692–696.

80. Sauret JM, Guitart AC, Rodríguez-Froján G, Cornudella R. Intermittent short-term negative pressure ventilation and increased oxygenation in COPD patients with severe hypercapnic respiratory failure. *Chest* 1991; 100: 455–459.

81. Montserrat JM, Martos JA, Alarcon A, Celis R, Plaza V, Picado C. Effect of negative pressure ventilation on arterial blood gas pressures and inspiratory muscle strength during an exacerbation of chronic obstructive lung disease. *Thorax* 1991; 46: 6–8.

82. Corrado A, De Paola E, Messori A, Bruscoli G, Nutini S. The effect of intermittent negative pressure ventilation and long-term oxygen therapy for patients with COPD. A 4-year study. *Chest* 1994; 105: 95–99.

83. Corrado A, De Paola E, Gorini M, *et al.* Intermittent negative pressure ventilation in the treatment of hypoxic hypercapnic coma in chronic respiratory insufficiency. *Thorax* 1996; 51: 1077–1082.

84. Corrado A, Gorini M, Ginanni R, *et al.* Negative pressure ventilation *versus* conventional mechanical ventilation in the treatment of acute respiratory failure in COPD patients. *Eur Respir J* 1998; 12: 519–525.

85. Simonds AK. Negative pressure ventilation in acute hypercapnic chronic obstructive pulmonary disease. *Thorax* 1996; 51: 1069–1070.

86. Gorini M, Ginanni R, Villella G, Tozzi D, Augustynen A, Corrado A. Non-invasive negative and positive pressure ventilation in the treatment of acute on chronic respiratory failure. *Intensive Care Med* 2004; 30: 875–881.

87. Todisco T, Baglioni S, Eslami A, *et al.* Treatment of acute exacerbations of chronic respiratory failure: integrated use of negative pressure ventilation and noninvasive positive pressure ventilation. *Chest* 2004; 125: 2217–2223.

88. Corrado A, Confalonieri M, Marchese S, *et al.* Iron lung *versus* mask ventilation in the treatment of acute on chronic respiratory failure in COPD patients: a multicenter study. *Chest* 2002; 121: 189–195.

89. Corrado A, Ginanni R, Villella G, *et al.* Iron lung *versus* conventional mechanical ventilation in acute exacerbation of COPD. *Eur Respir J* 2004; 23: 419–424.

90. Nava S, Confalonieri M, Rampulla C. Intermediate respiratory intensive care units in Europe: a European perspective. *Thorax* 1998; 53: 798–802.

91. Vitacca M, Natalini G, Cavaliere S, *et al.* Breathing pattern and arterial blood gases during Nd-YAG laser photoresection of endobronchial lesions under general anesthesia: use of negative pressure ventilation: a preliminary study. *Chest* 1997; 112: 1466–1473.

92. Natalini G, Cavaliere S, Vitacca M, Amicucci G, Ambrosino N, Candiani A. Negative pressure ventilation *versus* spontaneous assisted ventilation during rigid bronchoscopy. A controlled randomised trial. *Acta Anaesthesiol Scand* 1998; 42: 1063–1069.

93. Marino WD, Pitchumoni CS. Reversal of negative pressure ventilation-induced lower esophageal sphincter dysfunction with metoclopramide. *Am J Gastroenterol* 1992; 87: 190–194.

94. Levy RD, Cosio MG, Gibbons L, Macklem PT, Martin JG. Induction of sleep apnoea with negative pressure ventilation in patients with chronic obstructive lung disease. *Thorax* 1992; 47: 612–615.

CHAPTER 3

Management of acute respiratory failure in restrictive disorders (obesity excluded)

J.C. Winck, M. Gonçalves

Serviço de Pneumologia, Faculdade de Medicina do Porto, Porto, Portugal.

Correspondence: J.C. Winck, Serviço de Pneumologia, Faculdade de Medicina do Porto, Alameda Prof Hernâni Monteiro, 4200-319 Porto, Portugal. Fax: 351 225512215; E-mail: jwinck@hsjoao.min-saude.pt

Introduction

International surveys performed in intensive care units (ICUs) around the world in 1996 and 1998, showed that neuromuscular patients corresponded to 1.8–10% of patients receiving mechanical ventilation [1, 2]. An Italian survey of respiratory ICUs in 1997–1998 showed that chest wall and neuromuscular disorders accounted for 9% of patients admitted [3].

Restrictive disorders are the most-frequent indication for long-term home mechanical ventilation, with thoracic cage and neuromuscular patients accounting for 65% of patients ventilated at home in Europe [4].

Noninvasive ventilation (NIV) has been shown to be the first line intervention for acute respiratory failure (ARF) due to chronic obstructive pulmonary disease (COPD) [5]. In patients with ARF due to restrictive disorders, the evidence is lower; although published studies demonstrate positive results [6]. In fact, randomised clinical trials (RCT) of NIV in ARF tend to exclude patients with restrictive disorders. In the only RCT of NIV in ARF that included patients with neuromuscular diseases (NMDs; n=6), the authors did not discuss those patients because the group was too small for analysis [7].

While PORTIER et al. [8], in a prospective multicentre study of patients with acute-on-chronic respiratory failure (including 16.7% with restrictive disorders), suggested that the underlying disorder did not influence prognosis, ROBINO et al. [9], in a retrospective study with the largest sample of restrictive patients published to date (mainly with chest wall disorders (CWD)), suggested that effectiveness of NIV was less in this group of patients.

Recently, BANFI et al. [10] successfully managed seven patients with kyphoscoliosis (KS) with infection-related respiratory failure at home. In fact, by increasing daily duration of mechanical ventilation to >20 h, respiratory acidosis was corrected and the patients were returned to their baseline condition in 4 weeks.

It seems that respiratory failure due to these disorders needs a different approach from the more-common obstructive pulmonary diseases [9, 11].

ARF in chest wall disorders

Patients with severe KS and acute decompensation of respiratory failure, exhibit marked decrease of pulmonary compliance but, contrary to in COPD, increase in airway resistance and intrinsic positive end-expiratory pressure (PEEPi) seem to play only a

Eur Respir Mon, 2008, 41, 37–46. Printed in UK - all rights reserved. Copyright ERS Journals Ltd 2008; European Respiratory Monograph; ISSN 1025-448x.

secondary role [12]. Because cough is not impaired like in NMD, secretion management is not so critical in this context, and management of ARF may be easier.

Some case series have shown that ARF occurring in KS can be managed noninvasively, either through negative [13] or positive pressure ventilation [6, 14]. Recently BANFI *et al.* [10] have shown reversal of respiratory acidosis in KS patients with ARF, by increasing duration of home mechanical ventilation up to >20 h, both with volume and pressure-cycled ventilators.

ARF in neuromuscular disorders

In neuromuscular disorders, the normality of the respiratory function requires the integrity of three main respiratory muscles: 1) inspiratory muscles, responsible for ventilation; 2) expiratory muscles, involved in the ability to cough; and 3) bulbar muscles, that protect against the risk of aspiration [15]. Laryngeal weakness and swallowing dysfunction can lead to aspiration, which is the main reason for failure of noninvasive respiratory aids during ARF in NMD [16].

In patients with previous NMD, respiratory failure is commonly triggered by upper respiratory tract infections [17]. This can impair the three muscle components [11, 17]. Those patients normally present with rapid shallow breathing, tachycardia, accessory-muscle use, thoraco-abdominal asynchrony and orthopnoea. Blood gases, vital capacity, maximum inspiratory and expiratory pressures, and peak cough flow should be evaluated and used to give useful information about the integrity of the respiratory muscle system. In accord with the disease and objective parameters, the need for mechanical ventilation can be predicted. Hypercapnia is a late finding of impending ventilatory failure whereas hypoxaemia may suggest atelectasis and secretion encumbrance or pneumonia.

In order to avoid NMD patients being admitted to hospital with ARF, a regular follow-up of all chronic NMD patients with lung function evaluation, in order to establish domiciliary noninvasive respiratory aids, is fundamental [18]. Moreover a pro-active intervention with intensification of home mechanical assisted cough and NIV, guided by oxygen saturation, has been proposed by some authors [19]. In fact, this protocol reduces hospitalisation for NMD cases followed in specific outpatient clinics.

However, there will always be cases where ARF will be the presentation for NMD, especially those with a rapid evolution like amyotrophic lateral sclerosis (ALS) [20, 21]; apart from those patients, acute neuromuscular disorders (such as Guillain–Barré syndrome (GBS)) together with the ICU-acquired neuromuscular disorders are the most frequent NMD associated with ARF (table 1).

ARF in amyotrophic lateral sclerosis

Analysing a large US database, LECHTZIN *et al.* [22], reported that, in hospitalised ALS patients, mortality was 15%. According to conventional protocols, patients with

Table 1. – Major neuromuscular disorders (NMD) associated with acute respiratory failure

Motor Nerves	Neuromuscular junction	Myopathies	Spinal cord	Acquired NMD
Amyotrophic lateral sclerosis	Myasthenia gravis	Myotonic dystrophy	Trauma	Critical illness myoneuropathy
Guillain–Barré syndrome		Duchenne muscular dystrophy	Transverse myelitis	

ALS, who present acutely in respiratory failure and require endotracheal intubation and invasive ventilation, are rarely weaned and rarely return home [23].

If the cause of ARF is secretion encumbrance and assisted mucus clearance techniques are unavailable at home, a strict protocol of mechanical in-exsufflation (MIE) should be implemented (sometimes with a 5-min frequency), together with continuous NIV, until blood gases are normalised [24]. It should be noted that patients with NMD and excessive secretions/atelectasis may require the use of very frequent assisted-cough techniques, which require time-consuming care from nursing staff and respiratory therapists; this makes the help of family caregivers essential [25]. This will reverse the majority of cases [26]; however, some patients can be intubated for 24/48 h to rest and optimise secretion clearance with MIE through an endotracheal tube [24]. Subsequently it might be possible to extubate them directly with continuous NIV.

There are not many studies analysing the role of NIV in ARF due to ALS. In 2000, VIANELLO et al. [27] published the first study, prospectively comparing the efficacy of NIV combined with cricothyroidotomy ("minitracheostomy") and conventional mechanical ventilation via endotracheal tube in 14 patients with ARF and NMD (including three patients with ALS). Mean pH was 7.29 in both groups, mortality was lower and ICU stay was shorter in the NIV group compared with controls, suggesting that their "noninvasive ventilatory approach" could be a first-line intervention in this setting.

In 2005, VIANELLO et al. [28] evaluated the short-term outcomes of 11 NMD patients (including two patients with ALS), not as severely acidotic (mean pH of 7.36), with acute upper respiratory tract infections and tracheobronchial mucous encumbrance. Apart from NIV, they were submitted to MIE treatment in addition to standard physical therapy. The outcomes were compared with 16 historically matched controls, who had received chest physical therapy alone. The treatment failure (defined as the need for cricothyroidotomy or endotracheal intubation, despite treatment) was significantly lower in the MIE group than in the conventional chest physical treatments group (2 out of 11 and 10 out of 16 cases, respectively). No side effects were related to the use of MIE alone, while the need of bronchoscopy assisted suctioning was similar in the two groups (5 out of 11 and 6 out of 16 cases, respectively).

As noted by GONÇALVES and BACH in their commentary [25], some mistakes concerning the use of the MIE probably compromised the final results. Setting the machine at very low insufflation and exsufflation pressures (<30 cmH$_2$O), and forgetting the abdominal thrust during the exsufflation phase were reasons for suboptimal results. These low pressures have been shown not to be effective in lung models [29] as well as in clinical studies [30, 31] and accordingly, did not effectively avert bronchoscopy-assisted aspiration. Moreover, using the MIE 2.7 times a day as described may be insufficient. In fact, as mentioned before, during an acute episode of respiratory tract infection, MIE may have to be applied very frequently, and the only way to solve this problem is to allow the primary care providers or relatives to stay at the bedside to use it anytime as required [32].

SERVERA et al. [16] in a non-ICU setting, prospectively evaluated the efficacy of continuous NIV together with coughing aids (including MIE) to avoid endotracheal intubation for 17 patients with NMD during ARF. The studied group had a mean pH of 7.38 and included 11 patients with ALS (5 of which with bulbar dysfunction). There was treatment failure in 20.8% and mortality in 8.3% cases, significantly related with patients with severe bulbar impairment. The patients in which NIV and assisted coughing may be unsuccessful and those who cannot cooperate may have a more invasive approach: endotracheal intubation and mechanical ventilation followed by tracheostomy [33] or as VIANELLO et al. [34] proposed cricothyroidotomy. However, even in bulbar ALS patients, MIE should be tried, since HANAYAMA et al. [35] described an ALS woman with immeasurable peak cough flow (PCF), already with a gastrostomy, in which MIE was able to clear bronchial secretions and reverse ARF.

In the present authors' experience, with 11 consecutive nonbulbar ALS with ARF, noninvasive respiratory aids (*i.e.* continuous NIV and high-intensity mechanical assisted cough) had a success rate of 100%, with resolution of respiratory failure, and discharge after 8 days (fig. 1) [26]. With this protocol, MIE resolved atelectasis and none of those patients needed endotracheal intubation or fibreoptic bronchoscopy assisted aspiration (fig. 2).

Concerning the mode of noninvasive ventilation, it is preferable to use volume-cycled ventilators in assist control, with high tidal volumes, for sufficient lung expansion and to allow air-stacking for coughing [16, 26]. This can be performed during the day using a mouthpiece and at night with a nasal or oral interface. As soon as the patient learns to air-stack and can autonomously produce PCF above 160 L·min^{-1}, assisted coughing can be reduced in frequency, provided that oxygen saturation levels on the ventilator are >95% [36]. In the beginning, the patient will need continuous NIV but, at discharge, will return to the previous duration of home NIV [16, 26].

When patients with ALS under home mechanical ventilation need to be hospitalised due to ARF, there are some technical as well as ethical aspects that need to be considered. It needs to be confirmed if all noninvasive respiratory aids were optimised at home, if the patient has refused tracheostomy, if bulbar impairment is severe and if the risk of aspiration is high. Lung function status, previous to the decompensation, can be helpful in the decision making. Discussions about aggressiveness of resuscitation should have been carried out with the family and patient in a stable state [37].

Another issue is when nonbulbar patients with NMD are intubated because of failure of NIV or due to a more-conventional approach. In this context, it is a common attitude to gradually reduce the support of the ventilator until the patient is weaned. Unfortunately NMD patients with a pre-existing respiratory dysfunction often fail to wean from invasive ventilation and are almost invariably tracheostomised. MIE in these cases can be very successful to help clear secretions, first *via* the tube and, then, after the tube is removed *via* an oronasal mask, while the ventilation is delivered through noninvasive interfaces. MIE, applied in this circumstance, avoids mucus encumbrance,

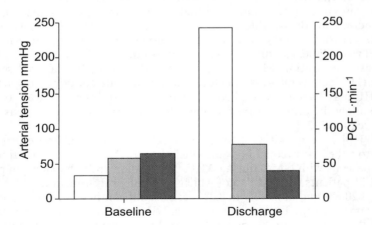

Fig. 1. – Outcomes of 11 patients with nonbulbar amyotrophic lateral sclerosis and acute respiratory failure. Peak cough flow (PCF; □), and arterial oxygen (Pa,O_2; ▨) and carbon dioxide (Pa,CO_2; ■) tension were measured. The length of stay was 7.9±8.9 days, at administration pH 7.37±1.3, Pa,O_2 7.69±1.12 kPa (57.8±8.4 mmHg), Pa,CO_2 8.61±3.47 kPa (64.7±26.1 mmHg) and 0 treatment failure. 1 mmHg = 0.133 kPa.

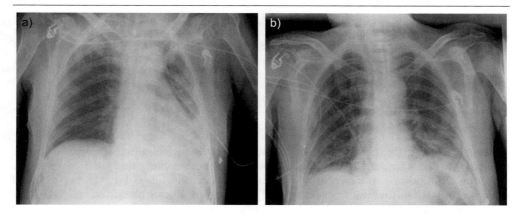

Fig. 2. – Resolution of left lower lobe atelectasis in one amyotrophic lateral sclerosis patient a) before and b) after mechanical in-exsufflation.

the need of blind suctioning through the nose and definitely tracheostomy for patients, who are ventilator dependent 24 h per day.

ARF in Guillain–Barré syndrome and in myasthenia gravis

In the developed world, GBS and myasthenia gravis (MG) account for the majority of cases of respiratory failure associated with NMD.

Although the use of NIV in this setting has not been extensively evaluated [38–40], it should be always attempted unless there is significant bulbar dysfunction. In fact, GBS and MG are similar to other NMDs where a noninvasive respiratory aids protocol has avoided endotracheal intubation [16, 26, 28]. The only difference is that contrary to the majority of ALS and NMD patients with ARF, those patients are naïve to NIV.

According to the literature, 25-50% of GBS patients and 15–27% MG patients require mechanical ventilation [41, 42]. A practical rule (the "20/30/40 rule") proposed by LAWN et al. [43] in which a vital capacity (VC) <20 mL·kg^{-1}, maximal inspiratory pressure $<$-30 cmH$_2$O and maximal expiratory pressure <40 cmH$_2$O were associated with progression to respiratory failure, may be useful in deciding whether to initiate ventilatory support. These simple bedside tests of respiratory function may be clinically generalisable to other neuromuscular conditions.

ARF in Guillain–Barré syndrome

GBS is an acute immune-mediated polyneuropathy, with an incidence of 0.6–2 cases per 100,000 inhabitants [44]. Mechanical ventilation was required in $\leq$50% of patients and was a risk factor for a poor outcome [45, 46]. Traditionally, patients are subjected to prolonged invasive ventilation, with a 49% incidence of atelectasis and 25% mortality [47]. Moreover, 7% of patients will need ventilatory support after 1 yr [46]. Recently, PEARSE et al. [38] used NIV for 2 weeks in a patient with respiratory failure secondary to GBS. In this patient with preserved bulbar function, NIV was applied continuously with a pressure support of 10 cmH$_2$O in the first days and withdrawn at 2 weeks, avoiding the complications of mechanical ventilation. However, WIJDICKS et al. [48] report the failure of bilevel ventilation in two cases of GBS. Those patients deteriorated under low levels of pressure support, presumably due to worsening hypoventilation and sputum retention.

So, it must be kept in mind that NIV can worsen gastric distension caused by disautomony and may contribute to poor tolerance and efficacy. However, with strict monitoring and trained staff, it is possible to apply NIV in this setting, especially if effective secretion clearance techniques [26, 31] are used rather than traditional chest physiotherapy or tracheal suctioning *via* nasopharyngeal airways, which are unpleasant and even deleterious to the patients.

ARF in myasthenia gravis

MG is the most frequent disease of the neuromuscular junction, characterised by the reduction in the number of acetylcholine post-synaptic receptors and, in 80% of cases, with the antibodies' antireceptors. The incidence of MG is 0.4 cases per 100,000 inhabitants [49]. Only a minority of cases will be diagnosed during an episode of ARF [50]; more commonly patients already diagnosed have an exacerbation of myasthenic weakness (myasthenic crisis (MC)) causing ARF [39, 40]. Contrary to GBS, monitoring of serial VC does not predict the necessity of ventilatory assistance due to the erratic nature of the variation [49].

Traditionally patients with MC are managed using endotracheal intubation and mechanical ventilation. Recent work from the Mayo Clinic showed that NIV can be an alternative [39, 51]. In fact, use of low span bilevel positive pressure ventilation prevented intubation in 70% of cases even in patients with bulbar weakness [51]. In a more representative series (60 episodes of MC in 52 patients), the same group confirmed that NIV was an effective treatment for ARF in MG, significantly reducing the ICU stay [39]. The only predictor of NIV failure was an arterial carbon dioxide tension exceeding 5.99 kPa (45 mmHg). This was somewhat contradicted by AGARWAL *et al.* [40] who described a patients with a MC and hypercapnic acidosis, successfully managed with higher levels of bilevel positive pressure ventilation.

Although the majority may be weaned from mechanical ventilation after a myasthenic crisis, some patients develop chronic respiratory failure and need long-term mechanical ventilation.

ARF in spinal cord injury

Demographic data from the US spinal cord injury (SCI) database in 1973–2003 show a significant increase in the percentage of cervical injuries and ventilator-dependent cases, with 6.8% of SCI patients requiring ventilation on discharge in 2000–2003 [52]. Most SCI patients who require ventilatory support undergo tracheostomy during their acute hospitalisation [53]. Despite improvements in SCI medical management, re-hospitalisation rates remain high, associated with respiratory complications [54]. Cervical spine injuries can be separated into higher-cervical cord injuries (levels C1 and C2) and mid- and lower-cervical cord injuries (C3 to C8). The former produce almost total respiratory muscle paralysis, while the latter have limited expiratory function. Lesions from C3-C5 cause also significant compromise of inspiration [53].

During the 1980s, survival for ventilatory dependent tetraplegic patients ranged from 63% at age 3 yrs [55] to 33% at age 5 yrs [56]. In those times, only 51% of SCI patients with C3 injury levels were able to be weaned [56]. Life expectancy was considerably improved in those successfully weaned [57].

High level tetraplegic patients are perfect candidates for noninvasive ventilatory assistance due to their young age, intact mental status and bulbar musculature [58]. In fact, BACH [59] suggested that patients with lesions under C1 level, can be managed by using noninvasive respiratory aids (up to continuous noninvasive IPPV and manually and mechanically assisted coughing) provided that they are able to generate assisted peak cough flow >160 L·min^{-1}.

It is recommended that all patients with acute SCI have their VC measured every 6 h during the first few days of admission. If symptoms or signs of impending ventilatory failure develop or VC decreases to <1500 mL, the patient should be placed on continuous oximetry monitoring and trained in using MIV and manually and mechanically assisted coughing [60].

When patients with SCI are tracheostomised, there will always be the potential for decannulation. Although this topic is beyond the scope of the present chapter, it must be emphasised that, even in patients with little ventilator-free breathing ability, a switch to NIV and "aggressive" mechanical insufflation–exsufflation can lead to successful decannulation [61].

Critical-illness myoneuropathy

ICU-acquired NMD is reported in 25% of patients who have been ventilated for ≥7 days [62]. This figure increases in patients with sepsis and severe acute asthma [63].

Normally, patients present with diffuse skeletal-muscle weakness and difficulty in weaning. ICU-acquired NMD is associated with a longer duration of mechanical ventilation, longer ICU stay and increased mortality [63]. Cough inefficacy and reduction in maximal respiratory pressures have been reported in these patients [64], suggesting the implementation of secretion-clearance techniques together with noninvasive ventilatory support could play a role [11]. Although studies reporting application of noninvasive respiratory aids in this context are lacking, in the present authors' experience, application of this protocol in ICU-acquired NMD has allowed decannulation and weaning in a significant number of patients (data not published).

Critical illness myoneuropathy has also been implicated in respiratory failure that develops after discharge from the ICU [64]. Recovery of peripheral and respiratory muscle function is highly variable, with some patients having persisting weakness at 2 yrs follow-up.

Summary

Although noninvasive ventilation (NIV) has an established role for stable patients with restrictive disorders and chronic respiratory failure, evidence from randomised clinical trials in the acute setting is lacking. However, based on the published studies, NIV associated with cough assistance is very effective in neuromuscular diseases (NMDs) with acute respiratory failure (ARF), especially those without significant bulbar dysfunction.

With evidence emerging for myasthenia gravis and Guillain–Barré syndrome, patients with ARF and pre-existing NMD (most already trained in NIV) are the best candidates for a noninvasive respiratory aids protocol.

Secretion-clearance techniques are critically important in managing NMD patients and they may be the weak link in the management of ARF!

Continuous volume cycled ventilation (through a nasal or oral interface) associated with high intensity mechanical in-exsufflation may be very effective in the hands of experienced staff with the proper protocols.

Keywords: Acute respiratory failure, mechanical in-exsufflation, neuromuscular disorders, noninvasive ventilation, secretion management.

References

1. Esteban A, Anzueto A, Alía I, *et al.* How is mechanical ventilation employed in the intensive care unit? An international utilization review. *Am J Respir Crit Care Med* 2000; 161: 1450–1458.
2. Esteban A, Anzueto A, Frutos F, *et al.* Characteristics and outcomes in adult patients receiving mechanical ventilation: a 28-day international study. *JAMA* 2002; 287: 345–355.
3. Confalonieri M, Gorini M, Ambrosino N, Mollica C, Corrado A, Scientific Group on Respiratory Intensive Care of the Italian Association of Hospital Pneumonologists. Respiratory intensive care units in Italy: a national census and prospective cohort study. *Thorax* 2001; 56: 373–378.
4. Lloyd-Owen SJ, Donaldson GC, Ambrosino N, *et al.* Patterns of home mechanical ventilation use in Europe: results from the Eurovent survey. *Eur Respir J* 2005; 25: 1025–1031.
5. Lightowler JV, Wedzicha JA, Elliott MW, Ram FS. Non-invasive positive pressure ventilation to treat respiratory failure resulting from exacerbations of chronic obstructive pulmonary disease: Cochrane systematic review and meta-analysis. *BMJ* 2003; 326: 185.
6. Finlay G, Concannon D, McDonnell TJ. Treatment of respiratory failure due to kyphoscoliosis with nasal intermittent positive pressure ventilation (NIPPV). *Ir J Med Sci* 1995; 164: 28–30.
7. Martin TJ, Hovis JD, Costantino JP, *et al.* A randomized, prospective evaluation of noninvasive ventilation for acute respiratory failure. *Am J Respir Crit Care Med* 2000; 161: 807–813.
8. Portier F, Defouilloy C, Muir JF. Determinants of immediate survival among chronic respiratory insufficiency patients admitted to an intensive care unit for acute respiratory failure. A prospective multicenter study. The French Task Group for Acute Respiratory Failure in Chronic Respiratory insufficiency. *Chest* 1992; 101: 204–210.
9. Robino C, Faisy C, Diehl J-L, Labrousse J, Guerot E. Effectiveness of non-invasive positive pressure ventilation differs between decompensated chronic restrictive and obstructive pulmonary disease patients. *Intensive Care Med* 2003; 29: 603–610.
10. Banfi P, Redolfi S, Robert D. Home treatment of infection-related acute respiratory failure in kyphoscoliotic patients on long-term mechanical ventilation. *Respir Care* 2007; 52: 713–719.
11. Winck JC, Gonçalves M. Muscles and lungs: fatal attraction, but time for intervention. *Monaldi Arch Chest Dis* 2005; 63: 121–3.
12. Conti G, Rocco M, Antonelli M, *et al.* Respiratory system mechanics in the early phase of acute respiratory failure due to severe kyphoscoliosis. *Intensive Care Med* 1997; 23: 539–544.
13. Sawicka EH, Spencer GT, Branthwaite MA. Management of respiratory failure complicating pregnancy in severe kyphoscoliosis: a new use for an old technique? *Br J Dis Chest* 1986; 80: 191–196.
14. Elliott MW, Steven MH, Phillips GD, Branthwaite MA. Non-invasive mechanical ventilation for acute respiratory failure. *BMJ* 1990; 300: 358–360.
15. Benditt JO. The neuromuscular respiratory system: physiology, pathophysiology, and a respiratory care approach to patients. *Respir Care* 2006; 51: 829–837.
16. Servera E, Sancho J, Zafra MJ, Catala A, Vergara P, Marin J. Alternatives to endotracheal intubation for patients with neuromuscular diseases. *Am J Phys Med Rehabil* 2005; 84: 851–857.
17. Poponick JM, Jacobs I, Supinski G, DiMarco AF. Effect of upper respiratory tract infection in patients with neuromuscular disease. *Am J Respir Crit Care Med* 1997; 156: 659–664.
18. Farrero E, Prats E, Povedano M, Martinez-Matos JA, Manresa F, Escarrabill J. Survival in amyotrophic lateral sclerosis with home mechanical ventilation: the impact of systematic respiratory assessment and bulbar involvement. *Chest* 2005; 127: 2132–2138.
19. Bach JR, Ishikawa Y, Kim H. Prevention of pulmonary morbidity for patients with Duchenne muscular dystrophy. *Chest* 1997; 112: 1024–1028.
20. Chen R, Grand'Masoin F, S MJ, Ramsay DA, Bolton CF. Motor neuron disease presenting as acute respiratory failure: a clinical and pathological study. *J Neurol Neurosurg Psychiatry* 1996; 60: 455–458.
21. de Carvalho M, Matias T, Coelho F, Evangelista T, Pinto A, Luís ML. Motor neuron disease presenting with respiratory failure. *J Neurol Sci 1996; Aug*, 139: Suppl. 117–122

22. Lechtzin N, Wiener CM, Clawson L, Chaudhry V, Diette GB. Hospitalization in amyotrophic lateral sclerosis: causes, costs, and outcomes. *Neurology* 2001; 56: 753–757.

23. Bradley MD, Orrell RW, Clarke J, *et al.* Outcome of ventilatory support for acute respiratory failure in motor neurone disease. *J Neurol Neurosurg Psychiatry* 2002; 72: 752–756.

24. Bach JR. Management of patients with neuromuscular disease. Philadelphia: Hanley & Belfus, 2004.

25. Goncalves MR, Bach JR. Mechanical Insufflation-exsufflation improves outcomes for Neuromuscular disease patients with repiratory tract infections. *Am J Phys Med Rehabil* 2005; 84: 89–91.

26. Gonçalves MR, Winck JC, Nadais G, Almeida J, Marques JA. Acute respiratory failure in Amyotophic lateral sclerosis: management with non-invasive respiratory aids. *Eur Respir J* 2004; 24: Suppl. 48, 314s.

27. Vianello A, Bevilacqua M, Arcaro G, Gallan F, Serra E. Non-invasive ventilatory approach to treatment of acute respiratory failure in neuromuscular disorders. A comparison with endotracheal intubation. *Intensive Care Med* 2000; 26: 384–390.

28. Vianello A, Corrado A, Arcaro G, *et al.* Mechanical insufflation-exsufflation improves outcomes for neuromuscular disease patients with respiratory tract infections. *Am J Phys Med Rehabil* 2005; 84: 83–88.

29. Sancho J, Servera E, Marín J, Vergara P, Belda FJ, Bach JR. Effect of lung mechanics on mechanically assisted flows and volumes. *Am J Phys Med Rehabil* 2004; 83: 698–703.

30. Bach JR. Update and perspective on noninvasive respiratory muscle aids. Part 2: The expiratory aids. *Chest* 1994; 105: 1538–1544.

31. Winck JC, Goncalves MR, Lourenco C, Viana P, Almeida J, Bach JR. Effects of mechanical insufflation-exsufflation on respiratory parameters for patients with chronic airway secretion encumbrance. *Chest* 2004; 126: 774–780.

32. Servera E, Sancho J, Gomez-Merino E, *et al.* Non-invasive management of an acute chest infection for a patient with ALS. *J Neurol Sci* 2003; 209: 111–113.

33. Bach JR, Bianchi C, Aufiero E. Oximetry and indications for tracheotomy for amyotrophic lateral sclerosis. *Chest* 2004; 126: 1502–1507.

34. Vianello A, Bevilacqua M, Arcaro G, Serra E. Prevention of pulmonary morbidity in patients with neuromuscular disorders: a possible role for permanent cricothyroid minitracheostomy. *Chest* 1998; 114: 346–347.

35. Hanayama K, Ishikawa Y, Bach JR. Amyotrophic lateral sclerosis. Successful treatment of mucous plugging by mechanical insufflation-exsufflation. *Am J Phys Med Rehabil* 1997; 76: 338–339.

36. Bach JR. Amyotrophic lateral sclerosis:predictors for prolongation of life by noninvasive respiratory aids. *Arch Phys Med Rehabil* 1995; 76: 828–832.

37. Oppenheimer EA. Treating respiratory failure in ALS: the details are becoming clearer. *J Neurol Sci* 2003; 209: 1–4.

38. Pearse RM, Draper A, Grounds RM. Non-invasive ventilation to avoid tracheal intubation in a patient with Guillain-Barré syndrome. *Br J Anaesth* 2003; 91: 913–916.

39. Seneviratne J, Mandrekar J, Wijdicks EF, Rabinstein AA. Noninvasive ventilation in myasthenic crisis. *Arch Neurol* 2008; 65: 54–58.

40. Agarwal R, Reddy C, Gupta D. Noninvasive ventilation in acute neuromuscular respiratory failure due to myasthenic crisis: case report and review of literature. *Emerg Med J* 2006; 23: e6.

41. Hughes RA, Wijdicks EF, Benson E, Cornblath DR, Hahn AF, Meythaler JM, *et al.* Supportive care for patients with Guillain-Barré syndrome. *Arch Neurol* 2005; 62: 1194–1198.

42. Mehta S. Neuromuscular disease causing acute respiratory failure. *Respir Care* 2006; 51: 1016–1021.

43. Lawn ND, Fletcher DD, Henderson RD, Wolter TD, Wijdicks EF. Anticipating mechanical ventilation in Guillain-Barré syndrome. *Arch Neurol* 2001; 58: 893–898.

44. Ropper AH. The Guillain-Barré syndrome. *N Engl J Med* 1992; 326: 1130–1136.

45. Ropper AH. Guillain-Barré Syndrome: management of respiratory failure. *Neurology* 1985; 35: 1662–1665.

46. Fletcher DD, Lawn ND, Wolter TD, Wijdicks EFM. Long-term outcome in patients with Guillain-Barré syndrome requiring mechanical ventilation. *Neurology* 2000; 54: 2311–2315.

47. Ali MI, Fernández-Pérez ER, Pendem S, Brown DR, Wijdicks EF, Gajic O. Mechanical ventilation in patients with Guillain-Barré syndrome. *Respir Care* 2006; 51: 1403–1407.

48. Wijdicks EF, Roy TK. BiPAP in early guillain-barré syndrome may fail. *Can J Neurol Sci* 2006; 33: 105–106.

49. Fitting J-W, Chevrolet JC. Acute respiratory failure due to neuromuscular disorders. *Rev Mal Respir* 1999; 16: 475–485.

50. Dushay KM, Zibrak JD, Jensen WA. Myasthenia gravis presenting as isolated respiratory failure. *Chest* 1990; 97: 232–234.

51. Rabinstein A, Wijdicks EF. BiPAP in acute respiratory failure due to myasthenic crisis may prevent intubation. *Neurology* 2002; 59: 1647–1649.

52. Jackson AB, Dijkers M, DeVivo MJ, Poczatek RB. A demographic profile of new traumatic spinal cord injuries: change and stability over 30 years. *Arch Phys Med Rehabil* 2004; 85: 1740–1748.

53. Mansel JK, Norman JR. Respiratory complications and management of spinal cord injuries. *Chest* 1990; 97: 1146–1152.

54. Cardenas DD, Hoffman JM, Kirshblum S, McKinley W. Etiology and incidence of rehospitalization after traumatic spinal cord injury: a multicenter analysis. *Arch Phys Med Rehabil* 2004; 85: 1757–1763.

55. Splaingard ML, Frates RC, Harrison GM, Carter RE, Jefferson LS. Home positive-pressure ventilation-twenty years' experience. *Chest* 1983; 84: 376–382.

56. Wicks AB, Menter RR. Long-term outlook in quadriplegic patients with initial ventilator dependecy. *Chest* 1986; 90: 406–410.

57. DeVivo MJ, Ivie CS. Life expectancy of ventilator dependent persons with spinal cord injuries. *Chest* 1995; 108: 226–232.

58. Bach JR, Alba A. Noninvasive options for ventilatory support of the traumatic high level quadriplegic patients. *Chest* 1990; 98: 613–619.

59. Bach JR. Continuous noninvasive ventilation for patients with neuromuscular disease and spinal cord injury. *Semin Respir Crit Care Med* 2002; 23: 283–292.

60. Bach JR, Hunt D, Horton JA. Traumatic tetraplegia: noninvasive respiratory management in the acute setting. *Am J Phys Med Rehabil* 2002; 81: 792–797.

61. Bach JR, Goncalves M. Ventilator weaning by lung expansion and decannulation. *Am J Phys Med Rehabil* 2004; 83: 560–568.

62. De Jonghe B, Sharshar T, Lefaucheur JP, *et al.* Paresis acquired in the intensive care unit: a prospective multicenter study. *JAMA* 2002; 288: 2859–2867.

63. Deem S. Intensive-care-unit-acquired muscle weakness. *Respir Care* 2006; 51: 1042–1052.

64. Latronico N, Guarneri B, Alongi S, Bussi G, Candiani A. Acute neuromuscular respiratory failure after ICU discharge. Report of five patients. *Intensive Care Med* 1999; 25: 1302–1306.

CHAPTER 4

NIV for acute hypercapnic respiratory failure in obese patients

A. Cuvelier, N. Amiot, B. Lamia, L.C. Molano, J-F. Muir

Pulmonary and Intensive Care Dept, Rouen University Hospital & UPRES EA 3830 (IFR MP23), Institute for Biomedical Research, University of Rouen, Rouen, France.

Correspondence: A. Cuvelier, Service de Pneumologie et Soins Intensifs Respiratoires, Hôpital de Bois-Guillaume, CHU de Rouen, 76031 Rouen, France. Fax: 33 232889094; E-mail: antoine.cuvelier@chu-rouen.fr

In the Western world, the prevalence of obese patients in intensive care units (ICU) is increasing. Additionally, morbid obesity has dramatic consequences on pulmonary function [1]. Therefore, respiratory physicians and intensivists are more likely to manage a larger number of acute hypercapnic respiratory failure (AHRF) episodes in patients with a body mass index (BMI) >30 kg·m^{-2}. Cor pulmonale is a major cause of ICU admission, which requires mechanical ventilation with higher mortality in obese compared with nonobese patients [2]. It is, therefore, surprising that experience of AHRF in obese patients has rarely been reported in the literature and, consequently, evidence-based guidelines remain to be established [3]. If there are very few data in the literature about noninvasive ventilation (NIV) in obese patients with hypoxaemic respiratory failure [4], there are cumulating reports that suggest that NIV plays a key role in the treatment of obese patients with AHRF [5].

AHRF in obese patients: epidemiological data

Clinical characteristics and specificities of obese patients hospitalised in ICUs are currently not well established. In a retrospective cohort study in obese and nonobese patients, it has been shown that obese patients had more major comorbidities than nonobese patients, with a higher prevalence of COPD, sleep respiratory disorders, cor pulmonale and pulmonary hypertension [2]. Similarly, obese patients had a higher prevalence of coronary heart diseases and systemic hypertension. In this study, it has been highlighted that pneumonia and hypoxaemic acute respiratory failure were the most frequent hospitalisation reasons for obese patients in the ICU [2]. Although both cohorts had the same severity at admission, mean length of hospital stay was longer in obese patients compared with nonobese patients. This more-prolonged stay was associated with a higher incidence of complications during ICU stay and a more prolonged weaning period [6]. A total of 12% of obese patients were tracheostomised compared with only 4% in nonobese patients.

KOENIG [7] found that the probability of inhalation pneumonia was increased in obese patients, especially during post-surgery, due to an increase in abdominal pressure, increased incidence of gastro-oesophageal reflux and an augmented gastric pH. This should be paralleled with physiopathological consequences of obesity with an increased respiratory work during weaning, due to increased airway resistance, a low thoracic compliance and a decreased efficacy of respiratory muscles. SHARP *et al.* [8] demonstrated in 1964 that respiratory work was 2–4-fold higher in obese patients.

Earlier studies found that morbid obesity was associated with higher mortality in the ICU but more-recent prospective data have questioned these results. EL-SOHL *et al.* [2] reported a 2-fold higher mortality in obese patients in the ICU (30 *versus* 17%) and these patients mostly die from bacterial infections, right heart failure, acute pancreatitis, pulmonary oedema and congestive heart failure. In their series, mortality in ventilated obese patients was 49% and BMI was considered an independent predictive factor of mortality. These authors also showed that morbid obesity was associated with prolonged mechanical ventilation [2, 9] and higher ICU length of stay [9], and that Acute Physiology and Chronic Health Evaluation (APACHE) II score was, in fact, not a satisfactory immediate prognosis index in these patients [2].

Physiopathology of AHRF in obese patients

In the present authors' experience, uncompensated respiratory acidosis in obese patients is the reason to hospitalise 20% of patients in their ICU. In these patients, uncompensated respiratory acidosis may be the consequence of an authentic acute alveolar hypoventilation or the consequence of an acute exacerbation of chronic pulmonary hypoventilation when the patients have daytime hypercapnia at stable state (the so-called "acute-on-chronic respiratory failure"). This distinction is usually not necessary because the triggering factors, physiopathology and management of both conditions are similar.

One or several triggering factors, such as pneumonia, pulmonary oedema, drug overdose and pulmonary embolism, may be identified, but their incidence does not seem to be higher than in a cohort of nonobese patients [2]. Conversely, a significantly higher proportion of obese patients present with cor pulmonale [2]. In the present authors' experience, no triggering factor has been identified in a majority of obese patients presenting with AHRF, which suggests the underlying responsibility of sleep related breathing disorders (SRBDs) that are associated with obesity [10, 11]. In a reference study, RABEC *et al.* suggest a simple classification of obese patients with AHRF according to their SRBD profile and their pulmonary comorbidity. At the present authors' centre, they routinely use the clinical approach according to RABEC *et al.* [12] that rationalises the management of the acute episode and the indication of domiciliary ventilation after discharge.

Obstructive sleep apnoeas

A definite diagnosis of obstructive sleep apnoea syndrome (OSAS) is provided by a ventilatory polygraphy or a polysomnography. The diagnosis of OSAS implies that the diurnal arterial carbon dioxide tension (Pa,CO_2) will be normalised when the patient is treated by continuous positive airway pressure (CPAP). The persistence of hypercapnia despite a well-performed CPAP treatment suggests an associated ventilatory or pulmonary disorder.

The incidence of AHRF in a cohort of OSAS patients remains unknown. ORDRONNEAU *et al.* [13] reported 25 patients in whom a diagnosis of OSAS was performed within 4 months after an ICU stay for AHRF. They were all invasively ventilated during 12 ± 2 days and discharged alive from ICU. These patients were compared with 182 other OSAS patients where the diagnosis of SRBDs was obtained during the routine activity of a sleep laboratory. Apnoea/hypopnoea index (AHI) at stable state was not different between the two groups but OSAS patients diagnosed after ICU stay had a more pronounced daytime hypoxaemia, more pronounced daytime hypercapnia and a higher percentage of the night spent with arterial oxygen saturation measured by pulse oximetry (Sp,O_2) <90% (59 ± 13 *versus* 39 ± 13%, respectively). Moreover, they were more susceptible to have low forced expiratory volume in one second (FEV1; 1.96 ± 0.5 *versus* 2.35 ± 0.8 L, respectively) and low FEV1/forced vital capacity (FVC; 65 ± 15 and 71 ± 11%, respectively) but this difference did not reach statistical significance. This study suggests that the severity of nocturnal desaturations is a better predictor of AHRF compared with apnoea/hypopnoea index (AHI) and that OSAS in COPD may also increase the risk of further AHRF. This last point has to be further evaluated in a large cohort of patients with this overlap syndrome.

Sleep alveolar hypoventilation

Alveolar hypoventilation and therefore daytime hypercapnia in obesity is currently explained by three mechanisms, which may overlap: decreased thoracic compliance, alteration of ventilatory control and increased upper airways resistance. Alveolar hypoventilation is the hallmark of the recently described obesity–hypoventilation syndrome (OHS), previously known as "Pickwickian" syndrome. This diagnosis is defined by the association of a BMI>30 kg·m^{-2} and a diurnal hypoventilation *i.e.* a daytime hypercapnia. When diagnosing OHS, most authors are very careful to exclude a concomitant chronic pulmonary disease that could also be responsible for chronic hypercapnia like COPD, thoracic deformation or neuromuscular disease. Clinicians should be aware that 80–90% of OHS patients have concomitant nocturnal hypoventilation and obstructive sleep apnoeas [14, 15]. Natural history of OHS is still poorly understood and the impact of associated OSAS in the development of chronic respiratory failure is still a subject of debate. Importantly, most of the current knowledge about the OHS has been assessed in patients indicated for nocturnal evaluation in a sleep laboratory, mainly because of suspected OSAS. Clinical assessments of chronic respiratory failure in a nonselected population of obese patients are more difficult to perform but may produce nonbiased information about the disease [16].

Incidence of AHRF appears to be high in a population of patients with OHS; KESSLER *et al.* [17] reported that about half of their OHS patients were hospitalised ≥1 time in the ICU before a definite diagnosis was performed. Moreover, the incidence of mechanical ventilation was high in their patients with most of them having had invasive ventilation.

Concomitant chronic obstructive pulmonary disease

Chronic obstructive pulmonary disease (COPD) is a very common diagnosis in the general population and is a major confounding factor when assessing pulmonary consequences of obesity. Currently, there is some evidence which suggests that COPD and obesity may act additively and perhaps synergistically in order to precipitate the development of chronic respiratory failure in obese patients.

COPD by itself is responsible for nocturnal hypoventilation and significant desaturations that appear during sleep stage 3–4 and are more pronounced during rapid eye movement (REM) sleep. These desaturations are attributed to a decreased activity of accessory respiratory muscles, decreased tidal volume during sleep (-20% during stage 3–4 non-REM sleep and -40% during REM sleep) and an increased dead space volume [18]. In COPD patients with obesity, this sleep pattern is added to the ventilatory consequences of obesity as previously described.

The overlap syndrome (concomitant COPD and OSAS) was identified in 1985 by FLENLEY [19]. This condition is now considered in the presence of the three following criteria: clinical history of COPD or emphysema, FEV1/FVC <70% and a definite diagnosis of OSAS [19]. Because OSAS and COPD are both prevalent diseases in the general population, it is therefore not surprising to find this association. The overlap syndrome is the final diagnosis in ~10–15% of OSAS patients investigated in a respiratory sleep laboratory, due to a high clinical suspicion of nocturnal respiratory events [20, 21].

The association of OSAS and COPD is not related to a specific clinical pattern compared with isolated OSAS, especially when considering diurnal hypersomnolence and dyspnoea. However, patients with overlap syndrome have more-severe nocturnal desaturations compared with OSAS or COPD patients. Moreover, the amplitude of these desaturations seems to be roughly similar to the addition of the desaturations due to OSAS and those due to COPD [22]; especially during REM sleep. Another specificity is that ~40% of patients with overlap syndrome in fact develop diurnal hypercapnia despite an obstructive airway pattern that is less severe than during COPD alone (as judged by the FEV1) [21]. This diurnal hypercapnia is correlated to the severity of the nocturnal desaturation [20] and is more-frequently accompanied by pulmonary hypertension than during isolated OSAS [20]. Inversely, pulmonary hypertension may be encountered at a stable state during OSAS and is not specifically associated to a coexisting COPD [23]. Pulmonary hypertension is a marker of sustained hypoxaemia and a major prognostic factor during chronic respiratory diseases. The incidence of acute respiratory failure (ARF) in a cohort of patients with overlap syndrome is currently not known but the previous study by ORDRONNEAU et al. [13] indicates that it is probably an important recruitment factor in ICU.

Evaluation of AHRF in obese patients

AHRF in obese patients is associated with respiratory encephalopathy, right heart failure with dyspnoea, peripheral oedema and diurnal hypersomnolence [24]. Chest radiograph often reveals cardiomegaly with interstitial or alveolar oedema with its "butterfly" pattern. This is frequent in obese patients who often have cardiac comorbidities or even a specific cardiomyopathy [25]. SRBDs may be clinically suspected during sleep with typical hypoventilation or even central apnoeas lasting 10–20 s. Some patients have obstructive apnoeas with ineffective breathing efforts followed by deep noisy inspirations. Nocturnal oximetry is not sufficiently sensitive to achieve a definite diagnosis of SRBDs, particularly as sleep is quite altered in patients in the ICU and because additional oxygen interferes with recording sleep data.

Ventilatory polygraphy and polysomnography

Performing polysomnography in the ICU, according to the quality criteria required, in a sleep laboratory is difficult and practically impossible. However, ventilatory polygraphs, even if not sensitive, produce highly specific information regarding SRBDs, whatever the sleep architecture. This approach has revolutionised the diagnosis of OSAS in stable state patients since the disease is no longer diagnosed in a sleep laboratory using electroencephalogram (EEG) but at home with simple-to-use ambulatory polygraphs, without assessment of sleep architecture. In the present authors' experience, hypoventilation or obstructive/central apnoeas are so prevalent in obese patients with AHRF that polysomnographies should be reserved only for clinical research.

Ventilatory polygraphs combine a transcutaneous oximetry, analysis of cardiac frequency, thoracic and abdominal movements by two impedance plethysmographic bands, and an analysis of nasal/mouth airflow with a dedicated sensor. Optionally, a body position sensor and a microphone in order to analyse tracheal sounds may be added. Nocturnal ventilatory polygraphy in the acute setting is not aimed at providing a quantitative analysis of SRBDs but is rather to help characterise the main nocturnal profiles (fig. 1). More-recent devices combine ventilatory assessments with a simplified EEG signal but their performance should still be evaluated in clinical practice. From the present authors' point of view, a sleep respiratory pattern in the ICU does not signify a definite diagnosis at stable state. For instance, the clinician should be aware that diagnosing hypoventilation in the ICU during AHRF does not signify that the patient has OHS at stable state. There is an apparent modification of ventilatory patterns in obese patients between acute and stable state. For instance, in the present authors' experience, a significant proportion of patients with hypoventilation during AHRF will not have daytime or even nocturnal hypoventilation after returning at stable state. Therefore, identifying sleep respiratory events in the ICU should not be confused with confirming a definite diagnosis of OHS, OSAS or OHS and OSAS [26]. All patients should be definitely diagnosed with a polysomnography in a sleep laboratory after returning to stable state, usually within the first three months after ICU discharge.

Apart from diagnosing the nocturnal respiratory pattern during AHRF, a potential benefit of polygraphy in ICU is to determine how the ventilator should be set in order to correct the nocturnal/daytime hypoventilation and/or the central/obstructive apnoeas that characterise these patients in AHRF. This approach will be discussed in the following paragraph of this chapter. Finally, the choice of a performing polygraph requires not only choosing a nonfragile and easy-to-set material but also effective software in order to interpret the data (fig. 1). The automatic interpretation of obstructive or central SRBD, based on the software, should never be definitive and a manual analysis by a trained physician is mandatory. In the present authors' experience, this work takes ~20–30 min per patient. Clearly, the performance of the software may vary from one model to the other and is one of the most relevant criteria when choosing one device over the other.

The optimal timing to perform polygraphy in the ICU is not clear. Some authors prefer short-term assessments for only 30–180 min [27, 28]. Due to a low sensibility

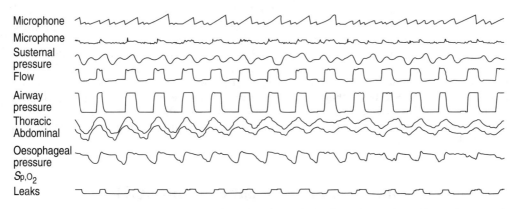

Fig. 1. – A representative polygraphic record under noninvasive ventilation in an obese patient with acute hypercapnic respiratory failure. An oesophageal record was simultaneously performed in order to assess possible asynchronies and identify poor patient–ventilator interactions. Sp,O_2: arterial oxygen saturation measured by pulse oximetry.

(polygraphy may be subnormal especially if the patient did not sleep during these minutes), the present authors suggest that full-night recordings in fact provide better assessments. In their experience, ventilatory polygraphy in spontaneous breathing is performed as soon as respiratory acidosis is controlled. The trained staff on call during the night provide an additional clinical judgment about sleep quality and respiration during sleep. Low-flow oxygen may be used if necessary but always maintained as low as possible in order to optimise the interpretation of the Sp,O_2 recording. The authors suggest that these polygraphic recordings during AHRF should never be performed outside the ICU (*i.e.* never in the ward or sleep laboratory).

Clinical results

The advantage of a rapid diagnosis of respiratory events in obese patients with AHRF has been confirmed by previous clinical studies, during a period where NIV or CPAP were not used in routine practice. In the 1970s, a diagnosis of Pickwickian syndrome was usually associated with 30–40% mortality, and clinicians were aware of the high incidence of carbonarcosis in these patients. More recently, BUCKLE *et al.* [27] reported their own experience regarding polysomnography in nine patients hospitalised in the ICU for hypoxaemic or hypercapnic respiratory failure. Their approach led to an aetiological diagnosis (six patients with OHS, two patients with neuromuscular disorder and one patient with COPD) and permitted to choose the most adapted therapeutics (CPAP, NIV and oxygen) in order to improve SRBD. According to these authors, performing polysomnography avoided endotracheal intubation in half of the patients. Moreover, this exploration helped to set and monitor the ventilatory settings.

RESTA *et al.* [28] detailed how they performed polysomnographies for at least 3 h in 14 obese patients hospitalised for AHRF, during the first 3–5 days after admission. A second polysomnographic assessment was performed at least 6 weeks after the AHRF episode in a sleep laboratory. A total of 10 (71.3%) patients had obstructive apnoeas or hypopnoeas and two (14.3%) patients had central apnoeas. A characteristic pattern of nocturnal hypoventilation was found in the majority of cases and was the sole SRBD pattern in only two (14.3%) patients. All patients required to be mechanically ventilated with low-flow oxygen; eight of them were discharged home with domiciliary CPAP and five patients with domiciliary pressure-cycled NIV.

Obviously, sleep hypoventilation is the major abnormality encountered in the great majority if not all obese patients with AHRF. However, neither the natural history of SRBD in obese patients nor the physiopathology of the AHRF episodes in these patients is clearly understood. The present authors suggest that a semiologic description of SRBD in the acute setting should not presume of a clinical diagnosis at stable state. Obviously, if a patient has nocturnal hypoventilation during AHRF, this does not signify that they have OHS at stable state. In the absence of further knowledge about natural history of SRBD, either in the acute or chronic settings, a definite pulmonary diagnosis in obese patients should be restricted to the chest physician according to clinical history, polysomnography and pulmonary function tests that will be performed after ICU discharge.

Mechanical ventilation in obese patients with AHRF

Due to the fact that hypercapnia and respiratory acidosis worsen under oxygen therapy alone, obese patients with AHRF should be managed by mechanical ventilation as soon as Pa,CO_2 rise >6.0 kPa and/or pH $\leq$7.35. Pa,CO_2 is one of the key parameter to be monitored by iterative arterial blood gas samplings and possibly by alternative less invasive methodologies like transcutaneous Pa,CO_2 [29, 30]. Pharmacological management by respiratory analeptics and/or diuretics is of minor clinical benefit in obese patients with AHRF.

There is a physiopathological rationale for using NIV in obese patients with AHRF, in order to decrease respiratory load, increase thoracic compliance, improve nocturnal alveolar hypoventilation and to reset respiratory centres. In a pioneering work, PANKOW et al. [31] have compared diurnal physiological respiratory parameters under spontaneous breathing and during bi-level NIV in 18 patients with BMI >40 mg·kg^{-1}. They considered three categories of patients: simple obesity (n=5), OSAS (n=7) and OHS (n=6). No significant difference was observed between each group; however, in all patients, an improvement of tidal volume and a decreased respiratory rate were observed under NIV in the OSAS and OHS groups. End-tidal carbon dioxide tension (PET,CO_2) was not modified in cases of simple obesity and OSAS but was decreased in OHS patients. An important result was that muscular activity was significantly reduced (~40%) in the three patient groups, indicating that NIV is able to decrease the load imposed to respiratory muscles in morbidly obese patients.

NIV: case series

SHIVARAM et al. [32] treated six patients with morbid obesity (159$\pm$19% of ideal weight) associated with OSAS and hospitalized for AHRF (pH 7.23$\pm$0.03, Pa,CO_2 of 10.6$\pm$0.5 kPa). All these patients were treated by CPAP with additional oxygen and their clinical status improved in the 24 h after mechanical ventilation was initiated. STURANI et al. [33] confirmed the benefit of noninvasive ventilation in six other obese patients (BMI 50.3$\pm$4.8 kg·m^{-2}) with AHRF and encephalopathy. Their patients were ventilated with a bi-level mode and a 10·min^{-1} backup frequency (inspiratory positive airway pressure (IPAP) 18 cmH$_2$0, expiratory positive airway pressure (EPAP) 7 cmH$_2$0). IPAP was progressively increased by 2 cmH$_2$0 increments, according to the clinical status. A 2–4 L·min^{-1} additional oxygen flow was necessary in most of the patients. These authors observed a rapid improvement of clinical status and arterial blood gases in <24 h, without requiring endotracheal intubation. Index of nocturnal respiratory events was 63$\pm$9 at the end of an ICU stay. In a retrospective study from the present authors' group, an immediate success was observed in 20 obese patients with AHRF and treated with bi-level NIV [26]. Two delayed NIV failures requiring endotracheal intubation were observed; 1 month later, polysomnography revealed OSAS in nine patients and OHS in 11 other patients who were treated by domiciliary NIV [26].

The most important experience was from RABEC et al. [12], who described the clinical evolution in 41 obese patients hospitalised for AHRF and treated by bi-level NIV (initial settings: IPAP 16 cmH$_2$0, EPAP 4 cmH$_2$0). A total of six patients had OSAS, 19 had OHS, four had COPD without OSAS and 10 had overlap syndrome (COPD plus OSAS). Mean age was 63$\pm$11 yrs, BMI was 42$\pm$9 kg·m^{-2}, pH at admission was 7.32$\pm$0.04, Pa,CO_2 was 9.4$\pm$1.7 kPa. 39 (95%) out of 41 patients were successfully treated by NIV without requiring endotracheal intubation. Mean Pa,CO_2 dropped to 6.7$\pm$0.8 kPa after 7 days of mechanical ventilation.

Case series concerning NIV in AHRF obese patients remain scarce, noncontrolled and have included only a small number of patients. By comparison with the major benefits of NIV prescribed in COPD patients hospitalised for AHRF [34, 35], the ability of NIV to prevent endotracheal intubation, decrease the number of complications and decrease the hospital length of stay in the obese patients with AHRF has still to be properly demonstrated. However, the therapeutic benefits in the previously mentioned studies were so remarkable that any future randomised studies might be considered as unethical. From the present authors' point of view, NIV is the first step when managing AHRF in obese patients and should be routinely considered outside the classical contraindications that imply immediate intubation (table 1).

NIV for AHRF in patients with OHS

Ventilatory assistance is aimed at improving alveolar hypoventilation and, therefore, positive inspiratory pressure will be the most important parameter to be established. Positive expiratory pressure does not provide any therapeutic effect, *per se*, since patients with OHS do not have associated obstructive apnoeas or hypopnoeas [36]. The optimal ventilatory mode is pressure support, using turbine-driven ventilators or ICU ventilators. A backup frequency rate is required in most cases, due of the likelihood of sleep central apnoeas. If a single circuit is used, it should be equipped with an expiratory valve or an intentional calibrated leak. In this previous case, a slight expiratory positive pressure is required in order to limit CO_2 rebreathing. Clinical series show that OHS patients with AHRF require high levels of inspiratory positive pressures (often >22 cmH_2O) due to low thoracic compliance in this disease. Another ventilatory mode in these patients is flow-preset mode that allows a better control of delivered volumes. AHRF in obese patients is one of the last medical situations where pressure support may be less effective than flow-preset modes. After discharge, most OHS patients are managed with nocturnal bi-level NIV without additional oxygen [37].

NIV for AHRF in obese patients with OHS + OSAS

Hypercapnia and even AHRF may reappear in some of these patients if discharged home with CPAP alone. Indeed, alveolar hypoventilation during AHRF is not always related to OSAS and it is therefore reasonable to use bi-level NIV on a first-line basis during AHRF episodes. Again, a backup frequency rate is highly suggested because of abnormal ventilatory control in some of these patients. In the present authors' experience, mean efficient expiratory positive pressure levels are usually 6–9 cmH_2O [26]. This critical pressure is aimed at stabilising upper airways and to prevent collapse during the subsequent inspirations. After improvement of alveolar hypoventilation, some of these patients may be switched to domiciliary CPAP (with or without additional oxygen), according to the results of a polysomnographic recording in the sleep laboratory. Finally, a limited number of overlap (OHS plus OSAS) patients may benefit from flow-preset domiciliary ventilation [38].

Table 1. – **Noninvasive ventilation (NIV) contraindications in obese patients with acute hypercapnic respiratory failure**

Ventricular arythmias
Bradycardia
Unstable haemodynamics
Respiratory encephalopathy that does not improve under NIV
Stridor or previously identified anatomic upper airways obstruction
Refractory hypoxaemia

NIV for AHRF in patients with overlap syndrome (COPD plus OSAS)

Bi-level noninvasive pressure support is the cardinal treatment for these patients [12] even though flow-preset ventilatory mode may be also successful in some patients. After discharge from the ICU, CPAP is still an option but some authors have found that CPAP is sometimes poorly tolerated and hypercapnia may reappear [39]. A majority of these patients are more comfortably treated by bi-level and even flow-preset NIV. Nocturnal oxygen therapy is required in the majority of these patients. The relatively high morbidity and mortality in patients with overlap syndrome after hospitalisation for AHRF [13] justifies early recognition of this morbid association and requires to regularly re-evaluate the treatment.

NIV: conclusion

The main specificities of ventilatory management of obese patients with AHRF are the following: the high efficiency of noninvasive bi-level mode, a back-up frequency rate, an additional oxygen therapy, higher inspiratory pressures if patients have overlap syndrome or OHS, elevated expiratory positive pressures if patients have pure or associated OSAS. When bi-level mode fails and if intubation criteria are not met (table 1) then the patient should be switched to a flow-preset mode [38, 40, 41]. Based on a relatively limited number of published reports, NIV failure rate in obese patients with AHRF varies from 0 to 36%, which is a better result than encountered in COPD patients with acute exacerbation. DUARTE et al. [42] found that patients failing with bi-level NIV have a greater BMI and this would be an argument in favor of switching to flow-preset mode. However, their study was a retrospective design and intubation criteria were not applied prospectively.

Invasive ventilation

Obese patients requiring invasive ventilation have prolonged ICU and hospital lengths of stay compared with patients managed by NIV [2, 42]. Clearly, intubation of an obese patient with AHRF in obese patients should be limited to those with NIV contraindications or NIV failure during an ICU stay (table 1). These situations have become rare in units that have developed SRBD evaluation and where clinical staff have been trained and developed expertise with NIV.

Endotracheal intubation may be a difficult procedure to perform in obese patients because of a short neck, a macroglossia and thickness of oropharyngeal soft tissues [43]. Clinicians should be aware of potential difficulty to expose the glottis during direct laryngoscopy, a situation that may be anticipated with the Mallampati clinical score that has been modified by SAMSOON and YOUNG [44]. Other tests predictive of a difficult intubation have been described [45]. Performing intubation is also difficult in patients who previously have had uvulo-palato-pharyngoplasty. Difficult intubation is associated with a non-negligible morbidity and mortality and one of the solutions is probably to guide the tube in the trachea with the aid of a fibrescope.

Invasive ventilation settings have some specificity in obese patients because of the increase of airway resistances and the decrease of thoracic compliances. Tidal volumes should not be set according to the real weight but rather based on ideal weight and secondarily adjusted according to airway pressures and serial arterial blood gas results. Trendelenburg posture improves mechanical ventilation in obese patients, by increasing tidal volume and by decreasing respiratory frequency [46]. A slight level of expiratory positive pressure is required in order to prevent segmental and sub-segmental atelectasis.

Otherwise, the ventilatory settings are similar to those prescribed in nonobese patients with flow-preset in sedated patients that are secondarily switched to pressure support as soon as sedation is stopped. Clearly, sedation duration should be shortened as much as possible and weaning protocols for benzodiazepines are of high clinical value [47]. During the weaning procedure, a cuff-leak test should be routinely performed, because of a frequent narrowing of the upper airways. Mechanical ventilation is therefore converted to NIV and, especially in patients in whom long-term NIV is indicated, according to sleep studies under spontaneous breathing. NIV has been shown to be effective in averting respiratory failure in severely obese patients when applied during the first 48 h post-extubation [48]. The benefits seem to be greater in obese patients having chronic hypercapnia at stable state [48].

Tracheostomy is now rarely performed in obese patients hospitalised for AHRF because of the rapid expansion of NIV procedures. In a long-term setting, tracheostomy may be indicated when NIV fails or is contra-indicated, mainly because of iterative inhalations. Tracheostomy is usually performed by percutaneous dilatation (Ciaglia technique). This technique has been evaluated in 13 obese patients and appears to be as easy and without additional complications to perform in obese than in nonobese patients [49]. On a long-term basis, rigid cannulas are often badly tolerated due to the short and thickened neck.

Summary

Acute hypercapnic respiratory failure in obese patients is an increasing cause of hospitalisation in intensive care units. Despite a few publications on this topic, noninvasive ventilation (NIV) has become the main modality of ventilatory assistance for these patients. NIV specificities are: efficacy of the bilevel mode, mandatory back-up frequency, additional oxygen therapy required, positive inspiratory pressures elevated in patients having obesity–hypoventilation syndrome (OHS) or associated COPD and obstructive sleep apneas (OSAS), positive expiratory pressure elevated in case of OSAS. Flow-preset mode should be tested in case of failure with bilevel mode. In patients with COPD or OHS, an associated nocturnal alveolar hypoventilation at stable state justifies to institute domiciliary NIV. The ventilatory settings will be set according to arterial blood gases and polysomnography a few months after discharge from AHRF.

Keywords: Acute respiratory failure, obesity, obesity-hypoventilation syndrome, overlap syndrome, sleep apnea.

Acknowledgements. The authors would like to thank R. Medeiros (University of Rouen, Rouen, France), for helpful assistance when editing the manuscript.

References

1. Jubber AS. Respiratory complications of obesity. *Int J Clin Pract* 2004; 58: 573–580.
2. El-Solh A, Sikka P, Bozkanat E, Jaafar W, Davies J. Morbid obesity in the medical ICU. *Chest* 2001; 120: 1989–1997.
3. Cuvelier A, Muir JF. Acute and chronic respiratory failure in patients with obesity-hypoventilation syndrome: a new challenge for noninvasive ventilation. *Chest* 2005; 128: 483–485.

4. Coimbra VR, Lara Rde A, Flores EG, Nozawa E, Auler JO Jr, Feltrim MI. Application of noninvasive ventilation in acute respiratory failure after cardiovascular surgery. *Arq Bras Cardiol* 2007;89, 270–6: 298–305.

5. Pastores SM. Morbidly obese patients with acute respiratory failure: don't reach for the endotracheal tube yet!. *Crit Care Med* 2007; 35: 956–957.

6. Tremblay A, Bandi V. Impact of body mass index on outcomes following critical care. *Chest* 2003; 123: 1202–1207.

7. Koenig SM. Pulmonary complications of obesity. *Am J Med Sci* 2001; 321: 249–279.

8. Sharp JT, Henry JP, Sweany SK, Meadows WR, Pietras RJ. The total work of breathing in normal and obese men. *J Clin Invest* 1964; 43: 728–739.

9. Akinnusi ME, Pineda LA, El Solh AA. Effect of obesity on intensive care morbidity and mortality: A meta-analysis. *Crit Care Med* 2008; 36: 151–158.

10. BaHammam A, Syed S, Al-Mughairy A. Sleep-related breathing disorders in obese patients presenting with acute respiratory failure. *Respir Med* 2005; 99: 718–725.

11. Casey KR, Cantillo KO, Brown LK. Sleep-related hypoventilation/hypoxemic syndromes. *Chest* 2007; 131: 1936–1948.

12. Rabec C, Merati M, Baudouin N, Foucher P, Ulukavac T, Reybet-Degat O. Management of obesity and respiratory insufficiency. The value of dual-level pressure nasal ventilation. *Rev Mal Respir* 1998; 15: 269–278.

13. Ordronneau J, Chollet S, Nogues B, Chailleux E. Sleep apnea syndrome in intensive care. *Rev Mal Respir* 1994; 11: 51–55.

14. Rabec CA. Obesity hypoventilation syndrome: what's in a name? *Chest* 2002; 122: 1498.

15. Weitzenblum E, Kessler R, Chaouat A. Obesity-hypoventilation syndrome. *Rev Mal Respir* 2008; 25: 391–403.

16. Nowbar S, Burkart KM, Gonzales R, Fedorowicz A, Gozansky WS, Gaudio JC, Taylor MR, Zwillich CW. Obesity-associated hypoventilation in hospitalized patients: prevalence, effects, and outcome. *Am J Med* 2004; 116: 1–7.

17. Kessler R, Chaouat A, Schinkewitch P, Faller M, Casel S, Krieger J, Weitzenblum E. The obesity-hypoventilation syndrome revisited: a prospective study of 34 consecutive cases. *Chest* 2001; 120: 369–376.

18. Douglas N. Sleep in patients with chronic obstructive pulmonary disease. *Clin Chest Med* 1998; 19: 115.

19. Flenley D. Sleep in chronic obstructive lung disease. *Clin Chest Med* 1985; 6: 51–61.

20. Chaouat A, Weitzenblum E, Krieger J, Ifoundza T, Oswald M, Kessler R. Association of chronic obstructive pulmonary disease and sleep apnea syndrome. *Am J Respir Crit Care Med* 1995; 151: 82–86.

21. Resta O, Foschino Barbaro MP, Brindicci C, Nocerino MC, Caratozzolo G, Carbonara M. Hypercapnia in overlap syndrome: possible determinant factors. *Sleep Breath* 2002; 6: 11–18.

22. Sanders MH, Newman AB, Haggerty CL, Redline S, Lebowitz M, Samet J, O'Connor GT, Punjabi NM, Shahar E. Sleep and sleep-disordered breathing in adults with predominantly mild obstructive airway disease. *Am J Respir Crit Care Med* 2003; 167: 7–14.

23. Bady E, Achkar A, Pascal S, Orvoen-Frija E, Laaban J. Pulmonary arterial hypertension in patients with sleep apnoea syndrome. *Thorax* 2000; 55: 934–939.

24. Fletcher EC, Shah A, Qian W, Miller CC 3rd. "Near miss" death in obstructive sleep apnea: a critical care syndrome. *Crit Care Med* 1991; 19: 1158–1164.

25. Wong C, Marwick TH. Obesity cardiomyopathy: pathogenesis and pathophysiology. *Nat Clin Pract Cardiovasc Med* 2007; 4: 436–443.

26. Cuvelier A, Beduneau G, Molano L, Stain J, Muir J. Instauration of NPPV in obese patients after ICU stay [Abstract]. *Am J Respir Crit Care Med* 2002; 165: A26.

27. Buckle P, Pouliot Z, Millar T, Kerr P, Kryger M. Polysomnography in acutely ill intensive care unit patients. *Chest* 1992; 102: 288–291.

28. Resta O, Guido P, Foschino Barbaro MP, Picca V, Talamo S, Lamorgese V. Sleep-related breathing disorders in acute respiratory failure assisted by non-invasive ventilatory treatment: utility of portable polysomnographic system. *Respir Med* 2000; 94: 128–134.

29. Cuvelier A, Grigoriu B, Molano LC, Muir JF. Limitations of transcutaneous carbon dioxide measurements for assessing long-term mechanical ventilation. *Chest* 2005; 127: 1744–1748.

30. Maniscalco M, Zedda A, Faraone S, Carratu P, Sofia M. Evaluation of a transcutaneous carbon dioxide monitor in severe obesity. Intensive Care Med 2008.

31. Pankow W, Hijjeh N, Schuttler F, Penzel T, Becker HF, Peter JH, von Wichert P. Influence of noninvasive positive pressure ventilation on inspiratory muscle activity in obese subjects. *Eur Respir J* 1997; 10: 2847–2852.

32. Shivaram U, Cash ME, Beal A. Nasal continuous positive airway pressure in decompensated hypercapnic respiratory failure as a complication of sleep apnea. *Chest* 1993; 104: 770–774.

33. Sturani C, Galavotti V, Scarduelli C, *et al.* Acute respiratory failure due to severe obstructive sleep apnea syndrome, managed with nasal positive pressure ventilation. *Monaldi Arch Chest Dis* 1994; 49: 558–560.

34. Lightowler JV, Wedzicha JA, Elliott MW, Ram FS. Non-invasive positive pressure ventilation to treat respiratory failure resulting from exacerbations of chronic obstructive pulmonary disease: Cochrane systematic review and meta-analysis. *BMJ* 2003; 326: 185.

35. Keenan SP, Sinuff T, Cook DJ, Hill NS. Which patients with acute exacerbation of chronic obstructive pulmonary disease benefit from noninvasive positive-pressure ventilation? A systematic review of the literature. *Ann Intern Med* 2003; 138: 861–870.

36. Mokhlesi B, Kryger MH, Grunstein RR. Assessment and management of patients with obesity hypoventilation syndrome. *Proc Am Thorac Soc* 2008; 5: 218–225.

37. Cuvelier A, Muir JF. Obesity-hypoventilation syndrome and noninvasive mechanical ventilation: new insights in the Pickwick papers? *Chest* 2007; 131: 7–8.

38. Piper A, Sullivan C. Effects of short-term NIPPV in the treatment of patients with severe obstructive sleep apnea and hypercapnia. *Chest* 1994; 105: 434.

39. de Miguel J, Cabello J, Sanchez-Alarcos JM, Alvarez-Sala R, Espinos D, Alvarez-Sala JL. Long-term effects of treatment with nasal continuous positive airway pressure on lung function in patients with overlap syndrome. *Sleep Breath* 2002; 6: 3–10.

40. Perez de Llano LA, Golpe R, Ortiz Piquer M, Veres Racamonde A, Vazquez Caruncho M, Caballero Muinelos O, Alvarez Carro C. Short-term and long-term effects of nasal intermittent positive pressure ventilation in patients with obesity-hypoventilation syndrome. *Chest* 2005; 128: 587–594.

41. Hans GA, Pregaldien AA, Kaba A, Sottiaux TM, Deroover A, Lamy ML, Joris JL. Pressure-controlled Ventilation Does Not Improve Gas Exchange in Morbidly Obese Patients Undergoing Abdominal Surgery. Obes Surg 2007.

42. Duarte AG, Justino E, Bigler T, Grady J. Outcomes of morbidly obese patients requiring mechanical ventilation for acute respiratory failure. *Crit Care Med* 2007; 35: 732–737.

43. Gonzalez H, Minville V, Delanoue K, Mazerolles M, Concina D, Fourcade O. The importance of increased neck circumference to intubation difficulties in obese patients. *Anesth Analg* 2008; 106: 1132–1136.

44. Samsoon GL, Young JR. Difficult tracheal intubation: a retrospective study. *Anaesthesia* 1987; 42: 487–490.

45. Hiremath AS, Hillman DR, James AL, Noffsinger WJ, Platt PR, Singer SL. Relationship between difficult tracheal intubation and obstructive sleep apnoea. *Br J Anaesth* 1998; 80: 606–611.

46. Fahy BG, Barnas GM, Nagle SE, Flowers JL, Njoku MJ, Agarwal M. Effects of Trendelenburg and reverse Trendelenburg postures on lung and chest wall mechanics. *J Clin Anesth* 1996; 8: 236–244.

47. Kress JP, Pohlman AS, O'Connor MF, Hall JB. Daily interruption of sedative infusions in critically ill patients undergoing mechanical ventilation. *N Engl J Med* 2000; 342: 1471–1477.

48. El-Solh AA, Aquilina A, Pineda L, Dhanvantri V, Grant B, Bouquin P. Noninvasive ventilation for prevention of post-extubation respiratory failure in obese patients. *Eur Respir J* 2006; 28: 588–595.

49. Mansharamani NG, Koziel H, Garland R, LoCicero J 3rd, Critchlow J, Ernst A.. Safety of bedside percutaneous dilatational tracheostomy in obese patients in the ICU. *Chest* 2000; 117: 1426–1429.

CHAPTER 5

NIV: indication in case of acute hypoxaemic respiratory failure (pulmonary oedema and immunosuppressed patients excluded)

M. Ferrer*,#, *A. Torres*#,¶

**Unidad de Cuidados Intensivos e Intermedios Respiratorios, Servei de Pneumologia, Hospital Clínic,* ¶*Institut d'Investigacions Biomèdiques August Pi i Sunyer (IDIBAPS), Universitat de Barcelona, and* #*Centre de Investigación Biomédica En Red-Entermedades Respiratorias (CibeRes, CB06/06/0028), Barcelona, Spain.*

Correspondence: M. Ferrer, Servei de Pneumologia, Hospital Clínic, Villarroel 170, 08036 Barcelona, Spain. Fax: 34 932275549; E-mail: miferrer@clinic.ub.es

Introduction

Based on controlled clinical trials that demonstrate a marked decrease in the needs for intubation, as well as improved morbidity and mortality, noninvasive ventilation (NIV) is now considered as a first-line ventilatory treatment in selected patients with severe exacerbation of chronic obstructive pulmonary disease (COPD) and hypercapnic respiratory failure [1–4]. The benefits of NIV appear to be the consequence of avoiding tracheal intubation and the associated morbidity and mortality. Morbidity includes an increased risk for ventilator-associated pneumonia (VAP) [5], ventilator-induced lung injury [6], increased needs of sedation that contribute to prolonged ventilation and complications of the upper airway related to prolonged translaryngeal intubation.

Other patients, who show benefits from the use of NIV, are those affected by acute cardiogenic pulmonary oedema (CPO). Both NIV and continuous positive airway pressure (CPAP) are equally effective in decreasing the needs for intubation and improving mortality in these patients [7, 8]. Finally, immunosuppressed patients have poor outcome when they develop pulmonary infiltrates and acute hypoxaemic respiratory failure (AHRF); in these patients, NIV seems to decrease the needs for intubation and the related morbidity and mortality [9, 10].

However, the role of NIV in other type of patient is still under debate. It is possible that other populations at risk of complications related to invasive mechanical ventilation may benefit from the use of NIV. However, the efficacy of NIV in patients with different types of AHRF is less evident from controlled clinical trials. The first problem in addressing patients with AHRF is the heterogeneity of this condition. Studies assessing the outcome of patients with AHRF, treated with NIV in the intensive care unit (ICU) identified up to nine different groups of patients, with substantial differences in outcomes among them (fig. 1) [11]. Moreover, the majority of clinical trials that have assessed the efficacy of NIV in patients with AHRF, studied mixed populations of patients, which resulted in controversial results when all trials were analysed together.

Therefore, the present chapter will analyse the role of NIV in the management of patients with AHRF from clinical trials with mixed and specific populations of patients.

Eur Respir Mon, 2008, 41, 60–71. Printed in UK - all rights reserved. Copyright ERS Journals Ltd 2008; European Respiratory Monograph; ISSN 1025-448x.

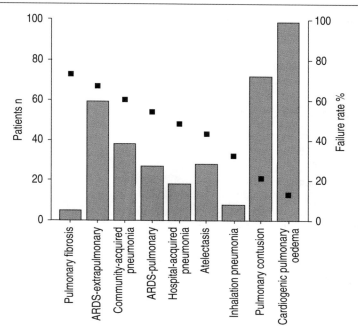

Fig. 1. – Causes of acute hypoxemic respiratory failure and frequency of noninvasive ventilation failure. Acute respiratory distress syndrome (ARDS) patients were divided into pulmonary and extra-pulmonary origin. ■: number of patients; ■: percentage of patients that required intubation. Adapted from [11].

Severe community-acquired pneumonia

Severe community-acquired pneumonia (CAP) is defined as those cases that require admission to an ICU. Direct admission to an ICU is required for patients with septic shock or acute respiratory failure (ARF) requiring invasive mechanical ventilation, defined as major severity criteria in the current Infectious Disease Society of America/ American Thoracic Society guidelines used to define severe CAP [12]. Admission to an ICU is also recommended for patients with other minor severity criteria (table 1). Among all criteria that define severe CAP, the need for invasive ventilation, severe arterial hypoxaemia and increased respiratory rate are related to AHRF.

Despite the fact that the main aspect in the management of patients with pneumonia is an appropriate initial empirical antimicrobial treatment, the supportive measures (respiratory failure, shock, renal failure and protection of the airways, among others) are also essential in patients with severe CAP. The background for the use of NIV in severe CAP is related to the presence of severe ARF. Invasive ventilation is indicated in case of life-threatening respiratory failure; however, invasive ventilation is associated with increased risk of severe complications. Since, in general, the main objective of NIV in severe ARF is help in overcoming the acute episode without the need for invasive mechanical ventilation; by avoiding tracheal intubation, morbidity and mortality with decrease in these patients (fig. 2).

NIV and pneumonia

Pneumonia in patients treated with NIV is persistently associated with poor outcome in the literature. The first study, which found this association, was a retrospective analysis of

Table 1. – Criteria for severe community-acquired pneumonia according to the Infectious Disease Society of America/American Thoracic Society guidelines adapted from [12]

Minor criteria
Respiratory rate[#] ≥ 30 breaths·min^{-1}
$Pa,O_2/FI,O_2$[#] ≤ 250
Multilobar infiltrates
Confusion/disorientation
Uraemia (blood urea nitrogen level ≥ 20 mg·dL^{-1})
Leukopoenia (WBC count $<4 \times 10^9$ cells·L^{-1})
Thrombocytopoenia (platelet count $<100 \times 10^9$ cells·L^{-1})
Hypothermia (core temperature $<36°C$)
Hypotension requiring aggressive fluid resuscitation
Major criteria
Invasive mechanical ventilation
Septic shock with the need for vasopressors

Pa,O_2: arterial oxgen tension; FI,O_2: inspiratory oxygen fraction; WBC: white blood cell. [#]: noninvasive ventilation can substitute for respiratory rate ≥ 30 breaths·min^{-1} or $Pa,O_2/FI,O_2$ ≤ 250.

59 episodes of ARF in 47 patients with COPD exacerbations. NIV was effective in 46 patients and failed in 13 patients, who required tracheal intubation and invasive mechanical ventilation [13]. Among others, a univariate analysis assessing predictors of NIV failure found pneumonia as the cause of exacerbation associated with a higher failure of NIV. In that study, pneumonia was the cause of 38% of unsuccessful episodes and 9% of successful episodes of ARF. While the failure rate of patients with other causes of exacerbation was 16%, the failure rate of patients with pneumonia was 56%.

A multinational study in 8 ICUs analysed the evolution of 356 patients, who received NIV for an episode of severe AHRF, in relation to the aetiology of the episode [11]. Among the different causes of AHRF, the highest rates of tracheal intubation corresponded to patients with acute respiratory distress syndrome (ARDS; 51%) and CAP (50%; fig. 1). A multivariate analysis of predictors of NIV failure found the presence of ARDS or CAP to be a significant and independent predictor of NIV failure, with an adjusted odds ratio of 3.75. Other independent predictors of NIV failure were age >40 yrs, higher scores of severity at ICU admission and worse hypoxaemia after 1 h of NIV treatment.

Another prospective study analysed 24 patients without underlying chronic respiratory disease who were treated with NIV because of severe CAP and ARF [14]. In general, the use of NIV was followed by a decrease in respiratory rate and increase in

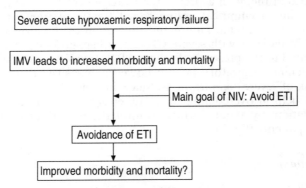

Fig. 2. – Rationale for using noninvasive ventilation (NIV) in severe acute hypoxaemic respiratory failure. IMV: invasive mechanical ventilation; ETI: endotracheal intubation.

arterial hypoxaemia after 30 mins, with return to the baseline values after NIV was removed. The overall intubation rate was 67% in these patients. Among others, advanced age and lower levels of arterial oxygenation were predictors for intubation. Likewise, intubation was associated with higher mortality and longer hospital stay. By contrast, those patients in whom NIV prevented intubation had a very favourable outcome. Due to the good outcome in these patients when tracheal intubation was avoided and the fact that the assessment of the efficacy of NIV resulted in minimal delay in intubation, the authors of that study suggested that these patients may undergo a trial of NIV with appropriate monitoring in order to avoid unnecessary delay in intubation.

This contrast between a favourable physiological response to NIV and a poor clinical evolution of patients with severe CAP was observed in another study in patients with severe AHRF, 18 with severe CAP and 15 with CPO [15]. Both groups had similar baseline levels of arterial hypoxaemia, respiratory rate and cardiac frequency. The improvement in arterial hypoxaemia and cardiac frequency was similar in both groups of patients, while respiratory frequency improved only in patients with CPO when NIV was applied. Likewise, the intubation rate was higher and the hospital stay was longer in patients with pneumonia.

In light of these results it can be concluded that, in patients with severe AHRF who need NIV, those whose cause of respiratory failure is pneumonia are among those with worse outcomes, even with similar levels of arterial hypoxaemia. However, prospective randomised clinical trials are needed in order to assess whether NIV is effective in patients with severe CAP.

Evidences on the efficacy of NIV in CAP

Few controlled trials have assessed the efficacy of NIV in patients with severe pneumonia. The only prospective randomised controlled trial in patients with severe CAP included 56 patients, who were allocated to receive conventional treatment with or without NIV [16]. That study demonstrated that patients who had received NIV together with conventional treatment had lower rate of tracheal intubation and a shorter stay in the intermediate care unit than those who received conventional treatment only (21 versus 50%, respectively; p<0.03); although the length of hospital stay and hospital mortality were similar between both groups. That study also showed, in a subset analysis, that the significant benefits of NIV occurred in patients with COPD and hypercapnic respiratory failure only; this subset of patients had also a lower mortality after 2 months (11 versus 63%, respectively; p=0.05). By contrast, patients with neither COPD nor hypercapnic respiratory failure did not benefit from NIV. Although those results were promising, the routine use of NIV in patients with CAP and without COPD has not been clearly established.

A more-recent prospective randomised controlled trial in patients with severe AHRF demonstrated that NIV decreased ICU mortality and the need for tracheal intubation, compared with high-concentration oxygen therapy [17]. Moreover, a subgroup analysis observed that patients with pneumonia as the cause of the episode of AHRF were those in whom NIV showed significant benefits; in this subset of patients, the benefits in decreasing tracheal intubation and ICU mortality remained. With regard to the other subsets of patients, there was a nonsignificant trend to a lower rate of NIV failure in patients with thoracic trauma, and NIV failure in patients from this study with CPO and ARDS was very low and high, respectively, without differences between patients treated with NIV and those from the control group [17]. In that study, the use of NIV resulted in a faster improvement of arterial hypoxaemia and tachypnoea, compared with high-concentration oxygen therapy (fig. 3). Likewise, NIV was also associated with a lower rate of septic shock and a trend to a lower incidence of hospital-acquired pneumonia.

In summary, patients with severe CAP, who receive NIV as a support for severe AHRG, are among those with the highest rate of NIV failure. For this reason, when NIV is indicated in these patients, they should be managed in a setting with appropriate resources in staff and equipment for a correct monitoring in order to detect evidences of NIV failure early and, therefore, avoid unnecessary delay in the intubation of patients. However, an appropriate selection of patients with severe CAP, and the addition of NIV to the standard treatment may decrease the likelihood to need intubation.

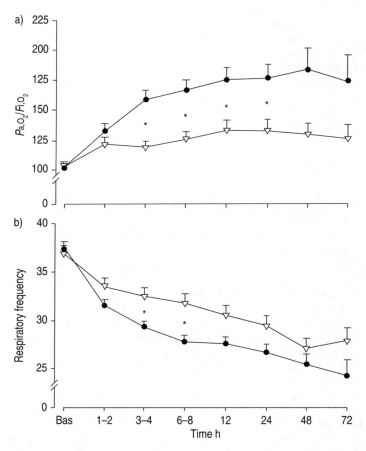

Fig. 3. – Time-course evolution (mean+SEM) of arterial hypoxaemia, as assessed by a) the arterial oxgen tension (P_{a,O_2})/inspiratory oxygen fraction (F_{I,O_2}) ratio and b) respiratory frequency in the noninvasive ventilation (NIV; ●) and control (▽) groups. Both variables improved with time in both groups. After Bonferroni correction, the improvement of the two variables was significantly greater in the NIV group after 3–4 h randomisation and remained significantly greater 6–8 and 24 h after randomisation for $P_{a,O_2}/F_{I,O_2}$ ratio and respiratory frequency, respectively. The number of patients under study at baseline (Bas), 1–2, 3–4, 6–8, 12, 24, 48 and 72 h were 51, 51, 50, 49, 44, 35, 21 and 12, respectively for the NIV group, and 54, 54, 52, 49, 44, 38, 20 and 15, respectively for the control group. The time-course decrease of patients corresponds to those meeting criteria to terminate the protocol. *: p<0.05 compared with the NIV and control groups. Adapted from [17].

ARDS

Patients with ARDS are among those with the worst outcome when they receive NIV as a support measure for severe AHRF, with high rates of NIV failure [11, 17, 18] and limited efficacy in different studies. The severity of arterial hypoxaemia and the frequent impairment of pulmonary mechanics in those patients may explain the high intubation rate shown in several studies, regardless of NIV use or not.

To date, there are no controlled clinical trials that have assesses the efficacy of NIV specifically in patients with acute lung injury (ALI)/ARDS. A prospective observational study in 54 patients with ALI, who received NIV, found that shock, metabolic acidosis and profound hypoxaemia predicted NIV failure [18]. In that study, the observed mortality of patients who failed NIV was higher than that predicted by the Acute Physiology and Chronic Health Evaluation (APACHE)-II score, suggesting that NIV should be used very cautiously, or not at all, in patients with predictors of NIV failure.

Another prospective multicentre cohort study investigated the application of NIV as a first-line intervention in 147 patients with early ARDS [19]. In that study, NIV improved hypoxaemia and avoided intubation in 54% of patients and avoidance of intubation was associated with a lower incidence of VAP and a lower ICU mortality rate. Intubation was more common in older patients and patients with higher severity scores or the need for a higher level of positive end-expiratory pressure of pressure support ventilation. The variables independently associated with NIV failure were higher severity scores and failure to improve hypoxaemia after 1 h of NIV.

Other causes of severe ARF

An important part of the first published series assessing the efficacy of NIV in patients with AHRF included patients with different causes of AHRF. There series could not establish the efficacy of NIV in this subset of patients and showed disparate results, mainly because of the heterogeneity of AHRF, since patients with CPO, ARDS and trauma were also included [20]. Moreover, some of these initial studies observed that the efficacy of NIV was limited in patients with AHRF of different origin, compared with patients with hypercapnic respiratory failure [21].

The first randomised clinical trial performed specifically in hypoxaemic patients compared NIV with tracheal intubation in 64 patients with severe AHRF and predefined criteria for initiating ventilatory support [22]. Among the patients who received NIV, only 31% required intubation. Likewise, the improvement in arterial oxygenation after the protocol was implemented was similar in patients from both groups; the incidence of severe infectious complications was lower in patients who received NIV compared with those who were initially intubated (3 *versus* 31%, respectively). There was also a trend to a lower ICU mortality and shorter length of stay [22].

In contrast with these favourable results, another controlled clinical trial assessed the efficacy of NIV in an emergency department for patients with ARF by different causes. That study did not find a decrease in the intubation rate of patients who received NIV [23]. It also found a trend towards a higher mortality in the group of patients treated with NIV (25 *versus* 0% in the control group), attributed to an unnecessary delay in tracheal intubation. That study included a small amount of patients and patients were unevenly distributed between the treatment and the control group, despite randomisation, in such a way that patients in the NIV group had higher severity scores than those in the control group [23]. However, that study highlighted that NIV may not be successful in every hospital setting because the expertise may differ from one institution to another.

Despite the fact that the evidence in the use of NIV in patients with AHRF is mainly favourable, more controlled clinical trials are needed to better establish and define what subsets of such a wide range of patients may benefit from using NIV.

The efficacy of NIV in patients with AHRF not due to CPO was assessed in a systematic review and meta-analysis [24]. That review found that the addition of NIV to standard care in this setting reduced the rate of tracheal intubation (absolute risk reduction 23%; 95% confidence interval (CI) 10–35%), ICU length of stay (absolute reduction 2 days; 95% CI 1–3 days), and ICU mortality (absolute risk reduction 17%; 95% CI 8–26%). However, trial results were significantly heterogeneous. The authors concluded that randomised trials suggest that patients with AHRF are less likely to require tracheal intubation when NIV is added to standard therapy but the effect on mortality is less clear and the heterogeneity found among studies suggests that effectiveness varies among different populations. As a result, that systematic review of the literature did not support the routine use of NIV in all patients with AHRF [24].

The efficacy of CPAP using face masks in patients with severe AHRF, compared with oxygen therapy, was assessed in a randomised controlled trial. The study consisted of patients with pneumonia, in 54% of the population, and pulmonary oedema, in the rest. The authors assessed the physiological benefits of CPAP, as well as the effect in decreasing the needs for tracheal intubation [25]. Despite the fact that patients receiving CPAP had an initially better improvement of arterial oxygenation and comfort than those who received oxygen therapy, there were no differences in the needs for tracheal intubation, hospital mortality and ICU length of stay (fig. 4).

The different clinical efficacy between NIV and CPAP may be explained by the results of a physiological study performed in 10 patients with severe AHRF of different origin. This study compared the short-term effect of CPAP at 10 cmH_2O (CPAP-10) and 2 combinations of NIV with pressure-support ventilation (PSV): an inspiratory support level of 10 cmH_2O with positive end-expiratory pressure (PEEP) of 10 cmH_2O (PSV 10-10) and an inspiratory support level of 15 cmH_2O with PEEP of 5 cmH_2O (PSV 15-5) [26]. Compared with spontaneous breathing, the respiratory frequency decreased with the highest levels of inspiratory support (PSV 15-5). By contrast, arterial oxygenation improved similarly with CPAP-10 and PSV 10-10, while this increase failed to reach statistical significance for PSV 15-5. Finally, the work of breathing decreased with both modalities of NIV but not with CPAP (fig. 5), although the highest reduction in dyspnoea was achieved with PSV 15-5. In summary, in patients with severe AHRF, it is necessary to combine NIV with PEEP in order to decrease the inspiratory effort; CPAP improves arterial oxygenation but does not unload the respiratory muscles. Moreover, high levels of inspiratory support are needed to ameliorate dyspnoea. These results explain why NIV with PEEP is preferred over CPAP in patients with severe AHRF, in general, particularly those with severe pneumonia.

ARF in the post-operative period

The respiratory function may be substantially modified during the post-operative period. These patients often develop atelectasis due to a decrease in the pulmonary volumes (vital capacity, functional residual capacity, tidal volume) and diaphragm dysfunction, which may last up to 7 days, with important deterioration in arterial oxygenation. Moreover, swallowing disorders and vomiting may cause aspiration during the post-operative period.

Both NIV and CPAP are frequently used in these clinical situations. Physiological studies have shown that CPAP is effective in improving arterial oxygenation after

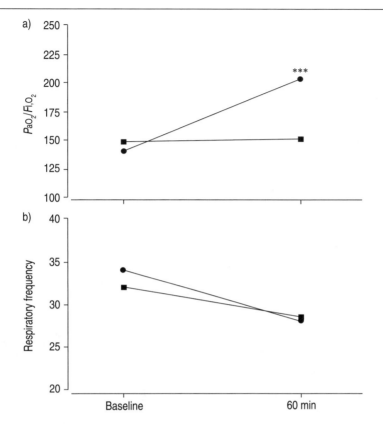

Fig. 4. – Initial evolution of a) the arterial hypoxaemia, assessed by the arterial oxygen tension (P_{a,O_2})/inspiratory oxygen fraction (F_{I,O_2}) ratio and b) the respiratory rate for patients treated with continuous positive airway pressure (CPAP) plus oxygen (●) compared with those treated with oxygen alone (■), from baseline to 60 min after the initiation of treatment. ***: $p<0.001$ for the CPAP plus oxygen group.

extubation without adverse haemodynamic effect, during post-operative period of cardiac or thoracic surgery [27]. This study, however, demonstrated that 9–10 cmH$_2$O is the minimal effective level of positive airway pressure for this purpose, since lower levels of airway pressure are not appropriately transmitted to the tracheal and thoracic cavity. The same authors had demonstrated that nasal CPAP improved arterial oxygenation and avoided reintubation in 90% of cases in patients who had worsening of arterial oxygenation after elective surgery [28]. By contrast, physiological studies in patients extubated after elective cardiac surgery have shown that NIV caused haemodynamic changes, with improvement in the cardiac index and without changes in systemic and pulmonary artery pressure or in arterial oxygenation [29].

Several randomised clinical trials have assessed the efficacy of NIV in post-operative ARF from different causes. In patients with solid organ transplantation and post-operative ARF, NIV improved arterial oxygenation and decreased the needs for tracheal intubation, compared with conventional treatment [9].

A physiological study in patients submitted to elective lung resection showed that, compared with standard medical therapy, the addition of NIV resulted in improved arterial oxygenation without changes in arterial carbon dioxide levels, dead space or pleural leaks [30]. A randomised controlled trial in patients who developed ARF during

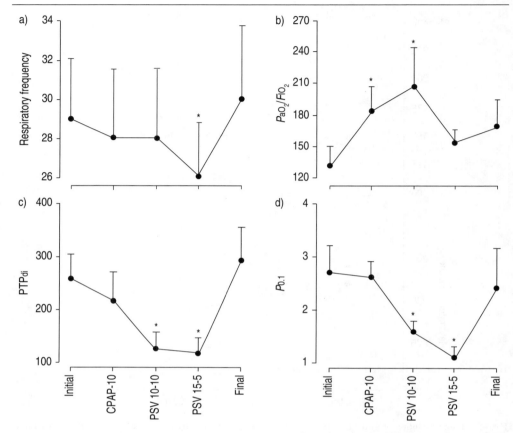

Fig. 5. – Average changes in respiratory variables (respiratory frequency, arterial hypoxaemia, assessed by the arterial oxygen tension ($Pa_{,O_2}$)/inspiratory oxygen fraction ($FI_{,O_2}$) ratio, work of breathing, assessed by the pressure-time product of the diaphragm (PTPdi) and the respiratory drive, assessed by the occlusion pressure ($P0.1$)) comparing the initial and final values during spontaneous breathing with the three ventilatory modalities. CPAP-10: continuous positive airway pressure of 10 cmH$_2$O; PSV 10-10: pressure-support ventilation (PSV) of 10 cmH$_2$O with positive end-expiratory pressure (PEEP) of 10 cmH$_2$O; PSV 15-5: PSV of 15 cmH$_2$O and PEEP of 5 cmH$_2$O. *: $p < 0.05$.

the post-operative period of lung cancer resection demonstrated that NIV was effective in decreasing the needs for tracheal intubation and improving hospital mortality [31]. The efficacy of NIV in those studies seems, however, related to the underlying diseases of patients rather than the post-operative respiratory complications.

In obese patients with restrictive ventilatory disorder undergoing gastroplasty, nasal NIV during the post-operative period improved diaphragm dysfunction and accelerated recovery of patients [32]. A prospective observational study in patients who had ARF after abdominal surgery showed that the use of NIV resulted in avoidance of intubation in 67% of cases [33]. Patients who required intubation had worse arterial oxygenation and more extended bilateral pulmonary infiltrates than those who escaped from intubation. In that study, arterial oxygenation and tachypnoea improved only in the non-intubated patients, with a reduction in the hospital stay and mortality, compared with the intubated patients. A randomised controlled trial in patients with ARF after major abdominal surgery compared the use of CPAP and oxygen therapy [34]. That study showed that CPAP reduced the rate of tracheal intubation, compared with oxygen therapy (1% *versus* 10%, respectively; p=0.005), as well as other severe complications, although the reduction of hospital mortality was not significant.

Summary

The randomised clinical trials of the literature suggest that patients with severe acute hypoxaemic respiratory failure have, in general, a lower likelihood of needing tracheal intubation when noninvasive ventilation, as a support for respiratory failure, is added to the standard medical treatment. However, the effects of noninvasive ventilation on mortality are less evident and the heterogeneity of the different published studies suggests that the efficacy may be different among different populations. Therefore, the results of the literature do not support the routine use of noninvasive ventilation in all patients with severe acute hypoxaemic respiratory failure.

Keywords: Acute hypoxaemic respiratory failure, acute respiratory distress syndrome, noninvasive ventilation, post-operative respiratory failure, severe pneumonia.

Support Statement: This chapter was supported by Centro de Investigación Biomédica En Red-Enfermedades Respiratorias (CibeRes, CB06/06/0028) and 2005 SGR 00822.

References

1. Mehta S, Hill NS. Noninvasive ventilation. *Am J Respir Crit Care Med* 2001; 163: 540–577.
2. Keenan SP, Sinuff T, Cook DJ, Hill NS. Which patients with acute exacerbation of chronic obstructive pulmonary disease benefit from noninvasive positive-pressure ventilation? A systematic review of the literature. *Ann Intern Med* 2003; 138: 861–870.
3. Peter JV, Moran JL, Phillips-Hughes J, Warn D. Noninvasive ventilation in acute respiratory failure – a meta-analysis update. *Crit Care Med* 2002; 30: 555–562.
4. Lightowler JV, Wedzicha JA, Elliott MW, Ram FS. Non-invasive positive pressure ventilation to treat respiratory failure resulting from exacerbations of chronic obstructive pulmonary disease: Cochrane systematic review and meta-analysis. *BMJ* 2003; 326: 185–189.
5. Girou E, Schortgen F, Delclaux C, *et al.* Association of noninvasive ventilation with nosocomial infections and survival in critically ill patients. *JAMA* 2000; 284: 2361–2367.
6. Meade MO, Cook DJ, Kernerman P, Bernard G. How to use articles about harm: the relationship between high tidal volumes, ventilating pressures, and ventilator-induced lung injury. *Crit Care Med* 1997; 25: 1915–1922.
7. Masip J, Roque M, Sánchez B, Fernández R, Subirana M, Expósito JA. Noninvasive ventilation in acute cardiogenic pulmonary edema: systematic review and meta-analysis. *JAMA* 2005; 294: 3124–3130.
8. Peter JV, Moran JL, Phillips-Hughes J, Graham P, Bersten AD. Effect of non-invasive positive pressure ventilation (NIPPV) on mortality in patients with acute cardiogenic pulmonary oedema: a meta-analysis. *Lancet* 2006; 367: 1155–1163.
9. Antonelli M, Conti G, Bufi M, *et al.* Noninvasive ventilation for treatment of acute respiratory failure in patients undergoing solid organ transplantation: a randomised trial. *JAMA* 2000; 283: 235–241.
10. Hilbert G, Gruson D, Vargas F, *et al.* Noninvasive ventilation in immunosuppressed patients with pulmonary infiltrates, fever, and acute respiratory failure. *N Engl J Med* 2001; 344: 481–487.
11. Antonelli M, Conti G, Moro ML, *et al.* Predictors of failure of noninvasive positive pressure ventilation in patients with acute hypoxemic respiratory failure: a multi-center study. *Intensive Care Med* 2001; 27: 1718–1728.

12. Mandell LA, Wunderink RG, Anzueto A, *et al.* Infectious Diseases Society of America/American Thoracic Society consensus guidelines on the management of community-acquired pneumonia in adults. *Clin Infect Dis* 2007; 44: Suppl. 2, S27–S72.

13. Ambrosino N, Foglio K, Rubini F, Clini E, Nava S, Vitacca M. Non-invasive mechanical ventilation in acute respiratory failure due to chronic obstructive pulmonary disease: correlates for success. *Thorax* 1995; 50: 755–757.

14. Jolliet P, Abajo B, Pasquina P, Chevrolet JC. Non-invasive pressure support ventilation in severe community-acquired pneumonia. *Intensive Care Med* 2001; 27: 812–821.

15. Domenighetti G, Gayer R, Gentilini R. Noninvasive pressure support ventilation in non-COPD patients with acute cardiogenic pulmonary edema and severe community-acquired pneumonia: acute effects and outcome. *Intensive Care Med* 2002; 28: 1226–1232.

16. Confalonieri M, Potena A, Carbone G, Porta RD, Tolley EA, Umberto Meduri G. Acute respiratory failure in patients with severe community-acquired pneumonia. A prospective randomized evaluation of noninvasive ventilation. *Am J Respir Crit Care Med* 1999; 160: 1585–1591.

17. Ferrer M, Esquinas A, Leon M, Gonzalez G, Alarcon A, Torres A. Noninvasive ventilation in severe hypoxemic respiratory failure: a randomized clinical trial. *Am J Respir Crit Care Med* 2003; 168: 1438–1444.

18. Rana S, Jenad H, Gay PC, Buck CF, Hubmayr RD, Gajic O. Failure of non-invasive ventilation in patients with acute lung injury: observational cohort study. *Crit Care* 2006; 10: R79.

19. Antonelli M, Conti G, Esquinas A, *et al.* A multiple-center survey on the use in clinical practice of noninvasive ventilation as a first-line intervention for acute respiratory distress syndrome. *Crit Care Med* 2007; 35: 18–25.

20. Meduri GU, Turner RE, Abou-Shala N, Wunderink R, Tolley E. Noninvasive positive pressure ventilation *via* face mask. First-line intervention in patients with acute hypercapnic and hypoxemic respiratory failure. *Chest* 1996; 109: 179–193.

21. Wysocki M, Tric L, Wolff MA, Millet H, Herman B. Noninvasive pressure support ventilation in patients with acute respiratory failure: a randomized comparison with conventional therapy. *Chest* 1995; 107: 761–768.

22. Antonelli M, Conti G, Rocco M, *et al.* A comparison of noninvasive positive-pressure ventilation and conventional mechanical ventilation in patients with acute respiratory failure. *N Engl J Med* 1998; 339: 429–435.

23. Wood KA, Lewis L, Von Harz B, Kollef MH. The use of noninvasive positive pressure ventilation in the emergency department: results of a randomized clinical trial. *Chest* 1998; 113: 1339–1346.

24. Keenan SP, Sinuff T, Cook DJ, Hill NS. Does noninvasive positive pressure ventilation improve outcome in acute hypoxemic respiratory failure? A systematic review. *Crit Care Med* 2004; 32: 2516–2523.

25. Delclaux C, L'Her E, Alberti C, *et al.* Treatment of acute hypoxemic nonhypercapnic respiratory insufficiency with continuous positive airway pressure delivered by a face mask: A randomized controlled trial. *JAMA* 2000; 284: 2352–2360.

26. L'Her E, Deye N, Lellouche F, *et al.* Physiologic effects of noninvasive ventilation during acute lung injury. *Am J Respir Crit Care Med* 2005; 172: 1112–1118.

27. Kindgen-Milles D, Buhl R, Loer SA, Müller E. Nasal CPAP therapy: effects of different CPAP levels on pressure transmission into the trachea and pulmonary oxygen transfer. *Acta Anaesthesiol Scand* 2002; 46: 860–865.

28. Kindgen-Milles D, Buhl R, Gabriel A, Böhner H, Müller E. Nasal continuous positive airway pressure: A method to avoid endotracheal reintubation in postoperative high-risk patients with severe nonhypercapnic oxygenation failure. *Chest* 2000; 117: 1106–1111.

29. Hoffmann B, Jepsen M, Hachenberg T, Huth C, Welte T. Cardiopulmonary effects of non-invasive positive pressure ventilation (NPPV) – a controlled, prospective study. *Thorac Cardiovasc Surg* 2003; 51: 142–146.

30. Aguiló R, Togores B, Pons S, Rubí M, Barbé F, Agustí AG. Noninvasive ventilatory support after lung resectional surgery. *Chest* 1997; 112: 117–121.

31. Auriant I, Jallot A, Hervé P, *et al.* Noninvasive ventilation reduces mortality in acute respiratory failure following lung resection. *Am J Respir Crit Care Med* 2001; 164: 1231–1235.
32. Joris JL, Sottiaux TM, Chiche JD, Desaive CJ, Lamy ML. Effect of bi-level positive airway pressure (BiPAP) nasal ventilation on the postoperative pulmonary restrictive syndrome in obese patients undergoing gastroplasty. *Chest* 1997; 111: 665–670.
33. Jaber S, Delay JM, Chanques G, *et al.* Outcomes of patients with acute respiratory failure after abdominal surgery treated with noninvasive positive pressure ventilation. *Chest* 2005; 128: 2688–2695.
34. Squadrone V, Coha M, Cerutti E, *et al.* Continuous positive airway pressure for treatment of postoperative hypoxemia: a randomized controlled trial. *JAMA* 2005; 293: 589–595.

CHAPTER 6

NIV for cardiogenic pulmonary oedema

A. Gray*, D. Schlosshan#, M.W. Elliott¶

*Dept of Respiratory Medicine, St James's University Hospital and #Dept of Cardiology, Leeds General Infirmary, Leeds, and ¶Dept of Emergency Medicine, Royal Infirmary of Edinburgh, Edinburgh, UK.

Correspondence: M.W. Elliott, Dept of Respiratory Medicine, St James's University Hospital, Beckett Street, Leeds, LS9 7TF, UK. Fax: 44 1132066042; E-mail: mwelliott@doctors.org.uk

The epidemiology of acute heart failure

Acute heart failure (AHF) is one of the leading causes of admission to hospital in Europe and the USA [1]. In the USA, >1 million patients are admitted to hospital resulting in 6.5 million bed-days [1]. European data suggest AHF admissions result in 1 million and 1.4 million bed-days, annually, in the UK and France, respectively [1]. Heart failure is the most common reason for admission in patients aged >65 yrs [2] and results in a considerable readmission rate to hospital [1, 2]. Most importantly, there is significant short- and long-term mortality [1, 2]. It is anticipated that the prevalence of heart failure will continue to rise [2, 3].

Definitions

Unlike acute coronary syndromes AHF is a generic term encompassing the "complex clinical syndrome that can result from any structural or functional cardiac disorder that impairs the ventricle to fill or eject blood" [4]. This has led to inconsistencies and lack of consensus on the definitions, epidemiology, pathophysiology and clinical management of AHF [2], as well as the development of relevant research outcomes [2, 5]. A number of professional bodies and authorities have attempted to address this by producing consensus statements [2, 4–7]. "Acute decompensated heart failure" is a clinical condition in which the patient, with known heart failure, has an acute or subacute deterioration in their symptoms requiring intervention. An international working group has recently defined these patients as presenting with an "AHF syndrome" [2]. Patients may present *de novo* or have previously recognised heart failure. These patients primarily present to hospital with signs and symptoms that relate to pulmonary congestion occurring as a result of elevated left ventricular filling pressures with the accompanying symptoms of dyspnoea and fatigue [8]. Cardiac output may be impaired or preserved. Patients have preserved left ventricular function and diastolic heart failure, are older and predominantly female [9, 10].

Epidemiology and patient characteristics

There is increasing information available from registries and surveys from Europe (EuroHeart Failure Survey I and II [11, 12], the Italian Acute Heart Failure Survey [13]

Eur Respir Mon, 2008, 41, 72–93. Printed in UK - all rights reserved. Copyright ERS Journals Ltd 2008; European Respiratory Monograph; ISSN 1025-448x.

and EFICA [14]) and North America (Acute Decompensated Heart Failure National Registry (ADHERE) [3] and Organized Program To Initiate life-saving treatment In hospitalized patients with Heart Failure (OPTIMIZE-HF) registries [15]) that enable a clearer understanding of the characteristics of patients admitted with AHF syndromes, including presenting symptoms and physiology including severity of illness, management strategies, use of resource and clinical outcomes. It is clear that populations, clinical management and outcomes vary considerably depending on setting and geographical location [2, 16].

The ADHERE [3] had data on approximately 105,000 heart failure patients from 274 hospitals in the USA up to 2004. The mean age of patients was 72 yrs and 52% were female. Common comorbidities included hypertension (73%), coronary heart disease (57%) and diabetes (44%). A total of 46% of patients had preserved left ventricular function. The median length of stay was 4.3 days and there was an in-hospital mortality rate of 4% and 5% received mechanical ventilation.

The EuroHeart failure II survey [12] reported on 3,580 patients with AHF from across Europe. The mean age was 69.9 yrs and 61% were male. A total of 37.1% had *de novo* heart failure. Pulmonary oedema accounted for 16.2% and hypertensive heart failure for 11.4% of admissions, as defined by the European Society of Cardiology 2005 guidelines. Over one-third of patients had preserved left ventricular function and 6.7% died during hospital admission. The median length of stay was 9 days and approximately one-half were admitted to coronary or critical care. A total of 13.9% received either noninvasive ventilation (NIV) or invasive ventilation, increasing to 31.5% if the patient was classified as having pulmonary oedema as the primary presenting condition. Ventilatory support was markedly more common in the EFICA study investigating the characteristics of 599 patients admitted with AHF to 60 critical care units in France [14]. In this study, 35% were endotracheally intubated and ventilated and 24% received noninvasive ventilatory support. However, these patients were sicker (4-week mortality was 27.4%) and had a significant rate of cardiogenic shock, compared with other studies.

An Italian national survey from 2004 [13] included 206 hospitals with cardiology services enrolled 2,807 patients in a 3-month period and characterised them according to the 2001 European Society of Cardiology Guidelines. The mean age was 73 yrs; 44% had *de novo* heart failure and in 49.6%, pulmonary oedema was the principal presenting symptom. A total of 89% of the patients had impaired left ventricular function. The median length of hospital stay was 9 days and there was a 7.3% in-hospital mortality rate, which increased to 12.8% by 6 months.

Heart failure classifications

As previously described, AHF is recognised to be a heterogeneous syndrome, which can be classified in a variety of ways depending upon clinical presentation, pathophysiological processes, previous or *de novo* heart failure or associated acute coronary syndrome. Clinical management should, therefore, be tailored towards this rather than a unified approach across the disease spectrum. GHEORGHIADE *et al.* [2] have recently classified patients presenting with AHF into eight groups and suggest that management should be targeted to the presenting symptoms (table 1). A similar classification suggested by the European Society of Cardiology [6] also includes subgroups of patients with hypertension, right heart failure, cardiogenic shock and isolated pulmonary oedema.

Table 1. – Clinical presentations of acute heart failure

Clinical presentation	Incidence[#]	Signs and symptoms	Characteristics
Elevated systolic blood pressure	>50%	Usually develop abruptly	Predominantly pulmonary (radiographic/clinical), rather than systemic, congestion due to rapid fluid redistribution from systemic to pulmonary circulation; many patients have preserved ejection fraction
Normal systolic blood pressure	>40%	Develop gradually (days or weeks) and are associated with significant systemic congestion	Despite high ventricular filling pressure, radiographic pulmonary congestion may be minimal because of pulmonary vasculaturelymphatics adaptation due to chronic elevated left atrial pressures
Low systolic blood pressure (<90 mm Hg)	<8%	Usually have a low cardiac output with signs of organ hypoperfusion	Many of those patients have advanced or end-stage heart failure
Cardiogenic shock	<1%	Rapid onset	Primarily complicating acute *Mycoplasma fulminant* myocarditis
Pulmonary oedema	<3%[¶]	Rapid or gradual onset	Clinical: severe dyspnoea, tachypnea, tachycardia and hypoxaemia, requiring immediate airway intervention. Radiographic: present in up to 80% of patients; often not associated with clinical pulmonary oedema
"Flash" pulmonary oedema	unknown	Abrupt onset	Precipitated by severe systemic hypertension. Uncorrected, respiratory failure and death ensue. Patients are easily treated with vasodilators and diuretics. After blood pressure normalisation and reinstitution of routine medications, patients can be discharged within 24 h
Isolated right heart failure	unknown	Rapid or gradual onset	Not well characterised; there are no epidemiological data (e.g., acute cor pulmonale, right ventricular infarct)
Acute coronary syndromes (~25% of acute coronary syndromes patients have signs/symptoms of heart failure)	unknown	Rapid or gradual onset	Many such patients may have signs and symptoms of heart failure that resolve after initial therapy or resolution of ischaemia
Post-cardiac surgery heart failure	unknown	Rapid or gradual onset	Occurring in patients with or without previous ventricular dysfunction, often related to worsening diastolic function and volume overload immediately after surgery

Reproduced from [2], with permission from the publisher. [#]: of all acute heart failure syndrome admissions; [¶]: incidence may be related to the definition used (clinical or radiographic).

Cardiopulmonary interactions and the effect of positive pressure ventilation

In order to understand possible mechanisms of benefits of positive pressure ventilation in patients with heart failure, it is first important to understand the interaction of the heart and lungs during normal respiration. As the heart is located within the thorax, there is a close and continuous interaction between changes in intracardiac pressures and intrathoracic pressure (PIT). During normal respiration, phasic changes in lung volume and PIT can simultaneously change most determinants of cardiac function including cardiac frequency, preload, contractility and afterload.

During spontaneous inspiration, PIT decreases and returns towards the baseline during expiration. The degree to which PIT and lung volume change is a function of airway resistance and both lung and chest wall compliance. Positive pressure ventilation induces opposite changes in PIT [17].

Circulatory components are affected by the PIT, depending on their location. The heart and the intrathoracic aorta lie within the thorax and are therefore affected by changes in PIT. The extrathoracic aorta lies outside the thorax and is consequently not affected by PIT but by atmospheric pressure; because of this anatomical relationship, PINSKY [18] described the heart within the thorax as "a pressure chamber within another pressure chamber". The difference between the pressure in the heart and the pressure surrounding the heart (*i.e.* PIT) affects both systemic venous return to the right ventricle (RV) and systemic outflow from the left ventricle (LV).

During inspiration, PIT decreases, thus reducing right atrial (RA) pressure. Therefore, the pressure gradient for venous return from the periphery to the right heart increases during inspiration leading to increased venous return and increased right diastolic volume [19]. As a result, RV stroke volume increases during inspiration [20, 21]. This effect is somewhat dampened by an increase in RV afterload caused by an increase in alveolar pressure [22]. Therefore, both RV preload and RV afterload are increased during inspiration, leading to an increase in RV diastolic volume [20, 21].

The effects of inspiration on left ventricular outflow are generally opposite. Normal inspiratory effort is accompanied by a fall in left ventricular stroke volume [23–25]. The magnitude appears to be related to the depth of inspiration, *i.e.* the increasing negativity of the pleural pressure [26]. BUDA *et al.* [26] and others [22, 27] proposed the following model to explain the relationship between PIT and left ventricular outflow during deep inspiration: increasing negativity of PIT during inspiration decreases the pressure surrounding the LV. During systole the inward contraction of the LV is impeded by the opposite force of the negative PIT. LV transmural pressure (Ptm) is calculated as follows:

$$P\text{tm}= P\text{LV} - P\text{IT} \qquad (1)$$

where PLV is the LV systolic pressure. The LV is therefore required to generate higher pressure to overcome the PIT in addition to the aortic diastolic pressure to eject blood during systole. Left ventricular afterload is therefore determined by the difference between aortic diastolic pressure (equal to PLV) and PIT. Therefore afterload increases not only through increasing aortic pressure but also through a fall in PIT. This increase in afterload leads to a decrease in stroke volume and increase in end-systolic volume.

In summary, there is a close interaction between determinants of cardiac function and changes in lung volumes and PIT. A fall in PIT during inspiration has opposing effects on the RV and LV. This acts to increase venous return to the right heart and decrease stroke volume for the left heart. During normal respiration, however, the net effect on the cardiovascular system is minimal. Conditions associated with large changes in PIT, however, are known to significantly affect cardiac performance and filling through these mechanisms.

Acute effects of NIV on the normal heart

Positive pressure ventilation significantly increases PIT and is therefore expected to affect cardiac haemodynamics through similar mechanisms, but in the opposite direction. The combined effect of positive pressure ventilation provided either by positive end-expiratory pressure (PEEP) or continuous positive airway pressure (CPAP) in a normal heart is to decrease right and left ventricular preload, increase RV afterload and decrease LV afterload. As the normal heart is largely preload dependent, the sum of these effects is such that cardiac output frequently falls with CPAP or PEEP [26, 28–30]. These effects can be exacerbated at higher levels of positive pressure ventilation and hypovolaemia.

Acute effects of NIV on cardiac haemodynamics in heart failure

Much of the work on heart failure in humans has been done in patients with chronic heart failure (CHF). In many cases, acute cardiogenic pulmonary oedema (CPO) occurs in patients with a background of CHF. Many of the principles in patients with CHF also apply in acute CPO. Following the pioneering studies in the 1970s on the haemodynamic effects of PIT on cardiac haemodynamics, PINSKY et al. [31] postulated that increases in PIT would have different effects on the failing heart compared to the normal heart. This hypothesis was based on the assumption that a failing heart is less sensitive to changes in preload and more sensitive to changes in afterload compared with a normal heart. The hypothesis was that the afterload lowering effects of positive PIT may have a beneficial effect on cardiac function in the failing heart. In an early study performed on anaesthetised dogs with left ventricular failure it was first observed that intermittent positive pressure ventilation led to improved cardiac function [31]. Subsequently, it was observed that phasic high PIT support applied to anaesthetised patients in cardiogenic shock augmented cardiac output, mean arterial pressure and ejection fraction, while LV filling remained unaltered [32]. Beneficial acute effects on cardiac output in humans with heart failure were also seen in other studies [33, 34].

BRADLEY et al. [35] demonstrated that CPAP at a level of 5 cmH$_2$O caused an increase in cardiac output of 30% in patients with CHF, caused by dilated cardiomyopathy and a pulmonary capillary wedge pressure (PPCW) >12 mmHg. Patients with a PPCW <12 mmHg however decreased their cardiac out put in response to CPAP. DE HOYOS et al. [36] extended these findings by the observation that 5–10 cmH$_2$O produced a dose-related augmentation in cardiac output when applied acutely to patients with CHF and elevated PPCW. In contrast, in both control subjects and patients with heart failure and normal PPCW (<12 mmHg) there was a dose-related decrease in cardiac and stroke volume indices, while on continuous positive airway pressure.

These studies and others [37] confirmed that LV filling was a strong determinant of augmented cardiac output and stroke volume in the failing heart in response to CPAP. It was postulated that patients with low LV preload are more preload dependent and that any decrease in preload caused by NIV, potentially leads to leftwards shift on the Frank–Starling curve and a fall in cardiac output.

NAUGHTON et al. [38] confirmed that CPAP has a significant effect on afterload in patients with CHF. The effects, of graduated CPAP from 0 to 10 cmH$_2$O, on PIT were studied and several important observations were made. The amplitude of the inspiratory oesophageal pressure amplitude was more negative than in healthy subjects, suggesting that patients with CHF needed to generate greater inspiratory force during inspiration; this, in turn resulted in greater LV transmural pressure in patients with CHF. CPAP significantly reduced negative oesophageal pressure swings and decreased LV transmural pressure in patients with CHF, without significant effects on cardiac index. LV transmural pressure and oesophageal pressure did not change significantly in healthy subjects in response to CPAP. From these observations, the authors concluded that, in patients with CHF, the inspiratory muscles generate greater force per breath, and the systolic oesophageal pressure contributes more to LV transmural pressure, than in healthy subjects. By increasing P_{IT} in patients with CHF, CPAP unloaded inspiratory muscles and reduced left ventricular afterload without compromising cardiac output. Similar observations were made by MEHTA *et al.* [39]. The short-term effect of CPAP at 10 cmH$_2$O on RV and LV volumes, determined by radionucleide angiography, in 22 patients with CHF was assessed and no significant reduction in left ventricular volumes was found, except in subset of patients with very large volumes. The authors concluded that any improvements of LV function as a result of NIV are, therefore, more likely to be due to the reduction of afterload by CPAP rather than preload.

The haemodynamic response to CPAP treatment seems to be quite variable. Other studies have shown little or no change in cardiac output in response to CPAP [40–43] despite high filling pressures. BARATZ *et al.* [40] examined the effect of nasal CPAP in 13 patients with acutely decompensated CHF, all of whom had P_{PCW} >12 mmHg. However, only seven out of the 13 patients showed a significant increase in cardiac output in response to CPAP. The authors noted that nonresponders had a high resting heart rate, lower ejection fraction and were more likely to have ischaemic cardiomyopathy. LISTON *et al.* [41] applied CPAP at 5 cmH$_2$O to patients with CHF and high filling pressures and observed a fall in cardiac output and increase in systemic vascular resitance. CPAP with a pressure of 10 cmH$_2$O induced significantly greater reductions in right and left ventricular volumes in patients with CHF caused by dilated cardiomyopathy than in those caused by ischaemic cardiomyopathy [39]. The authors postulated that the myocardial fibrosis and scarring associated with ischaemic cardiomyopathy could alter the compliance and, therefore, make the ventricles more resistant to the effects of NIV. Indeed, patients with idiopathic dilated cardiomyopathy often have higher left ventricular volumes and a more compliant ventricle than patients with ischaemic cardiomyopathy and possibly have more acute haemodynamic benefit to gain from NIV than patients with a less-compliant ventricle with smaller left ventricular volumes [44]. Nevertheless, several studies have demonstrated both acute and chronic haemodynamic benefits in patients with CHF caused by ischaemic cardiomyopathy [38, 45, 46].

The acute effects of CPAP on cardiac function appear to be significantly influenced by the underlying cardiac rhythm. KIELY *et al.* [47] compared the haemodynamic response to CPAP, in patients with CHF, in sinus rhythm (SR) and atrial fibrillation (AF). A significant difference was demonstrated in the response to CPAP, with a fall in cardiac index in the AF group and trend towards an increase in the SR group. It was postulated that patients with AF may be more sensitive to decreases in preload generated by CPAP.

Studies on the haemodynamic effects of bilevel ventilation on cardiac function are limited. ACOSTA *et al.* [48] first assessed the haemodynamic effects of bilevel ventilation at a level of 5 cmH$_2$O in 14 patients with stable CHF. The main findings included a significant increase in cardiac output, ejection fraction and end-diastolic volume, and a decrease in systemic vascular resistance. Using higher pressures, PHILIP-JOET *et al.* [37] demonstrated that bilevel ventilation had similar haemodynamic effects compared with CPAP in patients with CHF. However, bilevel ventilation appeared to be superior to CPAP in improving oxygenation and ventilation.

The current evidence suggests that bilevel ventilation acutely increases cardiac output in selected patients with CHF and elevated left ventricular filling pressures but reduces cardiac output in those whose filling pressures are normal. The net effect of NIV in patients with CHF is likely to be the result of a balance between the preload-reducing effect of NIV and the afterload-reducing effect of NIV; however, the response is variable (table 2).

Table 2. – Determinants of response of positive pressure

The effect of positive pressure depends on:
the aetiology of heart failure
baseline cardiac volumes
degree of diastolic dysfunction
compliance of the ventricle
the presence of right ventricular failure
rhythm
preload dependence

Effect of NIV on respiratory muscles and lung mechanics

The respiratory muscles in patients with CHF are abnormal; patients with CHF suffer from inspiratory muscles weakness [49–51]. Suggested explanations include reduction in respiratory muscle blood flow or generalised muscular atrophy and weakness related to cardiac cachexia [52]. Furthermore, the inspiratory muscles are exposed to an excessive load and have to generate a greater force per breath compared with healthy subjects [53]. NAUGHTON et al. [38] found that patients with optimally treated CHF had three- to four-fold greater inspiratory pleural pressure swings than healthy control subjects, probably due to reduced lung compliance caused by pulmonary congestion.

Several studies have shown that NIV has beneficial effects on respiratory muscles in patients with AHF and CHF. Application of 10 cmH$_2$O of CPAP to these patients, while awake, during regular breathing led to a 40% reduction in the amplitude of pleural pressure swings. This reflected unloading of inspiratory muscles, which was probably due to increased lung compliance secondary to extrathoracic redistribution of lung water [38, 42], and reported a significant reduction in the work of breathing, the pressure–time index of the respiratory muscles and the negative swings in PIT with CPAP at 10 cmH$_2$O in patients with CPO.

There are several mechanisms by which CPAP and PEEP improve respiratory parameters in patients with heart failure. CPAP has been shown to increase functional residual capacity and open collapsed or underventilated alveoli, thus decreasing right to left intrapulmonary shunt and improving oxygenation. Although CPAP and PEEP do not actively assist ventilation, the increase in functional residual capacity may also improve lung compliance and decrease the work of breathing by moving the patient on to a more compliant part of the pressure–volume curve [54–56]. Bilevel ventilation offers theoretical advantages over CPAP, by actively assisting ventilation while providing PEEP at the same time. This would be expected to be more efficient in reducing the work of breathing in these patients.

In summary, NIV can unload respiratory muscles, decrease the work of breathing and improve lung mechanics in these patients. It is likely that the individual responses to NIV vary considerably and depend upon several factors, including level of positive airway pressure provided, changes in the lung, airways, chest wall, and inspiratory and expiratory respiratory muscles.

NIV in acute CPO: the evidence

There has been a steady stream of published randomised trials investigating the effectiveness of NIV in the management of acute CPO over the last 20 yrs [57–72]. None has been powered to detect mortality benefit as the primary outcome and most have used a variety of surrogate end-points, such as physiological parameters, intubation or predefined treatment failure. Moreover, these trials have investigated the comparative effectiveness of: CPAP and standard oxygen therapy [59–63, 72]; NIV and standard oxygen therapy [57, 65]; NIV and CPAP [64, 69–71]; or either intervention (CPAP/NIV) compared with standard oxygen therapy alone [58, 66–68]. Almost all these trials, now numbering 25, have shown improvement in physiology or a reduction in endotracheal intubation rate or other surrogate markers of treatment failure in the NIV arm. One study by MEHTA *et al.* [69] was terminated prematurely due to an excess number of patients with acute myocardial infarction (MI) in the NIV arm. Other studies, specifically designed to address this issue, have not confirmed any relationship between NIV and MI rate [70]. Despite the lack of definitive mortality benefit NIV is increasingly used in clinical practice [73] and advocated by many specialty organisations [7, 74, 75]. In an attempt to determine whether a true mortality benefit exists, a number of authors have recently reviewed, assimilated and published systematic reviews with meta-analyses. The following section reviews the key meta-analyses and recent primary trials.

Systematic reviews and meta-analyses

There have been seven systematic reviews published since 2005 [63, 76–81]. MASIP *et al.* [81] identified 15 eligible randomised controlled trials comparing NIV with standard oxygen or with another type of NIV *i.e.* CPAP compared with NIV (table 3). Data from studies were extracted into a standardised data collection form by two independent reviewers and checked by a third. Methodological quality was assessed using a recognised scoring system [83]. The primary outcomes for the systematic review were in-hospital mortality and treatment failure as all included trials reported these outcomes. Treatment failure was inconsistently categorised and the authors defined this arbitrarily as the "need to intubate". Data on MI rate during hospital admission were collected and analysed. All other parameters, such as physiology, length of stay and critical care admission were not consistently reported across trials. There were six trials comparing only CPAP with standard oxygen therapy, two comparing only NIV with standard oxygen therapy, three trials with three trial arms (two interventions, CPAP or NIV) and three studies comparing CPAP with NIV. The majority of trials were single centre, based in intensive care units, emergency departments or both in 10 different countries and included small numbers of patients (n=26–130). The majority used full-face masks and CPAP (2.5–16 cmH$_2$O) and NIV levels (8–20 and 3–5 cmH$_2$O for inspiratory and expiratory, respectively) varied. There was considerable variation in the complexity of ventilator design. Only one study used mortality as a primary end-point. Methodological quality of the included trials was, in general, adequate. There were data on 727 patients for the comparison of NIV (CPAP or NIV) with standard oxygen. Patients receiving NIV had a significant reduction of in-hospital mortality (p<0.01; risk ratio 0.55; 95% confidence interval (CI) 0.40–0.78) and endotracheal intubation (p<0.01; risk ratio 0.48; 95% CI 0.32–0.57). Results remained significant if CPAP was analysed independently for both in-hospital mortality and need for intubation. NIV was shown to reduce mortality but not to a statistically significant level (p=0.07), which is likely to reflect the numbers of patients included in these trials (n=315), but remained significant for intubation (p=0.02). There was no difference in outcome between CPAP and NIV; however, these comparisons only included a total of 219 patients. There was no difference in MI rates between arms. Tests for heterogeneity and publication bias were insignificant. MASIP *et al.* [82] concluded that this meta-analysis demonstrated improved survival in patients receiving NIV and should now be considered first-line therapy in patients presenting with acute CPO.

Table 3. – Randomised studies, analysing noninvasive ventilation

First author [ref.]	Location	n#	Mask type	CPAP cmH$_2$O	IPAP/ EPAP cmH$_2$O	Primary outcomes	Other considerations
CPAP *versus* standard oxygen therapy							
RASANEN [59]	1 ICU in Finland	40	Full face	10		Clinical outcomes	
BERSTEN [60]	1 ICU in Australia	40 (39)	Full face	10		Intubation	
LIN [61]	1 ICU in Taiwan	100	Full face	2.5–12.5		Intubation, in-hospital mortality	Swan–Ganz catheterisation
TAKEDA [84]	1 ICU in Japan	30 (29)	Full face or nasal	4–10		Laboratory parameters	Measurement of plasma endothelin 1
KELLY [62]	1 ED and ICU in UK	58	Full face	7.5		Clinical outcomes, laboratory parameters	Measurement of plasma neurchormonal concentrations
L'HER [63]	4 EDs in France	89	Full face	7.5		48-h mortality	Elderly patients (age >75 yrs)
NPSV *versus* standard oxygen therapy							
MASIP [85]	1 ICU in Spain	40 (37)	Full face		20/5, mean	Intubation, resolution time	IPAP was adjusted to tidal volume
LEVITT [64]	1 ED in USA	38	Full face or nasal		8/3, initial	Intubation	Prematurely interrupted when [69] was published
NAVA [65]	5 EDs in Italy	130	Full face		14.5/6.1, mean	Intubation	*Post hoc* analysis in hypercapnic patients
Trials with three study groups							
PARK [66]	1 ED in Brazil	26	Full face and nasal	5–12.5	a/3, initial	Intubation	Full-face mask for CPAP and nasal for NPSV
CRANE [67]	2 EDs in UK	60	Full face	10	15/5 fixed	Success in ED (2 h), in-hospital mortality	Pre-hospital nitrates therapy evaluated
PARK [68]	1 ED in Brazil	83 (80)	Full face	10 initial up to 16	15/10 initial	Intubation	
CPAP *versus* NPSV							
MEHTA [69]	1 ED in USA	27	Full face and nasal	10	15/5 fixed	Intubation, physiological improvement	Prematurely stopped for higher rate of AM in NPSV group
BELLONE [70]	1 ED in Italy	36	Full face	10	15/5 initial	AM	Study restricted to patients with hypercapnia
BELLONE [71]	1 ED in Italy	46	Full face	10	15/5 initial	Resolution time	Primary end-point was AM rate, only nonischaemic APO

Data included in meta-analysis of MASIP *et al.* [81] and reproduced with permission from the publisher. CPAP: continuous positive airway pressure; IPAP: inspiratory positive airway pressure; EPAP: expiratory positive airway pressure; ICU: intensive care unit; ED: emergency department; NPSV: bilevel noninvasive pressure support ventilation; AM: acute myocardial infarction; APO: acute pulmonary oedema. #: data are presented as n (n finally included after withdrawal).

In another meta-analysis, PETER *et al.* [82] identified 23 eligible studies from 14 countries over an 18-yr period. Data assimilation of these trials, including the eight not included in the review by MASIP *et al.* [81], resulted in similar findings. Once again, the design of the systematic review was of a high standard. The primary outcomes chosen were, again, in-hospital mortality and the need for intubation and mechanical ventilation. Secondary outcomes included treatment failure, length of hospital stay, length of time

NIV was applied and MI rate. Figures 1, 2 and 3 detail the principal data synthesis for the review's primary comparisons. There was a significant reduction in mortality from those patients treated with CPAP (relative risk 0.59, 95% CI 0.28–0.90, number needed to treat was five; p=0.015). There was a trend towards improved survival with NIV. Both CPAP (relative risk 0.44, 95% CI 0.29–0.66, number needed to treat was six; p=0.0003) and NIV (relative risk 0.50, 95% CI 0.27–0.90, number needed to treat was seven; p=0.02) showed benefit when intubation was an outcome. There was no difference in any outcome when CPAP and NIV were compared. There was a trend towards an increase in MI rate with NIV but this was largely due to the weighting of the one study by MEHTA et al. [69]. PETER et al. [82] suggest that both NIV modalities are effective; although, due to the relatively small proportions of pulmonary oedema patients included in these trials their results are difficult to generalise. In addition, the authors felt that further work was required to define the relationship between PEEP and myocardial ischaemia better, as well as further trials in hypercapnic patients with acute CPO.

Recent primary trials

Two recent trials have been published or presented at international conferences since the results of the multiple systematic reviews. These may result in the reappraisal of the role of NIV in ACPO.

The 3CPO trial

The 3CPO trial [91], has recently completed recruitment across 26 emergency departments in the UK. This trial is larger than the combined experience of all previous

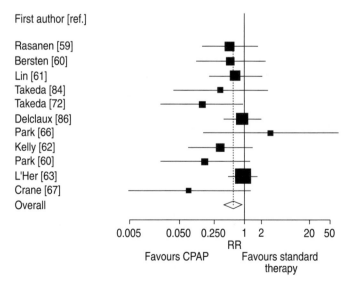

Fig. 1. – Pooled data of in-hospital mortality, comparing continuous positive airway pressure (CPAP) with standard therapy. Data are presented as relative risk (RR; ■), whiskers represent 95% confidence intervals (CI) and weight % is denoted by relative size. From top, RR (95% CI; weight %) were 0.50 (0.14–1.73; 10.4), 0.53 (0.11–2.55; 6.7), 0.67 (0.20–2.22; 10.9), 0.33 (0.04–2.85; 3.8), 0.14 (0.02–0.98; 4.7), 0.91 (0.39–2.14; 19.2), 3.30 (0.15–72.08; 1.9), 0.33 (0.07–1.45; 7.5), 0.16 (0.02–1.24; 4.1), 0.92 (0.48–1.76; 28.5) and 0.08 (0.00–1.28; 2.2), respectively. Overall RR (95% CI) was 0.59 (0.38–0.90). Reproduced from [82], with permission from the publisher.

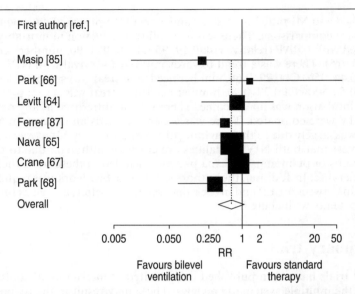

Fig. 2. – Pooled data of in-hospital mortality comparing bilevel ventilation with standard therapy. Data are presented as relative risk (RR; ■), whiskers represent 95% confidence intervals (CI) and weight % is denoted by relative size. From top, RR (95% CI; weight %) were 0.19 (0.01–3.71; 3.4), 1.38 (0.03–62.25; 2.1), 0.81 (0.19–3.51; 14.0), 0.50 (0.05–4.94; 5.8), 0.67 (0.25–1.77; 31.9), 0.83 (0.30–2.29; 29.5) and 0.32 (0.07–1.45; 13.3), respectively. Overall RR (95% CI) was 0.63 (0.37–1.10). Reproduced from [82], with permission from the publisher.

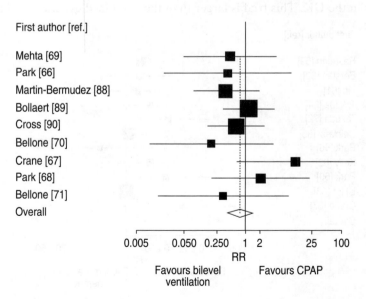

Fig. 3. – Pooled data of in-hospital mortality comparing bilevel ventilation with contiuous positive airway pressure (CPAP). Data are presented as relative risk (RR; ■), whiskers represent 95% confidence intervals (CI) and weight % is denoted by relative size. From top, RR (95% CI; weight %) were 0.46 (0.05–4.53; 7.9), 0.42 (0.02–8.91; 4.4), 0.38 (0.08–1.85; 16.4), 1.12 (0.33–3.79; 27.5), 0.62 (0.16–2.39; 22.4), 0.18 (0.01–3.63; 4.6), 11.00 (0.65–186.62; 5.1), 2.00 (0.19–20.77; 7.5) and 0.33 (0.01–7.68; 4.2), respectively. Overall RR (95% CI) was 0.75 (0.40–1.43). Reproduced from [82], with permission from the publisher.

published trials. In this multicentre open prospective randomised controlled trial patients were randomised to one of three treatment arms: standard oxygen therapy delivered by variable delivery oxygen mask with reservoir bag, CPAP (5–15 cmH$_2$O) or NIV (inspiratory pressure 8–20 cmH$_2$O, expiratory pressure 4–10 cmH$_2$O). The primary end-point for comparison between NIV and standard oxygen was 7-day mortality. The primary end-point for the comparison between CPAP and NIV was 7-day mortality or intubation. Patients were included if they were tachypnoeic (respiratory rate >20 breaths·min^{-1}) and acidotic (pH<7.35) at presentation. All other therapy was at the discretion of the treating clinician and there was no predefined treatment failure. In total, 1,069 patients (age 78±10 yrs; 43% male) were recruited to standard oxygen therapy (n=367), CPAP (10±4 cmH$_2$O; n=346) or NIV (inspiratory 14±5, expiratory 7±2 cmH$_2$O; n=356). The mean±SD duration of CPAP therapy was 2.2±1.5 h and NIV 2.0±1.3 h. There was no difference between 7-day mortality for standard oxygen therapy (9.8%) and NIV (9.5%; p=0.87). The combined end-point of 7-day death or intubation rate was similar irrespective of NIV modality (11.7 *versus* 11.1%, CPAP *versus* NIV respectively; p=0.81). In comparison with standard oxygen therapy, NIV was associated with greater reductions (treatment difference, 95% CI) in breathlessness (visual analogue score 0.7, 0.2–1.3; p=0.008), cardiac frequency (3 beats·min^{-1}, 1–6 beats·min^{-1}; p=0.004), acidosis (pH 0.03, pH 0.02–0.04; p<0.001) and hypercapnia (0.7 kPa, 0.4–0.9 kPa; p<0.001) at 1 h. There were no treatment-related adverse events and there were no differences in other secondary outcomes, such as MI rate, intubation, length of hospital stay or critical care admission rate.

In another trial [58], 120 patients were enrolled in three French emergency departments to either CPAP or NIV. Patients had either a clinical or radiological diagnosis of pulmonary oedema and two of the following three criteria: respiratory rate >30 breaths·min^{-1}; oxygen saturations <90% with standard oxygen delivered ≥5 L·min^{-1} by a variable delivery mask with reservoir; and/or use of accessory musculature. CPAP and NIV were delivered *via* a Boussignac system, which is a simple portable device. CPAP was increased to 10 cmH$_2$O, NIV to a tidal volume of 8–10 mL·kg^{-1} and expiratory pressure support was set at 5 cmH$_2$O. A combined primary end-point of death, MI or intubation in the first 24 h of hospital admission was used. Secondary outcomes included physiology, arterial gas analysis, length of hospital stay, in hospital mortality and work of breathing measured by the Patrick scale. Data from 109 patients were available for analysis. During the intervention, mean CPAP levels were 7.7 cmH$_2$O and for NIV 12/4.9 cmH$_2$O. There was no difference between interventions for any outcome. Respiratory distress and physiology improved in both arms. Only 3% of patients required intubation and one person died within the first 24 h. Exploratory analysis of patients with and without hypercapnia did not change the rate of improvement or the difference between interventions; ~50% were hypercapnic at presentation. It is of interest that 68 potentially eligible patients had noninvasive support applied in the prehospital setting and 11 were intubated.

Interpretation of the evidence

There are clear differences between the findings of recent meta-analyses reporting previous primary trials and the results of the 3CPO trial. All of the primary trials, previous pooled data [92, 93] and the recent systematic reviews concluded that NIV (CPAP or noninvasive positive pressure ventilation (NIPPV)) delivers clinical benefit compared with standard oxygen therapy. No data to date support the additional benefit if NIPPV over CPAP, despite the mechanistic advantages [43]. This is despite unequivocal correlation in early improvements in symptoms and surrogate measures of disease severity. Additionally, regardless of the theoretical advantages of NIPPV over CPAP, no trial to date has reported additional benefit with NIPPV. There are potential reasons why a true benefit may not have been detected [60]. Finally, despite continuing concerns [69, 82, 94] regarding the potential for an increase in MI rates in patients treated with NIPPV, the 3CPO trial has confirmed the safety of the intervention.

NIV (CPAP or NIPPV) compared to oxygen therapy alone

The 3CPO trial has shown no difference in short- or long-term mortality rates between standard oxygen therapy and NIV treatments in patients presenting to emergency departments with severe acute CPO. This was despite early improvements in symptoms and surrogate measures of disease severity. Specifically, there was no demonstrable difference in any primary or secondary outcome for the comparison between NIV and standard oxygen therapy, other than breathlessness measured by a visual analogue scale, physiology at 1 h (pulse rate) and arterial gas exchange parameters at 1 h (pH and arterial carbon dioxide tension).

These results are contrary to findings of the recent meta-analyses, despite similar improvements in physiological and gas-exchange variables. These meta-analyses and systematic reviews of immediate treatment with NIV in patients with acute CPO have reported up to a 47% reduction in mortality [82]. The 3CPO trial was adequately powered to assess this question and recruited more patients than the total combined experience of these analyses and reviews.

There are a number of potential reasons why the 3CPO trial findings do not support the results of the previous small randomised controlled trials and the conclusions drawn from multiple recent meta-analyses.

Patient populations

The population of patients recruited to the 3CPO trial may be different to those recruited to the ~25 small randomised controlled trial previously reported. In particular, there may be differences in age, severity of illness, comorbidities or underlying mechanisms of heart failure. This is unlikely for the following reasons. Based on previous studies, strict inclusion and exclusion criteria were applied in the 3CPO trial, enabling the 3CPO researchers to target the group of patients most likely to benefit from NIV *i.e.* those with respiratory distress and acidosis. Indeed, the recent trial by NAVA *et al.* [65] showed a reduction only in intubation rates in a hypercapnic subgroup. The baseline characteristics and event rates in the NIV arms were comparable to previous studies and demonstrated that the recruited patients had severe disease. There was no evidence of patient selection bias with identical 7-day mortality in nonrecruited patients (9.2%). This was further supported by the excellent recruitment rates of eligible patients when compared with those previously reported. There was also no obvious interaction between treatment intervention and disease severity, suggesting that those with milder disease did not obscure potential benefits in the sickest patients.

The 3CPO trial mortality was higher than registry data (6.7%, EURO HF survey [14]; 4%, ADHERE registry [3]) and participants were older and predominantly female. These discrepancies in mortality and patient characteristics are likely to relate to differing study populations. AHF registries include all patients with decompensated heart failure rather than only those with severe acute pulmonary oedema. Indeed, in the

EURO HF registry, only 16% of patients had a qualifying diagnosis of acute pulmonary oedema. Patient age, male-to-female ratio and comorbidities were also similar to previous primary trials with mean age of 75–80 yrs, a female preponderance and highly comparable comorbidities such as hypertension, ischaemic heart disease, diabetes, CHF and COPD.

It is likely that a significant number of patients, given the physiological, age and sex characteristics of the recruited patients, had relatively preserved systolic function, so called, diastolic heart failure [9, 10, 95] presenting with hypertension [2, 16], which might be more amenable to rapid pharmacological vasodilatation. As echocardiography was not routinely performed as part of the 3CPO trial protocol, it remains unclear, however, whether the rate of MI is consistent with previous trials. Indeed, even using the more traditional World Health Organization (WHO) criteria for MI definition, the index rates for MI are considerably higher than the recent large trial undertaken by MORITZ et al. [58]; despite this, in-hospital mortality is identical between the two trials.

Influence of co-treatments

Although not mandated, the 3CPO trial recommended a set of co-treatments for recruited patients. This specifically included buccal and intravenous nitrates; ~90% of patients received this intervention. It is possible that the cardiovascular beneficial effects of NIV in acute CPO has been masked by another treatment working (e.g. nitrates) by the same mechanism i.e. a reduction in preload and afterload [96–98]. Indeed, CRANE [97] identified pre-hospital nitrate as being the only factor associated with improved mortality in a UK observational study of patients with acute CPO. Co-treatments in previous small trials have often been incompletely characterised and documented. It is therefore unclear whether there is consistency in these treatments, across trials.

Inconsistency in the delivery of NIV

The 3CPO trial may have failed to reveal a difference in mortality between NIV and standard oxygen therapy because the intervention was ineffectively delivered. Over 80% of sites had previous experience of NIV prior to the trial beginning. There was a comprehensive training programme for all centres in order to ensure operator competence and consistency throughout the trial. PLANT et al. [99] have previous reported the safe application of NIV with ward-based staff after similar levels of training and less pre-trial experience and exposure to the intervention. A readily applied portable ventilator that allowed both modalities of ventilation to be delivered, as well as a tolerance for leaks around the facemask of up to 50 L·min^{-1}, was used in the 3CPO trial. Whilst unable to measure the inspired oxygen concentration, the circuit delivered an oxygen concentration up to 60%. This ventilator system was not as sophisticated as some systems used in previous trials but more than others, including that used in the recent trial by MORITZ et al. [58]. Mean pressures for both CPAP (10 cmH$_2$O) and NIPPV (inspiratory 14, expiratory 7 cmH$_2$O) are highly comparable with previous studies [81, 82]. Mean times of delivery of the intervention were a little over 2 h, suggesting that the patients were physiologically and symptomatically significantly better within this short time frame and again are similar to recent data from MORITZ et al. [58]. There was cross-over between interventions in all three arms of the 3CPO trial and these were analysed on an intention-to-treat basis. There were differing reasons with respiratory distress and hypoxia being more likely in the control arm and lack of patient tolerance in the two intervention arms. After these patients were removed from primary outcome analysis, there remained no significant difference between groups, although mortality rates were lower.

Differing thresholds for endotracheal intubation and critical care admission

Previous trials have indicated that the physiological improvement seen with NIV is translated into a reduction in tracheal intubation rates [81, 82]. Pooled data from the meta-analysis by PETER *et al.* [82] suggest that six patients need to be treated with CPAP and seven with NIPPV in order to avoid one patient being intubated and mechanically ventilated. In contrast, the 3CPO trial found no benefit in reducing intubation rates by NIV and this may reflect the relatively low intubation rates. Reasons for this are unclear but may reflect the differing patient populations, concomitant therapies and thresholds for intubation and mechanical ventilation across different countries, clinical environments and time periods. Intubation rates in the standard therapy arms varied from 35–65% in initial trials [59, 60] to 5–7% for recent trials in emergency department settings [62, 67], despite similar severity of illness, in-hospital mortality and length of hospital stay. Intubation rate in the intervention arms have also fallen considerably over time with some initial trials reporting intubation rate of up to 35%, whereas recent reports have consistently suggested rates of ~5%. Indeed, a recent large trial [58] reported a 3% intubation rate; almost identical to that in the 3CPO trial. Given that the present and previous trials were, by necessity, "open", there is real concern of treatment bias with a differing threshold for intervention according to treatment allocation; for example, patients on standard oxygen maybe more likely to undergo intubation than those already gaining the apparent benefit of NIV. Additionally, clinicians may persevere with patients slow to improve with NIV if they believe in its efficacy. It is important to note that intubation did not correlate with mortality in the 3CPO trial.

Interpretation of previous data

Recent meta-analyses and systemic reviews have been composed of numerous randomised clinical trials. However, individual trials were composed of small treatment group sizes that varied between nine and 65 patients with recruitment rates of only 10–30% (*c.f.* 62% randomised in the 3CPO trial). In the meta-analyses, the small total number of outcome events was well below the recommended threshold of 200 [100] and this limits the generalisability of their findings. There is real concern of reporting, publication and recruitment bias in individual published studies that will be compounded by pooled analysis. The discrepancy between the 3CPO trial results in the setting of a large multicentre randomised controlled trial, previous pooled data are not unique and the limitations of meta-analysis are well reported [101].

MI risk

MEHTA *et al.* [69] prematurely terminated their trial comparing CPAP with NIPPV because of the concerns of an increase in MI rate in the NIPPV arm. A subsequent study by BELLONE *et al.* [70] did not replicate this finding and demonstrated no effect of NIPPV on MI rate. The systematic review by PETER *et al.* [82] reported a weak relationship between the delivery of NIPPV and an increase in MI rate. This finding was largely the result of the weighting of the study by MEHTA *et al.* [69] in the pooled data. The 3CPO trial showed that there is no relationship between MI rate and the application of either CPAP or NIPPV.

Conclusions

NIV is widely used in North America, Europe and Australasia for patients with severe acute CPO. There are clear mechanistic reasons why these interventions work in acute pulmonary oedema. Indeed multiple small trials revealed that physiological parameters improve quickly with the use of NIV and this reduced endotracheal intubation and potentially in-hospital mortality. These findings have not been supported by the findings of a recent large multicentre clinical effectiveness trial, the 3CPO trial, which failed to show any clear benefit of NIV for patients with severe acute CPO in UK emergency departments other than early improvement in some physiological characteristics and patient symptoms.

Despite theoretical advantages for NIPPV over CPAP, no trial data support additional benefit of this modality. The 3CPO trial has unequivocally demonstrated the safety of both NIPPV and CPAP and clearly shows there is no increased risk of MI with NIPPV.

Continuous positive airway pressure should, therefore, be the noninvasive ventilation modality of choice. Continuous positive airway pressure equipment is, in general, less complex and cheaper and, therefore, has advantages over noninvasive positive pressure ventilation. In addition, a number of simple systems allow the delivery of 100% oxygen. Clearly if a department already has equipment in use or is using noninvasive positive pressure ventilation for other clinical conditions such as chronic obstructive pulmonary disease then this will influence the decision as to the ventilation mode and equipment type used for the management of patients with pulmonary oedema. Finally, in the majority of patients, medical therapy should be instigated as the primary treatment of severe acute cardiogenic pulmonary oedema and noninvasive ventilation reserved for those patients who have significant respiratory distress and failure or those not improving with standard medical therapy.

Summary

This chapter reviews the use of positive pressure ventilation (continuous positive airway pressure and bilevel) for patients with acute cardiogenic pulmonary oedema. The incidence at presentation to hospital, its pathophysiology and the physiological basis for the use of positive pressure ventilation is first discussed. Recent meta-analyses are presented, followed by the results of two recent clinical trials, the results of which conflict with the meta-analyses. Possible reasons for this discrepancy are explored.

Keywords: Bilevel ventilation, cardiogenic pulmonary oedema, continuous positive airway pressure, left ventricular failure, noninvasive ventilation.

References

1. Zannad F, Adamopoulos C, Mebazaa A, Gheorghiade M. The challenge of acute decompensated heart failure. *Heart Fail Rev* 2006; 11: 135–139.

2. Gheorghiade M, Zannad F, Sopko G, *et al.* Acute heart failure syndromes: current state and framework for future research. *Circulation* 2005; 112: 3958–3968.

3. Adams KF Jr, Fonarow GC, Emerman CL, *et al.* Characteristics and outcomes of patients hospitalized for heart failure in the United States: rationale, design, and preliminary observations from the first 100,000 cases in the Acute Decompensated Heart Failure National Registry (ADHERE). *Am Heart J* 2005; 149: 209–216.

4. Hunt SA, American College of Cardiology, American Heart Association Task Force on Practice Guidelines (Writing Committee to Update the 2001 Guidelines for the Evaluation and Management of Heart Failure). ACC/AHA 2005 guideline update for the diagnosis and management of chronic heart failure in the adult: a report of the American College of Cardiology/American Heart Association Task Force on Practice Guidelines (Writing Committee Update the 2001 Guidelines for the Evaluation and Management of Heart Failure). *J Am Coll Cardiol* 2005; 46: e1–e82.

5. Collins S, Storrow AB, Kirk JD, Pang PS, Diercks DB, Gheorghiade M. Beyond pulmonary edema: diagnostic, risk stratification, and treatment challenges of acute heart failure management in the emergency department. *Ann Emerg Med* 2008; 51: 45–57.

6. Nieminen MS, Bohm M, Cowie MR, *et al.* Executive summary of the guidelines on the diagnosis and treatment of acute heart failure: the Task Force on Acute Heart Failure of the European Society of Cardiology. *Eur Heart J* 2005; 26: 384–416.

7. Silvers SM, Howell JM, Kosowsky JM, Rokos IC, Jagoda AS, American College of Emergency Physicians. Clinical policy: Critical issues in the evaluation and management of adult patients presenting to the emergency department with acute heart failure syndromes. *Ann Emerg Med* 2007; 49: 627–669.

8. De Luca L, Fonarow GC, Adams KF Jr, *et al.* Acute heart failure syndromes: clinical scenarios and pathophysiologic targets for therapy. *Heart Fail Rev* 2007; 12: 97–104.

9. Owan TE, Hodge DO, Herges RM, Jacobsen SJ, Roger VL, Redfield MM. Trends in prevalence and outcome of heart failure with preserved ejection fraction. *N Engl J Med* 2006; 355: 251–259.

10. Aurigemma GP, Gaasch WH, Aurigemma GP, Gaasch WH. Clinical practice. Diastolic heart failure. *N Engl J Med* 2004; 351: 1097–1105.

11. Cleland JG, Swedberg K, Follath F, *et al.* The EuroHeart Failure survey programme – a survey on the quality of care among patients with heart failure in Europe. Part 1: patient characteristics and diagnosis. *Eur Heart J* 2003; 24: 442–463.

12. Nieminen MS, Brutsaert D, Dickstein K, *et al.* EuroHeart Failure Survey II (EHFS II): a survey on hospitalized acute heart failure patients: description of population. *Eur Heart J* 2006; 27: 2725–2736.

13. Tavazzi L, Maggioni AP, Lucci D, *et al.* Nationwide survey on acute heart failure in cardiology ward services in Italy. *Eur Heart J* 2006; 27: 1207–1215.

14. Zannad F, Mebazaa A, Juilliere Y, *et al.* Clinical profile, contemporary management and one-year mortality in patients with severe acute heart failure syndromes: The EFICA study. *Eur J Heart Fail* 2006; 8: 697–705.

15. Fonarow GC, Heywood JT, Heidenreich PA, Lopatin M, Yancy CW, ADHERE Scientific Advisory Committee and Investigators. Temporal trends in clinical characteristics, treatments, and outcomes for heart failure hospitalizations, 2002 to 2004: findings from Acute Decompensated Heart Failure National Registry (ADHERE). *Am Heart J* 2007; 153: 1021–1028.

16. Alla F, Zannad F, Filippatos G. Epidemiology of acute heart failure syndromes. *Heart Fail Rev* 2007; 12: 91–95.

17. Miro AM, Pinsky MR. Heart-lung interactions. *In*: Tobin MJ, ed. Principles and Practice of Mechanical Ventilation. New York, McGraw-Hill, 1994; pp. 647–671.

18. Pinsky MR. Recent advances in the clinical application of heart-lung interactions. *Curr Opin Crit Care* 2002; 8: 26–31.

19. Franklin DL, Van Citters RL, Rushmer RF. Balance between right and left ventricular output. *Circ Res* 1962; 10: 17–26.

20. Shabetai R, Fowler NO, Gueron M. The effects of respiration on aortic pressure and flow. *Am Heart J* 1963; 65: 525–533.

21. Santamore WP, Lynch PR, Meier G, Heckman J, Bove AA. Myocardial interaction between the ventricles. *J Appl Physiol* 1976; 41: 362–368.

22. Bromberger-Barnea B. Mechanical effects of inspiration on heart functions: a review. *Fed Proc* 1981; 40: 2172–2177.

23. Hoffman JI, Guz A, Charlier AA, Wilcken DE. Stroke volume in conscious dogs; effect of respiration, posture, and vascular occlusion. *J Appl Physiol* 1965; 20: 865–877.

24. Schrijen F, Ehrlich W, Permutt S. Cardiovascular changes in conscious dogs during spontaneous deep breaths. *Pflugers Arch* 1975; 355: 205–215.

25. Robotham JL, Lixfeld W, Holland L, MacGregor D, Bryan AC, Rabson J. Effects of respiration on cardiac performance. *J Appl Physiol* 1978; 44: 703–709.

26. Buda AJ, Pinsky MR, Ingels NB Jr, Daughters GT, Stinson EB, Alderman EL. Effect of intrathoracic pressure on left ventricular performance. *N Engl J Med* 1979; 301: 453–459.

27. Robotham JL, Rabson J, Permutt S, Bromberger-Barnea B. Left ventricular hemodynamics during respiration. *J Appl Physiol* 1979; 47: 1295–1303.

28. Cassidy SS, Robertson CH Jr, Pierce AK, Johnson RL Jr. Cardiovascular effects of positive end-expiratory pressure in dogs. *J Appl Physiol* 1978; 44: 743–750.

29. Fewell JE, Abendschein DR, Carlson CJ, Murray JF, Rapaport E. Continuous positive-pressure ventilation decreases right and left ventricular end-diastolic volumes in the dog. *Circ Res* 1980; 46: 125–132.

30. Jardin F, Farcot JC, Boisante L, Curien N, Margairaz A, Bourdarias JP. Influence of positive end-expiratory pressure on left ventricular performance. *N Engl J Med* 1981; 304: 387–392.

31. Pinsky MR, Summer WR, Wise RA, Permutt S, Bromberger-Barnea B. Augmentation of cardiac function by elevation of intrathoracic pressure. *J Appl Physiol* 1983; 54: 950–955.

32. Pinsky MR, Summer WR. Cardiac augmentation by phasic high intrathoracic pressure support in man. *Chest* 1983; 84: 370–375.

33. Pinsky MR, Marquez J, Martin D, Klain M. Ventricular assist by cardiac cycle-specific increases in intrathoracic pressure. *Chest* 1987; 91: 709–715.

34. Grace MP, Greenbaum DM. Cardiac performance in response to PEEP in patients with cardiac dysfunction. *Crit Care Med* 1982; 10: 358–360.

35. Bradley TD, Holloway RM, McLaughlin PR, Ross BL, Walters J, Liu PP. Cardiac output response to continuous positive airway pressure in congestive heart failure. *Am Rev Respir Dis* 1992; 145: 377–382.

36. De Hoyos A, Liu PP, Benard DC, Bradley TD. Haemodynamic effects of continuous positive airway pressure in humans with normal and impaired left ventricular function. *Clin Sci* 1995; 88: 173–178.

37. Philip-Joet FF, Paganelli FF, Dutau HL, Saadjian AY. Hemodynamic effects of bilevel nasal positive airway pressure ventilation in patients with heart failure. *Respiration* 1999; 66: 136–143.

38. Naughton MT, Rahman MA, Hara K, Floras JS, Bradley TD. Effect of continuous positive airway pressure on intrathoracic and left ventricular transmural pressures in patients with congestive heart failure. *Circulation* 1995; 91: 1725–1731.

39. Mehta S, Liu PP, Fitzgerald FS, Allidina YK, Douglas BT. Effects of continuous positive airway pressure on cardiac volumes in patients with ischemic and dilated cardiomyopathy. *Am J Respir Crit Care Med* 2000; 161: 128–134.

40. Baratz DM, Westbrook PR, Shah PK, Mohsenifar Z. Effect of nasal continuous positive airway pressure on cardiac output and oxygen delivery in patients with congestive heart failure. *Chest* 1992; 102: 1397–1401.

41. Liston R, Deegan PC, McCreery C, Costello R, Maurer B, McNicholas WT. Haemodynamic effects of nasal continuous positive airway pressure in severe congestive heart failure. *Eur Respir J* 1995; 8: 430–435.

42. Lenique F, Habis M, Lofaso F, Dubois-Rande JL, Harf A, Brochard L. Ventilatory and hemodynamic effects of continuous positive airway pressure in left heart failure. *Am J Respir Crit Care Med* 1997; 155: 500–505.

43. Chadda K, Annane D, Hart N, Gajdos P, Raphael JC, Lofaso F. Cardiac and respiratory effects of continuous positive airway pressure and noninvasive ventilation in acute cardiac pulmonary edema. *Crit Care Med* 2002; 30: 2457–2461.

44. Bulkley BH, Hutchins GM, Bailey I, Strauss HW, Pitt B. Thallium 201 imaging and gated cardiac blood pool scans in patients with ischemic and idiopathic congestive cardiomyopathy. A clinical and pathologic study. *Circulation* 1977; 55: 753–760.

45. Granton JT, Naughton MT, Benard DC, Liu PP, Goldstein RS, Bradley TD. CPAP improves inspiratory muscle strength in patients with heart failure and central sleep apnea. *Am J Respir Crit Care Med* 1996; 153: 277–282.

46. Tkacova R, Liu PP, Naughton MT, Bradley TD. Effect of continuous positive airway pressure on mitral regurgitant fraction and atrial natriuretic peptide in patients with heart failure. *J Am Coll Cardiol* 1997; 30: 739–745.

47. Kiely JL, Deegan P, Buckley A, Shiels P, Maurer B, McNicholas WT. Efficacy of nasal continuous positive airway pressure therapy in chronic heart failure: importance of underlying cardiac rhythm. *Thorax* 1998; 53: 957–962.

48. Acosta B, DiBenedetto R, Rahimi A, *et al.* Hemodynamic effects of noninvasive bilevel positive airway pressure on patients with chronic congestive heart failure with systolic dysfunction. *Chest* 2000; 118: 1004–1009.

49. Hammond MD, Bauer KA, Sharp JT, Rocha RD. Respiratory muscle strength in congestive heart failure. *Chest* 1990; 98: 1091–1094.

50. Mancini DM, Henson D, LaManca J, Levine S. Respiratory muscle function and dyspnea in patients with chronic congestive heart failure. *Circulation* 1992; 86: 909–918.

51. McParland C, Krishnan B, Wang Y, Gallagher CG. Inspiratory muscle weakness and dyspnea in chronic heart failure. *Am Rev Respir Dis* 1992; 146: 467–472.

52. Mancini DM, LaManca JJ, Donchez LJ, Levine S, Henson DJ. Diminished respiratory muscle endurance persists after cardiac transplantation. *Am J Cardiol* 1995; 75: 418–421.

53. Hughes PD, Hart N, Hamnegard CH, *et al.* Inspiratory muscle relaxation rate slows during exhaustive treadmill walking in patients with chronic heart failure. *Am J Respir Crit Care Med* 2001; 163: 1400–1403.

54. Katz JA. PEEP and CPAP in perioperative respiratory care. *Respir Care* 1984; 29: 614–629.

55. Katz JA, Marks JD. Inspiratory work with and without continuous positive airway pressure in patients with acute respiratory failure. *Anesthesiology* 1985; 63: 598–607.

56. Branson RD, Hurst JM, DeHaven CB Jr. Mask CPAP: state of the art. *Respir Care* 1985; 30: 846–857.

57. Masip J, Betbese AJ, Paez J, *et al.* Non-invasive pressure support ventilation *versus* conventional oxygen therapy in acute cardiogenic pulmonary oedema: a randomised trial. *Lancet* 2000; 356: 2126–2132.

58. Moritz F, Brousse B, Gellee B, *et al.* Continuous positive airway pressure versus bilevel noninvasive ventilation in acute cardiogenic pulmonary edema: a randomized multicenter trial. *Ann Emerg Med* 2007; 50: 666–675.

59. Rasanen J, Heikkila J, Downs J, Nikki P, Vaisanen I, Viitanen A. Continuous positive airway pressure by face mask in acute cardiogenic pulmonary edema. *Am J Cardiol* 1985; 55: 296–300.

60. Bersten AD, Holt AW, Vedig AE, Skowronski GA, Baggoley CJ. Treatment of severe cardiogenic pulmonary edema with continuous positive airway pressure delivered by face mask. *N Engl J Med* 1991; 325: 1825–1830.

61. Lin M, Yang YF, Chiang HT, Chiang BN, Cheitlin MD. Reappraisal of continuous positive airway pressure therapy in acute cardiogenic pulmonary edema. Short-term results and long-term follow-up. *Chest* 1995; 107: 1379–1386.

62. Kelly CA, Newby DE, McDonagh TA, *et al.* Randomised controlled trial of continuous positive airway pressure and standard oxygen therapy in acute pulmonary oedema; effects on plasma brain natriuretic peptide concentrations. *Eur Heart J* 2002; 23: 1379–1386.

63. L'Her E, Duquesne F, Girou E, *et al.* Noninvasive continuous positive airway pressure in elderly cardiogenic pulmonary edema patients. *Intensive Care Med* 2004; 30: 882–888.

64. Levitt MA. A prospective, randomized trial of BiPAP in severe acute congestive heart failure. *J Emerg Med* 2001; 21: 363–369.

65. Nava S, Carbone G, DiBattista N, *et al.* Noninvasive ventilation in cardiogenic pulmonary edema: a multicenter randomized trial. *Am J Respir Crit Care Med* 2003; 168: 1432–1437.

66. Park M, Lorenzi-Filho G, Feltrim MI, *et al.* Oxygen therapy, continuous positive airway pressure, or noninvasive bilevel positive pressure ventilation in the treatment of acute cardiogenic pulmonary edema. *Arq Bras Cardiol* 2001; 76: 221–230.

67. Crane SD, Elliott MW, Gilligan P, Richards K, Gray AJ. Randomised controlled comparison of continuous positive airways pressure, bilevel non invasive ventilation, and standard treatment in emergency department patients with acute cardiogenic pulmonary oedema. *Emerg Med J* 2004; 21: 155–161.

68. Park M, Sangean MC, Volpe MS, *et al.* Randomized, prospective trial of oxygen, continuous positive airway pressure, and bilevel positive airway pressure by face mask in acute cardiogenic pulmonary edema. *Crit Care Med* 2004; 32: 2407–2415.

69. Mehta S, Jay GD, Woolard RH, *et al.* Randomized, prospective trial of bilevel versus continuous positive airway pressure in acute pulmonary oedema. *Crit Care Med* 1997; 25: 620–628.

70. Bellone A, Monari A, Cortellaro F, Vettorello M, Arlati S, Coen D. Myocardial infarction rate in acute pulmonary edema: noninvasive pressure support ventilation versus continuous positive airway pressure. *Crit Care Med* 2004; 32: 1860–1865.

71. Bellone A, Vettorello M, Monari A, Cortellaro F, Coen D. Noninvasive pressure support ventilation *vs.* continuous positive airway pressure in acute hypercapnic pulmonary edema. *Intensive Care Med* 2005; 31: 807–811.

72. Takeda S, Nejima J, Takano T, *et al.* Effect of nasal continuous positive airway pressure on pulmonary edema complicating acute myocardial infarction. *Jpn Circ J* 1998; 62: 553–558.

73. Browning J, Atwood B, Gray A. Use of non-invasive ventilation in UK emergency departments. *Emerg Med J* 2006; 23: 920–921.

74. British Thoracic Society Standards of Care Committee. Non-invasive ventilation in acute respiratory failure. *Thorax* 2002; 57: 192–211.

75. Evans TW. International Consensus Conferences in Intensive Care Medicine: non- invasive positive pressure ventilation in acute respiratory failure. Organised jointly by the American Thoracic Society, the European Respiratory Society, the European Society of Intensive Care Medicine, and the Société de Réanimation de Langue Française, and approved by the ATS Board of Directors, December 2000. *Intensive Care Med* 2001; 27: 166–178.

76. Collins SP, Mielniczuk LM, Whittingham HA, Boseley ME, Schramm DR, Storrow AB. The use of noninvasive ventilation in emergency department patients with acute cardiogenic pulmonary edema: a systematic review. *Ann Emerg Med* 269, 48: 260–269.

77. Ho KM, Wong K. A comparison of continuous and bi-level positive airway pressure non-invasive ventilation in patients with acute cardiogenic pulmonary oedema: a meta-analysis. *Critical Care* 2006; 10: R49.

78. Winck JC, Azevedo LF, Costa-Pereira A, Antonelli M, Wyatt JC. Efficacy and safety of non-invasive ventilation in the treatment of acute cardiogenic pulmonary edema – a systematic review and meta-analysis. *Crit Care* 2006; 10: R69.

79. Agarwal R, Aggarwal AN, Gupta D, Jindal SK. Non-invasive ventilation in acute cardiogenic pulmonary oedema. *Postgraduate Med J* 2005; 81: 637–643.

80. Nadar S, Prasad N, Taylor RS, Lip GY. Positive pressure ventilation in the management of acute and chronic cardiac failure: a systematic review and meta-analysis. *Int J Cardiol* 2005; 99: 171–185.

81. Masip J, Roque M, Sanchez B, Fernandez R, Subirana M, Exposito JA. Noninvasive ventilation in acute cardiogenic pulmonary edema: systematic review and meta-analysis. *JAMA* 2005; 294: 3124–3130.

82. Peter JV, Moran JL, Phillips-Hughes J, Graham P, Bersten AD. Effect of non-invasive positive pressure ventilation (NIPPV) on mortality in patients with acute cardiogenic pulmonary oedema: a meta-analysis. *Lancet* 2006; 367: 1155–1163.

83. Jadad AR, Moore RA, Carroll D, *et al.* Assessing the quality of reports of randomized clinical trials: is blinding necessary? *Control Clin Trials* 1996; 17: 1–12.

84. Takeda S, Takano T, Oqawa R. The effect of nasal continuous positive airway pressure on plasma endothelin-1 concentrations in patients with severe cardiogenic pulmonary edema. *Anesth Analg* 1997; 84: 1091–1096.

85. Masip J, Betbesé AJ, Páez J, *et al.* Non-invasive pressure support ventilation *versus* conventional oxygen therapy in acute cardiogenic pulmonary edema: a randomized study. *Lancet.* 2000; 356: 2126–2132.

86. Delclaux C, L'Her E, Alberti C, *et al.* Treatment of acute hypoxemic nonhypercapnic respiratory insuffi ciency with continuous positive airway pressure delivered by a face mask: A randomized controlled trial. *JAMA* 2000; 284: 2352–2360.

87. Ferrer M, Esquinas A, Leon M, *et al.* Noninvasive ventilation in severe hypoxemic respiratory failure: a randomized linical trial. *Am J Respir Crit Care Med* 2003; 168: 1438–1444.

88. Martin-Bermudez R, Rodriguez-Portal JA, Garcia-Garmendia JL, *et al.* Non-invasive ventilation in cardiogenic pulmonay edema. Preliminary results of a randomized trial. *Intensive Care Med* 2002; 28: A255.

89. Bollaert PE, Sauder PH, Girard F, *et al.* Continuous positive airway pressure (CPAP) *versus* proportional assist ventilation (PAV) for noninvasive ventilation in cardiogenic pulmonary edema (CPE): a randomized study. *Am J Respir Crit Care Med* 2002; 165: B57.

90. Cross AM, Cameron P, Kierce M, *et al.* Non-invasive ventilation in acute respiratory failure: a randomised comparison of continuous positive airway pressure and bi-level positive airway pressure. *Emerg Med J* 2003; 20: 531–534.

91. Gray A, Goodacre S, Newby DE, *et al.* Noninvasive ventilation in acute cardiogenic pulmonary edema. *N Engl J Med* 2008; 359: 142–151.

92. Pang D, Keenan SP, COOK DJ, Sibbald WJ. The effect of positive pressure airway support on mortality and the need for intubation in cardiogenic pulmonary edema: a systematic review. *Chest* 1998; 114: 1185–1192.

93. Kelly C, Newby DE, Boon NA, Douglas NJ. Support ventilation *versus* conventional oxygen. *Lancet* 2001; 357: 1126.

94. Silvers SM, Howell JM, Kosowsky JM, Rokos IC, Jagoda AS. American College of Emergency Physicians. Clinical policy: Critical issues in the evaluation and management of adult patients presenting to the emergency department with acute heart failure syndromes. *Ann Emerg Med* 2007; 49: 627–669.

95. Bhatia RS, Tu JV, Lee DS, *et al.* Outcome of heart failure with preserved ejection fraction in a population-based study. *N Engl J Med* 2006; 355: 260–269.

96. Cotter G, Metzkor E, Kaluski E, *et al.* Randomised trial of high-dose isosorbide dinitrate plus low-dose furosemide versus high-dose furosemide plus low-dose isosorbide dinitrate in severe pulmonary oedema. *Lancet* 1998; 351: 389–393.

97. Crane SD. Epidemiology, treatment and outcome of acidotic, acute, cardiogenic pulmonary oedema presenting to an emergency department. *Eur J Emerg Med* 2002; 9: 320–324.

98. Graham CA. Pharmacological therapy of acute cardiogenic pulmonary oedema in the emergency department. *Emerg Med Australas* 2004; 16: 47–54.

99. Plant PK, Owen JL, Elliott MW. Early use of non-invasive ventilation for acute exacerbations of chronic obstructive pulmonary disease on general respiratory wards: a multicentre randomised controlled trial. *Lancet* 2000; 355: 1931–1935.

100. Flather MD, Farkouh ME, Pogue JM, Yusuf S. Strengths and limitations of meta-analysis: larger studies may be more reliable. *Control Clin Trials* 1997; 18: 568–579.

101. LeLorier J, Gregoire G, Benhaddad A, Lapierre J, Derderian F. Discrepancies between meta-analyses and subsequent large randomized, controlled trials. *N Engl J Med* 1997; 337: 536–542.

NIV: indication in case of acute respiratory failure and immunosuppression

G. Hilbert

Correspondence: G. Hilbert, Département de Réanimation Médicale, Hôpital Pellegrin, F 33076 Bordeaux, France. Fax: 33 556796122; E-mail: gilles.hilbert@chu-bordeaux.fr

Pulmonary complications are an important cause of illness in immunocompromised patients and contribute, to a large extent, to the mortality associated with various types of immunosuppression [1, 2]. Pulmonary infiltrates commonly appear following chemotherapy, solid-organ transplant and haematopoietic stem-cell transplantation. With the increasing use of these treatment modalities and the growing potency of immunosuppressive regimens, physicians will more-frequently be asked to evaluate and to care for these individuals. This more-specifically involves the physicians working in intensive care units (ICUs) when the respiratory failure occurs among these patients. Strategies for management include both a specific approach, in terms of diagnosis tools and treatment regimens used, and a symptomatic approach, in terms essentially of treatment of acute respiratory failure (ARF). Classically, these recipients require frequently intubation and mechanical ventilatory assistance. Too often, this intervention has been followed by further, ultimately fatal complications, including sepsis. Although invasive mechanical ventilation is highly effective and reliable in supporting alveolar ventilation [3, 4], endotracheal intubation is associated with numerous risks of complications [5]. Furthermore, in immunocompromised patients, mechanical ventilation is associated with a significant risk of death [6–10]. The outcome predictors that consistently predict poor outcome of haematopoietic stem-cell transplantation recipients admitted to the ICU were the need for mechanical ventilation and the presence of multiple organ system failure. ARF requiring mechanical ventilation increased the odds of death in the ICU by 55.6 times [11].

Thus, avoiding intubation should be an important objective in the management of hypoxaemic acute ARF in immunosuppressed patients.

Rationale for noninvasive ventilation

Above all, a key driving force behind the increasing use of noninvasive ventilation (NIV) has been the desire to avoid the complications of invasive ventilation. Patients may have been intubated before their transfer to ICU, or soon after their admission. In other patients, invasive ventilation can be performed after a failure of NIV. In immunocompromised patients, ARF has most often the features of acute lung injury (ALI) or acute respiratory distress syndrome (ARDS) mainly from pneumonia. Therefore, the ventilatory management of respiratory failure in these patients has to face one of the most-severe lung diseases. Although invasive mechanical ventilation is highly effective and reliable in supporting alveolar ventilation, endotracheal intubation is associated with numerous risks of complications. Complications of endotracheal intubation include upper airway injuries, tracheal stenosis, tracheomalacia, sinusitis and

Eur Respir Mon, 2008, 41, 94–109. Printed in UK - all rights reserved. Copyright ERS Journals Ltd 2008; European Respiratory Monograph; ISSN 1025-448x.

ventilator-associated pneumonia [5]. Furthermore, in immunocompromised patients, mechanical ventilation is associated with a significant risk of death [6–11]. Over the last years, overall survival rates of immunocompromised patients admitted to the ICU are improving, with, in part, the benefits of NIV in selected patients. This has led the best experts to defend the concept of "do everything that can be done". Even so, the negative impact of intubation and mechanical ventilation has been confirmed in several recent studies. In a recent study, in patients with haematological malignancy, the overall mortality in the ICU was 44%, only 12% in patients without mechanical ventilation but 74% among those under mechanical ventilation (p<0.001); multivariate analysis revealed mechanical ventilation and Simplified Acute Physiology Score (SAPS)II as independent prognostic factors of both ICU mortality and long-term survival [10]. In their literature review, SOUBANI et al. [11] clearly showed that the lower the percentage of patients receiving mechanical ventilation, the higher the survival rate.

On one hand, ARF was often seen by oncologists as a terminal stage of illness, this view being based on these studies indicating a very low survival rate, despite a heavy investment. On the other hand, a large proportion of these patients with ARF, was refused by physicians of ICUs, well aware that intubation with mechanical ventilation was a strong predictor of mortality in that population.

In the early 1990s, hospital survival for patients with HIV-related *Pneumocystis carinii* pneumonia and ARF, was very low (~20%). In a more-recent study on 155 HIV patients intubated and mechanically ventilated for ARF, hospital mortality was 62% and still 80% in patients who had previously received prophylaxis for *P. carinii* [12]. Thus, avoiding intubation must remain a major intent in managing hypoxaemic ARF in immunocompromised patients. NIV uses a tight-fitting face mask as an alternative interface between the patient and the ventilator in order to avoid these complications. In contrast to invasive ventilation, NIV leaves the upper airway intact, preserves airway defense mechanisms and allows patients to eat, drink, verbalise and expectorate secretions. The development of improved masks and ventilator technology have made this mode of ventilation acceptable. Several controlled studies have clearly demonstrated the benefits of NIV in acute exacerbations of chronic obstructive pulmonary disease (COPD) and, as stated in the conclusions of the recent international consensus conference considering the role of NIV in ARF, patients hospitalised for exacerbations of COPD with rapid clinical deterioration should be considered for NIV to prevent further deterioration in gas exchange, respiratory workload and the need for endotracheal intubation [13]. Starting from the good results obtained in patients with acute exacerbations of COPD, NIV is now being used to support those with hypoxaemic ARF, including those with ALI or ARDS. Nevertheless, in contrast to COPD patients with acute exacerbation, who constitute a relatively homogeneous group of patients, those with hypoxaemic ARF constitute a much more heterogeneous group. Overall, in patients with hypoxaemic ARF, experience is less extensive than in COPD patients. The consensus conference concluded that larger, controlled studies were required to determine the potential benefit of adding NIV to standard medical treatment in the avoidance of endotracheal intubation in hypoxaemic ARF [13].

Mechanisms of improvement with NIV in immunocompromised patients with ARF

In patients with hypoxaemic ARF, intrapulmonary shunt and ventilation-perfusion imbalances may cause life-threatening hypoxaemia. Moreover, high work of breathing from increased alveolar dead space and reduced respiratory system compliance may cause ventilatory failure with hypercapnia and respiratory acidosis. When employed during episodes of hypoxaemic ARF, the goal of NIV is to ensure an adequate arterial oxygen tension (Pa,O_2) until the underlying problem can be reversed.

Numerous case series and reports have shown that continuous positive airway pressure (CPAP) [14–20] and NIV [21] improve oxygenation, reduce respiratory rate and lessen dyspnoea in hypoxaemic ARF. KESTEN et al. [17] applied 10 cmH$_2$O of nasal CPAP in 9 subjects with P. carinii pneumonia and AIDS, all of whom had presented with bilateral pulmonary infiltrates and hypoxaemia. Nasal CPAP, for 20 mins, without supplemental oxygen increased mean Pa,O_2 from 56 to 68 mmHg and decreased the calculated alveolar–arterial oxygen gradient from 48 to 34 mmHg. CONFALONIERI et al. [21] have compared NIV with invasive mechanical ventilation in AIDS patients with P. carinii pneumonia. Changes in arterial blood gas and respiratory rate were comparable in the two groups of patients during the first 72 h of the study.

Several prospective controlled studies, comparing CPAP or NIV with standard medical treatment, have shown that the use of these methods of ventilation in hypoxaemic ARF was associated with prompt improvement in pulmonary gas exchange as determined by arterial blood gases obtained within the first few hours [22–25]. ANTONELLI et al. [22] conducted a prospective, randomised trial of NIV compared with endotracheal intubation with conventional mechanical ventilation in 64 patients with hypoxaemic ARF who required mechanical ventilation. A total of 7 (22%) of the 32 patients randomised to NIV had ARDS of varied aetiology. The patients in the two groups had a similar initial change in Pa,O_2/inspiratory oxygen fraction (FI,O_2): within the first hour of ventilation, 20 (62%) patients in the NIV group and 15 (47%) patients in the conventional ventilation group had an improvement in Pa,O_2/FI,O_2. Their Pa,O_2/FI,O_2 ratios increased significantly from 116 ± 24 to 230 ± 76 mmHg with NIV and from 124 ± 25 to 211 ± 68 mmHg with conventional ventilation. In a study comparing NIV with standard treatment using supplemental oxygen administration in recipients of solid organ transplantation with hypoxaemic ARF, 7 (22%) of 32 patients randomised to NIV had ARDS of varied aetiology [23]. Within the first hour of treatment, 14 (70%) patients in the NIV group and only 5 (25%) patients in the standard treatment group improved their Pa,O_2/FI,O_2 ratio. In another randomised controlled trial, the physiological effects of CPAP versus standard oxygen therapy were compared in 123 patients with hypoxaemic ARF and Pa,O_2/FI,O_2 ≤ 300 due to bilateral pulmonary oedema, 102 of them with ALI [24]. After 1 h of treatment, median Pa,O_2/FI,O_2 was greater with CPAP (203 versus 151; p=0.02). In a prospective, randomised trial of NIV, compared with standard medical treatment with supplemental oxygen in immunosuppressed patients with hypoxaemic ARF, initial improvement in Pa,O_2/FI,O_2 was observed in 46% of the NIV group and in 15% of the standard group (p=0.02) [25]. Even if NIV was used intermittently, in a sequential mode, the protocol of NIV used in that study achieved significantly higher rates of improvement in gas exchange abnormalities than in patients with standard treatment. Reducing work of breathing during noninvasive ventilation sessions may also allow respiratory muscles to be more efficient during nonassisted breaths.

NIV can improve the pathophysiology of hypoxaemic respiratory failure. Mechanisms of improvement can include the beneficial effects of positive end-expiratory pressure (PEEP) on distribution of extravascular lung water, on alveolar recruitment of under ventilated alveoli by increasing lung volume at end expiration and in early treatment of atelectasis. In addition, improvements in ventilation/perfusion ratios or even shunt undoubtedly occur in patients with ARDS, in whom the application of expiratory pressure should have an effect similar to that of PEEP in invasively ventilated patients. By lowering left ventricular transmural pressure, CPAP may reduce afterload and increase cardiac output, making it an attractive modality for therapy of acute pulmonary oedema. Even if CPAP alone is able to improve lung mechanics in patients with ARF and decrease work of breathing compared with unsupported ventilation [26], the addition of pressure support (PS) has a positive effect in reducing work of breathing and maintaining a tidal volume compatible with adequate alveolar ventilation.

Clinical studies

The main studies on NIV in immunocompromised patients with hypoxaemic ARF are reported in table 1.

Nonrandomised studies

CPAP has been used successfully for years to correct severe hypoxaemia in immunocompromised patients with hypoxaemic ARF [17, 18, 20, 29]. GREGG et al. [18] studied the efficacy of CPAP in 10 AIDS patients with pneumonia and avoided intubation in seven of them. BEDOS et al. [29] reported data for 110 consecutive patients with ARF secondary to AIDS-related *P. carinii* pneumonia and who were admitted to an ICU within 24 h after their hospital admission. CPAP was used initially in 66 (60%) patients and failed in 22 (32%) patients who received mechanical ventilation; 20 of those 22 patients died. These data suggest that CPAP with a face mask could be a safe and effective means of providing ventilatory support to patients with severe *P. carinii* pneumonia and probably avoids intubation and its high mortality rate in a subgroup of less-acutely ill patients. Among the 64 neutropenic patients with febrile acute hypoxaemic normocapnic respiratory failure treated by CPAP, in addition to standard therapy, in the study by HILBERT et al. [20], CPAP was efficient in only 25% of cases. The enrolled patients were critically ill, with a $Pa,O_2/FI,O_2$ ratio of 128 ± 32, and with a high SAPS II and more than two organ dysfunctions, explaining, in part, the poor results obtained. Nevertheless, all the responders and only four nonresponders survived their ICU stay. More recently, CONFALONIERI et al. [21] have compared NIV with invasive mechanical ventilation in AIDS patients with *P. carinii* pneumonia-related ARF, needing mechanical ventilation. A

Table 1. – Studies examining the effectiveness of NIV in immunocompromised patients with hypoxaemic acute respiratory failure

First author [ref]	Patients n	Details	Mask ventilatory mode	Intubation rate %
TOGNET [27]	18	Haematological plus neutropenia	Nasal PS- PEEP	67
CONTI [28]	16	Haematological intubation criteria	Nasal PS-PEEP	31
BEDOS [29]	66	*Pneumocystis carinii* pneumonia	Facial CPAP	32
HILBERT [20]	64	Haematological, neutropenia	Facial CPAP	75
AZOULAY [30]	48	Cancer plus haematological	PS-PEEP	56
CONFALONIERI [21]	24	*Pneumocystis carinii*, pneumonia case–control study	Facial PS-PEEP	33
ROCCO [31]	38	Immunosuppressed patients, case–control study	Helmet *versus* facial PS-PEEP	42
ANTONELLI [23][#]	40	Solid organ transplantation, $Pa,O_2/FI,O_2 \leq 200$	Facial PS-PEEP	20/70[¶]
HILBERT [25][#]	52	Immunosuppressed patients, $Pa,O_2/FI,O_2 \leq 200$	Facial PS-PEEP	46/77[¶]

PS: Pressure Support; PEEP: positive end-expiratory pressure; CPAP: continuous positive airway pressure; Pa,O_2: arterial oxygen tension; FI,O_2: inspiratory oxygen fraction. [#]: prospective, randomised, controlled study; [¶]: noninvasive ventilation/standard medical treatment related to the aetiology of hypoxaemic acute respiratory failure.

total of 24 patients treated with NIV by a facial mask were matched with 24 patients treated with invasive ventilation by endotracheal intubation. Use of NIV avoided intubation in 67% of patients. Even if the existence of criteria of ARDS was not reported, all the patients were at a very advanced stage of ARF, since they presented criteria of intubation. The NIV-treated group had a lower mortality in the ICU, the hospital and within 2 months of study entry. Differences in mortality between the two groups disappeared after 6 months. The findings of that study provided further support for applying NIV in AIDS patients with severe *P. carinii* pneumonia-related ARF as a first-line therapeutic choice; however, randomised controlled trials are required to confirm these results.

TOGNET *et al.* [27] have reported their experience of NIV in 18 haematological patients with ARF which occurred before, during or just after therapeutic aplasia. NIV, with a PS mode and preferably a nasal mask, was performed intermittently: 12 patients were ultimately intubated and died; seven needed intubation within 3 h following admission (because of the inability of NIV to provide adequate ventilation in six patients); and six patients were not intubated and were discharged. CONTI *et al.* [28] have evaluated treatment with NIV by nasal mask as an alternative to endotracheal intubation and conventional mechanical ventilation in 16 patients with haematological malignancies complicated by ARF and having intubation criteria (at inclusion, $Pa,O_2/FI,O_2$ of 87 ± 22). NIV was delivered *via* nasal mask using a BiPAP ventilator: five patients died in the ICU following complications independent of the respiratory failure and 11 were discharged from the ICU in stable condition after a mean stay of 4.3 ± 2.4 days and were subsequently discharged from the hospital. Thus, NIV proved to be feasible and appropriate for the treatment of respiratory failure in haematological patients who were at high risk of intubation-related complications. AZOULAY *et al.* [30] retrospectively studied a cohort of patients with solid or haematological cancer admitted to the ICU for ARF. The first group of 132 patients was admitted in the period 1990–1995 while the second group, composed of 105 patients, was admitted in 1996–1998. The types of cancer were equally distributed among the two groups. The survival rate in the period 1996–1998 was significantly higher than in the previous period. In a matched-pair analysis of cancer patients requiring mechanical ventilation support, the mortality among NIV patients was significantly lower than in conventionally ventilated patients (43.7 *versus* 70.8%; p=0.008) [30]. Univariate analyses of the patients' characteristics, co-morbidity and type of malignancy did not show that any significant association with 30-day mortality. However, in the multivariate analysis, two variables were found to predict ICU outcome: higher SAPS II at admission was associated with an increased mortality rate whereas the use of NIV during the 1996–1998 period was associated with a marked improvement in survival. Another study compared NIV with invasive intubation and ventilation for this patient group [32]. In that retrospective study, 27 patients, who received NIV, were matched for SAPS II with 52 patients who required immediate intubation on a 1:2 basis. In contrast to several earlier reports, the authors could not demonstrate the presence of a survival benefit for the use of NIV. Indeed, treatment with NIV successfully averted the need for intubation in eight (31%) patients, five (62.5%) of whom survived their hospital stay; this last rate was similar to this recorded in patients who required immediate intubation. Nevertheless, these results must be taken cautiously because hypoxaemic ARF was dramatically more severe in the NIV group than in the invasive ventilation group (median $Pa,O_2/FI,O_2$ ratio 71 *versus* 141, respectively; p<0.001).

More recently, a case-control study on a total of 34 patients was performed to evaluate the effectiveness of early administration of CPAP through a helmet, in haematological malignancy patients with ARF [33]. Each patient was treated by CPAP outside an ICU, directly in the haematological ward. The authors described a success rate as high as possible in patients ventilated with the helmet, while eight NIV failures were registered in the group ventilated with a face mask because of an intolerance of this interface.

Prospective randomised controlled studies

ARF in patients undergoing solid organ transplantation

Organ transplantation has become a therapy for an increasing population of patients with end-stage organ failure. Although preventing rejection remains the principle focus in improving overall survival statistics, pulmonary complications following transplantation are responsible for most morbidity and contribute substantially to the mortality associated with various organ transplantation procedures.

ANTONELLI et al. [23] studied solid organ transplant recipients with hypoxaemic ARF and compared NIV delivered through a face mask with standard treatment using oxygen supplementation to avoid endotracheal intubation and decrease duration of ICU stay. NIV resulted in lower intubation rates (20 versus 70%; p=0.002), less fatal complications (20 versus 50%; p=0.05) and reduced ICU stay and mortality (20 versus 50%; p=0.05). However, hospital mortality did not differ between NIV and standard therapy groups. In a subgroup analysis, patients with ARDS randomised to NIV had an intubation rate of 38 versus 86% in the standard treatment group (p=0.08).

Immunosuppressed patients with pulmonary infiltrates, fever and ARF

HILBERT et al. [25] hypothesised that the intermittent use of NIV at an early stage of hypoxaemic ARF would reduce the need for endotracheal intubation and the incidence of complications. In a prospective, randomised, controlled study, the efficacy of noninvasive ventilation delivered intermittently through a mask was compared with that of standard medical treatment with supplemental oxygen and no ventilatory support in patients with immunosuppression from various causes in whom hypoxaemic ARF had been precipitated by pulmonary infiltrates and fever [25].

The immunosuppression could have been caused by neutropenia, after chemotherapy or bone marrow transplantation in patients with haematological cancers, drug-induced immunosuppression, in organ-transplant recipients or as a result of corticosteroid or cytotoxic therapy for a nonmalignant disease, or AIDS.

The patients were selected and exclusion criteria were: a requirement for emergent intubation for cardiopulmonary resuscitation, respiratory arrest or a rapid deterioration in neurological status with a Glasgow Coma Scale score ≤ 8; a haemodynamic instability or electrocardiogram instability; COPD; a cardiac origin of the respiratory failure, which was established by physical signs, chest radiograph and echocardiogram; an arterial carbon dioxide tension (Pa,CO_2) >55 mmHg, with acidosis (pH <7.35); failure of greater than two new organs; uncorrected bleeding diathesis; and tracheotomy, a facial deformity or recent oral, esophageal or gastric surgery. Patients were randomly assigned to receive either standard treatment (26 patients) or standard treatment plus NIV through a face mask (26 patients). It is important to underline that randomisation was made at an early stage of the respiratory failure, long before the patients were headed for intubation.

NIV was delivered through a face mask, in a discontinuous mode, with a protocol close to that previously described in COPD patients, i.e., periods of NIV lasted ≥ 45 mins and alternated every 3 h with periods of spontaneous breathing [34, 35]. Between periods of ventilation, patients breathed oxygen spontaneously while arterial oxygen saturation (Sa,O_2) was continuously monitored. NIV was automatically resumed when Sa,O_2 was <85% or when dyspnoea worsened, as evidenced by a respiratory rate of >30 breaths·min^{-1}.

During the first 24 h, NIV was administered for a mean of 9 ± 3 h. Subsequently, the mean duration of NIV was 7 ± 3 h·day^{-1}. The mean duration of NIV was 4 ± 2 days.

The rates of initial and sustained improvement in $Pa,O_2/FI,O_2$ and other outcomes in both groups are reported in table 2. In the NIV group, compared with standard therapy, fewer patients required endotracheal intubation (12 versus 20; p=0.03) and there were fewer complications (13 versus 21; p=0.02). Overall, with NIV, there were improvements in mortality in the ICU (10 versus 18; p=0.03) and in total in-hospital mortality (13 versus 21; p=0.02).

Comments on the randomised controlled studies

Neutropenia in patients with haematological malignancies was the most frequent type of immunosuppression in patients included in the study [25]. If NIV avoided intubation in only 47% of neutropenic patients, this rate was significantly higher than in the standard treatment group (7%; p=0.02). Very high rates of mortality are recorded in patients with haematological malignancies admitted to an ICU, more particularly if they are neutropenic and if intubation and mechanical ventilation are necessary [2, 4–9, 36]. The risk of complications of invasive mechanical ventilation is related to the duration of ventilatory support [36, 37]. Recent prospective trials have shown the advantage of NIV in significantly reducing the incidence density of nosocomial pneumonia, compared with conventional intubation and positive pressure ventilation. It is important to note that ventilator-associated pneumonia was associated with in-ICU death in 100% of cases in both randomised controlled studies dealing with immunocompromised patients [23, 25].

In the study by ANTONELLI et al. [23], the eight ARDS patients randomised to NIV had an intubation rate of 37.5% and a mortality rate of 37%. Few studies have reported on the application of NIV in ARDS. In another study by the same group, seven out of 32 patients randomised to NIV had ARDS. A total of four out of the seven patients with ARDS avoided intubation and survived, while three patients required intubation and died. Only one trial exclusively enrolled patients with ALI/ARDS; ROCKER et al. [38], in

Table 2. – Outcome variables in the study by HILBERT et al. [25]

	Noninvasive ventilation group[#]	Standard treatment group[#]	p-value
Patients requiring intubation	12 (46)	20 (77)	0.03
Intubation per sub-population			
Hematologic malignancy and neutropenia	8/15 (53)	14/15 (93)	0.02
Drug-induced immunodepression	3/9 (33)	5/9 (56)	0.32
AIDS	1/2 (50)	1/2 (50)	
ICU deaths	10 (38)	18 (69)	0.03
ICU deaths per sub-population			
Hematologic malignancy and neutropenia	7/15 (47)	13/15 (87)	0.02
Drug-induced immunodepression	3/9 (33)	4/9 (44)	0.50
AIDS	0/2 (0)	1/2 (50)	
Length of stay in ICU days	7±3	10±4	0.06
Hospital deaths	13 (50)	21 (81)	0.02
Hospital deaths per sub-population			
Hematologic malignancy and neutropenia	8/15 (53)	14/15 (93)	0.02
Drug-induced immunodepression	4/9 (44)	6/9 (67)	0.32
AIDS	1/2 (50)	1/2 (50)	

Data are presented as n (%), n/N total or mean±SD. ICU: intensive care unit. [#]: n=26.

an uncontrolled study, reported the outcome of 12 episodes of ALI/ARDS in 10 patients treated with NIV. Overall success rate for NIV trials was 50%. In detail, avoidance of intubation was achieved on six (66 %) out of nine occasions when NIV was used as the initial mode of assisted ventilation; it failed after three episodes of planned (1) or self (2) extubation. These encouraging results showed that NIV should be considered as a treatment option for patients in stable condition in the early phase of ALI/ARDS. The studies published to date should provide the rationale for prospective randomised studies.

Both trials showed that early application of NIV was well tolerated and helped avert the need for endotracheal intubation and improved the outcomes in selected immunocompromised patients with hypoxaemic ARF [23, 25]. The authors used intermittent NIV, since the onset of management [25] or after the first 24 h of treatment [23], at a less advanced stage of hypoxaemic ARF than in other studies that assessed the value of NIV in patients, who met the criteria for intubation [22, 28]. On the basis of the present author's previous experience, NIV is used in a sequential mode [20, 34, 35]. This mode is a discontinuous mode, with some specificity, *i.e.*, the predetermination of the duration of the ventilation sessions and of the time between the NIV sessions. One of the potential advantages of the sequential approach are an harmonious distribution of NIV sessions, a better acceptance and tolerance for the patients and a better management by nursing staff. The protocol of sequential ventilation is appreciated by staff and has contributed to the standardisation of techniques of NIV in the ICU. It has not been necessary to modify the organisation of the present author's unit since the introduction of these new techniques.

Both randomised controlled studies dealing with immunocompromised patients have several limitations [23, 25]. It is impossible to eliminate bias when a study cannot be blinded, and the studies included only selected patients with immunosuppression who were treated in a single ICU. Furthermore, all the patients in the study by HILBERT *et al.* [25] were transferred to the ICU directly from medical wards. Some oncology units are set up as mini–ICUs and only patients, whose condition is unstable are transferred to a typical ICU. Further studies are needed in order to refine the process of selecting patients for treatment with NIV.

NIV as a means of assisting ventilation during fibreoptic bronchoscopy

It is important to establish the specific causes of an immunocompromised patient's pulmonary disease, so that specific therapy can be instituted. Furthermore, a positive diagnosis and a well adapted treatment could be the main determinants in the improved outcome of immunosuppressed patients managed with NIV [25]. Consequently, fibreoptic bronchoscopy and bronchoalveolar lavage are major tools in diagnosing diffuse infiltrates that often occur in association with fever and new onset of respiratory symptoms in immunosuppressed patients [25, 39, 40].

Nevertheless, although there is no absolute contraindication to this procedure, severe hypoxaemia is an accepted contraindication to fiberoptic bronchoscopy in nonintubated patients. The American Thoracic Society recommends avoiding bronchoalveolar lavage in patients who are breathing spontaneously with hypercapnia and/or hypoxaemia that cannot be corrected to a Pa,O_2 of ≥ 75 mmHg with supplemental oxygen.

In a study of eight immunosuppressed patients with suspected pneumonia and $Pa,O_2/FI,O_2$ of ≤ 100, ANTONELLI *et al.* [41] assessed the feasibility and safety of fibreoptic bronchoscopy with NIV. They found that NIV during bronchoscopy was well-tolerated, significantly improved the $Pa,O_2/FI,O_2$ ratio, and successfully avoided the need for endotracheal intubation. Another recent study, including 46 patients, suggested that the application of another noninvasive interface, *i.e.*, the laryngeal mask airway, also appears to be a safe and effective alternative to intubation for accomplishing bronchoscopy with bronchoalveolar lavage in immunosuppressed patients with suspected pneumonia and severe hypoxaemia ($Pa,O_2/FI,O_2 \leq 125$) [42]. In a recent prospective randomised trial on 26 patients, NIV was shown superior to conventional oxygen supplementation in preventing gas exchange deterioration, and with better haemodynamic tolerance, during fiberoptic bronchoscopy in patients with less severe forms of hypoxaemia ($Pa,O_2/FI,O_2 < 200$) [43]. In that study, PS was 15–17 cmH$_2$O, PEEP was set at 5 cmH$_2$O and FI,O_2 at 0.9; the session of NIV was begun 10 min before the fibreoptic bronchoscopy and continued for at least 30 min after the procedure. The present author currently has the same approach.

Equipment and techniques: particulars in immunocompromised patients

The time suitable to appreciate improvement in the patient or, conversely, failure of NIV treatment, may depend on many factors. The lack of ARF resolving at 1–2 h makes it possible to individualise the patients for whom the efforts to try improving adaptation and outcome must be most important. Thus, consider if it could be possible to ameliorate several factors that can improve adaptation of the patient on NIV and the outcome of the technique. This reasoning is helpful within the first few hours of NIV, when the patient needs to adapt, and also later, when prolonged ventilation is required.

Many factors may be improved. Some of them are well known and similar to those considered when PS with PEEP is used in intubated patients; several others are more specific to NIV.

Interface

NIV can be administered to immunocompromised patients with different types of interface. The patient interface most commonly employed is a full-face or nasal mask secured firmly, but not tightly, with a headstrap [13]. The full-face mask delivers higher ventilation pressures with fewer leaks, requires less patient cooperation and permits mouth breathing. However, it is less comfortable, increases the dead space, impedes communication and limits oral intake. The nasal mask needs patient nasal passages and requires mouth closure to minimise air leaks. The leaks through the mouth decrease alveolar ventilation and may decrease the efficacy of NIV in reducing the work of breathing. Furthermore, high flows of gas passing through the nose in case of mouth leaks can markedly increase nasal resistance and thus further reduce the efficacy of nasal NIV [44].

Patients may develop complications related to the use of NIV such as skin necrosis, gastric distention, nosocomial pneumonia or evidence of barotrauma (pneumothorax, pneumomediastinum, pneumoperitoneum or pulmonary interstitial emphysema). Data from the literature and observations from the present author's practice, suggest a highest incidence of facial-skin breakdown and/or intolerance of the interface in the subgroup of patients with hypoxaemic ARF and haematological malignancies. The incidence of pressure necrosis of the skin over the nasal bridge reached 31% in an uncontrolled study [28]. Three patients were excluded from the study by HILBERT *et al.* [20], because they refused to keep the facial mask during the first CPAP session. The reason was acute stress in one case and major painful mucositis in two cases. A bad tolerance of CPAP was reported in five other patients enrolled in this study and who were intubated. Mask intolerance because of pain, discomfort or claustrophobia may require discontinuation of NIV and endotracheal intubation.

Various modifications are available to minimise this complication, such as use of forehead spacers or the addition of a thin plastic flap that permits air sealing with less mask pressure on the nose. Straps that hold the mask in place are also important for patient comfort and many types of strap assemblies are available. Most manufacturers provide straps that are designed for use with a particular mask. More points of attachment add to stability and strap systems with Velcro fasteners are useful.

There is no evidence to support the use of particular patient interface devices in patients with hypoxaemic ARF [13]. Nevertheless, clinical experience suggests that full-face masks improve efficacy by reducing leaks and are more appropriate for use in the setting of severe hypoxaemic ARF. As shown in table 1, a facial mask was used preferentially in the studies examining the efficacy of NIV in immunocompromised patients with hypoxaemic ARF.

The fact that most NIV failures are due to technical problems, justifies the recent studies which evaluated new interface devices. Attempting to improve tolerability of patients, ANTONELLI et al. [45] adopted a transparent helmet made from latex-free polyvinyl chloride, which allowed patients to see, read and speak, as an interface during NIV. They conducted a prospective trial, with a matched control group, in order to investigate the efficacy of NIV using the helmet to treat patients with hypoxaemic ARF. Six (18%) patients in the helmet group and 9 (13%) patients in the facial mask group had ARDS. A total of eight (24%) patients in the helmet group and 21 (32%) patients in the facial mask group failed NIV and were intubated. No patients failed NIV because of intolerance of the technique in the helmet group compared with eight (38%) patients in the mask group (p=0.047). Complications related to the technique (skin necrosis, gastric distension and eye irritation) were fewer in number in the helmet group compared with the standard mask group (no patients *versus* 14 (21%) patients, respectively; p=0.002). The helmet allowed the continuous application of NIV for a longer period of time (p=0.05). The authors concluded that NIV by helmet successfully treated hypoxaemic ARF with better tolerance and fewer complications than facial mask NIV. The helmet is very popular in Italy and excellent results have been reported with the administration of CPAP through a helmet in haematological malignancy patients with ARF [33]. A better tolerance of the helmet, compared with a conventional interface, was also found in a case-control study [31]. However, this interface can be responsible for an increased work of breathing and dyspnoea [46], a potential risk of CO_2 rebreathing, to be carefully weighed against the major benefits achieved respecting the integrity of the face. In practice, in many units, including the present author's, the helmet is used in the second or even third line, as an alternative to face mask in case of intolerance responsible for skin lesions, with a risk of failure of the method.

Ventilatory modes

One of the main differences between management of COPD patients and of patients with hypoxaemic ARF is the place of CPAP in the therapeutic armamentarium of physicians treating patients with hypoxaemic ARF. Pressures commonly used to deliver CPAP to patients with hypoxaemic ARF range from 5 to 15 cmH_2O. Such pressures can be applied using a wide variety of devices including CPAP valves connected to a compressed gas source, small portable units used for home therapy of obstructive sleep apnoea and ventilators designed for use in the ICU. Depending on the critical care ventilator selected, CPAP may be administered using "demand", "flow-by" or "continuous flow" techniques, with imposed work differing slightly between them. CPAP is widely used in the belief that it may reduce the need for intubation and mechanical ventilation in patients with acute hypoxaemic respiratory insufficiency. Nevertheless, to the present author's knowledge, although several studies have shown the ability of the method to improve hypoxaemia, only one randomised study has demonstrated that the use of CPAP reduces the need for endotracheal intubation in patients with severe hypercapnic cardiogenic pulmonary oedema [47]. A recent study showed that, compared with standard oxygen therapy, CPAP neither reduced the need for intubation nor improved outcomes in patients with hypoxaemic ARF [24]. Alternatively, positive results have been reported in randomised controlled studies where PS and PEEP was used [23, 25]. During PS ventilation, the ventilator is triggered by the patient and delivers a set pressure for each breath and cycles to expiration either when it senses a fall in inspiratory flow rate below a threshold value, or at a preset time. Noninvasive PS ventilation offers the potential of excellent patient–ventilator synchrony, reduced diaphragmatic work and improved patient comfort.

The choice of NIV with PS and PEEP, rather than CPAP, a technique previously systematically used in hypoxaemic ARF in the present author's ICU [20], has undoubtedly contributed to the good results recently reported in immunosuppressed patients [25]. In the present author's practice, after the mask had been secured, the level of PS is progressively increased and adjusted for each patient to obtain an expired tidal volume of 7–10 mL·kg of body weight^{-1} and a respiratory rate of fewer than 25 breaths·min^{-1}. PEEP is repeatedly increased by 2 cmH$_2$O, up to a level of 10 cmH$_2$O, until the F_{I,O_2} requirement is 70% or less. The F_{I,O_2} is adjusted to maintain S_{a,O_2} above 90%. Ventilator settings are adjusted on the basis of continuous monitoring of S_{a,O_2}, clinical data and measurements of arterial blood gases. Studies comparing the impact on clinical outcome of CPAP and PS plus PEEP, in patients with hypoxaemic ARF, should be useful. For the moment, and looking forward to the results of further studies, PS ventilation plus PEEP could be the ventilatory mode recommended for treatment with NIV of hypoxaemic ARF.

Many factors must be considered when PS plus PEEP is used. Some of them are well known (*e.g.*, inspiratory trigger sensitivity, inspiratory flow) and close to those considered when this ventilatory mode is used in intubated patients. Several others are more specific to NIV: *e.g.*, the negative impact of leaks on work of breathing with a risk of patient–ventilator asynchrony [48]. Gas leaks around the mask or from the mouth limit the efficacy of the device make monitoring of tidal volume difficult and may prevent adequate ventilatory assistance in patients who require high inspiratory airway pressures and represent an important cause of failure. Leaks may also indicate low compliance or ventilation close to total lung capacity. Thus, particular attention should be paid to the leaks during application of NIV in patients with hypoxic ARF. In a study on six patients with ALI due to AIDS-related opportunistic pneumonia, a time-cycled expiratory trigger provided a better patient–machine interaction than a flow-cycled expiratory trigger, in the presence of air leaks during NIV [48]. Another possibility is to modify the threshold of flow cut-off.

The present author believes that the first hours of delivering NIV, with careful attention to mask fit, patient comfort and patient–ventilator synchrony, represent a critical opportunity to improve outcome.

Predictive factors of NIV outcome

In the randomised study by HILBERT *et al.* [25], the effect on outcomes of the presence and the absence of a final diagnosis of the cause of pneumonitis with respiratory failure was studied. In the NIV group, the patients with a final diagnosis had significant lower rates for intubation (p=0.03), death in the ICU (p=0.04) or in the hospital (p=0.006). So, a positive diagnosis and a well-adapted treatment could be the main determinants in the improved outcome of immunosuppressed patients managed with NIV.

In a prospective study, variables predictive of NIV failure were investigated in 354 patients with hypoxaemic ARF, 37 of them with immunosuppression [49]. Multivariate analysis identified age >40 yrs (odds ratio (OR) 1.72, 95% confidence interval (CI) 0.92–3.23), SAPS II ≥ 35 (OR 1.81, 95% CI 1.07–3.06), the presence of ARDS or community-acquired pneumonia (OR 3.75, 95% CI 2.25–6.24) and a $Pa,O_2/FI,O_2 \leq 146$ after 1 h of NIV (OR 2.51, 95% CI 1.45–4.35) as factors independently associated with failure of NIV.

Nevertheless, in practice, it can be difficult to predict an individual outcome and decide promptly to withdraw the noninvasive ventilatory support, keeping in mind the poor prognosis of intubation in numerous patients [50]. Alternatively, it is crucial to do all that can be done to attempt to optimise the technical aspects which are crucial for a successful application of NIV.

Even though learning techniques of NIV is described as simple in some studies, it is essential and education must be continuous; this allows better indications of the techniques and optimises the technical aspects and monitoring, to guarantee that intubation is not delayed when the method fails. Indeed, the use of NIV with a delay in reintubation can lead to excess mortality and the moment of reintubation should not be delayed if it becomes necessary. Undoubtedly, ARF in immunocompromised patients is one of the indications of NIV that requires experience and a good control of the technique; this justifies, in this indication, practising NIV in the ICU.

Conclusions

Starting from the good results obtained in patients with acute exacerbations of COPD, NIV is now being used to support those with hypoxaemic ARF, certain of them with immunosuppression.

A reduction in the incidence of nosocomial infection is a consistent and important advantage of NIV compared with invasive ventilation and is probably one of the most important advantages of avoiding endotracheal intubation using NIV. ARF in immunocompromised patients is a recognised indication of NIV and, according to recent international recommendations (of level I), NIV should be used whenever possible in this indication to reduce the risk of nosocomial pneumonia [37]. Above all, NIV makes it possible to reduce the mortality of the patients of oncohaematology with ARF.

Given the risks of serious complications and death associated with intubation, the relative safety of appropriately applied NIV should change the approach to ventilation in immunocompromised patients with respiratory failure; patients in whom respiratory distress develops should be treated conventionally with oxygen and other indicated therapies and should be monitored closely; if moderate-to-severe respiratory distress develops with tachypnoea and hypoxaemia, NIV should be initiated unless there are contraindications [50]. The early involvement of ICUs in immunocompromised patients care, and the better definitions of patients who require ICU admission will probably play a major role in the future.

The experiences gradually acquired by the different units, the regular training of the personnel, further technological advances and future research, will position noninvasive ventilation more accurately in the therapeutic armamentarium of physicians dealing with immunocompromised patients with acute respiratory failure and are likely to improve the conditions for performing noninvasive ventilation in the future.

Summary

Mechanical ventilation is an independent prognostic factor of mortality in immunocompromised patients; thus, to avoid intubation must remain a major objective in this pathology. After several studies showing the feasibility, two prospective randomised and controlled studies demonstrated that noninvasive ventilation (NIV) made it possible to improve the outcome in selected immunocompromised patients admitted in intensive care unit.

Acute respiratory failure (ARF) in immunocompromised patients is a recognised indication of NIV and, according to recent international recommendations (of level I), should be used whenever possible in this indication to reduce the risk of nosocomial pneumonia. Above all, NIV makes it possible to reduce the mortality of the patients of onco-haematology with ARF. The prognosis is still improved when a diagnosis of pneumonitis can be retained and the bronchoscopy can be carried out directly under NIV among the more hypoxaemic patients.

Undoubtedly, ARF in immunocompromised patients belongs to the indications of NIV which require experiment and a good control of the technique justifying, in this indication, the practice of NIV in intensive care units.

Keywords: Critical care, immunocompromised, intermittent positive pressure ventilation, noninvasive ventilation, respiratory failure, ventilation.

References

1.   Masur H, Shelhamer J, Parrillo JE. The management of pneumonias in immunocompromised patients. *JAMA* 1985; 253: 1769–73.
2.   Estopa R, Torres Marti A, Kastanos N, Rives A, Agusti-Vidal A, Rozman C. Acute respiratory failure in severe hematologic disorders. *Crit Care Med* 1984; 12: 26–28.
3.   Tobin MJ. Advances in mechanical ventilation. *N Engl J Med* 2001; 344: 1986–1996.
4.   The ARDS Network. Ventilation with lower tidal volumes as compared with traditional tidal volumes for acute lung injury and the acute respiratory distress syndrome. *N Engl J Med* 2000; 342: 1301–1308.
5.   Stauffer JL. Complications of translaryngeal intubation. *In*: Principles and practice of mechanical ventilation. Tobin MJ, ed. New York, Dekker Inc., 1994; pp. 711–747.
6.   Ewig S, Torres A, Riquelme R, *et al.* Pulmonary complications in patients with haematological malignancies treated at a respiratory intensive care unit. *Eur Respir J* 1998; 12: 116–122.
7.   Gruson D, Hilbert G, Portel L, *et al.* Severe respiratory failure requiring ICU admission in bone marrow transplant recipients. *Eur Respir J* 1999; 13: 883–887.
8.   Bach PB, Schrag D, Nierman DM, *et al.* Identification of poor prognostic features among patients requiring mechanical ventilation after hematopoietic stem cell transplantation. *Blood* 2001; 98: 3234–3240.
9.   Rañó A, Agustí C, Benito N, *et al.* Prognostic factors of non-HIV immunocompromised patients with pulmonary infiltrates. *Chest* 2002; 122: 253–261.

10. Kroschinsky F, Weise M, Illmer T, et al. Outcome and prognostic features of ICU treatment in patients with hematological malignancies. *Intensive Care Med* 2002; 28: 1294–1300.

11. Soubani AO, Kseibi E, Bander JJ, et al. Outcome and prognostic factors of hematopoietic stem cell transplantation recipients admitted to a medical ICU. *Chest* 2004; 126: 1604–1611.

12. Curtis JR, Yarnold PR, Schwartz DN, Weinstein RA, Bennett CL. Improvements in outcomes of acute respiratory failure for patients with human immunodeficiency virus-related *Pneumocystis carinii* pneumonia. *Am J Respir Crit Care Med* 2000; 162: 393–398.

13. Organized jointly by the American Thoracic Society, the European Respiratory Society, the European Society of Intensive Care Medicine, and the Société de Réanimation de Langue Française, and approved by ATS Board of Directors, December. International Consensus Conferences in Intensive Care Medicine: noninvasive positive pressure ventilation in acute respiratory failure. *Am J Respir Crit Care Med 2001* 2000; 163: 283–291.

14. Greenbaum DM, Millen JE, Eross B, Snyder JV, Grenvik A, Safar P. Continuous positive airway pressure without tracheal intubation in spontaneously breathing patients. *Chest* 1976; 69: 615–621.

15. Smith RA, Kirby RR, Gooding JM, Civetta JM. Continuous positive airway pressure (CPAP) by face mask. *Crit Care Med* 1980; 8: 483–485.

16. Covelli HD, Weled BJ, Beekman JF. Efficacy of continuous positive airway pressure administered by face mask. *Chest* 1982; 81: 147–150.

17. Kesten S, Rebuck AS. Nasal continuous positive airway pressure in *Pneumocystis carinii* pneumonia. *Lancet* 1988; 2: 1414–1415.

18. Gregg RW, Friedman BC, Williams JF, McGrath BJ, Zimmerman JE. Continuous positive airway pressure by face mask in *Pneumocystis carinii* pneumonia. *Crit Care Med* 1990; 18: 21–24.

19. Brett A, Sinclair DG. Use of continuous positive airway pressure in the management of community acquired pneumonia. *Thorax* 1993; 48: 1280–1281.

20. Hilbert G, Gruson D, Vargas F, et al. Noninvasive continuous positive airway pressure in neutropenic patients with acute respiratory failure requiring intensive care unit admission. *Crit Care Med* 2000; 28: 3185–3190.

21. Confalonieri M, Calderini E, Terraciano S, et al. Noninvasive ventilation for treating acute respiratory failure in AIDS patients with *Pneumocystis carinii* pneumonia. *Intensive Care Med* 2002; 28: 1233–1238.

22. Antonelli M, Conti G, Rocco M, et al. A comparison of noninvasive positive-pressure ventilation and conventional mechanical ventilation in patients with acute respiratory failure. *N Engl J Med* 1998; 339: 429–435.

23. Antonelli M, Conti G, Bufi M, et al. Noninvasive ventilation for treatment of acute respiratory failure in patients undergoing solid organ transplantation: a randomized trial. *JAMA* 2000; 283: 235–241.

24. Delclaux C, L'Her E, Alberti C, et al. Treatment of acute hypoxemic nonhypercapnic respiratory insufficiency with continuous positive airway pressure delivered by a face mask: a randomized controlled trial. *JAMA* 2000; 284: 2352–2360.

25. Hilbert G, Gruson D, Vargas F, et al. Noninvasive ventilation in immunosuppressed patients with pulmonary infiltrates, fever, and acute respiratory failure. *N Engl J Med* 2001; 344: 481–487.

26. Katz JA, Marks JD. Inspiratory work with and without continuous positive airway pressure in patients with acute respiratory failure. *Anesthesiology* 1985; 63: 598–607.

27. Tognet E, Mercatello A, Polo P, et al. Treatment of acute respiratory failure with non-invasive intermittent positive pressure ventilation in haematological patients. *Clin Intensive Care* 1994; 5: 282–288.

28. Conti G, Marino P, Cogliati A, et al. Noninvasive ventilation for the treatment of acute respiratory failure in patients with hematologic malignancies: a pilot study. *Intensive Care Med* 1998; 24: 1283–1288.

29. Bédos JP, Dumoulin JL, Gachot B, et al. *Pneumocystis carinii* pneumonia requiring intensive care management: survival and prognostic study in 110 patients with human immunodeficiency virus. *Crit Care Med* 1999; 27: 1109–1115.

30. Azoulay E, Alberti C, Bornstain C, *et al.* Improved survival in cancer patients requiring mechanical ventilatory support : impact of noninvasive mechanical ventilatory support. *Crit Care Med* 2001; 29: 519–525.

31. Rocco M, Dell'Utri D, Morelli A, *et al.* Noninvasive ventilation by helmet or face mask in immunocompromised patients: a case-control study. *Chest* 2004; 126: 1508–1515.

32. Depuydt PO, Benoit DD, Vandewoude KH, Decruyenaere JM, Colardyn FA. Outcome in noninvasively and invasively ventilated hematologic patients with acute respiratory failure. *Chest* 2004; 126: 1299–1306.

33. Principi T, Pantanetti S, Catani F, *et al.* Noninvasive continuous positive airway pressure delivered by helmet in hematological malignancy patients with hypoxemic acute respiratory failure. *Intensive Care Med* 2004; 30: 147–150.

34. Hilbert G, Gruson D, Gbikpi-Benissan G, Cardinaud JP. Sequential use of noninvasive pressure support ventilation for acute exacerbations of COPD. *Intensive Care Med* 1997; 23: 955–961.

35. Hilbert G, Gruson D, Portel L, Gbikpi-Benissan G, Cardinaud JP. Non-invasive pressure support ventilation in COPD patients with postextubation hypercapnic respiratory insufficiency. *Eur Respir J* 1998; 11: 1349–1353.

36. Rubenfeld GD, Crawford SW. Withdrawing life support from mechanically ventilated recipients of bone marrow transplants: a case for evidence based guidelines. *Ann Intern Med* 1996; 125: 625–633.

37. American Thoracic Society; Infectious Diseases Society of America. Guidelines for the management of adults with hospital-acquired, ventilator-associated, and healthcare-associated pneumonia. *Am J Respir Crit Care Med* 2005; 171: 388–416.

38. Rocker GM, Mackenzie MG, Williams B, Logan PM. Noninvasive positive pressure ventilation: successful outcome in patients with acute lung injury/ARDS. *Chest* 1999; 115: 173–177.

39. Stover DE, Zaman MB, Hajdu SI, Lange M, Gold J, Armstrong D. Bronchoalveolar lavage in the diagnosis of diffuse pulmonary infiltrates in the immunosuppressed host. *Ann Intern Med* 1984; 101: 1–7.

40. Gruson D, Hilbert G, Valentino R, *et al.* Utility of fiberoptic bronchoscopy in neutropenic patients admitted to intensive care unit with pulmonary infiltrates. *Crit Care Med* 2000; 28: 2224–2230.

41. Antonelli M, Conti G, Riccioni L, Meduri GU. Noninvasive positive-pressure ventilation *via* face mask during bronchoscopy with BAL in high-risk hypoxemic patients. *Chest* 1996; 110: 724–728.

42. Hilbert G, Gruson D, Vargas F, *et al.* Bronchoscopy with bronchoalveolar lavage *via* the laryngeal mask airway in high-risk hypoxemic immunosuppressed patients. *Crit Care Med* 2001; 29: 249–255.

43. Antonelli M, Conti G, Rocco M, *et al.* Noninvasive positive-pressure ventilation *vs.* conventional oxygen supplementation in hypoxemic patients undergoing diagnostic bronchoscopy. *Chest* 2002; 121: 1149–1154.

44. Richards GN, Cistulli PA, Ungar RG, Berthon-Jones M, Sullivan CE. Mouth leak with nasal continuous positive airway pressure increases nasal airway resistance. *Am J Respir Crit Care Med* 1996; 154: 182–186.

45. Antonelli M, Conti G, Pelosi P, *et al.* New treatment of acute hypoxemic respiratory failure: noninvasive pressure support ventilation delivered by helmet – a pilot controlled trial. *Crit Care Med* 2002; 30: 602–608.

46. Racca F, Appendini L, Gregoretti C, *et al.* Effectiveness of mask and helmet interfaces to deliver noninvasive ventilation in a human model of resistive breathing. *J Appl Physiol* 2005; 99: 1262–1271.

47. Bersten AD, Holt AW, Vedig AE, Skowronski GA, Baggoley CJ. Treatment of severe cardiogenic pulmonary edema with continuous positive airway pressure delivered by face mask. *N Engl J Med* 1991; 325: 1825–1830.

48. Calderini E, Confalonieri M, Puccio PG, Francavilla N, Stella L, Gregoretti C. Patient–ventilator asynchrony during noninvasive ventilation: the role of expiratory trigger. *Intensive Care Med* 1999; 25: 662–667.

49. Antonelli M, Conti G, Moro ML, *et al.* Predictors of failure of noninvasive positive pressure ventilation in patients with acute hypoxemic respiratory failure: a multi-center study. *Intensive Care Med* 2001; 27: 1718–1728.
50. Hill NS. Noninvasive ventilation for immunocompromised patients. *N Engl J Med* 2001; 344: 522–524.

NIV: indication in case of acute respiratory failure in children

O. Nørregaard

Danish Respiratory Centre West, Arhus University Hospital, Arhus, Denmark.

Correspondence: O. Norregaard, Danish Respiratory Centre West, Arhus University Hospital, Norrebrogade 44, Arhus, 8000, Denmark. Fax: 45 89492900; E-mail: oleno@as.oae.dk

Respiratory failure is a major cause of morbidity and mortality around the world [1]. In certain conditions, such as neuromuscular diseases, it is the most frequent cause of death; and not just in the poorer parts of the world. Previously, respiratory failure would either not have been treated, or would have been treated with intubation in the acute setting or tracheostomy for chronic conditions.

During the last couple of decades, noninvasive ventilation (NIV) techniques have increasingly been added to the armamentarium for the treatment of acute respiratory failure (ARF) as well as for long-term respiratory insufficiency. The drawbacks of invasive ventilation and the increasingly obvious advantages of NIV both account for this development.

Both intubation and tracheostomy are associated with a number of adverse effects [2] and, in the paediatric population, complication rates as high as 40% have been reported [3], including accidental extubation, atelectasis, tissue damage, postintubation stridor, bronchopulmonal dysplasia, bronchial tube blockage [4], nosocomial infections and difficulties with sedation [5].

NIV applied to adults in the acute setting has seen favourable outcomes, including reduced intubation rates, decreased complication rates, increased survival and decreased stay at the intensive care unit and at the hospital [6].

With respect to the use of NIV in children in ARF, the 10-yr old consensus report is still almost true in stating that "At present, nasal mask ventilation in young children must be considered an investigational technique for research and/or use only by experienced centres. Further to our knowledge ... there are no generally accepted guidelines" [7].

NIV for ARF in the paediatric population has been used only to a very small extent. Increasingly, however, during the last few years, the use has been expanding and data supporting the technique in children are emerging. Experience has typically been restricted to case series and has mainly dealt with long-term use of NIV [8]. The recent development in NIV for paediatric ARF does, however, give hope for a new and supplementary mode of treatment in infants and children with acute respiratory distress.

Physiology and symptoms

Although children and adults share a number of basic respiratory characteristics, the paediatric pulmonary function is in many ways more vulnerable and prone to incompensation. The neonate is characterised by a relatively stiff lung and a very

Eur Respir Mon, 2008, 41, 110–132. Printed in UK - all rights reserved. Copyright ERS Journals Ltd 2008; European Respiratory Monograph; ISSN 1025-448x.

compliant chest wall. In order to maintain a functional residual capacity (FRC) of 40% of total lung capacity instead of the unmodified only 15%, the neonate introduces a number of compensating mechanisms, including laryngeal breaking [9], maintenance of the post-inspiratory tone in the muscles of the chest wall [10] and a respiratory frequency fast enough to allow only incomplete deflation. The very compliant chest wall impedes the neonate's ability to generate adequate tidal volumes [11], increases the work of breathing (WOB) [12] by constantly wasting force on chest wall deformation instead of generating alveolar ventilation [13] as an effective pump would, contributes to fatigue [14] and accentuates growth retardation [15]. The mechanics of the respiratory system are further challenged by high flow resistance of the nasal airway, in particular in infants where it contributes almost half of the airway resistance [16]. The small airways of young children are very sensitive to any further narrowing (e.g., caused by secretions, oedema, adenoids or even a minor displacement of the mask used for NIV) that, based on the Bernoulli principle, will generate a vicious cycle of increased narrowing and subsequent increased WOB. In addition, a small zone of apposition of the diaphragm [13], horizontal ribs and in the young immature muscles [17] with a lower fraction of fatigue-resistant fibres, all limit the endurance of the respiratory system.

In the preterm baby, disturbed alveolarisation [18] and the absence of pores of Kohn, Lambert and Martin, do not allow collateral air flow to happen at the bronchoalveolar level thus impeding aeration and favouring the creation of atelectasis [19]. Expiratory flows are obstructed due not only to the small dimensions of the airways but also to the altered compliance of the airways and the low FRC generating airway closure during tidal breathing. Furthermore, submucosal glands occupy a larger proportion of the airway wall in babies and children without respiratory disease than in adults. This relative gland hypertrophy could, theoretically, when proportionally increased in bronchial disease, contribute markedly to mucus hypersecretion and airflow obstruction [20]. The mucins in respiratory tract secretions from children without respiratory disease share similar macromolecular properties to the mucins in sputum from patients with chronic bronchitis [21], except they are more acidic [22] possibly indicating that secretions in children are more viscous than adult respiratory secretions.

An integral part of the paediatric respiratory scenario is that the metabolic rate is twice that of the adult leading to a ratio of alveolar ventilation:FRC of 5:1 in the infant and 1.5:1 in the adult [23] obviously increasing the risk of hypoxaemia; any parenchymal pulmonary disease will increase this further. If the ensuing risk of acidosis and the associated deleterious effect on muscle function, and, in the neonate, particularly the preterm, the risk of foetal circulation, are additionally taken into consideration, the risk of incompensation becomes obvious.

The hypoxaemic ventilatory response is attenuated in the infant [24]; apnoeas are more frequent than in the adult and linked to rapid eye movement (REM) sleep, which is more abundant the younger the child is. Muscle tone is particularly low during REM sleep, generating a further decrease in FRC and in the power of the respiratory pump while the flow resistance of the airways and WOB increase. Any generated increase in respiratory frequency will increase the dead space:tidal volume ratio.

If, at any time, these mechanisms will generate a load that exceeds the total competence of the respiratory system, the system will incompensate and to a varying degree produce symptoms. In the acute setting, symptoms can vary from mild-to-moderate respiratory distress to a comatose child in respiratory arrest, as outlined in table 1.

Conditions associated with increased risk of ARF are numerous and include immaturity of the respiratory pacemaker and the pulmonary tissue, impaired ability to cough, incompetent ability to swallow, retained secretions, scoliosis, neuromuscular

Table 1. – Clinical characteristics of a child with acute respiratory failure

Increased respiratory frequency or bradypnea
Wheezing
Expiratory grunting
Decreased or absent breath sounds
Flaring of nostrils
Paradox breathing
Intercostal retractions
Use of accessory muscles
Fatigue
Sweating
Dehydration
Dyspnoea
Bradycardia or tachycardia
Anxiety
Agitation
Headache
Confusion
Coma

disease and bronchial hyper-reactivity/asthma. Infection is often a common final pathway in many conditions leading to ARF.

Commonly, respiratory failure is classified as either type I or II, although this is not an exhaustive terminology. Characteristics of respiratory failure type I and II are presented in table 2. In addition to symptoms, a number of physiological criteria for respiratory insufficiency have been defined, as presented in table 3.

Other indicators of the respiratory state of an individual have included rapid shallow breathing index, maximal inspiratory pressure, maximal sniffing pressure, pulse transit time [25] and breathing intolerance index (i.e. $(t_I/t_{tot}) \times (V_T/VC)$, where t_I is the inspiratory time; t_{tot}, the total time for one breath; V_T, the tidal volume; and VC, the vital capacity [26]).

Treatment

The overall goal of NIV in ARF is to restore the balance between the load on the respiratory system and that system's competence by unloading the failing respiratory pump, in particular typically during sleep or sedation. More specifically, central objectives are to decrease WOB, to increase oxygenation and ventilation, and to rest and

Table 2. – Characteristics of respiratory failure type I and II

Type I	Type II
Hypoxaemia (low P_{a,O_2})	Normal-to-low P_{a,O_2}
Normal-to-low P_{a,CO_2}	Hypercapnia (high P_{a,CO_2})
V'/Q' mismatch	
Clinical examples of type I and II respiratory failure	
Atelectasis	Neuromuscular disease
Status asthmaticus	Obesity
Pneumonia	Scoliosis
Cystic fibrosis	Other restrictive pulmonary disease
	Impaired respiratory drive

P_{a,O_2}: arterial oxygen tension; P_{a,CO_2}: arterial carbon dioxide tension; V'/Q': ventilation/perfusion ratio.

Table 3. – Values for pulmonary function and arterial bood gasses associated with respiratory insufficiency

Pa,CO_2 >6.0 kPa,
Sa,O_2 <97% on room air
VC <15 mL·kg^{-1} body weight (if the child can co-operate)
PCEF <180 L·min^{-1} (if the child can co-operate)

Pa,CO_2: arterial carbon dioxide tension; Sa,O_2: arterial oxygen saturation; VC: vital capacity; PCEF: peak cough expiratory flow.

comfort the child. In adults, NIV has been shown to reduce transdiaphragmatic pressure, the pressure–time index and consequently WOB, and to increase VT [27–29].

It is very important to remember that NIV should always be preceded and accompanied by relevant therapy aiming at reversing the process that generated ARF, i.e. surfactant in preterms, antibiotics for infections, broncholytic agents in asthma, vasoactive drugs in left ventricular failure etc.

While supplemental oxygen may serve as an adjunct in hypoxaemic respiratory failure, it is critical to understand that failure of the respiratory pump, as is typically but not exclusively seen in respiratory failure type II, is not corrected by oxygen alone and may, in some cases, be aggravated by it.

Monitoring

It is of pivotal importance to monitor implemented treatment. Just as timing of initiating treatment is important, so is the recognition of the proper time to terminate failing NIV treatment and convert to endotracheal ventilation. Some of the studies with poor outcome from NIV in adults with ARF have pointed to delay in the recognition of unsuccessful NIV as the reason for failure [30].

Monitoring ongoing NIV is in principle based on the same parameters that defined ARF, and will typically include arterial oxygen saturation (Sa,O_2), carbon dioxide levels, either as trancutaneous tensions or by means of end-tidal capnography [31]. However, although capnography is informative in several ways, it is not reliable in an open noninvasive respiratory assist system. Arterial blood gases, respiratory frequency and child–ventilator synchrony, in addition to clinical parameters such as pulse, sweating, peripheral perfusion and mental state, constitute additional relevant parameters to monitor. Recorded continuous monitoring including transcutaneous gas-exchange parameters, thoraco-abdominal bands and mask pressure (fig. 1) will offer a valuable tool in determining the state and dynamics of the child in response to changes in pathology and to various interventions and, in particular, visualise child–ventilator synchrony or asynchrony (fig. 2). Visualisation of the pressure tracings during the expiratory phase will add to the understanding of whether mask-related rebreathing may be part of the explanation if hypercapnia is present. The combined picture of pressure tracings, thoraco-abdominal movements, oxygen saturation and carbon dioxide tension will also help to localise leaks (fig. 3). In the paediatric intensive care unit, additional monitoring could include continuous recording of airway pressure and flow in order to characterise pulmonary mechanics, continuous invasive blood pressure (arterial and central venous), venous oxygen saturation (Sv,O_2), central temperature and lactate. Full polysomnography (including electroencephalogram (EEG), electro-oculogram (EOG) and electromyogram (EMG)) will typically be performed in less-acute settings.

Educated staff, familiar with the sometimes complex equipment and professional in handling children, a prerequisite for success in these often delicate matters.

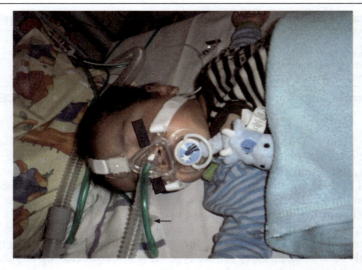

Fig. 1. – Transparent nasal mask with green line (arrow) for continuous pressure tracing. Note the visible and unobstructed nostrils and head gear that allows for sweating.

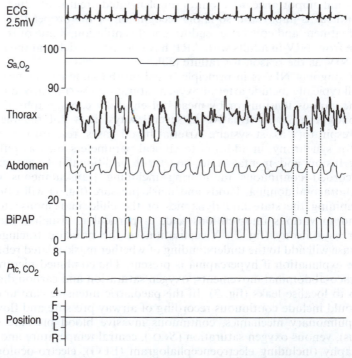

Fig. 2. – Monitoring of a noninvasively ventilated child with continuous tracings of mask pressure and thoraco-abdominal movements. Note the child–ventilator dyssynchrony and thoraco-abdominal paradox (----), and child–ventilator synchrony and reduced thoraco-abdominal paradox pattern (·····). Sa,O_2: arterial oxygen saturation; BiPAP: bilevel positive airway pressure; Ptc,CO_2: transcutaneous carbon dioxide tension; F: front; B: back; L: left; R: right.

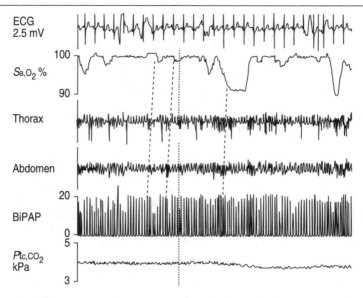

Fig. 3. – Decrease in mask pressure associated with reduced movements of thorax and abdomen preceding oxygen desaturations. The pattern is compatible with leaks. Sa,O_2: arterial oxygen saturation; BiPAP: bilevel positive airway pressure; Ptc,CO_2: transcutaneous carbon dioxide tension.

Modalities

NIV often refers to positive pressure-targeted ventilation, but it should also include positive volume-targeted ventilation, negative pressure ventilation and, in a wider sense, it seems justified to include continuous positive airway pressure (CPAP), supplementary oxygen and some of the technologies used for clearing of secretions.

Achieving minute ventilation from NIV, when applied as positive pressure ventilation, depends on the mechanical characteristics of the respiratory system, such as compliance, resistance, auto-positive end-expiratory pressure (auto-PEEP), ventilatory frequency, leakage and ventilator–patient interaction. The inspiratory and expiratory trigger function, usually sensed as either pressure or flow changes in the system, is of fundamental importance. Flow-triggering has in some investigations been found to superior to pressure-triggering [32]; an insensitive trigger will increase the WOB, while a too-sensitive trigger may introduce auto-triggering, possibly leading to patient–ventilator dyssynchrony and unintentional hyperventilation. Trigger adjustment will depend upon ventilator brand and model. In children and infants with a weak or reduced pulmonary function, inspiratory flows generated by the patient may be too small to activate the trigger, in particular in the case of an interposed humidifier, resulting in controlled ventilation, regardless, to some extent, of the setting [33]. Some products include the possibility to set a timeframe for inspiration in order to optimise pressure delivery and to counteract distorted inspiratory–expiratory ratios. The expiratory trigger (adjustable or not) will, in some models, work purely as a function of time or as a function of a predefined decline in inspiratory flow before changing to expiratory positive airway pressure (EPAP). In the latter case, leaks will lead the machine to prolong the inspiratory phase well beyond the point where the user has ceased to inspire, thus contributing to child–ventilator asynchrony, increased WOB with the risk of reappearance of respiratory failure, discomfort, possible gastric distension and, in the worst case, aspiration to the lungs. Newer models increasingly try to combine the pressure-targeted mode with an assurance of a desired minute ventilation [34], and recently some brands have introduced the servo-principle into portable machines.

Oxygen, if needed, is typically bled into the single hose system or directly into the mask. Due to the high flow rates in these pressure-targeted respiratory assist devices, it is usually not possible to achieve an inspired oxygen fraction (FI,O_2) >0.5 even with flow rates of 5–10 L·min^{-1}.

The bilevel pressures can be delivered in spontaneous (patient-driven) mode, in a spontaneous/timed mode or in a purely timed mode.

These ventilators/respiratory assist devices are widely used. Patient comfort seems to be an important feature in favour of the pressure-targeted machines, as there is no convincing evidence that these machines work better than volume-targeted or *vice versa*, apart from the pressure-targeted machines better ability to cope with leaks. Among the pressure-targeted machines' characteristics and quality does vary considerably [35].

Servo-ventilators increasingly being used in intensive care units have been working in the pressure-targeted mode for NIV in acute paediatric cases. These ventilators are generally more advanced than the portable machines, including more-elaborate monitoring of pressure, flow, volume, compliance and other parameters in order to assess patient–ventilator interaction; they use a double hose system for optimal carbon dioxide-elimination and the newer models are increasingly capable of dealing with leaks. Some of the newer models are able to support the infant's spontaneous inspiration, breath by breath, respecting as well the initiation as the termination of the breath and consequently optimising patient–ventilator synchrony [36]. The problem of leaks is still not totally eliminated. A more detailed review of the technicalities and specifications of various paediatric intensive care ventilators is beyond the scope of the present chapter, as is a comprehensive algorithm for setting the ventilators.

There are data, [37] though, which suggest that easily measurable clinical parameters, such as respiratory frequency and comfort rating, are comparable with more-sophisticated and invasive techniques, as a guide in setting the ventilator for paediatric ventilation.

Volume-targeted ventilators deliver a set flow to the user's airways for a preset time interval or in response to an inspiratory effort, terminating when a preset volume has been delivered. Leaks have been a problem with this technique and, unless the machine is able to deliver a V_T up to twice that, which is needed for an intubated patient, reduced V_T and patient discomfort may occur [38]. Limited maximal inspiratory flow to sufficiently support spontaneous respiratory efforts is also a disadvantage. The use of these ventilators for NIV in paediatric ARF seems to be decreasing (while it seems that there is still some use in the long-term setting).

Negative pressure ventilators repeatedly apply a negative pressure to the trunk or part of it by means of a tank, a suit or a shell to imitate the physiological negative inspiratory pressure swings. Theoretically this should be advantageous in children with right heart failure, which indeed has been shown in the post-operative setting. The machines are cumbersome, though, they interfere with patient care and are associated with skin injury and obstructive apnoeas (that can be counteracted by positive airway pressure) [39, 40]. The use of these devices is, at present, limited.

Mechanical insufflation–exufflation applies, by means of a mechanical pump (Cough-Assist®) *via* a nasal mask, mouth piece or full face mask (or a tracheostomy), pressures in the range of 10–40 cmH$_2$O cycling between positive and negative pressures [41], that can each be set at a desired value. The machine can operate in an automatic or manual mode. The latter facilitates patient–machine co-operation. The rationale is to expand the lungs, loosen secretions, increase compliance and perform a noninvasive suctioning manoeuvre to eliminate secretions.

Interfaces

The interface plays a crucial role in NIV with respect to comfort, success or failure of NIV and to adverse effects, not least in the paediatric population. Development of paediatric interfaces is still far from complete and much work needs to be performed before a wide range of well-performing products for all age groups are readily available. Optimisation includes issues, such as how easy it is to mount the mask on the child, quality of the head gear, safety aspects, material transparency and hygienic aspects.

Available interfaces at present include nasal masks (fig. 1), nasal plugs (fig. 4) or cannulas, oral interfaces, full face masks (covering mouth and nose or as a hybrid between an oral interface and nasal prongs) and helmets. Some of these products come either as standard products or can be custom made [42, 43]; for younger children and infants especially, one often has to rely on custom-made interfaces because of the paucity of industrial products in that field.

When applying a mask to a child with ARF, there are at least three major considerations: 1) maximal comfort for the child; 2) verification that the mask works, (*i.e.*, it is in place and allows free delivery of pressure or volume during inspiration and expiration); and 3) the mask should not have adverse effects, such as major leaks, in particular not in the orbital region, carbon dioxide rebreathing, gastrointestinal inflation, skin abrasions or necrosis. Additionally, a fourth issue of dead space and the role the interface plays in the child's ability to trigger the ventilator and/or the risk of re-breathing should also be kept in mind.

Leaks are a major issue in NIV (fig. 3) [44]; they carry the risk of reduced alveolar ventilation, child–ventilator dyssynchrony, increased nasal resistance, irritation to the eyes, disturbed sleep and comfort and, ultimately, rejection of the treatment. Additionally, leaks may tempt the clinician to tighten the head gear too much, resulting in pressure marks or even breakdown of the skin at various prominences like the nasal bridge. In the dilemma between leaks and tight straps, the clinician should usually accept some leakage if no other option is available.

Nasal masks are often chosen in children, even after the child is no longer an obligatory nose breather. Particular paediatric facial anatomy, the risk of aspiration,

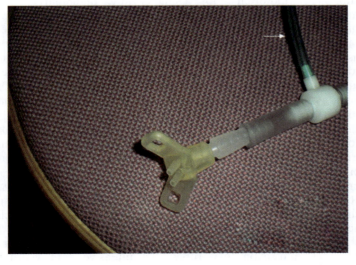

Fig. 4. – Binasal canula with green line (arrow) for continuous pressure recording during noninvasive ventilation.

problems with co-operation and proper fitting of full face masks in a chubby toddler may be part of the explanation as well as the added dead space of full face masks. The latter issue is complex. Recent data from a bench study [45] indicated the importance of the flow-sensitive dynamic dead space (contrary to static dead space which seems much-less important), stressing the importance of continuous flow during the whole expiratory phase and of optimal positioning of the exhalation ports diametrically opposite the inspiratory port, typically over the nasal bridge, as it probably facilitates laminar flow in that position. The position of the exhalation port as well as the mask design also seems to affect carbon dioxide rebreathing [46], at least in adult models, where the mask with the smallest volume and with the exhalation port placed within the mask demonstrated less rebreathing than alternative designs.

To what extent these findings are applicable in real life is still not known, although there are recent data documenting the use of helmet ventilation in hypercapnic neuromuscular paediatric patients [47], in hypoxaemic infants [48] and preterm babies [49].

Masks should preferably be made of transparent material that allows easy inspection of the nostrils to ensure that they are not partly or totally occluded by secretions or from dislocation of the mask. The risk is particular high in the very small, as even minor displacements of the mask may interfere with unobstructed delivery of flow or pressure. This very simple but very important point should have a very high priority among attendants. It also emphasises the importance of proper head-gear that will keep the interface in place. This is a challenge in infants with a rounded and smooth scull moving the head around during sleep or awake; even more so because a too tight fixation of the cap may produce impressions on the soft cranial bony structures and add to the compression of the maxillar bone. This is a serious adverse effect [50, 51] in long-term NIV in children (fig. 5). To what extent it is a problem related to ARF remains to be documented; however, in many cases, ARF will occur in children who already are using long-term NIV and who may already have acquired facial flattening.

The mask material should be soft and follow the facial contours. Owing to the dynamics of these contours as a result of growth, weight changes and pressure from the interface, mask fitting is an ongoing process. In case of acute on chronic failure, the mask used at home may turn out to be outdated and not optimal in the acute setting. As a rule of thumb, one should often choose a smaller rather than a larger mask for proper fitting. In case of oral leaks, a full face mask or an added chin strap may be an alternative. In neonates, a pacifier ("dummy") may serve the same purpose very well. If facial masks are not attractive nasal pillows or cannulas may be useful as an alternative, or as a means to alternate between different interfaces during a treatment to minimise and spread adverse effects. If a custom made mask is used for the first time in a child, it is recommendable to check the pressure drop across the inner cushion if that is part of the mask design, as the resistance through the apertures may vary from one individual mask to another.

Appropriate headgear should be a concern and, in small children, custom made versions are often preferable. The material should be soft, allow for sweating (or keep the head warm, whichever is relevant) and have a surface that is not too smooth, in order to stabilise interface position.

If skin injuries are present or if facial contours pose a challenge to acceptable mask fit and leak limitation, the helmet may prove effective, even in paediatric [52] patients. The helmet also eliminates the problems with difficult fixation of masks in the child and may become attractive in the neonate [49].

The helmet, in contrast to most systems using a mask or prongs, works by means of separate inspiratory and expiratory tubes like intensive care ventilators (fig. 6). Rebreathing can be regulated by the volume of the helmet and the fresh gas flow.

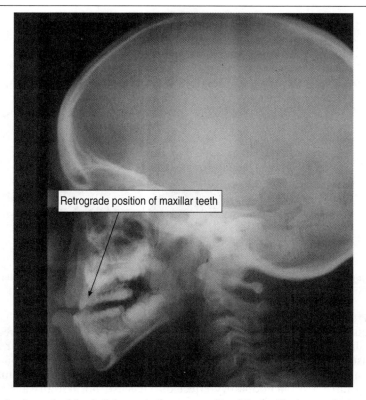

Retrograde position of maxillar teeth

Fig. 5. – Lateral radiograph of the skull demonstrating compression of the maxillar bone and retrograde position of maxillar teeth as a result of noninvasive ventilation of a child. Note relative protrusion of mandibular teeth. This may obstruct the normal antegrade development of the maxillar bone.

The fraction of inspired oxygen, the temperature, the humidity and the inspiratory and expiratory pressures can likewise be adjusted to the requirements of the user. The use of a helmet neither precludes judicious sedation nor the use of a nasogastric tube. The helmet must be made of transparent material, must contain a safety valve to prevent asphyxia and a port for handling and examination of the patient. Drawbacks of the helmet include the risk of a high level of noise, some difficulty in handling the patient, rebreathing and a tight fit without causing skin lesions.

Nasal prongs have primarily been used for infants and preterm infants [53] and have in general been well tolerated.

Humidification

Dryness is a common complaint from users of NIV [54]. Without humidification, the relative humidity in the NIV circuit is substantially lower (16.3–26.5%) than the ambient relative humidity (27.6–31.5%) [55]. The unidirectional flow prevents the recovery by the nasal mucosa of one third of the water delivered through the airflow leading to an increase of nasal resistance. If that provokes an increase in oral breathing and associated leaks, an increase of up to six-fold in nasal resistance has been observed [56]. Considering that the area of any tube is reduced by the radius of the fourth power, any

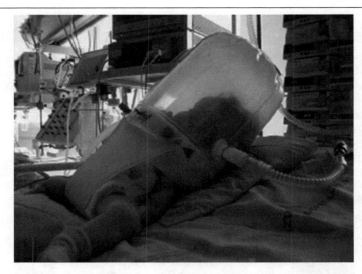

Fig. 6. – Helmet for noninvasive positive pressure ventilation of infants with acute respiratory failure. Reproduced from [48] with permission from the publisher.

retention of secretions or crusts will potentially start a vicious circle based on the Bernoulli equation and generate an increase of WOB in addition to increased risk of decreased pulmonary compliance and atelectasis [57]. Patients at particular risk include those with asthma, cystic fibroses, cilia dysfunction and other with copious secretions. This should aggressively be avoided and humidification is one of the means, which, in addition may have a bronchodilatory effect on, at least, normal airways [58]. Heated humidifiers are much-more effective than passover versions and often more comfortable too. Compared with the use of heat and moisture exchanger (HME) inserts, heated humidifiers in adults are associated with significantly less WOB and indices of patient effort and an increased efficiency of NIV [59]. Heated humidification increases the relative and absolute humidity to acceptable levels during NIV [55]. Heated humidification during nasal NIV in normal adults also attenuates the adverse effects of mouth leaks on effective VT and nasal resistance and improves overall comfort [60]. To what extent these oberservations can be applied to the paediatric population has still not been determined but, intuitively, they would probably be even more important in the younger children. The addition of a humidifier, however, would probably add to the resistance of the system and adversely interfere with triggering. There hardly seems to be a place for HME in infants and younger children. A meta-analysis of the risk of endotracheal tube occlusion with a HME versus a heated humidifier (HH) favoured the HH by a relative risk factor of 3.84. [61].

Sedation and pain management

No recommendations for sedation and pain management are currently available; however, it seems that these agents are presently used more liberally, maybe as a result of increasing professionalism, better back-up facilities and increasing awareness of the problem in paediatric intensive care units compared with a decade ago. Midazolam in the range of 0.15 mg·kg^{-1} has been used in some studies [48], opiates and chloral hydrate [62] or oral clonidine [63] in others.

Setting

Units taking care of children with ARF should be able to handle this potentially life threatening condition in a professional manner or have very close and free access to a department able to do that, which in practice will be an intensive care unit or preferably a paediatric intensive care unit. The staff should be trained and sufficient in number [64], intubation facilities and extensive monitoring equipment readily available. The condition of the child should define the setting. When different units are involved a predefined algorithm for referrel between units is recommendable.

Although the child may be sedated (to some degree) or, because of the respiratory failure (and possibly concomitant disease), not totally aware of the situation, it should be the ambition to create an environment that is adjusted to specifically comfort and fulfil also the psychological and emotional needs of a child. Educated staff and well structured work routines and the use of protocols have proven favourable [33].

Selection criteria

Clinical characteristics of respiratory insufficiency and failure and associated blood gasses have been outlined in tables 1 and 3.

As there are no generally accepted criteria specifically for initiating NIV in a neonate or an older child with ARF, many clinicians will often use a combination of these and other characteristics, the clinical setting and personal experience. Recent data from a prospective study may provide some additional guidance with respect to the course of NIV-treatment and CPAP-treatment [62] in predominantly young children with acute hypoxaemic (type I) or hypercapnic (type II) respiratory failure. An $F_{I,O_2} > 80\%$ after 1 h of NIV, predicted failure to respond to the treatment, with a sensitivity of 56% and an specificity of 83%. In spite of significant improvement in blood gasses, cardiac frequency and respiratory frequency in both groups (*i.e.* responders and nonresponders) these parameters could not significantly predict the course, although the responders tended to have a lower respiratory frequency than the nonresponders.

Contraindications

Contraindications are not defined and some would argue that the proper term for contraindications should be conditions where the true effect of NIV has not yet been tested. Generally, if NIV is not accepted or is not able to oxygenate and ventilate the patient in a satisfactory manner, alternative modes should be applied, *i.e.* usually intubation or tracheostomy. Copious secretions or bulbar malfunction may preclude the application of NIV [65]. Children with severe facial malformations, facial burns or trauma may be difficult to apply a mask or an oral interface to, but with the advent of the helmet another alternative has been added to the armamentarium beside negative pressure ventilation. Difficulties with co-operation, in the acute setting can to some extent, be overcome with judicious sedation. The need for ventilatory assistance around the clock does not, in the acute setting, preclude NIV, to some extent contrary to long-term ventilation. Obviously, a dramatically sick child with multi-organ failure, unstable circulation and/or impending respiratory failure would not be a candidate for NIV; at least not at present.

Outcome

Published reports on the results of NIV applied to infants and children with ARF are not very abundant, not very systematic and not very old. The goal is to summarise what is known about the topic related to specific pathologies to the limited extent this is possible from the available data.

Mixed populations

One of the largest and earliest studies from an ICU comprised retrospective data from 28 children, of whom none suffered from neuromuscular disease, with a median age of 8 yrs treated *via* a nasal mask with BiPAP®-settings of inspiratory/expiratory positive airway pressure (IPAP/EPAP)=12/6 cm H_2O supplied with oxygen as needed for 72 h as treatment for acute hypoxaemic failure (type 1), most frequently originating from pneumonia. Pa,CO_2 decreased from 6.0 to 5.2 kPa (p< 0.01), respiratory frequency from 45 to 33 breaths·min^{-1} and $Pa,O_2/FI,O_2$ increased from 141 to 280. Adverse effects were minor and included skin abrasions of the bridge of the nose [66].

Almost 10 years ago, PADMAN *et al.* [67] published a prospective study, which included 34 critically ill children (mean age 11 yrs) from a paediatric ICU with a range of underlying medical conditions such as pneumonia (13 individuals), stridor, reactive airway disease, asthma, post-operative hypoventilation with atelectasis, acute chest syndrome and sleep-aggravated breathing disorder (10 individuals). They were ventilated with bilevel devices, using IPAP/EPAP settings of 7–12/3–5 cmH$_2$O for a median duration of 6 days using nasal masks and humidifiers. After 72 h of ventilatory support, Pa,CO_2 was reduced from 8.4 to 6.1 kPa (p<0.05), bicarbonate concentrations from 30 to 24 mM (p<0.01) and respiratory frequency from 39 to 25 breaths·min^{-1} (p<0.04). Three (8.8%) required intubation. Adverse effects were limited to skin breakdown over the nasal bridge in four patients.

A recent study [62] from a paediatric ICU investigated the treatment of 42 children with a median age of 2.5 yrs (range 0.01–18 yrs) with acute hypoxaemic and hypercapnic respiratory failure caused by pneumonia (n=14), viral infections (n= 4), postoperative repair of congenital heart disease (n=11), Hyaline membrane disease (n=3) and miscellaneous conditions (n=10). NIV was applied for ~20 h *via* nasal or full face masks using a bilevel technique in assisted spontaneous breathing in 50% of the group and CPAP in the other 50%. Settings were unclear. Some were sedated with opiates, midazolam or chloral hydrate and analgesics as needed. A total of 24 responded to the therapy and 18 had to be intubated. Both groups improved significantly with respect to respiratory frequency, pH and Pa,CO_2 after 8 h, but none of these parameters was descriminative. The only predictive parameter was FI,O_2 after 1 h of NIV (0.48 in responders and 0.80 in nonresponders). The authors speculate that complication rate and co-operation with the ventilator may have been decisive factors for success or failure.

A contemporary, smaller Spanish study [68] of 23 children with a mean age of 37 months suffering from acute hypoxaemic failure (n=14), acute hypercapnic failure (n=4) or post-extubation failure (n=6) demonstrated a reduction in respiratory frequency from 45 to 34 breaths·min^{-1} and a pulse reduction from 148 to 122 after NIV treatment using mostly full face masks and a mixture of ICU ventilators and "specific noninvasive ventilators". Five were intubated, three of whom were aged <6 months.

A group of 15 children aged between 1 month and 5 yrs suffering from hypoxaemic ARF with $Pa,O_2/FI,O_2$ <300 for a variety of reasons (mostly post-extubation after major surgery) were in a feasibility study (uncontrolled) exposed to CPAP treatment *via* a helmet. CPAP level ranged between 5 and 10 cmH_2O, inspiratory gas flows were 30 $L \cdot min^{-1}$ and measurements were performed after 2 h of CPAP use. Insignificant improvements in oxygenation and carbon dioxide removal were noted in most of the children; however, two had to be intubated. There were no skin lesions, conjunctivitis, epistaxis or gastric distension reported [48].

Children with neuromuscular diseases

One study [69] from the late 1990s, applied a combined treatment of NIV and expiratory support (manual and assisted coughing) in the paediatric ICU prospectively to 10 children aged 12–20 yrs suffering primarily from neuromuscular disease (primarily Duchenne's muscular dystrophy), all without ventilator-free time. Six were originally intubated. Most of the children used BiPAP® with IPAP/EPAP settings of 24/3 cmH_2O. Outcome data were limited but it was reported that the four patients who originally used NIV continued treatment successfully and that the others were all extubated, mostly to a mouthpiece or a nasal mask. Patient co-operation was reported to be critical for treatment success.

A recent Italian study [47] in 10 children with an age range from 3 months to 12 yrs suffering from various neuromuscular diseases with ARF, used a mixture of face masks and helmets in combination with a very-sensitive flow-triggered ICU ventilator with a preset inspiratory time in order to minimise leaks. Sedation and pain relief were administered as needed. Treatment was successful in eight patients. Hypercapnic failure patients (Pa,CO_2 range of 48–94 mmHg) normalised their carbon dioxide values during 6-8 h of treatment, and $Pa,O_2/FI,O_2$ ratio increased from a median value of 75 to 240. No intubations and no severe complications occurred. The authors conclude that even "... life-threatening respiratory distress and very young age should not preclude NPPV [noninvasive positive-pressure ventilation] application in the PICU [paediatric ICU] setting."

Another study included 11 children of very-young age (6–26 months) with severe skeletal and bulbar weakness suffering from spinal muscular atrophy (SMA) type one [33]. Before extubation, they received inspiratory/expiratory pressures of 25–40 cmH_2O. Following extubation, they were managed according to a well defined protocol with IPAP/EPAP settings of >14/3 cmH_2O, that proved to be superior to nonprotocol treatment. Following the acute scenario, two required continuous NIV, six only nocturnal NIV, two were tracheostomised and one was lost at follow-up.

Children with airway diseases

Considering that asthma is the most common cause for hospital admission in childhood [70], any improvement from NIV in this area would be of major interest. A recent American study [71] confirmed for the first time, in a prospective manner, data from a previous nonprospective study [72] and a case series [73] reporting benefits from NIV in the acute setting. A total of 20 children with a median age of 48 months (range 2 months to 14 yrs) entered a cross-over study of bilevel support for 2 hours with an IPAP/EPAP setting of 10/5 cmH_2O via a nasal or full face mask combined with broncholytic inhalations, humidification, oxygen and standard therapy. NIV was associated with a decrease in respiratory frequency from 49 ± 14 to 32 ± 6 breaths$\cdot min^{-1}$ ($p<0.0001$) and a decrease in total Clinical Asthma Score (CAS) from 5.4 ± 1.2 to 2.1 ± 1.0 $p<0.0001$). After discontinuation of NIV, an increase in respiratory frequency and CAS reappeared. NIV was not associated with significant changes in Sa,O_2 nor in transcutaneous carbon dioxide tension. The findings are compatible with an unloading effect of NIV (although maybe incompletely, as cardiac frequency did not change), and emphasises the importance of choosing valid and relevant parameters for monitoring. The study did not report how fast clinical changes could be observer (within the 2-h time frame) nor does it comment on the issue of back-up rate and patient–ventilator synchrony. Three patients did not tolerate NIV, two of whom were aged <1 yr.

These findings were, to some extent, confirmed in a larger retrospective study including 83 children, with a median age of 8 yrs, in status asthmaticus refractory to conventional pharmacological treatment and designated for admission to the paediatric ICU [74]. A total of 73 tolerated nasal BiPAP® and concurrent continuous inhaled β-2 agonists for an average of 5.8 h. There was an "immediate" improvement with 77% of patients showing a 24% decrease in respiratory frequency (none experienced an increase) and 88% an improved oxygenation. Only two patients required intubation. A total of 22% were admitted directly to ward service, and none of these was subsequently transferred to the paediatric ICU. Intolerance to the mask was established within 10 min, and more often in the younger chidren. No adverse effects were observed. The study did not report data on BiPAP®-settings or on patient–ventilator synchrony.

Children with malignant diseases

Two minor case series [52, 75] have reported successful treatment of respiratory distress associated with malignant haematologic disease.

Infants

Administration of oxygen [76], CPAP and nasal intermittent positive pressure ventilation (IPPV; i.e. NIV) in preterm infants could be categorised as being somewhere in a grey zone between treatment of acute and/or chronic respiratory failure, thus justifying a comment as perceived in an acute perspective.

The use of oxygen administration via a nasal cannula, in preterm infants, shares some of the problems associated with CPAP use in older children. Studies have documented that flows of 2 L·min^{-1} using a 0.3 cm nasal cannula produced a mean pressure of 9.8 cmH$_2$O in infants of 30 weeks gestation studied at aged 28 days [77]. This, and other studies, has drawn the attention to oxygen administration as a form of respiratory support. Along with the benefits of this treatment one should be aware of the inherent risks of lung overexpansion and desiccated nostrils as a result of a nonheated and nonhumidified flow.

A Cochrane review [78] comparing nasal IPPV and nasal CPAP for the treatment of apnoea of prematurity concluded that nasal IPPV was a potentially beneficial treatment for apnoea in premature babies and, based on two small studies, that delivery via nasal prongs may be more effective than CPAP alone. The need for further research is underlined.

The Cochrane review by DE PAOLI et al. [79] concluded that short binasal prong devices were more effective than single prongs in reducing the likelihood of the short-term adverse outcomes of re-intubation and respiratory failure after extubating preterm infants to nasal CPAP, and also in treating preterm infants for respiratory distress syndrome as evidenced by reduction in oxygen requirements and respiratory frequency.

Recently a clinical study [80] compared the effect of nasal BiPAP with nasal CPAP on gas exchange in preterm babies. A total of 20 babies with a weight of 445–1,810 g (12 weighed <1,100 g) were subjected to four sessions, each lasting 1 h in a cross-over scenario between CPAP of 4–6 cmH$_2$O and bilevel ventilation with IPAP/EPAP settings of 8–10/4–6, a back up rate of 30 and an inspiratory:expiratory ratio of 1:3, both treatments delivered *via* a short binasal prong. During nasal BiPAP® sessions, a significant increase in oxygen saturation and transcutaneous oxygen tension were seen along with a significant decrease in transcutaneous carbon dioxide tension and respiratory frequency.

Later AGHAI *et al.* [81] compared, in a cross-over design in 15 infants with a body weight of $1,367 \pm 325$ g treatment with nasal CPAP of 5 cmH$_2$O with three levels of bi-level ventilatory support (10, 12 and 14 cmH$_2$O) in assist-control mode *via* largest possible nasal prongs. Data were collected over a maximum period of 30 s after 5 min of stabilisation. Inspiratory and resistive WOB decreased with high bi-level ventilation.

This trend was supported in a very-recent study, of 15 preterm babies of 972 ± 215 g, which compared NCPAP of 5.3 cmH$_2$O, delivered *via* binasal prongs, with bilevel pressure support ventilation of 7.9 cmH$_2$O above CPAP for 2 h after 15 min of stabilisation [82]. Maximal inspiratory time was limited to 0.45 s, and trigger sensitivity was adjusted in each child to achieve minimal response delay without auto-triggering. Peak and minute inspiratory efforts were significantly reduced as were indices of chest wall asynchrony (reduction in phase shift angle) during bilevel ventilation pointing to an effective unloading of the patient's respiratory pump; however, no difference was found with respect to VT, minute ventilation, carbon dioxide tension or hypoxaemic episodes. The extent of patient–ventilator synchrony was not specifically commented upon by the authors.

A comparable reduction of resistive WOB, respiratory frequency and phase angle (respiratory asynchrony) was noted during the use of variable-flow CPAP compared with bubble nasal CPAP of 4 to 8 cmH$_2$O delivered *via* binasal prongs to supine preterm infants of 1,042 g suffering from mild respiratory distress [53]. Data were collected over 30 s epochs. Both systems resulted in a decreased inspiratory WOB.

Whether the unloading of the neonate has any long-term consequences is unknown. It is interesting to speculate, though, whether it would result in a better neurologic outcome than, for instance, the long-term results of high-frequency oscillatory ventilation where an excess of children with abnormal neurodevelopmental status was the result [83].

Nasal prongs have been the standard interface for neonatal CPAP. With the advent of helmets for ventilatory support, this option has been investigated in a neonatal ICU where the outcome in 20 very low birth weight infants (815 g) exposed for 90 min to conventional CPAP and 90 min to CPAP delivered *via* a helmet was compared [49]. Neonatal Infant Pain Scale (NIPS) scores were significantly lower when infants were on the helmet than when they were on nasal CPAP (0.26 and 0.63, respectively) whereas no difference was found in the other parameters monitored, such as Sa,O$_2$, transcutaneous catbon dioxide tension, respiratory frequency, cardiac frequency, level of CPAP and temperature.

Children with other conditions

Dengue haemorrhagic fever can develop into dengue shock syndrome (DSS), a septic condition involving alveolar oedema, increased vascular permeability with development to ARDS and associated high mortality. A Vietnamese study [84] documented, in 37 children with DSS pleural effusions (92%) and interstitial pulmonary oedema (33%), and aged 1–11 yrs, that the addition of 6 cm of CPAP to conventional therapy significantly reduced respiratory frequency and significantly improved responsiveness to treatment (13/19 *versus* 4/18, respectively; p<0.01).

NIV has, in case studies, been applied to children with various other acute conditions like burns [85], traumatic tetraplegia [86] and peri-operatively in relation to scoliosis surgery in neuromuscular patients [87], with favourable results.

Negative pressure ventilation

Negative pressure ventilation (NPV) for children with ARF has been administered for several decades but is still not widely used and not much has been published in recent years. Older studies demonstrated that NPV was associated with a lower incidence of pneumothoraces and bronchopulmonary dysplasia than IPPV [88]. In the post-operative setting after correction of tetralogy of Fallot, NPV has been accompanied by an increase in pulmonary blood flow of 65% [89]. A more-recent controlled study over a period of 4 yrs in 244 neonates suffering from respiratory distress syndrome compared negative pressure support of -4– -6 cmH$_2$O with standard therapy including CPAP of 4 cmH$_2$O and demonstrated that the need for intubation was slightly less in the group receiving negative pressure support compared with the control group (86 *versus* 91%, respectively) [90]. Partly fuelled by public concerns about mortality and neonatal morbidity as a result of that treatment, a follow-up assessment study of part of the ventilated population was performed recently [91]. The results from 65 complete pairs from the original study were available and showed no significant difference in full IQ between the two groups. However, performance IQ was better in the group treated with NPV and scores on language production and visuospatial skills were significantly higher in that group compared to the group that had received standard treatment. The authors argued that future trials should be designed with long-term outcomes in mind; a point of view that deserves very high priority and which can only be strongly supported.

Another NPV study, using a chest cuirass, proved successful in a case series of critically ill infants aged 4–16 months exposed to -18– -30 cmH$_2$O in conjunction with 30 cmH$_2$O [92].

A recent study in two different paediatric ICUs comprising 52 infants with a mean age of 34 weeks, suffering from bronchiolitis-related apnoea, compared the results from treatment with noninvasive NPV ranging from -4– -25 cmH$_2$O when applied as intermittent NPV with those from the treatment with PPV either *via* prongs or a tube [93]. Pressures during PPV were not presented. The use of NPV was associated with a significantly reduced rate of intubation compared with the non-NPV regimen (26 *versus* 86%, respectively), a significantly shorter paediatric ICU stay (2 *versus* 7 days, respectively) and a reduced use of sedation (52 *versus* 86%, respectively). Some of the limitations of that study included its retrospective nature, the clinical practice in two paediatric ICUs, the comparability of the two populations and the use of CPAP at the NPV-paediatric ICU. One can thus only agree with the authors' proposal for a randomised, prospective controlled trial.

A recent Cochrane review by SHAH *et al.* [94] on hypoxaemic respiratory failure in children concluded, based on the only study included [95], that continuous negative extrathoracic pressure applied to 33 infants suffering from bronchiolitis reduced oxygen requirements to <30% within 1 h.

Position

Ventilation of children and neonates in the prone position has been associated with improvement in oxygenation [96], whereas improvement with respect to other parameters such as ventilator-free days has been difficult to demonstrate [97]. These studies were performed on intubated patients. It has not been possible to identify studies combining NIV and prone position. Although it may pose an increased workload and complexity of manoeuvres, there are good physiological arguments for an attempt.

Secretion clearance

If data regarding NIV for children ARF are scarce, the data for noninvasive secretion clearance in that group are even more so. MISKE et al. [98] concluded from a retrospective study in the nonacute setting that inexsufflation in children with a median age of 11.3 yrs was safe, reasonable well tolerated, but that the effectiveness with respect to reducing lower respiratory tract infections could not be determined. BACH [99] showed that the use of inexsufflator in a group of children suffering from SMA type 1 with ARF was followed by a considerable reduction of incidents of re-intubation. Additionally, the use of the inexsufflator as an adjunct in male children with Duchenne's muscular dystrophy on long-term NIV, in order to prevent respiratory tract infections was followed by fewer hospitalisations compared with the group who did not follow the specified protocol.

Other studies have confirmed benefits of the inspiratory/expiratory technique applied to children as it has generated greater increases in peak cough flow than other standard cough augmentation techniques [100].

Summary

After some years with increasing use of long-term noninvasive ventilation (NIV) of children with chronic diseases, NIV has, within the very last few years, been emerging as an option for treating children and infants with acute respiratory failure. The prevalent modality is positive pressure ventilation and continuous positive airway pressure, although negative pressure ventilation has been practised. The techniques appear feasible, safe and effective to varying degrees. Data are still very scarce and much research is needed to identify indications, contraindications, best techniques, best modalities, best interfaces and best scenarios. Investigations with long-term follow-up are strongly needed.

Keywords: Acute respiratory failure, children, continuous positive airway pressure, infants, noninvasive ventilation.

References

1. Mulholland K. Global burden of acute respiratory infections in children: implications for intervention. *Pediatr Pulmonol* 2003; 36: 469–474.
2. Konrad F, Schreiber T, Brecht-Knaus D, Giorgieff M. Mucociliary transport in ICU patients. *Chest* 1994; 105: 237–241.
3. Donnelly MJ, Lacey PD, Maguire AJ. A twenty year (1971–1990) review of tracheostomies in a major pediatric hospital. *Int J Pediatr Otorhinolaryngol* 1996; 35: 1–9.

4. Rivera R, Tibbals J. Complications of endotracheal intubation and mechanical ventilation in infants and children. *Crit Care Med* 1992; 20: 193–199.
5. Craven DE, Kunches LM, Kilinsky V, Lichtenberg DA, Make B, McCabe WR. Risk factors for pneumonia in patients receiving mechanical ventilation. *Am Rev Respir Dis* 1986; 133: 792–796.
6. Lightowler JV, Wedzicha JA, Elliott MW, Ram FS. Non-invasive positive pressure ventilation to treat respiratory failure resulting from exacerbation of chronic obstructive pulmonary disease: Cochrane systematic review and meta-analysis. *BMJ* 2003; 326: 185–187.
7. Make BJ. Mechanical ventilation beyond the intensive care unit: report of a consensus conference of the American College of Chest Physicians. *Chest* 1998; 113: 289S–344S.
8. Norregaard O. Noninvasive ventilation in children. *Eur Respir J* 2002; 20: 1332–1342.
9. Mortola JP, Fisher JT, Smith JB, Fox GS, Week S, Willis D. Onset of respiration in infants delivered by caesarean section. *J Appl Physiol* 1982; 52: 716–724.
10. Lopes J, Muller NL, Bryan MH, Bryan AC. Importance of inspiratory muscle tone in maintenance of FRC in the newborn. *J Appl Physiol* 1981; 51: 830–834.
11. Hagan R, Bryan AC, Bryan MH, Gulston G. Neonatal chest wall afferents and regulation of respiration. *J Appl Physiol* 1977; 42: 362–367.
12. Guslits BG, Gaston SE, Bryan MH, England SJ, Bryan AC. Diaphragmatic work of breathing in premature infants. *J Appl Physiol* 1987; 62: 1410–1415.
13. Hershenson MB. The respiratory muscles and the chest wall. *In*: Beckerman RC, Brouilette RT, Hunt CE, eds. Respiratory Control Disorders in Infants and Children. Baltimore, Williams and Wilkins, 1992; pp. 28–46.
14. Muller N, Gulston G, Cade D. Diaphragmatic muscle fatigue in the newborn. *J Appl Physiol* 1977; 46: 688–695.
15. Howard SE. Diaphragmatic work of breathing in infants with chronic lung disease. MSc thesis, York University, Toronto ON, Canada, 1987.
16. Hall GL, Hantos Z, Wildhaber JH, Sly PD. Contribution of nasal airways to low frequency respiratory impedance. *Thorax* 2002; 57: 396–399.
17. Keens TG, Bryan AC, Levison H. Developmental patterns of muscle fiber types in human ventilatory muscle. *J Appl Physiol* 1978; 44: 909–913.
18. Hjalmarson O, Sandber K. Abnormal lung function in healthy preterm infants. *Am J Respir Crit Care Med* 2002; 165: 83–87.
19. Menkes H, Gardiner A, Gamsu G, Lampert J, Macklem PT. Influence of surface forces on collateral ventilation. *J Appl Physiol* 1971; 31: 544–549.
20. Field WE. Mucous gland hypertrophy in babies and children aged 15 years or less. *Br J Dis Chest* 1968; 62: 11–18.
21. Thornton DJ, Davies JR, Kraayenbribk M, Richardson PS, Sheelan JK, Carlstedt J. Mucus glycoproteins from "normal" human tracheobronchial secretion. *Biochem J* 1990; 265: 179–186.
22. Davies JR, Hovenberg HW, Linden CJ, *et al.* Mucus in airway secretions from healthy and chronic bronchitic patients. *Biochem J* 1996; 313: 431–439.
23. Berry FA. Inhalation agents in paediatric anaesthesia. *Clin Anaesthesiol* 1985; 3: 515–537.
24. Davidson-Ward SL, Bautista DB, Keens TG. Hypoxic arousal responses in normal infants. *Pediatr Pulmonol* 1989; 7: 276A.
25. Pagani J, Villa MP, Calcagnini G, *et al.* Pulse transit time as a measure of inspiratory effort in children. *Chest* 2003; 124: 1487–1493.
26. Koga T, Watanabe K, Sano M, Ishikawa Y, Bach JR. Breathing intolerance index: A new indicator for ventilator use. *Am J Phys Med Rehabil* 2006; 85: 24–30.
27. Brochard L, Isabey D, Piquet J. Reversal of acute exacerbations of chronic lung disease by inspiratory assistance of a face mask. *N Engl J Med* 1990; 323: 1523–1530.
28. Brochard L, Harf A, Lorino H. Inspiratory pressure support prevents diaphragmatic fatigue during weaning from mechanical ventilation. *Am Rev Respir Dis* 1989; 139: 513–521.
29. Carrey Z, Gottfried SB, Levy RD. Ventilatory muscle support in respiratory failure with nasal positive ressure ventilation. *Chest* 1990; 97: 150–158.

30. Wood KA, Lewis L, Von Harz B, Kollef MH. The use of noninvasive positive pressure ventilation in the emergency department. Results of a randomized clinical trial. *Chest* 1998; 113: 1339–1346.

31. Hess DR. Monitoring during mechanical ventilation. *Paediatric Respir Rev* 2006; 7: Suppl. 1, S37–S38.

32. Nava S, Ambrosino N, Bruschi C, Confalonieri M, Rampulla C. Physiological effects of flow and pressure triggering during non-invasive mechanical ventilation in patients with chronic obstructive disease. *Thorax* 1997; 52: 249–254.

33. Bach JR, Niranjan V, Weaver B. Spinal muscular atrophy type I. A non-invasive respiratory management approach. *Chest* 2000; 117: 100–105.

34. Storre JH, Seuthe B, Fiechter R, *et al.* Average volume-assured pressure support in obesity hypoventilation. *Chest* 2006; 130: 815–821.

35. Battisti A, Tassaux D, Janssens J-P, Michotte J-B, Jaber S, Jolliet P. Performance characteristics of 10 home mechanical ventilators in pressure-support mode. *Chest* 2005; 127: 1784–1792.

36. Dimitriou G, Greenough A, Laubscher B, Yamaguchi N. Comparison of airway pressure triggered and airflow triggered ventilation in very immature infants. *Acta Pediatr* 1998; 87: 1256–1260.

37. Fauroux B, Nicot F, Essouri N, *et al.* Setting of non-invasive pressure support in young patient with cystic fibrosis. *Eur Respir J* 2004; 24: 624–630.

38. Elliott M, Moxham J. Noninvasive mechanical ventilation by nasal or face mask. *In*: Tobin MJ, ed. Principles of mechanical ventilation. New York, McGraw-Hill, 1994: pp. 427–454.

39. Hill NS. Clinical application of body ventilators. *Chest* 1986; 90: 897–905.

40. Hill NS, Redline S, Carskadon M. Sleep-disordered breathing in patients with Duchenne's muscular dystrophy using negative pressure ventilators. *Chest* 1992; 102: 1656–1662.

41. Segal MS, Salomon A, Herschfus JA. Alternating positive-negative pressures in mechanical respiration (the cycling valve device employing air pressures). *Dis Chest* 1954; 25: 640–648.

42. Schonhofer B, Sortor-Leger S. Equipment needs for non-invasive ventilation. *Eur Respir J* 2002; 20: 1029–1036.

43. Antonelli M, ContiG, Pelosi P, et al. New treatment of acute hypoxemic respiratory failure: non-invasive pressure support ventilation delivered by helmet – a pilot controlled trial. *Crit Care Med* 2002; 30: 602–608.

44. Teschler H, Stampa J, Ragette R, *et al.* Effect of mouth leaks on effectiveness of nasal bilevel ventilatory assistance and sleep architecture. *Eur Respir J* 1999; 14: 1251–1257.

45. Saatci E, Miller DM, Stell IM, Lee KC, Moxham J. Dynamic dead space in face masks used with noninvasive ventilators: a lung model. *Eur Respir J* 2004; 23: 129–135.

46. Schettino GPP, Chatmongkolchart S, Hess DR, Kacmarek RM. Position of exhalation port and design of mask affect CO_2 rebreathing during non-invasive positive pressure ventilation. *Crit Care Med* 2003; 31: 2178–2182.

47. Piastra M, Antonelli M, Caresta E, Chiaretti A, Polidori G, Conti G. Noninvasive ventilation in childhood acute neuromuscular respiratory failure : a pilot study. *Respiration* 2006; 496: 791–798.

48. Codazzi D, Nacoti M, Passoni M, Bonanomi E, Sperti LR, Fumagalli R. Continuous positive airway pressure with modified helmet for treatment of hypoxemic acute respiratory failure in infants and a preschool population: A feasibility study. *Pediatr Crit Care Med* 2006; 7: 455–460.

49. Trevisanuto D, Grazzina N, Doglioni N, Ferrarese P, Marzari F, Zanardo V. A new device for administration of continuous positive airway pressure in infants: comparison with standard nasal CPAP continuous positive airway pressure system. *Intensive Care Med* 2005; 31: 859–864.

50. Fauroux B, Lavis JF, Nicot F, *et al.* Tolerance of nasal masks used for positive pressure ventilation in children. *Eur Respir J* 2004; 24: Suppl. 48, 474S.

51. Fauroux B, Lavis J-F, Nicot F, *et al.* Facial side effects during noninvasive positive pressure ventilation in children. *Intensive Care Med* 2005; 31: 965–969.

52. Piastra M, Antonelle M, Chiaretti A, *et al.* Treatment of acute respiratory failure by helmet-delivered non-invasive pressure support ventilation in children with acute leucemia: a pilot study. *Intensive Care Med* 2004; 30: 472–476.

53. Liptsen E, Aghai ZH, Pyon KE, *et al.* Work of breathing during nasal continuous airway pressure in preterm infants: a comparison of bubble *vs* variable-flow devices. *Journal of Perinatology* 2005; 25: 453–458.

54. Waters KA, Everett FM, Bruderer JW. Obstructive sleep apnea: the use of nasal CPCP in 80 children. *Am J Respir Crit Care Med* 1995; 152: 780–785.

55. Holland AE, Deheny L, Buchan C, Wilson JF. Efficacy of a heated Passover humidifier during non-invasive ventilation: a bench study. *Respir Care* 2007; 52: 38–44.

56. Hayes MJ, McGregor FB, Roberts DN, Schroter RC, Pride NB et al. Continuous nasal positive airway pressure with a mouth leak: effect on nasal mucosal blood flux and geometry. *Thorax* 1995; 50: 1179–1182.

57. Branson RD. The effects of inadequate humidity. *Respir Care Clin N Am* 1998; 4: 199–214.

58. Carbone JE, Marini JJ. Bronchodilatory effect of warm air inhalation during quiet breathin. *West J Med* 1984; 140: 398–402.

59. Lellouche F, Maggiore SM, Deye N, *et al.* Effect of the humidification device on the work of breathing during noninvasive ventilation. *Intensive Care Med* 2002; 11: 1582–1589.

60. Tuggey JM, Delmastro M, Elliott MW. The effect of mouth leak and humidification during non-invasive ventilation. *Respir Med* 2007; 10: 1874–1879.

61. Hess DR. And now for the rest of the story. *Respir Care* 2002; 47: 696–699.

62. Bernet V, Hug MI, Frey B. Predictive factors for the success of noninvasive mask ventilation in infants and children with acute respiratory failure. *Pediatr Crit Care Med* 2005; 6: 660–664.

63. Bhatt JM, Pimhak R, Mayer A. Oral clonidine as a sedative agent to establish children on non-invasive ventilation. *Chest* 2006; 130: 1369.

64. Plant PK, Owen JL, Parrott S, Elliot MW. Cost effectiveness of ward based non-invasive ventilation for acute exacerbation of chronic obstructive pulmonary disease: Economic analysis of randomised controlled trials. *BMJ* 2003; 326: 956.

65. Teague WG. Long term mechanical ventilation in infants and children. *In*: Hill NS, ed. Lung Biology in Health and Disease Volume 152: Long Term Mechanical Ventilation. New York, Marcel Dekker, 2001; p. 186.

66. Fortenberry JD, Del Toro J, Jeffersom LS, Evey L, Haase D. Management of paediatric acute hypoxemic respiratory unsufficiency with bilevel positive pressure (BiPAP) nasal mask ventilation. *Chest* 1995; 108: 1059–1064.

67. Padman R, Lawless ST, Kettrick RG. Noninvasive ventilation via bilevel positive airway pressure support in paediatric practice. *Crit Care Med* 1998; 26: 169–173.

68. Villanueva M, Espunes P, Solas LA, *et al.* Noninvasive ventilation in a pediatric intensive care unit. *An Pediatr Anales de pediatria (Barcelona, Spain: 2003)* 2005; 62: 13–19.

69. Niranjan V, Bach JR. Noninvasive management of pediatric neuromuscular ventilatory failure. *Crit Care Med* 1998; 26: 2061–2065.

70. Rasmussen F, Taylor DR, Flannery EM, *et al.* Risk factors for hospital admission from asthma from childhood to young adulthood: A longitudinal population study. *J Allergy Clin Immunology* 2002; 110: 220–227.

71. Thill PJ, McGuire JK, Baden HP, *et al.* Noninvasive positive pressure ventilation in children with lower airway obstruction. *Pediatr Crit Care Med* 2004; 5: 337–342.

72. Akingbola OA, Simakajornboon N, Hadley EF Jr, *et al.* Noninvasive positive-pressure ventilation in pediatric status asthmaticus. *Pediatr Crit Care Med* 2002; 3: 181–184.

73. Teague WG, Lowe E, Dominick J, Lang D. Noninvasive positive pressure ventilation (NIPPV) in critically ill children with status asthmaticus. *Am J Respir Crit Care Med* 1998; 157: 452A.

74. Beers SL, Abramo TJ, Bracken A, Wiebe RA. Bilevel positive airway pressure in the treatment of status asthmaticus in pediatrics. *Am J Emerg Med* 2007; 25: 6–9.

75. Cogliati AA, Conti G, Tritapepe L, *et al.* Noninvasive ventilation in the treatment oc acute respiratory failure induced by all-trans retinoic (retinoic acid syndrome) in children with acute promyelocytic leukaemia. *Pediatr Crit Care Med* 2002; 3: 70–73.

76. Finer NN. Nasal cannula use in the preterm infant: oxygen or pressure? *Pediatrics* 2005; 116: 1216–1217.

77. Locke RG, Wolfson MR, Schaffer TH, *et al.* Inadvertent administration of positive end-distending pressure during nasal cannula flow. *Pediatrics* 1993; 91: 135–138.

78. Lemyre B, Davies PG, De Paoli AG. Nasal intermittent positive pressure ventilation (NIPPV) versus nasal continuous positive airway pressure (NCPAP) for apnea of prematurity. *The Cochrane Database of Systematic Reviews* 2002; Issue 1. Art. No: CD002272. DOI:10.1002/14651858.CD002272.

79. De Paoli AG, Davis PG, Faber B, Morley CJ. Devices and pressure sources for administration of nasal continuous positive airway pressure (NCPAP) in preterm neonates. *The Cochrane Database of Systematic Reviews* 2002, Issue 3. Art, No.: CD2977. DOI:10.1002/14651858.CD002977.

80. Migliori C, Motta M, Angeli A, Chirico G. Nasal bilevel vs. positive airway pressure in preterm infants. *Pediatr Pulmonol* 2005; 40: 426–430.

81. Aghai ZH, Saslow JG, Hakhia t, et al. Synchronized nasal intermittent positive pressure ventilation (SNIPPV) decreases work of breathing (WOB) in premature infants with respiratory distress syndrome (RDS) compared to nasal continuous positive airway pressure (NCPAP). *Pediatr Pulmonol* 2006; 41: 875–881.

82. Ali N, Claure N, Alegria X, D'Ugard C, Organero R, Bancalari E. Effects of non-invasive pressure support ventilation (NI-PSV) on ventilation and respiratory effort in very low birth weight infants. *Pediatr Pulmonol* 2007; 42: 704–710.

83. The HiFi Study Group. High-frequency oscillatory ventilation compared with conventional mechanical ventilation in the treatment of respiratory failure in preterm infants. *N Engl J Med* 1989; 320: 88–93.

84. Cam BV, Tuan DT, Fonsmark L, *et al.* Randomized comparison of oxygen mask treatment vs nasal continuous airway pressure in Dengue shock syndrome with acute respiratory failure. *J Tropical Pediatr* 2002; 48: 335–339.

85. Smailes TS. Noninvasive positive pressure ventilation in burns. *Burns* 2002; 28: 795–801.

86. Bach JR, Hunt D, Horton JA. Traumatic tetraplegia. Noninvasive respiratory management in the acute setting (case study). *Am J Phys Med Rehabil* 2002; 81: 792–797.

87. Bach JR, Sabhaewal S. High pulmonary risk scoliosis surgery. Role of non-invasive ventilation and related techniques. *J Spinal Disord Tech* 2005; 18: 527–530.

88. Monin PJP, Cashore WJ, Hakanson DO, Oh W. Assisted ventilation of the neonate – comparison between positive and negative respirators. *Pediatr Res* 1976; 10: 464.

89. Shekerdemian LS, Bush A, Shore DF, *et al.* Cardiorespiratory response to negative pressure ventilation after tetralogy of Fallot repair: a hemodynamic tool for patients with low output states. *J Am Coll Cardiol* 1999; 33: 549–555.

90. Samuels MP, Raine J, Wright T. Continuous negative extrathoracic pressure in neonatal respiratory failure. *Paediatrics* 1996; 98: 1154–1160.

91. Telford K, Waters L, Vyas H, Manktelow BN, Draper ES, Marlow N. Outcome after neonatal continuous negative-pressure ventilation: follow-up assessment. *Lancet* 2006; 367: 1080–1085.

92. Klonin H, Bowman B, Peters M. Negative pressure ventilation via chest cuirass to decrease ventilator-associated complications in infants with acute respiratory failure: a case series. *Respir Care* 2000; 45: 486–490.

93. Al-balkhi A, Klonin H, Marinaki K, *et al.* Review of treatment of bronchiolitis related apnoea in two centers. *Arch Dis Child* 2005; 90: 288–291.

94. Shah PS, Ohlsson A, Shah JP. Continuous negative extrathoracic pressure or continuous positive pressure for acute hypoxemic respiratory failure in children. *The Cochrane Database of Systematic Reviews* 2008, Issue 3, Art. No.: CD003699.pub2. DOI:10.1002/14651858.CD003699.pub3.

95. Hartmann H, Jawad MH, Noyes J, *et al.* Negative extrathoracic pressure ventilation in central hypoventilation syndrome. *Archives of Disease in Childhood* 1994; 70: 418.23.

96. Wells DA, Gillies D, Fitzgerald DA. Positioning for acute respiratory distress in hospitalised infants and children. *Cochrane Database Syst Rev* 2005; 2: CD003645.

97.   Curley MA, Hibberd PL, Fineman LD, *et al.* Effect of prone positioning on clinical outcomes in children with acute lung injury: A randomized controlled trial. *JAMA* 2005; 294: 229–237.
98.   Miske LJ, Hickey EM, Kolb SM, Weiner DJ, Panitch HB. Use of the mechanical In-Exsufflator in pediatric patients with neuromuscular disease and impaired cough. *Chest* 2004; 125: 1406–1412.
99.   Bach JR, Ishikawa Y, Kim H. Prevention of pulmonary morbidity for patients with Duchenne muscular dystrophy. *Chest* 1997; 112: 1024–1028.
100. Chatwin M, Ross E, Hart N, *et al.* Cough augmentation with mechanical insufflation/exsufflation in patients with neuromuscular weakness. *Eur Respir J* 2003; 21: 502–508.

CHAPTER 9

NIV: use during the pre-hospital management of patients with acute respiratory failure

F. Thys*, S. Spencer*, F. Verschuren*, N. Delvau*, J. Roeseler#, F. Templier¶

*Emergency Dept. and #Physical Therapy, Cliniques Universitaires Saint-Luc, Université Catholique de Louvain, Brussels, Belgium and ¶SAMU 92, SMUR Garches, Hôpital Raymond Poincaré, Hôpitaux de Paris, Paris, France.

Correspondence: F. Thys, Service des Urgences, Cliniques Universitaires Saint-Luc, Université Catholique de Louvain, Avenue Hippocrate 10, B-1200 Brussels, Belgium. Fax: 32 27641620; E-mail: frederic.thys@uclouvain.be

Introduction

Over the past 20 or so years, the relevance of noninvasive ventilation (NIV) modes, for the management of acute respiratory failure (ARF) in intensive care, has been demonstrated in reducing both intubation rate and mortality. Selected indications for NIV are now widely accepted. Considering acute pulmonary oedema, associated or not with hypercapnia, NIV reduces the intubation rate, probably mortality too, with a similar benefit when using continuous positive airway pressure (CPAP) or bilevel positive airway pressure (BiPAP) [1]. The use of BiPAP decreases mortality associated with ARF in chronic obstructive pulmonary disease (COPD) patients, while CPAP has failed to show any benefits in this group of patients. For all other causes of ARF, indications as to the use of NIV are still controversial or under trial.

Several clinical trials have shown the feasibility and the efficacy of NIV in the early management of patients with ARF in the emergency department [2–7]. Furthermore, a series of clinical trials performed in an emergency room setting showed a positive impact of NIV on clinical improvement and gas exchange and also a reduction of endotracheal intubations [2, 4, 8, 9]. Two randomised controlled trials specifically assessed the efficacy of NIV in preventing endotracheal intubation [10, 11]. Those two trials had inclusion criteria for a variety of ARF causes. One study showed a 15% rate of intubation [10], while the second showed a high rate of treatment failure in the BiPAP group with 44% of intubation and a higher in-hospital mortality [11]. This shows the danger of an indiscriminate use of NIV. Actually, the analysis of the latter study demonstrates that the lack of relevant inclusion criteria, the choice of an inappropriate ventilator/patient interface and delayed intubation in cases of BiPAP treatment failure are always detrimental for the patient [12]. However, in the current context, for properly selected patients, NIV is successfully used on a daily basis in many emergency departments, allowing a significant reduction of endotracheal intubation rate, length of in-hospital stay, and mortality.

Alternatively, to the best of the present authors' knowledge, there is no evidence today to support the use of NIV in the treatment of ARF caused by an acute cardiogenic hypercapnic pulmonary oedema or secondary to an exacerbation of COPD in the context of pre-hospital care. Empirically, the possibility of treating a patient with ARF

Eur Respir Mon, 2008, 41, 133–142. Printed in UK - all rights reserved. Copyright ERS Journals Ltd 2008; European Respiratory Monograph; ISSN 1025-448x.

promptly, with an effective approach, should further increase the benefits of NIV and, thus, further improve patients' outcome. In the pre-hospital setting, endotracheal intubation (ETI) is often difficult and associated with a high morbidity and mortality; even if this analysis must be related to the operator's experience [13–15]. Avoiding ETI in the pre-hospital life support could have a significant, relevant and very positive clinical impact. However, the use of NIV in pre-hospital life support requires various constraints to be solved with regard to the specific environment, the equipment and the operators' training. It is, therefore, paramount to know whether it is useful to offer NIV management in this setting.

In this chapter, a summary of the currently available studies is given and expanded with the present authors' own expertise in addressing this question. It must be mentioned that, at the time of writing, searching the international database MEDLINE, 2,613 references to NIV were found, among which, only 117 are related to its use in emergency medicine and only 12 concern pre-hospital care.

Pre-hospital use of CPAP and acute cardiogenic pulmonary oedema

Several relevant randomised control trials were conducted within emergency departments and looked at the management of acute cardiogenic pulmonary oedema [9, 16–21]. There is currently strong evidence to support the use of CPAP for this indication, showing that its use decreases the rate of intubation and improves survival rates, even in the elderly population. There is no satisfactory evidence to encourage the use of BiPAP for this indication, even when confronted with an acute cardiogenic hypercapnic pulmonary oedema.

The few published trials performed in the pre-hospital setting for the use of CPAP in the management of acute cardiogenic pulmonary oedema often offer only low-level evidence. Five uncontrolled nonrandomised observational trials, including a total of ~715 patients suffering from acute cardiogenic pulmonary oedema were published. Despite the low level of evidence, all the results tend towards similar conclusions when using CPAP in pre-hospital care [22–25] and sometimes by paramedics [22, 23, 26]: clinical improvement and gas-exchange improvement. Measured in four trials, intubation rates varied between 0 and 8.9% in pre-hospital settings and between 10 and 37% in the first few hours [22, 23, 25]; these values were close to in-hospital trials rates (0–33%), with the same disparity [1]. The highest rate of endotracheal intubation was found in one of the two trials, in which paramedics used NIV. Only one of these trials mentioned that CPAP was on site immediately and continuously, including during handling and transfer on the stretcher [25]. When detailed, drugs given in association with NIV did not include a high dose of nitrates, even though nitrates are included in the current recommended treatment [27]. No adverse effects due to CPAP were reported. One of these trials, which was prospective monocentric and nonrandomised, compared the CPAP group with a control group. Knowing the bias and the limits of this methodology, a significant benefit of NIV management with regard to the intubation rate is still observed; 8.9% (CPAP group) *versus* 23.2% (control group) and also in terms of respiratory rate, cardiac frequency and dyspnoea score [26]. Following a first unpublished pilot study [28], a recently published randomised trial including 124 patients compared two different approaches: 15 mins of CPAP followed by standard drug therapy for the subsequent 15 mins (group A) *versus* 15 mins of standard drug therapy followed by 15 mins of association with CPAP (group B) [29]. A reduction of the intubation rate, a lower frequency of resort to inotropes and a decrease of mortality were significantly (p≤0.005) in favour of group A. The applied inspiratory oxygen fraction (F_{I,O_2}) was not specified. In the pilot study, it was limited to 35%, such that F_{I,O_2} was unlikely to be adequate for group B patients. CPAP was systematically interrupted at 30 min, irrespective of the clinical course of the patient, without explanation from authors, and clinical deterioration was observed in both groups, although worse for group B patients. The medication used was not detailed. That study, with a proper methodology, is the first pre-hospital randomised trial and it carries an essential message about the importance of early management of acute cardiogenic pulmonary oedema with CPAP, in pre-hospital care, to reduce both endotracheal intubation rate and secondary morbidity. This message is even more relevant when addressing patients' management by Emergency Medical Services-type systems, considering the high failure rate of intubation by paramedics. Surprisingly, in that trial, lower in-hospital mortality in the early CPAP group was observed, without explanation, despite a comparable clinical status on admission.

In conclusion, all these data, associated with the results of in-hospital trials, support the use of CPAP for patients suffering from acute cardiogenic pulmonary oedema, with a major benefit, whether in the hospital or pre-hospital setting.

Pre-hospital use of BIPAP and COPD exacerbation

Based on the available literature, it is correct to recommend the early use of BiPAP for management of patients with COPD exacerbation in the emergency room; under certain conditions, this could be extended to hypercapnic ARFs [10, 11, 30–33]. Current evidence suggests that the early use of BiPAP improves clinical parameters and reduces recourse to invasive ventilation, morbidity and length of in-hospital stay. However, identifying patients who have the best-expected benefit is vital. Patients with an arterial pH <7.30 seemed to be the ones who benefit most from this approach [34].

The first two studies published on the pre-hospital use of BiPAP are not very convincing (due to a very low level of evidence). In the first one, North-American paramedics applied BiPAP for acute cardiogenic pulmonary oedema, once in the ambulance and for 15 mins only [35]. The principal benefits were the ease for the rescue team and the absence of intervention time increase. The second study talked about the use of a noninvasive mode of ventilation on seven patients with acute respiratory failure by a French pre-hospital team [36]. Gas-exchange parameters appeared to improve, but arterial pH and carbon dioxide remained unchanged. One patient was intubated before admission due to a rapid deterioration despite NIV. The ventilator was a second-generation pneumatic type, without expiratory spirometry, not delivering a proper spontaneous ventilation mode with inspiratory support (controlled cycles with a set pressure), the pressure elevation gradient was set and low, with a minimum F_{I,O_2} of ~60%. A German randomised prospective monocentric trial investigating patients with ARF caused by acute cardiogenic pulmonary oedema recruited 23 patients and compared standard treatment with standard treatment plus BiPAP with oxygen saturation on admission as the primary end-point. The BiPAP group showed a sharper improvement in their pre-hospital arterial oxygen saturation measured by pulse oximetry (S_{p,O_2}). This trial is more a feasibility assessment of this approach as it does not compare BiPAP with the recommended pre-hospital management (*i.e.* CPAP). Regarding that study, the present authors regret the poor choice of primary end-point and a drug therapy (*i.e.* low dose of sublingual nitrates), which does reflect current recommendations [37]. A recent French monocentric prospective observational study recruited three groups of patients (acute cardiogenic pulmonary oedema, COPD exacerbation and other causes of ARF) initially sorted on treatment history and clinical criteria. In 138 patients, the intubation rate (pre- and in-hospital) was 26%, significantly higher for the "other ARF" group [38]. That observational and nonrandomised trial confirmed the feasibility of pre-hospital BiPAP use with a failure rate similar to rates measured during in-hospital studies. Therefore, it is highly likely that early BiPAP use is beneficial. The main reason for NIV failure is when the cause of ARF is neither COPD exacerbation nor acute cardiogenic pulmonary oedema; another reason is when there is an audible air leakage. None of these trials properly assessed the benefit–risk ratio for BiPAP use in the challenging pre-hospital setting. Considering the weakness of these studies, it seems too early to recommend BiPAP for routine pre-hospital use, even if this technique holds promise when applied to selected patients by experienced operators.

Specific constraints of pre-hospital NIV use

As a reminder, in the emergency room, the time required by the medical team to start BiPAP ventilation is not always compatible with the ever-increasing number of patients to treat simultaneously. In each emergency room, the annual number of patients eligible for BiPAP is not always high enough to warrant initial and continuous training for the medical staff. Resorting to a downstream hospital ward, which is able to admit a patient on NIV from the emergency room, varies widely, which in turn creates a high variability of the offer–demand ratio.

The pre-hospital setting is a very challenging environment; however, the medical team is dedicated to a single patient. This has a very positive impact on NIV set-up. In the present authors' experience, the handling and transfer of a patient during pre-hospital management is an important cause of air leakage and mal-positioning of the patient–ventilator interface. This is less of a problem with free-flow CPAP. The stretcher-handling phase puts the patient at risk, it causes added stress and fatigue and it is a suboptimal situation should rapid-sequence induction intubation be required.

Equipment: selection criteria

CPAP equipment

A CPAP device should not increase the breathing work and must allow maintenance of a positive inspiratory pressure [39]. The maximum FI,O_2 delivered needs to be high. In 2001, the French Anaesthesiology and Intensive Care Association (SFAR) recommended that any pre-hospital intervention vehicle should, as standard on-board equipment, have a device allowing spontaneous ventilation with a continuous positive expiratory pressure to be performed, without giving any other details as to specifications [40]. Recent recommendations following the Scientific Sessions of the French pre-hospital intervention teams (SAMU) advise the use of a no-valve free-flow system [41]. Whether regarding flow generators using the Venturi effect (Whisperflow[TM]; Philips Respironics, Murrysville, PA, USA) or at the Boussignac CPAP device[TM] (Vygon, Ecouen, France), they have the required performances and specifications for pre-hospital use [42–45]. Pressure modulation with flow generators requires multiple valves; by contrast, the Boussignac CPAP device[TM] offers easy modulation and monitoring. Flow generators use a lot of oxygen, often compelling operators to lower the FI,O_2. In some studies, because of high generator burn, FI,O_2 was limited to 35%. FI,O_2 delivered by the Boussignac CPAP device[TM] is, in comparison, much higher and oxygen consumption is lower [46]. The poor FI,O_2 modulation with this device is not an issue when treating cases of acute cardiogenic pulmonary oedema. To resort to a multiple-valve generator, even a sophisticated one, does seem justified. The more complex operational application is not rewarded by any benefits in terms of performance. Some devices even increase breathing work (*i.e.* through ineffective inspiratory trigger, hard-to-switch valves, failure to maintain inspiratory pressure).

BiPAP equipment

The device used must have the same performances as an intensive-care ventilator. Essential specifications are: appropriate ventilation mode, perfect inspiratory and expiratory triggers, fast pressurization capability with an adjustable gradient, wide range of FI,O_2, air-leakage balance and expiratory spirometry. For pre-hospital applications, the ventilator has to be a portable light-weight device with long-duration operational autonomy (with regard to power and medical gases). Home turbine-type or NIV-dedicated ventilators are an alternative. They usually meet pre-hospital requirements, especially modern devices [47, 48], even if this is still under discussion [49]. Second-generation pneumatic ventilators are not efficient enough to deliver satisfactory NIV. The new, versatile ventilators designed for ventilation in emergency medicine (Élisée 250^{TM}, Saime, Savigny le Temple, France; Oxylog 3000^{TM}, Dräger Medical, Lübeck, Germany; Newport HT50^{TM}, Newport Medical Instruments, Newport Beach, CA, USA) are developing the pre-hospital market. Turbine technology seems more appropriate. The usability of these ventilators by emergency physicians must be taken into account and, in this respect, they are not all equivalent [50].

Operator's training

Some studies demonstrate the difficulty, in the pre-hospital setting, of making an appropriate aetiologic diagnosis when confronted with a patient with ARF. This is an even bigger challenge for paramedics [51] and an essential step in identifying NIV indications and, as a consequence, avoiding inappropriate use of this technique.

NIV training is generally insufficient among members of pre-hospital intervention teams; this has been shown for BiPAP use [41]. There is a strong demand for teaching, especially hands-on training. In the present authors' experience, the learning curve is much faster for CPAP than for BiPAP. In CPAP clinical trials, the duration of the prerequisite training varied from 2 h to a day whereas, in BiPAP training, basic physiology reminders applied to mechanical ventilation are required. For the theoretical aspects and practical exercises, a minimum of 10 h is necessary. The operational implementation of BiPAP use, by an initially inexperienced team, requires significant coaching and a continuous training scheme.

The present authors believe that training is the main limiting factor for the application of this technique, preventing the routine use of NIV in pre-hospital care.

Inventory of the "real world"

In 2002, in Belgium, NIV was used in 49% of emergency departments. When it was not used, declared reasons included lack of adequate equipment (71%), lack of training (32.7%), and lack of time for the medical or nursing staff (22.8%), despite the fact that in these units, only 3.8% of doctors had doubts about the efficacy of NIV. When this mode of ventilation was used, supervision of patients under NIV during the first hour was assumed by a doctor–nurse tandem (54.5%), by a nurse only (19.6%) or by a doctor only (8.6%). NIV was continued for >4 h in a third of the cases. Devices used were either intensive-care ventilators (21.7%) or home mechanical ventilators (54.5%) or both types (23.9%) [52]. CPAP use in pre-hospital care remains marginal. The same applies to BiPAP which, when used, reflects the in-hospital experience of the team.

In 2001, in France, 40% of pre-hospital intervention vehicles had a CPAP device on-board; two thirds of these were inappropriate and failed to meet pre-hospital requirements. One in five intervention teams stated that they were able to provide NIV, two thirds with a second-generation pneumatic ventilator, known to be inadequate for this purpose, and one third with an intensive-care ventilator, not designed for portability [53]. In 2006, a rise in the proportion of vehicles carrying an NIV device was noted, but not always with the efficiency required for BiPAP use. Among the 69 teams interviewed, 79% declared having at least one on-board CPAP device (85% using a Boussignac CPAP system^{TM} and 64% using the CPAP mode on a pneumatic ventilator) and 56% of them said they had a ventilator able to provide BiPAP (66% with a second-generation pneumatic ventilator). Half of them could provide both CPAP and BiPAP and 15% had no NIV device. For those using NIV in the pre-hospital setting, operational implementation varied widely, indications were not always appropriate and the NIV systems used were not always adequate and validated.

Potential recommendations

In- and pre-hospital trials for the application of CPAP in the treatment of acute cardiogenic pulmonary oedema show a major expected benefit for the patient. Additionally, its usability by emergency physicians is very good, even in the pre-hospital environment. Therefore, the present authors recommend that all doctors should be trained in the use of CPAP in the pre-hospital setting, with free-flow devices and following clear clinical guidelines like those recently recommended [41]: Immediate CPAP application when confronted with a moderate to severe acute cardiogenic pulmonary oedema (dyspnoea with accessory muscles activity and/or respiratory rate >35 cycles·min^{-1} and/or an Sp,O_2 <90% when applying a reservoir mask with high-flow oxygen, the standard drug therapy must be started simultaneously); and delayed CPAP application when confronted with an initially mild acute cardiogenic pulmonary oedema not improving under standard drug therapy.

COPD exacerbation seems to be an interesting indication for the use of NIV in the pre-hospital setting. However, the benefit–risk ratio for BiPAP use in this context is still unknown. Further clinical trials are necessary before any recommendations could be made with regard to routine pre-hospital application, not to mention the difficulty of making a correct diagnosis prior to the identification of an appropriate NIV indication. In the meantime, it seems reasonable to implement BiPAP with highly-trained teams using proper equipment. When on-board gas exchange analysers are not available, the present authors recommend obtaining an arterial blood sample before BiPAP use, in order to measure the pH on admission to the emergency room, validating the indication and allowing for biological follow-up.

Prior to the implementation of NIV in the pre-hospital setting or to its implementation in the emergency room, the following prerequisites are essential: trained staff with an experience of CPAP or BiPAP use; available equipment and staff at all time; and quick access to intubation if necessary and adequate monitoring. Local guidelines must be designed to avoid inappropriate use of NIV and for the early identification of NIV failure avoiding detrimental intubation delays [12, 54].

It is paramount, in the pre-hospital setting, to identify quickly patients who will not improve under NIV. It as been shown that early assessment (after 30–60 mins) following NIV application, makes it possible, based on simple criteria, to identify potential failures of the technique. Thus, a patient under NIV, with a respiratory rate >20 cycles·min^{-1} or with a pH ≤ 7.35, has a high risk of requiring endotracheal intubation. A Glasgow coma scale score <13 after 1 h of NIV must also be considered as a sign of inappropriate NIV indication or NIV failure [32, 55]. It is even more important to take all these elements into account when talking of NIV in the pre-hospital setting; they must be integrated in the context of handling and transport of an unstable patient with ARF.

Conclusions

An early start of efficient management is vital when treating ARF. NIV has its role in this context for specific indications. Theoretically, its operational implementation in the pre-hospital setting should bring additional benefits with regard to the outcome for ARF patients.

Pre-hospital CPAP use is highly relevant in the management of patients with acute cardiogenic pulmonary oedema. Availability of efficient and portable devices, as well as short training time to use them properly, justifies the use of CPAP in the pre-hospital setting. Conversely, it is too early to recommend routine BiPAP use, even if this technique, mastered and for appropriate indications, is promising. Early identification of NIV failure is performed through simple criteria. Development of strict clinical guidelines should be emphasised in order to provide NIV to a larger patient population when indicated.

Training and experience of operators are the current limiting factors of this approach. Technical ventilation equipment constraints are reduced with the arrival of new ventilators, which are ergonomic, efficient and with a better operational autonomy.

It is important and challenging to design multicentric randomised trials to assess if it useful or pointless to perform noninvasive ventilation in the pre-hospital setting. In the present authors' experience, pre-hospital noninvasive ventilation use becomes more beneficial as the distance between the patient's location and the hospital is greater.

Summary

An early start of efficient management is vital when treating acute respiratory failure. Noninvasive ventilation (NIV) has its role in this context, for specific indications. Currently, NIV has not yet been established in pre-hospital emergency medicine. Training and experience of operators are the current limiting factors of this approach. Technical ventilation equipment constraints are reduced with the arrival of new ventilators, as they are more ergonomic and efficient and have a better operational autonomy. Recognising the pathophysiology of acute respiratory insufficiency, treatment with NIV seems superior in comparison to treatment with oxygen and medication only for specific indications. The advantages of NIV may lead to reduced morbidity and mortality, as long as attention is paid to possible contraindications. In the present chapter, the authors propose a summary of the currently available studies and confront it with their expertise, helping to clear up this question.

Keywords: Acute respiratory failure, continuous positive airway pressure, noninvasive ventilation, out-of-hospital emergency management, pre-hospital setting.

References

1. Masip J, Roque M, Sánchez B, Fernández R, Subirana M, Expósito JA. Noninvasive ventilation in acute cardiogenic pulmonary edema: systematic review and meta-analysis. *JAMA* 2005; 294: 3124–3130.
2. Pollack C Jr, Torres MT, Alexander L. Feasibility study of the use of bilevel positive airway pressure for respiratory support in emergency department. *Ann Emerg Med* 1996; 27: 189–192.
3. Sacchetti AD, Harris RH, Paston C, Hernandez Z. Bi-level positive pressure support system use in acute congestive congestive heart failure: preliminary case series. *Acad Emerg Med* 1995; 2: 714–718.
4. Thys F, Roeseler J, Delaere S, *et al.* Two-level non-invasive positive pressure ventilation in the initial treatment of acute respiratory failure in an emergency department. *Eur J Emerg Med* 1999; 6: 207–214.
5. Nava S, Carbone G, DiBattista N, *et al.* Noninvasive ventilation in cardiogenic pulmonary edema: a multicenter randomized trial. *Am J Respir Crit Care Med* 2003; 168: 1432–1437.
6. Crane SD, Elliott MW, Gilligan P, Richards K, Gray AJ. Randomised controlled comparison of continuous positive airways pressure, bilevel non-invasive ventilation, and standard treatment in emergency department patients with acute cardiogenic pulmonary oedema. *Emerg Med J* 2004; 21: 155–161.
7. Yosefy C, Hay E, Ben-Barak A, *et al.* BiPAP ventilation as assistance for patients presenting with respiratory distress in the department of emergency medicine. *Am J Respir Med* 2003; 2: 343–347.
8. Poponick JM, Renston JP, Bennett RP, Emerman CL. Use of a ventilatory support system (BiPAP) for acute respiratory failure in the emergency department. *Chest* 1999; 116: 166–171.
9. Park M, Sangean MC, Volpe Mde S, *et al.* Randomized, prospective trial of oxygen, continuous positive airway pressure, and bilevel positive airway pressure by face mask in acute cardiogenic pulmonary edema. *Crit Care Med* 2004; 32: 2407–2415.
10. Thys F, Roeseler J, Reynaert M, Liistro G, Rodenstein DO. Noninvasive ventilation for acute respiratory failure: a prospective randomised placebo-controlled trial. *Eur Respir J* 2002; 20: 545–555.
11. Wood KA, Lewis L, Von Harz B, Kollef MH. The use of noninvasive positive pressure ventilation in the emergency department: results of a randomized clinical trial. *Chest* 1998; 113: 1339–1346.
12. Sottiaux T. Noninvasive positive pressure ventilation in the emergency room. *Chest* 1999; 115: 301–303.
13. Guyette FX, Greenwood MJ, Neubecker D, Roth R, Wang HE. Alternate airways in the prehospital setting (resource document to NAEMSP position statement). *Prehosp Emerg Care* 2007; 11: 56–61.
14. Combes X, Jabre P, Jbeili C, *et al.* Prehospital standardization of medical airway management: incidence and risk factors of difficult airway. *Acad Emerg Med* 2006; 13: 828–834.
15. Newton A, Ratchford A, Khan I. Incidence of adverse events during prehospital rapid sequence intubation: a review of one year on the London Helicopter Emergency Medical Service. *J Trauma* 2008; 64: 487–492.
16. Mehta S, Jay GD, Woolard RH, *et al.* Randomized, prospective trial of bilevel *versus* continuous positive airway pressure in acute pulmonary edema. *Crit Care Med* 1997; 25: 620–628.
17. Crane SD, Elliott MW, Gilligan P, Richards K, Gray AJ. Randomised controlled comparison of continuous positive airways pressure, bilevel non-invasive ventilation, and standard treatment in emergency department patients with acute cardiogenic pulmonary oedema. *Emerg Med J* 2004; 21: 155–161.
18. Cross AM, Cameron P, Kierce M, Ragg M, Kelly AM. Non-invasive ventilation in acute respiratory failure: a randomised comparison of continuous positive airway pressure and bi-level positive airway pressure. *Emerg Med J* 2003; 20: 531–534.
19. Bellone A, Monari A, Cortellaro F, Vettorello M, Arlati S, Coen D. Myocardial infarction rate in acute pulmonary edema: noninvasive pressure support ventilation versus continuous positive airway pressure. *Crit Care Med* 2004; 32: 1860–1865.

20. L'Her E, Duquesne F, Girou E, *et al.* Noninvasive continuous positive airway pressure in elderly cardiogenic pulmonary edema patients. *Intensive Care Med* 2004; 30: 882–888.

21. Bellone A, Vettorello M, Monari A, Cortellaro F, Coen D. Noninvasive pressure support ventilation *vs.* continuous positive airway pressure in acute hypercapnic pulmonary edema. *Intensive Care Med* 2005; 31: 807–811.

22. Gardtman M, Waagstein L, Karlsson T, Herlitz J. Has an intensified treatment in the ambulance of patients with acute severe left heart failure improved the outcome? *Eur J Emerg Med* 2000; 7: 15–24.

23. Kosowsky JM, Stephanides SL, Branson RD, Sayre MR. Prehospital use of continuous positive airway pressure (CPAP) for presumed pulmonary edema: a preliminary case series. *Prehosp Emerg Care* 2001; 5: 190–196.

24. Kallio T, Kuisma M, Alaspää A, Rosenberg PH. The use of prehospital continuous positive airway pressure treatment in presumed acute severe pulmonary edema. *Prehosp Emerg Care* 2003; 7: 209–213.

25. Templier F, Dolveck F, Baer M, Chauvin M, Fletcher D. 'Boussignac' continuous positive airway pressure system: practical use in a prehospital medical care unit. *Eur J Emerg Med* 2003; 10: 87–93.

26. Hubble MW, Richards ME, Jarvis R, Millikan T, Young D. Effectiveness of prehospital continuous positive airway pressure in the management of acute pulmonary edema. *Prehosp Emerg Care* 2006; 10: 430–439.

27. Cotter G, Metzkor E, Kaluski E, *et al.* Randomised trial of high-dose isosorbide dinitrate plus low-dose furosemide versus high-dose furosemide plus low-dose isosorbide dinitrate in severe pulmonary oedema. *Lancet* 1998; 351: 389–393.

28. Plaisance P, Adnet F, Degardin F, *et al.* [Benefit of continuous positive airway pressure (CPAP) in the treatment of acute cardiogenic pulmonary edema in out-of-hospital management] Intérêt de la pression intra-thoracique positive permanente au masque (CPAP) dans le traitement des oedèmes aigus du poumon d'origine cardiogénique en médecine pré-hospitalière. *Ann Fr Anesth Réanim* 1994; 13: Suppl., R99.

29. Plaisance P, Pirracchio R, Berton C, Vicaut E, Payen D. A randomized study of out-of-hospital continuous postive airway pressure for acute cardiogenic pulmonary oedema: physiological and clinical effects. *Eur Heart J* 2007; 28: 2895–2901.

30. Ram FS, Picot J, Lightowler J, Wedzicha JA. Non-invasive positive pressure ventilation for treatment of respiratory failure due to exacerbations of chronic obstructive pulmonary disease. *Cochrane Database Syst Rev* 2004; 3: CD004104.

31. Celikel T, Sungur M, Ceyhan B, Karakurt S. Comparison of noninvasive positive pressure ventilation with standard medical therapy in hypercapnic acute respiratory failure. *Chest* 1998; 114: 1636–1642.

32. Poponick JM, Renston JP, Bennet RP, Emerman CL. Use of a ventilatory support system (BiPAP) for acute respiratory failure in the emergency department. *Chest* 1999; 116: 166–171.

33. Collaborative Research Group of Noninvasive Mechanical Ventilation for Chronic Obstructive Disease. Early use of non-invasive positive pressure ventilation for acute exacerbations of chronic obstructive pulmonary disease: a multicenter randomized controlled trial. *Chin Med J* 2005; 118: 2034–2040.

34. Keenan SP, Powers CE, McCormack DG. Noninvasive positive-pressure ventilation in patients with milder chronic obstructive pulmonary disease exacerbations: a randomized controlled trial. *Respir Care* 2005; 50: 610–616.

35. Craven RA, Singletary N, Bosken L, Sewell E, Payne M, Lipsey R. Use of bilevel positive airway pressure in out-of-hospital patients. *Acad Emerg Med* 2000; 7: 1065–1068.

36. Fort PA, Boussarie C, Hilbert G, Habachi M. [Prehospital noninvasive ventilation. Study of importance and feasibility (7 cases)]. *Presse Med* 2002; 31: 1886–1889.

37. Weitz G, Struck J, Zonak A, Balnus S, Perras B, Dodt C. Prehospital noninvasive pressure support ventilation for acute pulmonary edema. *Eur J Emerg Med* 2007; 14: 276–279.

38. Bruge P, Jabre P, Dru M, *et al.* An observational study of noninvasive positive pressure ventilation in an out-of-hospital setting. *Am J Emerg Med* 2008; 26: 165–169.

39. Gherini S, Peters RM, Virgilio RW. Mechanical work on the lungs and work of breathing with positive end-expiratory pressure and continuous positive airway pressure. *Chest* 1979; 76: 251–256.

40. [Consensus statement on the modalities of out-of-hospital care in management of patients in serious condition] Recommandations concernant les modalités de la prise en charge médicalisée préhospitalière des patients en état grave. Paris, Sfar Eds, 2001.

41. Templier F, Thys F, Durand JS, Jardel B. [Oxygen therapy and ventilatory assistance] Oxygénothérapie et supports ventilatoires. *In:* [Acute Dyspnea] Dyspnée aiguë. Journées scientifiques de Samu de France, Deauville 2004. Paris, SFEM editions, 2005; pp. 87–158.

42. Gibney RT, Wilson RS, Pontoppidan H. Comparison of work breathing on high gas flow and demand valve continuous airway pressure systems. *Chest* 1982; 82: 692–695.

43. Beydon L, Chassé M, Harf A, Lemaire F. Inspiratory work of breathing during spontaneous ventilation using demand valves and continuous flow systems. *Am Rev Respir Dis* 1988; 138: 300–304.

44. Fu C, Caruso P, Lucatto JJ, de Paula Schettino GP, de Souza R, Carvalho CR. Comparison of two flow generators with a noninvasive ventilator to deliver continuous positive airway pressure: a test lung study. *Intensive Care Med* 2005; 31: 1587–1591.

45. Leman P, Greene S, Whelan K, Legassick T. Simple lightweight disposable continuous positive airways pressure mask to effectively treat acute pulmonary oedema: randomized controlled trial. *Emerg Med Australas* 2005; 17: 224–230.

46. Templier F, Dolveck F, Baer M, Chauvin M, Fletcher D. [Laboratory testing measurement of FIO_2 delivered by Boussignac CPAP system with an input of 100% oxygen]. *Ann Fr Anesth Reanim* 2003; 22: 103–107.

47. Patel RG, Petrini MF. Respiratory muscle performance, pulmonary mechanics, and gas exchange between the BiPAP S/T-D system and the Servo Ventilator 900C with bilevel positive airway pressure ventilation following gradual pressure support weaning. *Chest* 1998; 114: 1390–1396.

48. Battisti A, Tassaux D, Janssens JP, Michotte JB, Jaber S, Jolliet P. Performance characteristics of 10 home mechanical ventilators in pressure-support mode: a comparative bench study. *Chest* 2005; 127: 1784–1792.

49. Schönhofer B, Sortor-Leger S. Equipment needs for noninvasive mechanical ventilation. *Eur Respir J* 2002; 20: 1029–1036.

50. Templier F, Miroux P, Dolveck F, *et al.* Evaluation of the ventilator-user interface of 2 new advanced compact transport ventilators. *Respir Care* 2007; 52: 1701–1709.

51. Taylor DM, Bernard SA, Masci K, MacBean CE, Kennedy MP. Prehospital noninvasive ventilation: a viable treatment option in the urban setting. *Prehosp Emerg Care* 2008; 12: 42–45.

52. Vanpee D, Delaunois L, Lheureux P, *et al.* Survey of non-invasive ventilation for acute exacerbation of chronic obstructive pulmonary disease patients in emergency departments in Belgium. *Eur J Emerg Med* 2002; 9: 217–224.

53. Douge G, Allaire H, Leroux C, *et al.* [Ventilatory support devices used in out-of-hospital care: National Survey] Matériels de support ventilatoire utilisés par les SMUR: Enquête nationale. *Rev SAMU* 2003; 351–355.

54. Elliott MW, Confalonieri M, Nava S. Where to perform noninvasive ventilation? *Eur Respir J* 2002; 19: 1159–1166.

55. Merlani PG, Pasquina P, Granier JM, Treggiari M, Rutschmann O, Ricou B. Factors associated with failure of noninvasive positive pressure ventilation in the emergency department. *Acad Emerg Med* 2005; 12: 1206–1215.

CHAPTER 10

NIV for weaning from mechanical ventilation and post-extubation ARF

C. Girault

Medical Intensive Care Unit, Rouen University Hospital Charles Nicolle and GRHV Research Group, UPRES-EA 3830 IFRMP.23, Institute for Biomedical Research, Rouen University Hospital, Rouen, France.

Correspondence: C. Girault, Service de Réanimation Médicale, Hôpital Charles Nicolle, Centre Hospitalier Universitaire-Hôpitaux de Rouen, 1 rue de Germont, 76031 Rouen, France. Fax: 33 232888314; E-mail: Christophe.Girault@chu-rouen.fr

Introduction

Due to its clinical efficacy in the initial management of acute respiratory failure (ARF) [1], noninvasive ventilation (NIV) has been widely used in intensive care units (ICUs) during the past 15 yrs, particularly in France [2]. At the same time, indications of NIV have been extended to the period following intubation, first for difficult weaning/ extubation from endotracheal mechanical ventilation (ETMV) and, secondly, for the management of post-extubation acute respiratory failure (ARF) [3, 4]. In this last indication, termed "post-extubation NIV", two situations should be clearly distinguished, according to the type of patients involved (medical or surgical) as well as the NIV strategy considered: either to prevent the occurrence of a post-extubation ARF in patients at risk of extubation failure ("preventative strategy") or to treat a post-extubation ARF and avoid re-intubation when this complication occurs ("curative strategy"; fig. 1).

In the present chapter, only medical conditions are addressed and surgical or post-operative patients are excluded. NIV is considered as the application of pressure support ventilation (PSV) with positive end-expiratory pressure (PEEP), bilevel positive airway pressure (BiPAP) or continous positive airway pressure (CPAP).

Physiopathological rationale for applying NIV for weaning and post-extubation ARF

Although weaning and extubation periods have to be clearly distinguished chronologically [5], their respective failure, however, can be due to closely related mechanisms (table 1). Among the main physiopathological determinants of weaning or extubation failure, the imbalance between the capacity to generate sufficient strength and efficient gas exchange and the ventilatory workload imposed on respiratory muscles is considered as the main mechanism of weaning failure [6]. In addition to respiratory muscle performance, weaning/extubation failure can be related to an inadequate cardiovascular response during the transition from ETMV to spontaneous breathing (SB), mainly due to left ventricular dysfunction [7]. Prediction of weaning/extubation outcome can also be difficult, despite numerous available predictive criteria [8]. Furthermore, although the SB trial tolerance is considered as one of the optimal criteria

Eur Respir Mon, 2008, 41, 143–153. Printed in UK - all rights reserved. Copyright ERS Journals Ltd 2008; European Respiratory Monograph; ISSN 1025-448x.

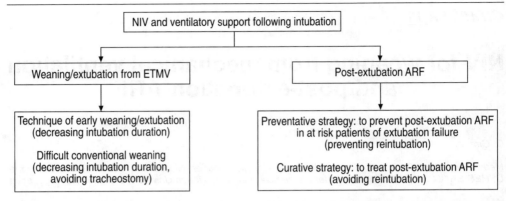

Fig. 1. – Role and objectives of noninvasive ventilation (NIV) for weaning/extubation and post-extubation acute respiratory failure (ARF). ETMV: endotracheal mechanical ventilation.

to assess the weaning or "deventilation" capability or even extubation, inspiratory effort can be significantly increased following extubation leading to failure [9]. Finally, as predictive factors of extubation failure are less well established and valuable at bedside, than those of weaning, *per se* (table 1), it appears useful to identify populations at risk of reintubation [5, 9, 10].

NIV application for weaning and during the post-extubation ARF period includes the following main objectives: to counteract the different physiopathological factors of weaning/extubation failure; to aid physicians with difficulties in predicting results of the weaning/extubation process; and, finally, to treat or prevent the occurrence of a post-extubation ARF, which is sometimes not foreseeable. In this way, NIV can meet the physiological objectives of any types of mechanical ventilation (decrease in the work of

Table 1. – Main physiopathological determinants of weaning or extubation failure

Weaning
  Pulmonary gas exchange impairment
  Imbalance between imposed respiratory workload and muscles capacity
    Increased ventilation
    Increased elastic or resistive load
    Dynamic hyperinflation, PEEPi
  Central respiratory drive impairment (sedation)
  Diaphragmatic dysfunction (critical illness neuro-myopathies)
  Inadequate cardio-circulatory response by LV dysfunction
    Sudden changes in LV pre- and afterload conditions
    Myocardial ischaemia
  Psychological factors (delirium, anxiety, depression)
  Metabolic or nutritional factors, anaemia
Extubation
  LV dysfunction
  Obstruction, increased upper airways resistance (oedema, inflammation, *etc.*)
  Bronchial hypersecretion, swallowing disorders
  Diaphragmatic paralysis, dysfunction (critical illness neuro-myopathies)
  Hypoxemia, atelectasis
  Consciousness disorders, encephalopathy
  Psychological factors (delirium, anxiety, depression)
  Metabolic, nutritional factors, anaemia

PEEPi: intrinsic positive end-expiratory pressure; LV: left ventricular.

breathing, improvement in the breathing pattern, gas exchange and dyspnoea) not only in patients with chronic obstructive pulmonary disease (COPD) [11] but also in non-COPD patients with a good haemodynamic tolerance [12]. It has also been demonstrated that noninvasive PSV was better tolerated but as effective as invasive PSV in reducing the work of breathing, improving breathing pattern and gas exchanges, compared with a T-piece SB trial in ventilator-dependant COPD patients [13]. Finally, it should be kept in mind that NIV is as efficient and beneficial when it is applied to hypercapnic ARF [14], a situation which frequently occurs in cases of weaning or extubation failure [5, 10].

Clinical rationale for applying NIV for weaning and post-extubation ARF

Weaning from ETMV should be considered as a true challenge for ICU clinicians. In practice, they have to find the optimal compromise between the risks of an overly prolonged ETMV (particularly nosocomial pneumonia) and those of a too-early weaning and extubation process [5, 10]. Therefore, any strategy with the aim of reducing morbidity and mortality of prolonged ETMV or reintubation appears relevant and should be developed in order to improve prognosis of patients.

Although the majority of patients can be rapidly and easily withdrawn from ETMV, up to 25% of them will require a gradual weaning procedure and 4% of them will be considered as "unweanable" with conventional techniques [15, 16]. These weaning difficulties, related to the underlying status, may reach up to 40% of cases in COPD patients [17]. Although closely related to application modalities of weaning techniques [15, 16], the time devoted to difficult weaning, may, in fact, reach up to 41% of the total ETMV duration and more than half of ICU stay in patients with COPD, cardiac failure or neurological problems [18]. In addition, in order to reduce the ETMV duration, any weaning strategy should ideally be implemented in specific protocols, locally adapted by ICU teams, including sedation and its withdrawal [5, 19].

Predicting weaning/extubation outcome, however, may be difficult, particularly in weaker patients. Re-intubation would, thusly, be necessary in 5–25% of cases within 48–72 h of a scheduled extubation despite the success in a SB trial [10, 20]. Re-intubation may also be necessary in 37% of cases reported in 3–16% of intubated patients [21]. Nevertheless, this should be reduced to the minimum number acceptable. Although re-intubation may reflect the severity of the underlying status, it is considered, in fact, as an independent risk factor of nosocomial pneumonia, which increases lengths of stay as well as intra-hospital mortality that may reach up to 30–40% in re-intubated patients [10, 20]. Moreover, the increased mortality could be more related to the re-intubation delay than to the cause of re-intubation itself [10]. Finally, the following conditions are now well recognised as risk factors of extubation failure: chronic respiratory failure (CRF), congestive heart failure, neuromuscular diseases, sedation and/or prolonged ETMV, elderly patients, denutrition or other co-morbidities [5, 10]. Therefore, it appears conceptually of interest to apply NIV following intubation in order to reduce the risks of prolonged ETMV and those of potential re-intubation in cases of post-extubation ARF. The efficacy and clinical benefit of NIV in the initial management of ARF, mainly hypercapnic [4, 14], as well as the decrease of nosocomial infections and antibiotics consumption in ICU with NIV are, finally, strong arguments for proposing this type of NIV strategy [22].

Table 2. – Main results of prospective randomised studies evaluating noninvasive ventilation (NIV) for weaning and post-extubation acute respiratory failure (ARF) in a medical population

First author [ref.]	Patients n	Intubation duration days	Total duration of MV days	Weaning success %	Post-extubation ARF n	Re-intubation n	Complications# n	ICU stay days	In-hospital stay days	ICU mortality %	In-hospital mortality %
Weaning/extubation¶											
Nava [26]	25/25		10±7/16±12**	54/13 (day 21)**			0/7*	15±5/24±13**			8/28 (day 60)**
Girault [27]	17/16	4.5±2/7.7±4**	11.5±5/3.5±1§,***	76.5/75		4/4	6/9	12±7/14±7	27±14/27±13	0/22.5	0/22.5 (day 90)
Ferrer [28]	21/22	9.5±8/20±13**	11.4±8/20±13**	85/40 (day 21)**		3/6	5/16**	14±9/25±12**	28±14/41±21***	10/41*	25/55 (day 90)*
Preventative strategy for post-extubation ARF+											
Jiang [29]	47/46						13/7					
Nava [30]	48/49	6.1±7/7.4±6					4/12*		9±5/11±15	23±16/25±21	6/18**	12/18
Ferrer [31]	79/83	6±4/7±5				13/27*	9/18		11±8/13±11	30±23/29±18	3/14*	16/23
Curative strategy for post-extubation ARF+											
Keenan [32]	39/42	3.8±4/5±4					28/29	16/17	15±1/19±25	32±25/30±28	15/24	31/31
Esteban [33]	114/107	7/8f					55/51		18/18f		25/14*	

Data are presented as value (as stated in the table) for NIV/control. MV: mechanical ventilation (intubation and/or NIV); ICU: intensive care unit. #: including nosocomial pneumonia; ¶: control group was invasive conventional weaning; +: control group was oxygen therapy; §: devoted to the weaning period; f: median. *: p≤0.05; **: p≤0.01; ***: p≤0.001.

Clinical results

NIV and weaning/extubation from ETMV

Noncontrolled clinical studies, conducted in difficult-to-wean CRF patients with conventional techniques, have suggested the feasability and interest of NIV in facilitating weaning and extubation, even decannulation, from prolonged ETMV [23–25]. The role of NIV as a weaning and extubation technique from ETMV has been specifically evaluated only very recently (table 2).

The first prospective randomised study compared extubation immediately relayed with NIV to conventional weaning in 50 ventilated COPD patients for hypercapnic ARF, after the first 48 h of ETMV and a first SB trial failure [26]. The results clearly demonstrated the benefit of NIV in reducing total duration of mechanical ventilation, length of ICU stay, occurrence of nosocomial pneumonia, increased weaning success on day 21 and decreased mortality on day 60 (table 2). The second randomised controlled trial was conducted using a similar methodology in 33 CRF patients from various aetiologies [27]. Results confirmed, in part, those of the Italian study, *i.e.* weaning with NIV allowed an earlier extubation, an average of 3 days, with no increase in the risk of weaning failure and no burden of short and medium-term mortality, compared with invasive conventionnal weaning (table 2). As reported in a previous study [26], the two weaning techniques similarly improved gas exchange compared with an SB trial. In contrast, if NIV allowed a reduction in the daily duration of ventilatory support with a trend towards a decrease in the rate of complications, NIV did not decrease the total duration of ventilatory support devoted to weaning nor the lengths of stay in the second trial [27]. Discrepancies in results could be explain by a smaller population in the second study, the respective modalities of NIV applied more or less continuously, as well as the type and severity of the underlying CRF in both studies [26, 27]. Nevertheless, the French study suggested that NIV may, in fact, allow extubation earlier but not necessarily to "de-ventilate" CRF patients more rapidly, according to their severity [27]. The third study evaluated the role of NIV in comparison with conventional weaning in 43 persistent SB trial-failure patients during three consecutive days [28]. The impressive results of that study, which was stopped based on interim analysis data, are summarised in table 2. Weaning with NIV also reduced the need for tracheostomy (5 *versus* 59%; p<0.001). In multivariate analysis, conventional weaning was found to be an independent risk factor of ICU (odds ratio (OR) 6.6, 95% confidence intervals (CI) 1.1–38.8; p=0.035) and 3-month (OR 3.5; 95% CI 1.2–9.6; p=0.018) mortality. Age >70 yrs (OR 5.1; 95% CI 1.7–15; p=0.003) and hypercapnia (arterial carbon dioxide tension (Pa,CO_2) >45 mmHg) during the SB trial (OR 5.8; 95% CI 1.8–18.7; p=0.003) were also found as independent risk factors for the 3-month mortality.

Based on these three randomised trials [26–28], early extubation relayed with NIV appears, therefore, to be a reliable, safe and beneficial weaning technique in difficult-to-wean CRF patients, mainly those with COPD. In addition, the study by FERRER *et al.* [28] strongly suggested that NIV may be more beneficial as weaning difficulties are important and hypercapnia occurs during the SB attempts. All these results should be confirmed with those of the VENISE trial [34], a French multicentre study which randomised >200 CRF patients between three weaning strategies, including NIV. Furthermore, the role of NIV for early weaning/extubation from ETMV has been strongly suggested by a recent meta-analysis [35] and this indication can now be considered in COPD patients [4, 5].

Also in the weaning process from ETMV, the benefit of NIV recently reported for decannulation of tracheostomised COPD patients should be prospectively validated [36].

Except for COPD patients, few clinical data are currently available for weaning/extubation from ETMV with NIV. In a prospective noncontrolled study, NIV allowed early successful extubation in only 13 (56%) out of 22 patients with post-traumatic ARF, who did not meet standard weaning criteria [37]. NIV has also been found to be as effective to early extubate 13 (87%) out of 15 non-COPD patients, mainly surgical, based on criteria that did not usually permit weaning, which suggested that extubation would have failed without NIV [12]. Finally, two cases of successful weaning with NIV have been reported in patients ventilated for acute respiratory distress syndrome after failure of conventional techniques [38].

NIV and post-extubation ARF

Preventative strategy. Prior to the occurrence of post-extubation ARF, NIV should be considered earlier following extubation, particularly in patients at risk for extubation failure, *i.e.* for re-intubation (table 3). A randomised study showed that untimely application of NIV, following immediate extubation, could be hazardous in nonselected patients, with a trend towards an increase in the re-intubation rate compared with oxygen therapy alone [29]. Nevertheless, the study methodology was debatable with a high rate of self-extubation (40%). Two prospective randomised studies have recently compared the use of "preventative NIV" with standard treatment using nasal oxygen in patients having passed a successful SB trial but being considered at risk for extubation failure (table 2) [30, 31]. The study by NAVA *et al.* [30] showed that NIV significantly decreased the need for re-intubation compared with oxygen therapy alone. Overall, in uni- and multivariate analysis, not re-intubating was shown to significantly improve survival ($p < 0.001$), allowing patients who benefit from NIV, therefore, to indirectly reduce their ICU mortality ($p = 0.01$). FERRER *et al.* [31] recently confirmed these positive results. That study demonstrated that "preventative NIV" allowed to avoid the occurrence of post-extubation ARF with no negative impact on re-intubation rate, despite a longer delay in the ARF occurrence for the NIV group (41 ± 19 *versus* 25 ± 21 h; $p = 0.022$). This benefit of NIV was associated with a decrease in ICU mortality (3 *versus* 14%; $p = 0.015$). A planned stratification also demonstrated that benefit on 3-month survival ($p = 0.006$) was only observed in hypercapnic patients during the SB trial ($P_{a,CO_2} > 45$ mmHg).

"Preventative NIV" has also been applied recently in a case–control study conducted in obese patients (BMI ≥ 35 kg·m^{-2}) [39]. Main results showed that NIV significantly decreased the absolute risk of post-extubation ARF by 16%, as well as the ICU ($p < 0.001$) and in-hospital ($p = 0.007$) length of stay, compared with an historic control group. Moreover, a benefit of in-hospital mortality ($p = 0.02$) was observed only in the sub-group of hypercapnic patients.

Table 3. – Risk factors for extubation failure to apply post-extubation preventative noninvasive ventilation in medical patients

Age >65 yrs
APACHE II score >12 (on the day of extubation)
Congestive heart failure
More than one co-morbidity (other than congestive heart failure)
More than one consecutive SB trial failure
Post-extubation $P_{a,CO_2} > 45$ mmHg
Ineffective cough
Post-extubation stridor (without the need for immediate re-intubation)
Obesity (BMI ≥ 35 kg·m^{-2})

APACHE: Acute Physiology and Chronic Health Evaluation; SB: spontaneous breathing; P_{a,CO_2}: arterial carbon dioxide tension; BMI: body mass index. Data taken from [30, 31, 39].

Finally, these three studies demonstrated that "preventative NIV", applied early following extubation in medical patients considered at risk of re-intubation (table 3), allows prevention of the occurrence of post-extubation ARF, decreases the re-intubation risk and may improve, therefore, the morbidity and mortality of patients. Although not addressed in the present chapter, similar encouraging results have been recently demonstrated in thoraco-abdominal [40] and pulmonary [41] post-operative patients.

Curative strategy. The feasibility and benefit of NIV have been suggested by MEDURI *et al.* [42] in this indication for >15 yrs, in seven out of 18 COPD patients, who developed an ARF following self-extubation. Later, a case–control study showed that "curative NIV" allowed avoidance of reintubation, decreased mechanical ventilation duration as well as ICU length of stay in 30 COPD patients exhibiting hypercapnic ARF, within 72 h post-extubation, compared with an historic control group [43]. Although standard treatment could have been considered sufficient, it has been further suggested that NIV could be more cost-effective than nasal oxygen therapy, by avoiding re-intubation in 52 (72%) out of 72 post-traumatic patients with severe hypoxaemia within 24 h post-extubation [44].

With the exception of a surgical context [45–48], only two prospective randomised studies have been conducted to date in medical patients (table 2) [32, 33]. The first, a single centre trial, reported no benefit of "curative NIV" on the re-intubation incidence compared with standard treatment [32]. Nevertheless, no deleterious effects of NIV were reported on patient outcome. The second, a multicentre study involving 221 patients (20% post-operative ARF) and later stopped based on intermediate analysis data, showed that NIV did not avoid re-intubation but rather significantly increased ICU mortality in this group [33]. This result could be explain by a longer re-intubation delay in the NIV group (12 *versus* 2.5 h; p=0.02) and the difference of mortality observed in this group when re-intubation was needed (38 *versus* 22%; p=0.06). Surprisingly, the success rate of NIV (with no re-intubation) used as rescue therapy in the control group (75%) was found to be higher than that observed for the NIV group (52%).

These negative results [32, 33] are somewhat surprising as they are discordant with those reported in clinical practice [49, 50]. The interpretation must take into account, however, that both studies were conducted in heterogeneous populations, suffering mainly from hypoxaemic ARF, including only 10–12% of COPD patients respectively, and sometimes performed by only a few experienced centres with NIV [32, 33]. Nevertheless, promising results could be still considered with "curative NIV" in a more-selected population, such as COPD patients [43]. In this population, some useful answers could be given by results of a French multicentre study [34]. For instance, current results should prompt clinicians to be cautious in using "curative NIV" routinely in the management of post-extubation ARF in medical ICU patients, in order to not delay re-intubation. Lastly, to the present author's knowledge and except for observational series [42, 49, 50], no prospective data are available regarding the specific role of "curative NIV" following self-extubation.

Role and limits of NIV application for weaning and post-extubation ARF

The benefit of NIV as a weaning/extubation technique from ETMV can only be considered if "de-ventilation" is not possible (ventilatory dependence after one or more SB trial failures) although the maintenance of endotracheal prothesis appears no longer necessary. In cases of post-extubation ARF, this benefit may be theoretically understood if "re-ventilation" is necessary but re-intubation is not immediately required. Also, prevention of post-extubation ARF with NIV should not be systematic and assume previously to identify patients at risk of extubation failure (table 3)

For the management of weaning/extubation with NIV, available data involve selected populations, mainly COPD patients [26–28]. Therefore, the use of NIV in this indication, as an alternative to conventional weaning techniques, may now be considered [4, 5]. For the management of post-extubation ARF with NIV ("post-extubation NIV") current available data should be interpreted according to the population involved (medical or surgical) as well as the type of strategy considered (preventative or curative NIV). In contrast to post-operative patients [40, 41, 45–48], only preventative NIV can be currently recommended in medical ICU patients, due to the significant risk of delaying re-intubation when ARF occurs in post-extubation in this population [33]. In addition, medical patients with hypercapnia during an SB trial could be more susceptible to benefit from NIV for weaning/extubation or to prevent post-extubation ARF [28, 31, 39]. Therefore, this hypercapnia could be considered as a simple objective and a useful criterion for clinicians in considering NIV in these situations.

Finally, whatever the indication, the main predictive factors of NIV failure should always be evaluated and identified [1, 4]. In all cases, NIV for weaning and post-extubation ARF requires good control of the technique, in order to not delay the re-intubation time and to be able to re-intubate patients at all times. Under these conditions, therefore, weaning and post-extubation NIV can only be applied in ICUs with a skilled care team competent with the technique.

Conclusion

Since the last international consensus conference [1], the management of weaning/extubation and post-extubation ARF with NIV may now be considered in ICU patients [4, 5]. Current data clearly demonstrate a clinical benefit of NIV as a weaning/extubation technique in cases of initial or persistent difficult weaning, mainly in COPD patients. For post-extubation ARF management, the benefit of NIV has only been demonstrated, to date, when it has been applied according to a preventative strategy in selected at risk patients, contrasting with the potential deleterious effect of a curative strategy in medical patients. However, further studies are warranted in more-selected populations for this indication. Hypercapnia during or following an SB trial appears to be a useful criterion for applying NIV for weaning and preventing post-extubation ARF. Currently, due to different clinical results, clinicians should clearly distinguish these three types of chronological NIV applications following intubation for ARF [3]. As for other indications, it should kept in mind that NIV, applied to weaning/extubation from ETMV or post-extubation ARF, needs rigorous analysis of the risks and benefits for patients, in order to not unnecessarily delay the re-intubation time. Furthermore, acquired experience with the technique remains as one of the key factors for the success of NIV in these clinical situations.

Summary

The clinical efficacy of noninvasive ventilation (NIV) in the initial management of acute respiratory failure (ARF) led to it being recently proposed as a noninvasive ventilatory strategy following intubation. In this condition, three different indications should be distinguished with potentially different results: NIV application for difficult weaning/extubation from endotracheal mechanical ventilation (ETMV) to reduce the duration of intubation (weaning/extubation strategy); NIV application for post-extubation ARF ("post-extubation NIV"), either to prevent ARF occurrence in patients at risk ("preventative strategy") or to avoid reintubation when this complication occurs ("curative strategy"). Current data show a clinical benefit of NIV, in terms of medical patients' morbi-mortality, for the preventive as well as the weaning/extubation strategies, mainly in cases of underlying chronic obstructive pulmonary disease. In contrast, the more controversial results observed with NIV for treating post-extubation ARF should lead the clinician to be cautious in this indication. In all cases, NIV applied for weaning from ETMV and post-extubation ARF can only be considered with an experienced team and should not unnecessarily delay the re-intubation time.

Keywords: Acute respiratory failure, endotracheal mechanical ventilation, extubation, noninvasive ventilation, weaning.

Acknowledgements. The author thanks Richard Medeiros, Rouen University Hospital Medical Editor, for his expert advice in editing the manuscript.

References

1. International Consensus Conference in Intensive Care Medicine. Noninvasive positive pressure ventilation in acute respiratory failure. *Am J Respir Crit Care Med* 2001; 163: 283–291.
2. Demoule A, Girou E, Richard JC, Taille S, Brochard L. Increased use of noninvasive ventilation in French intensive care units. *Intensive Care Med* 2006; 32: 1747–1755.
3. Nava S, Navalesi P, Conti G. Time of non-invasive ventilation. *Intensive Care Med* 2006; 32: 361–370.
4. [Consensus conference on non invasive positive pressure ventilation in acute respiratory failure (excluding newborn infants)]. Conférence de Consensus Commune SFAR, SPLF, SRLF 2006; pp. 13–20.
5. Boles JM, Bion J, Connors A, *et al.* Weaning from mechanical ventilation. Statement of the sixth international consensus conference on intensive care medicine. *Eur Respir J* 2007; 29: 1033–1056.
6. Laghi F, Tobin MJ. Disorders of the respiratory muscles. *Am J Respir Crit Care Med* 2003; 168: 10–48.
7. Richard C, Teboul JL, Archambaud F, Hebert JL, Michaut P, Auzepy P. Left ventricular function during weaning of patients with chronic obstructive pulmonary disease. *Intensive Care Med* 1994; 20: 181–186.
8. Meade M, Guyatt G, Cook D, *et al.* Predicting success in weaning from mechanical ventilation. *Chest* 2001; 120: 400S–424S.
9. Mehta S, Nelson DL, Klinger JR, Buczko GB, Levy MM. Prediction of postextubation work of breathing. *Crit Care Med* 2000; 28: 1341–1346.
10. Rothaar RC, Epstein SK. Extubation failure: magnitude of the problem, impact on outcomes, and prevention. *Curr Opin Crit Care* 2003; 9: 59–66.
11. Girault C, Richard JC, Chevron V, *et al.* Comparative physiologic effects of noninvasive assist-control and pressure support ventilation in acute hypercapnic respiratory failure. *Chest* 1997; 111: 1639–1648.
12. Kilger E, Briegel J, Haller M, *et al.* Effects of noninvasive positive pressure ventilation support in non-COPD patients with acute respiratory insufficiency after early extubation. *Intensive Care Med* 1999; 25: 1374–1380.

13. Vitacca M, Ambrosino N, Clini E, et al. Physiological response to pressure support ventilation delivered before and after extubation in patients not capable of totally spontaneous autonomous breathing. *Am J Respir Crit Care Med* 2001; 164: 638–641.

14. Demoule A, Girou E, Richard JC, Taille S, Brochard L. Benefits and risks of success or failure of noninvasive ventilation. *Intensive Care Med* 2006; 32: 1756–1765.

15. Brochard L, Rauss A, Benito S, et al. Comparison of three methods of gradual withdrawal from ventilatory support during weaning from mechanical ventilation. *Am J Respir Crit Care Med* 1994; 150: 896–903.

16. Esteban A, Frutos F, Tobin MJ, et al. A comparison of four methods of weaning patients from mechanical ventilation. *N Engl J Med* 1995; 332: 345–350.

17. Nava S, Rubini F, Zanott N, et al. Survival and prediction of successful ventilator weaning in COPD patients requiring mechanical ventilation for more than 21 days. *Eur Respir J* 1994; 7: 1645–1652.

18. Esteban A, Alia I, Ibanez J, Benito S, Tobin MJ, Spanish Lung Failure Collaborative Group. Modes of mechanical ventilation and weaning. A national survey of Spanish hospitals. *Chest* 1994; 106: 1188–1193.

19. Girard TD, Kress JP, Fuchs BD, et al. Efficacy and safety of a paired sedation and ventilator weaning protocol for mechanically ventilated patients in intensive care (Awakening and Breathing Controlled trial): a randomised controlled trial. *Lancet* 2008; 371: 126–134.

20. Esteban A, Alia I, Tobin MJ, et al. Effect of spontaneous breathing trial duration on outcome of attempts to discontinue mechanical ventilation. *Am J Respir Crit Care Med* 1999; 159: 512–518.

21. Chevron V, Ménard JF, Richard JC, Girault C, Leroy J, Bonmarchand G. Unplanned extubation: risk factors of development and predictive criteria for reintubation. *Crit Care Med* 1998; 26: 1049–1053.

22. Girou E, Shortgen F, Delclaux C, et al. Association of noninvasive ventilation with nosocomial infections and survival in critically ill patients. *JAMA* 2000; 284: 2361–2367.

23. Udwadia ZF, Santis GK, Steven MH, Simonds AK. Nasal ventilation to facilitate weaning in patients with chronic respiratory insufficiency. *Thorax* 1992; 47: 715–718.

24. Goodenberger DM, Couser Jl, May JJ.. Successful discontinuation of ventilation *via* tracheostomy by substitution of nasal positive pressure ventilation. *Chest* 1992; 102: 1277–1279.

25. Restrick LJ, Scott AD, Ward EM, Feneck RO, Cornwell WE, Wedzicha JA. Nasal intermittent positive-pressure ventilation in weaning intubated patients with chronic respiratory disease from assisted positive-pressure ventilation. *Respir Med* 1993; 87: 199–204.

26. Nava S, Ambrosino N, Clini E, et al. Noninvasive mechanical ventilation in the weaning of patients with respiratory failure due to chronic obstructive pulmonary disease. *Ann Intern Med* 1998; 128: 721–728.

27. Girault C, Daudenthun I, Chevron V, Tamion F, Leroy J, Bonmarchand G. Noninvasive ventilation as a systematic extubation and weaning technique in acute on chronic respiratory failure. A prospective randomized controlled study. *Am J Respir Crit Care Med* 1999; 160: 86–92.

28. Ferrer M, Esquinas A, Arancibia F, et al. Non-invasive ventilation during persistent weaning failure. A randomised-controlled trial. *Am J Respir Crit Care Med* 2003; 168: 70–76.

29. Jiang JS, Kao SJ, Wang SN. Effect of early application of biphasic positive airway pressure on the outcome of extubation in ventilator weaning. *Respirology* 1999; 4: 161–165.

30. Nava S, Gregoretti C, Fanfulla F, et al. Noninvasive ventilation to prevent respiratory failure after extubation in high risk patients. *Crit Care Med* 2005; 33: 2465–2470.

31. Ferrer M, Valencia M, Nicolas JM, Bernadich O, Badia JR, Torres A. Early noninvasive ventilation averts extubation failure in patients at risk: a randomized trial. *Am J Respir Crit Care Med* 2006; 173: 164–170.

32. Keenan SP, Powers C, McCormack DG, Block G. Noninvasive positive-pressure ventilation for post-extubation respiratory distress. A randomized controlled trial. *JAMA* 2002; 287: 3238–3244.

33. Esteban A, Frutos-Vivar F, Ferguson ND, et al. Noninvasive positive-pressure ventilation for respiratory failure after extubation. *N Engl J Med* 2004; 350: 2452–2460.

34. Girault C, Chajara A, Dachraoui F, *et al.* VENISE: Non-invasive ventilation for the weaning of mechanical ventilation in acute-on-chronic respiratory failure patients. A prospective randomised controlled and multicenter trial]. *Rev Mal Respir* 2003; 20: 940–945.

35. Burns KE, Adhikari NK, Meade MO. A meta-analysis of noninvasive weaning to facilitate liberation from mechanical ventilation. *Can J Anaesth* 2006; 53: 305–315.

36. Quinnell TG, Pilsworth S, Shneerson JM, Smith IE. Prolonged invasive ventilation following acute ventilatory failure in COPD: weaning results, survival, and the role of noninvasive ventilation. *Chest* 2006; 129: 133–139.

37. Gregoretti C, Beltrame F, Lucangelo U, *et al.* Physiologic evaluation of noninvasive pressure support ventilation in trauma patients with acute respiratory failure. *Intensive Care Med* 1998; 24: 785–790.

38. Windisch W, Storre JH, Matthys H, Sorichter S, Virchow JC. Weaning from mechanical ventilation by long-term nasal positive pressure ventilation in two patients with acute respiratory distress syndrome associated with pneumococcal sepsis. *Respiration* 2002; 69: 464–467.

39. El Solh AA, Aquilina A, Pineda L, Dhanvantri V, Grant B, Bouquin P. Noninvasive ventilation for prevention of postextubation respiratory failure in obese patients. *Eur Respir J* 2006; 28: 588–595.

40. Kindgen-Milles D, Muller E, Buhl R, *et al.* Nasal-continuous positive airway pressure reduces pulmonary morbidity and length of hospital stay following thoracoabdominal aortic surgery. *Chest* 2005; 128: 821–828.

41. Perrin C, Jullien V, Venissac N, *et al.* Prophylactic use of noninvasive ventilation in patients undergoing lung resectional surgery. *Respir Med* 2007; 101: 1572–1578.

42. Meduri GU, Abou-Shala N, Fox RC, Jones CB, Leeper KV, Wunderink RG. Noninvasive face mask mechanical ventilation in patients with acute hypercapnic respiratory failure. *Chest* 1991; 100: 445–454.

43. Hilbert G, Gruson D, Portel L, Gbikpi-Benissan G, Cardinaud JP. Noninvasive pressure support ventilation in COPD patients with postextubation hypercapnic respiratory insufficiency. *Eur Respir J* 1998; 11: 1349–1353.

44. Munshi IA, DeHaven B, Kirton O, Sleeman D, Navarro M. Reengineering respiratory support following extubation avoidance of critical care unit costs. *Chest* 1999; 116: 1025–1028.

45. Auriant I, Jallot A, Hervé P, *et al.* Noninvasive ventilation reduces mortality in acute respiratory failure following lung resection. *Am J Respir Crit Care Med* 2001; 164: 1231–1235.

46. Antonelli M, Conti G, Bufi M, *et al.* Noninvasive ventilation for treatment of acute respiratory failure in patients undergoing solid organ transplantation. A randomized trial. *JAMA* 2000; 283: 235–241.

47. Jaber S, Delay JM, Chanques G, *et al.* Outcomes of patients with acute respiratory failure after abdominal surgery treated with noninvasive positive pressure ventilation. *Chest* 2005; 128: 2688–2695.

48. Squadrone V, Coha M, Cerutti E, *et al.* Continuous positive airway pressure for treatment of postoperative hypoxemia: a randomized controlled trial. *JAMA* 2005; 293: 589–595.

49. Meduri GU, Turner RE, Abou-Shala N, Wunderink R, Tolley E. Noninvasive positive pressure ventilation *via* face mask: first-line intervention in patients with acute hypercapnic and hypoxemic respiratory failure. *Chest* 1996; 109: 179–193.

50. Girault C, Briel A, Hellot MF, *et al.* Non-invasive mechanical ventilation in clinical practice: a two-year experience in a medical intensive care unit. *Crit Care Med* 2003; 31: 552–559.

CHAPTER 11

NIV for acute respiratory failure: modes of ventilation and ventilators

F. Vargas*, A. Thille[#,¶], A. Lyazidi[#,¶], L. Brochard[#,¶,+]

*Medical Intensive Care Unit, Pellegrin-Tripode Teaching Hospital, Bordeaux, [#]Medical Intensive Care Unit, AP-HP, Albert Chenevier Henri Mondor Teaching Hospital, [¶]Inserm U 841, and [+]Université Paris 12, Créteil, France.

Correspondence: L. Brochard, Réanimation Médicale, Centre Hospitalier Albert Chenevier Henri Mondor, 51 Av. du Maréchal de Lattre de Tassigny, 94010 Créteil Cedex, France. Fax: 33 142079943; E-mail: Laurent.brochard@hmn.aphp.fr

Introduction

In acute respiratory failure (ARF), mechanical ventilation is used to achieve acceptable levels of arterial blood oxygenation with an adequate inspiratory oxygen concentration, to reduce the work and oxygen cost of breathing by unloading the respiratory muscles and, eventually to reduce dyspnoea. In patients with ARF, the rationale for using noninvasive ventilation (NIV) is not different from that for using invasive mechanical ventilation. NIV includes various techniques but the modality most frequently used is noninvasive positive pressure ventilation. Positive airway pressure may be obtained by controlling inspiratory flow and volume (volume-controlled ventilation) or directly, by delivering a positive pressure (pressure-controlled ventilation). The latter can be obtained in different ways: first, by delivering inspiratory positive airway pressure; secondly, by delivering inspiratory and expiratory positive airway pressures at different levels to deliver a bilevel positive airway pressure ventilation; and finally, by delivering inspiratory and expiratory positive airway pressure at a comparable level to realise a continuous positive airway pressure (CPAP). The present chapter will focus on the modes of ventilation frequently used during NIV. Success of NIV is strongly associated with good tolerance which can be related to patient, interface, ventilator and ventilator setting. Others modes of ventilation, developed in order to improve the patient–ventilator interaction, will be briefly described. Positive pressure ventilators have evolved over the past several decades, with increasing capabilities to enhance ventilator responsiveness to patient breathing demands and improved alarm and monitoring systems. NIV can be performed using both intensive care unit (ICU) ventilators and those specifically dedicated for NIV. Their merits and limitations are discussed in the last paragraph.

CPAP

Description

CPAP is a technique of artificial ventilatory support widely used in the ICU [1], particularly in neonates and infants in whom it was first applied. CPAP represents the

Eur Respir Mon, 2008, 41, 154–172. Printed in UK - all rights reserved. Copyright ERS Journals Ltd 2008; European Respiratory Monograph; ISSN 1025-448x.

application of a constant level of positive pressure at the airway opening during spontaneous breathing [2]. Therefore, CPAP is a technique of ventilatory artificial support for patients with ARF who are able to sustain spontaneous breathing activity. However, no breath is really "actively" assisted and CPAP is often not considered as a mode of ventilatory support because it does not result in active ventilator support. From the patient's work of breathing (WOB) and oxygenation standpoints, it does provide a ventilatory assistance, however, which can achieve the goals of ventilation, as described above. CPAP results in a higher mean intrathoracic pressure than unassisted spontaneous breathing but a lower pressure than positive pressure mechanical ventilation and positive end-expiratory pressure (PEEP). Mean airway pressure increases, with possible beneficial effects on atelectasis and improvement in oxygenation; lung compliance can increase, reducing WOB and the presence of intrinsic PEEP (PEEPi) can be counterbalanced with a partial reduction of the inspiratory effort. An advantage of CPAP over modes of mechanical ventilatory assistance is that CPAP does not require patient–ventilator synchronisation.

Physiological effects

Oxygenation and WOB. CPAP raises intrathoracic pressure, usually decreases arteriovenous shunting, improves oxygenation and dyspnoea [3, 4], and lessens WOB in patients with cardiogenic pulmonary oedema [5]. In patients with ARF without chronic obstructive pulmonary disease (COPD), CPAP increases functional residual capacity and displaces ventilation up from the lower flat portion of the respiratory system volume–pressure curve into a more-linear portion. Through this mechanism, CPAP improves oxygenation and reduces WOB. KATZ and MARKS [3] found that CPAP alone reduced the transpulmonary WOB in intubated patients, indicating an improvement in respiratory mechanics. However, L'HER et al. [6] could not find any significant effect of CPAP on respiratory effort in patients with acute lung injury, in contrast with marked reduction under pressure-support ventilation (PSV). This differs from the results of studies in cardiogenic pulmonary oedema and some other conditions [7–10]. Physiological and clinical studies in patients with cardiogenic pulmonary oedema suggested that PSV was comparable with or slightly superior to CPAP alone, in terms of the decrease in respiratory effort [11, 12]. DELCLAUX et al. [13] evaluated whether CPAP, compared with conventional medical treatment and oxygen alone, produced physiological benefits and reduced the need for endotracheal intubation in nonhypercapnic patients with acute lung injury. Despite a favourable early physiologic response to CPAP in terms of comfort and oxygenation, no benefits in terms of outcome variables were found. This failure of noninvasive CPAP to provide clinical benefits may be ascribable to the absence of an effect on respiratory effort, as demonstrated.

Tidal volume. In conditions where it tended to increase lung volume, above normal functional residual capacity, CPAP has been shown to increase expiratory muscle recruitment, an effect that may contribute to reduce tidal volume, by worsening mechanical conditions [10, 14]. Indeed, tonic expiratory muscle recruitment may tend to limit tidal excursion and tidal volume by decreasing chest wall and respiratory system compliance.

Haemodynamic effects. Positive pressure ventilation increases intrathoracic pressure and pressure in the right atrium. Venous return to the right heart is, therefore, reduced. This reduction of preload becomes especially important in patients with respiratory insufficiency, associated with deep and heavy breathing, resulting in large negative intrathoracic pressure swings and an elevated venous return. Positive pressure ventilation counterbalances this effect with a reduction of right heart preload. Increase of intrathoracic pressure decreases left ventricular transmural pressure and transmural pressure of the thoracic aorta. These effects result in a relevant reduction of the left ventricular afterload. This combined reduction of pre-load and afterload may result in different effects on cardiac output. Patients with advanced cardiac insufficiency do not show decreases of cardiac output under positive pressure ventilation. In contrast to the normal heart, the cardiac output of the failing heart is predominantly dependent on afterload changes. Studies using CPAP in patients with stable chronic heart failure have shown that the greatest increase in cardiac output is found in those patients with higher filling pressures [15]. CPAP may improve cardiac function through a decrease in the amplitude of negative pleural swings [5]. CHADDA et al. [12] found no evidence that CPAP and noninvasive PSV (NPSV) resulted in similar cardiac or haemodynamic effects, producing similar reductions in right and left ventricular pre-load, mediated by similar effects on intrathoracic pressure.

Coronary perfusion. On one hand, an increase in intrathoracic pressure has been shown to be associated with reduced coronary perfusion in animals; on the other hand, myocardial oxygen consumption might be reduced by the lowered pre-load and afterload of the heart and by reduction of the oxygen cost of breathing, knowing that more than 30% of oxygen consumption can come from the respiratory muscles during respiratory failure. No myocardial ischaemia should be expected under positive pressure ventilation, especially when a spontaneous breathing activity is maintained. The ventilatory pump is unloaded during ventilation, and the high blood flow can be redistributed to the heart, kidneys and brain, improving the clinical situation of the patient. An initial clinical trial found more ischaemic heart episodes from using PSV than using CPAP but it was difficult in that small study to differentiate pure randomisation imbalance from true physiological effect [11]. Several interpretations were proposed, including a faster decrease in arterial carbon dioxide tension (Pa,CO$_2$) with PSV. These effects were not confirmed in further studies but raised caution in the use of ventilatory support in patients with ischaemic diseases [12, 16].

PEEPi. In patients with ARF, due to exacerbation of airflow obstruction, CPAP counterbalances PEEPi, thus reducing the inspiratory threshold load significantly [8]. Until the level of set CPAP is lower than PEEPi, there is no significant change in the end-expiratory lung volume (EELV) as a consequence of expiratory flow limitation. When CPAP approaches the value of PEEPi or even greater, EELV increases and pulmonary hyperinflation worsens with deleterious consequence on the pressure generating capacity of the respiratory muscles. It was recently shown that, in stable patients with COPD who have measurable PEEPi, the application of CPAP has minimal effects on the inspiratory threshold load until CPAP levels greatly exceed PEEPi [17]. At these pressures, a reduction in the indices of respiratory muscle effort is obtained at the expense of substantial increases in lung volume, as well as expiratory muscle recruitment.

Main indications

Cardiogenic pulmonary oedema. Noninvasive respiratory assistance, in particular CPAP, has a strong pathophysiological rationale in patients with acute cardiogenic oedema. Three recent meta-analyses [18–20] showed that CPAP is effective in reducing the intubation rate in acute cardiac pulmonary oedema. CPAP and NPSV seem to result in very similar effects, both on physiological end-points and for clinical outcome, and

CPAP can be recommended as a first-line treatment. However, patients with left ventricular insufficiency and cardiogenic pulmonary oedema often suffer from a weakness or insufficiency of the ventilatory pump. This can be identified by a growing Pa,CO_2. These patients with hypercapnia are at increased risk of being intubated [21]. If CPAP is not powerful enough in this situation or if the application of CPAP does not reach beneficial effect, then noninvasive positive pressure ventilation should be considered [22].

The post-operative period. In the postoperative period, loss in lung volume, diaphragm dysfunction and oxygenation impairment, secondary to occurrence of atelectasis, may be the main pathophysiological pathways of respiratory complications. CPAP may be a useful adjunct in this setting. A recent randomised study showed that application of CPAP in the early postoperative period (arterial oxygen tension (Pa,O_2)/inspiratory oxygen fraction (FI,O_2) <300) in patients undergoing high-risk abdominal surgery was successful to prevent reintubation and complications compared with standard application of a Venturi mask [23]. Several other studies have shown beneficial effects on the main physiological variables when PEEP was applied in the early postoperative period after high-risk abdominal surgery [24].

Settings and interfaces

Relatively low continuous positive pressures (5–10 cmH$_2$O) seem to be enough to achieve the described effects. The level can be adjusted based upon the clinical response and tolerance. Oxygen can be adjusted to reach a better peripheral oxygenation (arterial oxygen saturation (Sa,O_2) >90%). To be effective (*i.e.*, to effectively reduce inspiratory and expiratory efforts), however, CPAP must work with airway pressure remaining constant at the PEEP level selected during the whole respiratory cycle [25]. Airway inspiratory fluctuations are mainly due to an insufficient gas delivery related to the individual need of flow during inspiration, because of inadequate CPAP systems or valves [25, 26].

Face masks are the most commonly used interfaces for CPAP. Alternatively, the helmet has been used to apply pressure at the airway opening without touching the face and it has been reported to be tolerated by patients with acute respiratory failure. Face masks and helmets, however, are two fundamentally different devices with respect to CO_2 elimination. A recent study performed by TACCONE *et al.* [27] demonstrated that the helmet can predispose to CO_2 rebreathing, depending on the flow settings, and should not be used to deliver CPAP with a ventilator. Helmet CPAP seems acceptable in terms of CO_2 rebreathing with a continuous high-flow system [27].

NPSV

Introduction

Pressure support is the most frequently used ventilatory mode during NIV [28]. Success of NIV is strongly associated with good clinical tolerance [28, 29] which can be related to patient, interface, ventilator and/or ventilator settings. A specific problem during NIV is the presence of leaks around the mask, which lead to discomfort and patient–ventilator asynchrony; therefore, further worsening the clinical situation. Two asynchronies can be directly caused by leaks during NIV: prolonged inspiration due to inspiratory leaks [30] and autotriggering due to expiratory leaks. An optimal adjustment of ventilatory settings may improve WOB, comfort and patient–ventilator synchrony, promoting the success of NIV.

Patient–ventilator asynchrony during NIV

Patient–ventilator asynchrony is defined as a mismatch between the patient's neural inspiratory time and the ventilator insufflation time. Whereas the detection of subtle asynchrony may require investigations such as oesophageal pressure measurement or diaphragmatic electromyography, several patterns of major asynchrony can be recognised by a trained clinician simply by examining flow and airway-pressure tracings (Figs 1–3) [31]. Major patient–ventilator asynchrony is common in clinical practice but the real incidence during a NIV session is poorly known. A recent multicentre study evaluated the incidence of patient–ventilator asynchrony during a 30-min session of NIV and was reported as an abstract [32]. A total of 60 patients were evaluated, recording diaphragmatic electromyographic activity in order to accurately measure the patients' inspiratory time. Frequent asynchrony counting for >10% of the respiratory efforts was present in 26 (43%) patients. Prolonged insufflation, due to delayed cycling, was the most frequent asynchrony, present in 25% of the patients. Ineffective triggering, autotriggering, double triggering and short cycle, due to premature cycling, were present in several of the patients. Not only the magnitude of leaks, but also the level of pressure support which could further increase inspiratory leaks, was significantly associated with frequent asynchrony [32].

Prolonged inspiration. When large leaks occur during inspiration, the ventilator continues to insufflate because the delivered flow remains above the cycling criterion (also referred to as expiratory trigger value), so that cycling off does not occur. In this situation, the patient attempts to expire and can fight against the ventilator because the expiratory valve remains closed, generating ineffective efforts during persistent insufflation (fig. 1). The magnitude of delayed cycling and the number of ineffective breaths are directly associated to the magnitude of leaks [32]. This problem is much more prevalent when using an ICU ventilator with no NIV mode but may occur also with NIV dedicated ventilators. Several adjustments can eliminate prolonged inspiration by reducing either the leaks or the ventilator insufflation time. First, mask position should be adjusted to minimise leaks around the mask. Secondly, limiting the total inspiratory pressure should be considered, reducing the pressure support and/or PEEP level. Persistent leaks indicate a need for limiting the ventilator insufflation time by increasing the expiratory trigger and/or reducing the maximal inspiratory time. Increasing the expiratory trigger ≥50% allows the ventilator to cycle off adequately [33]. CALDERINI *et al.* [30] reported that adjusting the maximal inspiratory time to 0.8–1.2 s also improved patient–ventilator synchrony, reducing the work of breathing and improving comfort. Most of the new-generation ICU ventilators and many NIV dedicated ventilators allow adjustment of the expiratory trigger or maximal inspiratory time.

Autotriggering. Expiratory leaks can generate a pressure drop below the external PEEP level or a drop in expired bias flow, simulating the patient's effort and triggering a ventilator breath. Autotriggering may promote a short cycle or a flow distortion since the patient does not generate effort and fight the ventilator (fig. 2). This source of autotriggering can be eliminated by increasing the bias flow and lowering the inspiratory trigger sensitivity [34], so that a stronger inspiratory effort is required to trigger the ventilator. Careful adjustment of the settings should avoid ineffective triggering, which, however, is sometimes difficult to detect.

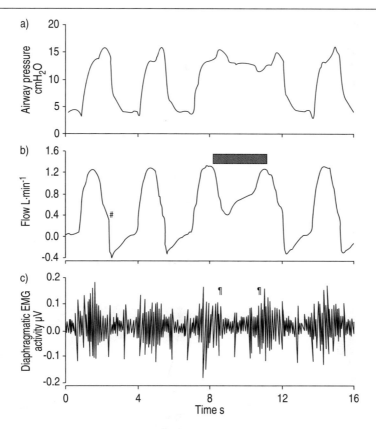

Fig. 1. – Ineffective efforts during persistent insufflation. a) Airway pressure, b) flow and c) the diaphragmatic electromyography are shown. When large leaks occur during inspiration, the ventilator continues to insufflate because the delivered flow remains above the value of the expiratory trigger (#), so that cycling off does not occur. In this situation, the patient attempts to expire (¶) and could fight the ventilator because the expiratory valve remains closed, generating ineffective efforts. ■: leaks.

Dose of ventilatory support.

Excessive ventilatory support. Ineffective triggering is a frequent asynchrony observed during invasive mechanical ventilation [35], as well as during NIV [32]. These ineffective breaths are mainly promoted by excessive ventilatory support, *i.e.* high pressure support levels. However, the mechanism generating ineffective triggering in NIV and in intubated patients is different. During invasive ventilation, this asynchrony is promoted by large tidal volumes, long insufflation time and reduced expiratory time, generating dynamic hyperinflation at the time of attempted triggering. During NIV, ineffective breaths mainly occur during prolonged insufflations due to inspiratory leaks [30, 32, 36]. In both cases, ineffective triggering is a marker of inadequately high pressure support level and an excessive dose of ventilation.

Insufficient ventilatory support. During PSV, if the pressure support level is too low or the cycling-off criterion is reached too early, the ventilator stops insufflation and opens the expiratory valve while the patient's inspiratory effort continues [37]. This produces an initial drop in airway pressure and flow distortion, followed by an increase related to patient inspiration, resulting in a characteristic contour (fig. 3). This asynchrony is

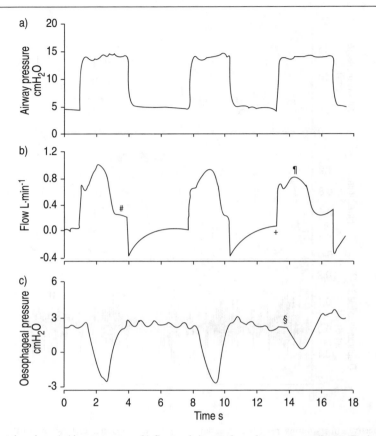

Fig. 2. – Auto-triggering. a) Airway pressure, b) flow and c) oesophageal pressure are shown. Expiratory leaks (#) can generate a pressure drop to less than the external positive end-expiratory pressure level, simulating a patient's effort and triggering a ventilator breath. Auto-triggering may promote a flow distortion (¶) since the patient does not generate effort and fight the ventilator. +: start of ventilator insufflation; §: start of patient's effort.

observed, especially in patients recovering from acute lung injury with a high ventilatory demand and a restrictive respiratory mechanics [31, 37]. If the patient's effort continues far beyond the end of the ventilator inspiratory time, a second ventilator insufflation can be triggered. In this case, double triggering is detected as two consecutive ventilator cycles separated by a very short or absent expiratory period.

Optimisation of ventilatory settings during NPSV

Adjusting the inspiratory trigger. The triggering phase contributes <10% of the patient's total effort to breathe [38]. Flow triggering has been shown to slightly reduce the effort needed to trigger the ventilator compared with pressure triggering [38]. Moreover, a less sensitive trigger could be associated with a higher incidence of ineffective triggering events [35]. These data indicate that a sensitive flow trigger should be used, to take full advantage of patient's efforts without inducing autotriggering. Autotriggering is a frequent asynchrony during NIV and a flow triggering set around 3 L·min^{-1} (when possible settings range 0.5–10 L·min^{-1}, for instance) could represent an

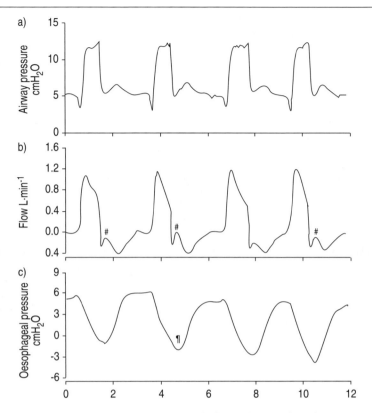

Fig. 3. – Insufficient ventilatory support. a) Airway pressure, b) flow and c) oesophageal pressure are shown. During pressure support ventilation, if the pressure support level is too low or cycling-off criterion is reached too early, the ventilator stops insufflation and opens the expiratory valve while patient's inspiratory effort continues. This produces an initial drop in airway pressure and flow distortion, followed by an increase related to patient inspiration, resulting in a characteristic contour ($^\#$). ¶: end of patient's effort.

optimal adjustment, being sensitive enough and avoiding auto-triggering. Some ventilators self-adjust trigger sensitivity as a function of leaks.

Adjusting the pressure support level. The main objective is to individually titrate pressure support level in order to obtain an expiratory tidal volume at least of 6 mL·kg^{-1}. A first approach starts with a higher pressure support level (~20 cmH$_2$O) and reduces it step by step if the patient is intolerant. The goal of this strategy is a rapid alleviation of respiratory distress but it may also promote discomfort due to excessive assistance and leaks. A second approach starts with a low pressure support level (~8 cmH$_2$O) and raises it gradually to the target tidal volume and adequate ventilatory assistance. This strategy may improve comfort and maximise patient tolerance by avoiding leaks at initiation of NIV. Then, analysis of flow and airway pressure tracings of the ventilator allows detection of signs of under-assistance (fig. 3) as well as signs of over-assistance and leaks (fig. 1).

Adjusting the pressurisation rate. Although pressurisation velocity depends on ventilator performance, the pressure rise time is adjustable on the new-generation ICU ventilators and on many NIV dedicated ventilators. A low pressurisation rate can lead to excessive patient inspiratory effort whereas a very fast pressure rise may result in overshoot termination, promoting leaks and generating patient discomfort [39]. The ideal rise time should be titrated as the fastest pressurisation rate that is not associated with overshoot. A longer rise time is sometimes necessary to avoid premature cycle termination, related to high pressure overshoot.

Adjusting PEEP. External PEEP has been shown to decrease ineffective triggering in patients with auto-PEEP [40] by reducing the work of breathing needed to trigger the ventilator [41–43]. The levels of dynamic PEEPi measured during NIV in patients with ARF are often relatively low (≤ 3 cmH$_2$O) in hypoxaemic patients [44], as well as in hypercapnic patients [45]. Consequently, an initial adjustment of PEEP around 3 cmH$_2$O should be sufficient to facilitate triggering of the ventilator and will participate in avoiding leaks by limiting maximal inspiratory pressure. However, a higher level of PEEP may be necessary in order to avoid obstructive apnoea during sleep or to improve oxygenation in case of severe hypoxaemia [44].

Adjusting the insufflation time. During PSV, the insufflation time depends partly on the patient's inspiratory effort but often tends to be longer than the patient's neural inspiratory time, leading to delayed cycling and prolonged insufflations [46]. After an initial high peak inspiratory flow (which depends on the magnitude of the patient's effort, the level of set pressure and the respiratory system resistance), the flow decreases according to the time constant of the respiratory system, down to a cycling off value, allowing expiration. In case of leaks, flow could remain greater than this cycling off criterion (also referred to as expiratory trigger) lengthening insufflation time. Although frequently set at 25% of peak inspiratory flow on many ICU ventilators, this value is now often adjustable (5–70%) resulting in changes in ventilator insufflation time. TASSAUX *et al.* [33] evaluated the impact of a reduced insufflation time on asynchrony and WOB in patients with COPD during invasive ventilation. Increasing this expiratory trigger improved patient–ventilator synchrony, decreasing ineffective efforts without changing diaphragmatic energy expenditure and alveolar ventilation. During NIV, the usual expiratory trigger of 25% could be increased up to 50% in case of leaks, generating prolonged insufflation, especially in patients with obstructive lung disease [30].

Other modes of NIV

Volume targeted ventilation

During volume targeted ventilation, the ventilator delivers a set flow, inspiratory time and tidal volume at each breath, and inflation pressure may vary. Compared with PSV, volume targeted ventilators are rarely used in ARF due to some important disadvantages and have rarely been applied [47]. High peak mask pressures during volume targeted modes may cause more discomfort in terms of leaks, risk of gastric distension, pressure sores and skin necrosis. NIV can be performed using assist-control ventilation (ACV) where the patient can drive the respiratory rate: the ventilator delivers a positive pressure breath at a preset tidal volume in response to the patient's inspiratory effort or at a preset rate if no effort occurs within the preselected time period. ACV may deliver volumes less that are less reliable in case of leaks. Controlled modes may be preferred in patients with apnoea and hypopnoeas or unstable ventilatory drive (pressure or volume targeted modes), and volume targeted ventilation will be preferred in cases of unstable respiratory mechanics, overloaded respiratory muscles and failure of pressure targeted modes to augment spontaneous breathing before endotracheal intubation. Comparisons between different modes in NIV have rarely been performed. Studies comparing PSV with ACV modes in patients with ARF found no differences with respect to short-term physiological end-points [48–51]. ACV mode resulted in a higher respiratory muscle rest but PSV was more comfortable and showed better leak compensation [51].

Proportional assist ventilation

Proportional assist ventilation (PAV) is a mode of synchronised partial ventilatory support in which the ventilator pressure output is proportional to instantaneous patient effort [52]. This is a partial ventilatory assistance based in matching the ventilatory support with neural output of the respiratory centre. The patient should receive more mechanical assistance when the demand is higher and less support when the demand is lower, thus achieving a better patient–ventilator interaction. The ventilator amplifies the patient's inspiratory effort based on the analysis of flow and volume which are transformed into a certain amount of pressure based on the equation of motion of the respiratory system. The intensity of this amplification, therefore, depends on the respiratory system elastance (through volume assist) and resistance (through flow assist), which is required to be known. Noninvasive estimation of these measurements have been used mainly for NIV. Elastance is estimated by progressive increase of the volume assist until over assistance occurs with excessive volume and pressure. The resistance assist is determined by looking for the optimal comfort with different peak flows [53, 54]. NIV was considered to be an application in which PAV should provide better comfort and synchrony and it has been shown to be effective in achieving the goal of NPSV in studies of patients with ARF [52, 55]. However, no significant systematic superiority over NIV in the PSV mode was found when the two modes of assistances were compared [56–58]. Elastance, resistance and PEEPi are difficult to measure in patients with partial support ventilation and noninvasive methods are not extensively validated for NIV [59, 60]. Another disadvantage is that ventilator leak compensations can produce large positive pressure favouring instability.

Neural trigger and cycling off during PSV

NPSV provides safe and effective assistance to patients with ARF due to various causes [29, 61]. However the patient's tolerance to the technique is a critical factor in determining success of avoiding endotracheal intubation. One of the key factors determining tolerance to NPSV is optimal synchrony between the patient's spontaneous breathing activity and the ventilator's settings, known as the patient–ventilator interaction [30, 62]. As described, optimal patient–ventilator synchrony can prove very difficult to achieve due to the presence of leaks and depending on the type of interface which can interfere with various aspects of ventilator function [36, 63]. Patient–ventilator synchrony during NPSV can be compromised when using conventional pneumatic triggering, with the ventilator-delivered inspiratory support starting long after the patient's inspiratory effort. The switch from inspiration to expiration (cycling-off) should, ideally, coincide with the end of the patient's inspiratory effort. However large asynchronies can be observed during NPSV at the end of inspiration, with the ventilator cycling off either too early or too late relative to the end of the patient's inspiratory effort [33, 46, 64]. A possible solution is to replace the pneumatic triggering with neural triggering and cycling off using the diaphragm electrical activity. The electrical activity of the inspiratory muscles can be used as an index of the inspiratory neural drive [65]. Detection and quantification of the electrical activity of the crural diaphragm (EAdi) by means of an oesophageal array of bipolar electrodes has been validated in humans [66, 67]. Crural EAdi has been shown to accurately express global diaphragm activation [46, 67–69]. The array of bipolar electrodes can be mounted on a feeding tube, which is routinely introduced in critically ill patients. Cycling on and off are determined directly by the EAdi. MOERER et al. [70] have realised a physiologic study, in seven healthy volunteers. The aim of that study was to compare synchrony between inspiratory effort and ventilator assist during neurally or pneumatically triggered and cycled-off NPSV delivered with the helmet interface. Triggering and cycling off delays, wasted efforts and breathing comfort were determined during restricted breathing efforts with various combinations of pressure support levels and respiratory rates. During pneumatic triggering and cycling off, patient–ventilator synchrony was progressively more impaired with increasing respiratory rate and levels of pressure. During neural triggering and cycling off, effect of increasing respiratory rate and levels of pressure support on patient–ventilator synchrony was minimal. Breathing comfort was higher during neural triggering than during pneumatic triggering. The authors concluded that in healthy volunteers, trigger effort and breathing comfort with a helmet interface is considerably less impaired during with neural triggering and cycling off, compared with conventional pneumatic triggering and cycling off. Because the ventilator is triggered directly by EAdi, the synchrony between neural and mechanical inspiratory time is guaranteed at both the onset and the end of inspiration. From a clinical standpoint, patients needing NPSV often have no gastric probe. Whether adding an oesophageal catheter for mask ventilation will be acceptable in patients with ARF, needs to be confirmed in critically ill patients needing NPSV.

Noninvasive neurally adjusted ventilatory assist

The mode referred to as neurally adjusted ventilatory assist (NAVA) uses the electrical activity of the diaphragm to control not only the timing but also the amount of pressure delivered. The ventilator is triggered, limited and cycled-off directly by EAdi. The EAdi is measured by a multiple array oesophageal electrode. For accurate measurement, the active region of the diaphragm is determined by cross correlating the signals obtained along the electrode array [71]. The processed signal is then transferred to the ventilator unit to regulate the ventilator the ventilatory support, which is therefore instantaneously applied in relation to EAdi [72]. In other words the EAdi is multiplied by a number in order to determine the support level (NAVA gain). During NAVA, the positive airway pressure reflects the EAdi and this relationship is not altered by variations in tidal volume and end expiratory lung volume [71]. The patient–ventilator synchrony is guaranteed at both the onset and the end of inspiration. The cycling-off is commonly set at 80% of peak inspiratory activity (EAdi). The amount of support provided corresponds instantaneously to the ventilatory demand, irrespective of variations in muscle length or contractility. NAVA can almost abolish transdiaphragmatic pressure swings while maintaining synchrony between inspiratory neural effort and ventilatory assist [73]. The use of neural control of mechanical ventilation has the capability of enhancing the synchrony between mechanical ventilation and respiratory muscle activity, improving patient comfort. Another advantage is that NAVA should not be affected by leaks. Recently, BECK et al. [74] have evaluated, in rabbits, whether NAVA can deliver assist in synchrony and proportionally to EAdi with a leaky noninvasive interface. The main result is that NAVA can be effective in delivering NIV, even when the interface is excessively leaky, and can unload the respiratory muscles while maintaining synchrony with the subject's demand [74]. However, only studies on animals and healthy subjects have been carried out. It remains to be determined whether NAVA can maintain adequate levels of support and adequate patient–ventilator interaction in different kinds of respiratory failure, especially with NIV.

Ventilators

How to generate CPAP?

Many systems can be used commonly to deliver CPAP: one of the most frequently used consists in a high flow generator producing an air/oxygen mixture by Venturi effect, with an additional source of O2 and a mechanical expiratory valve. An inspiratory reservoir and a CPAP water valve can also be used, or a standard mechanical ICU ventilator in CPAP mode. The Boussignac CPAP device is a small cylindrical plastic adaptor that fits onto a modified face mask. The system uses the incoming flow of oxygen to generate a turbulent virtual pressure valve in the open expiratory side of the mask. The gas is accelerated and enters circumferentially into the open-ended cylinder generating air entrainment and positive pressure. The rate of flow will determine the amount of pressure achieved. A flow of 15 $L \cdot min^{-1}$ allows producing a pressure between 5 to 6 cmH_2O and a flow of 25 $L \cdot min^{-1}$ a pressure greater than 10 cmH_2O. This simple and cheap device can be safely and effectively used in emergency wards [75, 76]. Regarding the use of new generation of ICU ventilators, low levels of imposed workload are now required for CPAP but substantial differences in terms of performance have been demonstrated on bench study [77].

Which ventilator for NPSV: ICU or specific NIV ventilators?

NPSV can be delivered using both ICU ventilators and ventilators specifically dedicated to NIV. In a recent survey from North America [78], these specific NIV ventilators were the most frequently used ventilators accounting for two-thirds of cases whereas CPAP generator represented ~30% and ICU ventilators <5%. By contrast, a recent French survey in ICUs found that an ICU ventilator was used in ~80% of the cases whereas NIV and home ventilators represented <20% of the cases [28].

Table 1 presents the characteristics of the main ICU ventilators, including NIV dedicated ventilators, with regard to their specific features for delivering NIV. The main advantage of the NIV ventilator is its ability to work in presence of leaks. Indeed, it has been found that the trigger function of NIV ventilators was more effective than ICU ventilators in the presence of leaks [79]. However, it is important to underline the fact that major differences may exist in terms of performances between NIV ventilators [80, 81]. Although some NIV ventilators exhibit trigger function and pressurisation capacity close to ICU ventilators in bench studies without leaks [81–83], performances of these devices remain sometimes lower than new generation of ICU ventilators [84, 85].

The main advantages of an intensive care unit ventilator are often a better monitoring capability and its ability to continue invasive mechanical ventilation and full ventilatory support in the case of endotracheal intubation. A new generation of intensive care unit ventilators exhibit high performances on bench testing [85] but can become less efficient in presence of leaks [79, 86]. Recently, many manufacturers have developed a "mode" specifically designed for noninvasive ventilation. This mode is supposed to detect leaks and automatically adjust both the inspiratory trigger, to avoid auto-triggering, and the expiratory cycling criterion or ventilator insufflation time, to avoid prolonged inspiration [86]. These new capabilities may improve patient–ventilator synchrony and noninvasive

Table 1. – Characteristics of the main intensive care unit ventilators regarding their noninvasive ventilator capabilities

Ventilator	Manufacturer	Gas source	Available NIV mode	Range inspiratory trigger	Range expiratory trigger %	Range inspiratory times s
Esprit Vision	Respironics (Murrysville, PA, USA)	Turbine Turbine	Automatic/manual Automatic	-20– -0.1 cmH$_2$O, 0.5–20 L·min^{-1} Automatic	Automatic, 10–45 Automatic	0.1–9.9 0.5–3
PB 840	Tyco (Carlsbad, CA, USA)	Pressurised	Manual	0.2–20 L·min^{-1}	1–80	0.4–3
Elisée 350	Resmed (North Ryde, Australia)	Turbine	Automatic/manual	Automatic, -1– -5 cmH$_2$O	Automatic, 10–90	1–3
Avea Vela	Viasys Healthcare (Conshohocken, PA, USA)	Compressor Turbine	Manual Manual	0.1–20 L·min^{-1} 1–8 L·min^{-1}	5–45 5–40	0.2–5 0.3–
Extend	Taema (Antony, France)	Pressurised	Manual	1–20 L·min^{-1} , 0.1–5 cmH$_2$O	1–70	0.3–3.5
Servo i	Maquet (Solna, Sweden)	Pressurised	Manual	0–100%, -20–0 cmH$_2$O	1–40	
Savina Evita 4	Dräger (Lübeck, Germany)	Turbine Pressurised	Automatic Automatic	1–15 L·min^{-1} 0.3–15 L·min^{-1}	Automatic Automatic	0.2–10 0.1–10
Engstrom	General Electric (Fairfield, CO, USA)	Pressurised	Manual	1–9 L·min^{-1}, -1– -10 cmH$_2$O	5–50	0.25–15
Galiléo	Hamilton (Rhäzuns, Switzerland)	Pressurised	Manual	0.5–10 mbar, 0.5–15 L·min^{-1}	10–40	0.1–3
E500	Newport medical instruments (Costa Mesa, CA, USA)	Pressurised	Automatic/manual	0–5 cmH$_2$O, 0.6–2 L·min^{-1}	Automatic, 5–55	0.1–5

% are relative to the inspiratory peak flow.

ventilation tolerance but results are still heterogeneous [86]. Technical differences demonstrated among ventilators on lung model studies have been shown to have clinical consequences in terms of the patient's effort [38, 86, 87]. It is, therefore, likely that these new noninvasive ventilation modes will allow a higher efficacy of noninvasive ventilation with these ventilators but clinical studies remain to be performed.

Summary

Continuous positive airway pressure (CPAP) is a technique of artificial ventilatory support widely used in the intensive care unit (ICU). CPAP raises intrathoracic pressure, decreases arteriovenous shunting and improves oxygenation and dyspnoea. An advantage of CPAP over modes of mechanical ventilatory assistance is that CPAP does not require patient–ventilator synchronisation. However, pressure support is the most frequently used ventilatory mode during noninvasive ventilation (NIV). A specific problem during noninvasive pressure support ventilation (NPSV) is the presence of leaks around the mask, which lead to discomfort and patient–ventilator asynchrony. An optimal adjustment of ventilatory settings may improve comfort, work of breathing and patient–ventilator interaction, promoting the success of NIV. Other modes of ventilation, developed in order to improve the patient–ventilator interaction can be used during NIV. The proportional assist ventilation is a partial ventilatory assistance based in matching the ventilatory support with neural output of the respiratory centre. No significant systematic superiority over NPSV was found when the two modes of assistance were compared. The neurally adjusted ventilatory assist (NAVA) mode uses the electrical activity of the diaphragm (EAdi). The ventilator is triggered, limited and cycled off directly by EAdi. Neural triggering and cycling off guarantee an optimal patient–ventilator interaction at both the onset and the end of inspiration. The NAVA mode can unload the respiratory muscles; however, only studies on animals and healthy subjects have been carried out. NPSV can be delivered using both ICU ventilators and ventilators specifically dedicated to NIV. Recently, many manufacturers have developed a "mode" specifically designed for NIV. This mode detects leaks and automatically adjusts both the inspiratory and expiratory trigger. These new capabilities may improve patient–ventilator synchrony and NIV tolerance but results are still heterogenous.

Keywords: Continuous positive airway pressure, mechanical ventilation, noninvasive ventilation, pressure support, ventilators.

References

1. Rossi A, Ranieri MV. Positive end-expiratory pressure. *In*: Tobin JM, ed. Principles and Practice of Mechanical Ventilation. New York, McGraw-Hill, 1994; p. 259.
2. Organized jointly by the American Thoracic Society, the European Respiratory Society, the European Society of Intensive Care Medicine, and the Société de Réanimation de Langue Française, and approved by ATS Board of Directors, December. International Consensus Conferences in Intensive Care Medicine: noninvasive positive pressure ventilation in acute Respiratory failure. *Am J Respir Crit Care Med 2001* 2000; 163: 283–291.

3. Katz JA, Marks JD. Inspiratory work with and without continuous positive airway pressure in patients with acute respiratory failure. *Anesthesiology* 1985; 63: 598–607.

4. Lin M, Yang YF, Chiang HT, Chang MS, Chiang BN, Cheitlin MD. Reappraisal of continuous positive airway pressure therapy in acute cardiogenic pulmonary edema. Short-term results and long-term follow-up. *Chest* 1995; 107: 1379–1386.

5. Lenique F, Habis M, Lofaso F, Dubois-Randé JL, Harf A, Brochard L. Ventilatory and hemodynamic effects of continuous positive airway pressure in left heart failure. *Am J Respir Crit Care Med* 1997; 155: 500–505.

6. L'Her E, Deye N, Lellouche F, *et al.* Physiologic effects of noninvasive ventilation during acute lung injury. *Am J Respir Crit Care Med* 2005; 172: 1112–1118.

7. Goldberg P, Reissmann H, Maltais F, Ranieri M, Gottfried SB. Efficacy of noninvasive CPAP in COPD with acute respiratory failure. *Eur Respir J* 1995; 8: 1894–1900.

8. Nava S, Ambrosino N, Rubini F, *et al.* Effect of nasal pressure support ventilation and external PEEP on diaphragmatic activity in patients with severe stable COPD. *Chest* 1993; 103: 143–150.

9. Maitre B, Jaber S, Maggiore S, *et al.* Continuous positive airway pressure during fiberoptic bronchoscopy in hypoxemic patients: a randomized double-blind study using a new device. *Am J Respir Crit Care Med* 2000; 162: 1063–1067.

10. Petrof BJ, Calderini E, Gottfried SB. Effect of CPAP on respiratory effort and dyspnea during exercise in severe COPD. *J Appl Physiol* 1990; 69: 179–188.

11. Mehta S, Jay GD, Woolard RH, *et al.* Randomized, prospective trial of bilevel *versus* continuous positive airway pressure in acute pulmonary edema. *Crit Care Med* 1997; 25: 620–628.

12. Chadda K, Annane D, Hart N, Gajdos P, Raphaël JC, Lofaso F. Cardiac and respiratory effects of continuous positive airway pressure and noninvasive ventilation in acute cardiac pulmonary edema. *Crit Care Med* 2002; 30: 2457–2461.

13. Delclaux C, L'Her E, Alberti C, *et al.* Treatment of acute hypoxemic nonhypercanic respiratory insufficiency with continuous positive airway pressure delivered by a face mask: a randomized controlled trial. *JAMA* 2000; 284: 2352–2360.

14. Wakai Y, Welsh MM, Leevers AM, Road JD. Expiratory muscle activity in the awake and sleeping human during lung inflation and hypercapnia. *J Appl Physiol* 1992; 72: 881–887.

15. Bradley TD, Holloway RM, McLaughlin PR, Ross BL, Walters J, Liu PP. Cardiac output response to continuous positive airway pressure in congestive heart failure. *Am Rev Respir Dis* 1992; 145: 377–382.

16. Bellone A, Monari A, Cortellaro F, Vettorello M, Arlati S, Coen D. Myocardial infarction rate in acute pulmonary edema: noninvasive pressure support ventilation *versus* continuous positive airway pressure. *Crit Care Med* 2004; 32: 1860–1865.

17. O'Donoghue FJ, Catcheside PG, Jordan AS, Bersten AD, McEvoy RD. Effect of CPAP on intrinsic PEEP, inspiratory effort, and lung volume in severe stable COPD. *Thorax* 2002; 57: 533–539.

18. Masip J, Roque M, Sánchez B, Fernández R, Subirana M, Expósito JA. Noninvasive ventilation in acute cardiogenic pulmonary edema: systematic review and meta-analysis. *JAMA* 2005; 294: 3124–3130.

19. Peter JV, Moran JL, Phillips-Hughes J, Graham P, Bersten AD. Effect of non-invasive positive pressure ventilation (NIPPV) on mortality in patients with acute cardiogenic pulmonary oedema: a meta-analysis. *Lancet* 2006; 367: 1155–1163.

20. Winck JC, Azevedo LF, Costa-Pereira A, Antonelli M, Wyatt JC. Efficacy and safety of non-invasive ventilation in the treatment of acute cardiogenic pulmonary edema – a systematic review and meta analysis. *Crit Care* 2006; 10: R69.

21. Masip J, Páez J, Merino M, *et al.* Risk factors for intubation as a guide for noninvasive ventilation in patients with severe acute cardiogenic pulmonary edema. *Intensive Care Med* 2003; 29: 1921–1928.

22. Nava S, Carbone G, DiBattista N, *et al.* Noninvasive ventilation in cardiogenic pulmonary edema: a multicenter randomized trial. *Am J Respir Crit Care Med* 2003; 168: 1432–1437.

23. Squadrone V, Coha M, Cerutti E, *et al.* Continuous positive airway pressure for treatment of postoperative hypoxemia. *JAMA* 2005; 293: 589–595.

24. Ferreyra GP, Baussano I, Squadrone V, *et al.* Continuous positive airway pressure for treatment of respiratory complications after abdominal surgery: a systematic review and meta-analysis. *Ann Surg* 2008; 247: 617–626.

25. Kacmarek RM Mang H, Barker N, *et al.* Effects of disposable or interchangeable positive end-expiratory pressure valves on work of breathing during the application of continuous positive airway pressure. *Crit Care Med* 1994; 22: 1219–1226.

26. Pelosi P, Chiumello D, Calvi E, *et al.* Effects of different continuous positive airway pressure devices and periodic hyperinflations on respiratory function. *Crit Care Med* 2001; 9: 1683–1689.

27. Taccone P, Hess D, Caironi P, Bigatello LM. Continuous positive airway pressure delivered with a "helmet": Effects on carbon dioxide rebreathing. *Crit Care Med* 2004; 32: 2090–2096.

28. Demoule A, Girou E, Richard JC, Taillé S, Brochard L. Increased use of noninvasive ventilation in French intensive care units. *Intensive Care Med* 2006; 32: 1747–1755.

29. Carlucci A, Richard JC, Wysocki M, *et al.* Noninvasive *versus* conventional mechanical ventilation. An epidemiologic survey. *Am J Respir Crit Care Med* 2001; 163: 874–880.

30. Calderini E, Confalonieri M, Puccio PG, Francavilla N, Stella L, Gregoretti C. Patient–ventilator asynchrony during noninvasive ventilation: the role of expiratory trigger. *Intensive Care Med* 1999; 25: 662–667.

31. Georgopoulos D, Prinianakis G, Kondili E. Bedside waveforms interpretation as a tool to identify patient–ventilator asynchronies. *Intensive Care Med* 2006; 32: 34–47.

32. Vignaux L, Vargas F, Roeseler J, *et al.* Patient-ventilator asynchrony during non-invasive pressure support ventilation. *Am J Respir Crit Care Med* 2008; 177: A263.

33. Tassaux D, Gainnier M, Battisti A, Jolliet P. Impact of expiratory trigger setting on delayed cycling and inspiratory muscle workload. *Am J Respir Crit Care Med* 2005; 172: 1283–1289.

34. Imanaka H, Nishimura M, Takeuchi M, Kimball WR, Yahagi N, Kumon K. Autotriggering caused by cardiogenic oscillation during flow-triggered mechanical ventilation. *Crit Care Med* 2000; 28: 402–407.

35. Thille AW, Rodriguez P, Cabello B, Lellouche F, Brochard L. Patient–ventilator asynchrony during assisted mechanical ventilation. *Intensive Care Med* 2006; 32: 1515–1522.

36. Schettino GP, Tucci MR, Sousa R, Valente Barbas CS, Passos Amato MB, Carvalho CR. Mask mechanics and leak dynamics during noninvasive pressure support ventilation: a bench study. *Intensive Care Med* 2001; 27: 1887–1891.

37. Tokioka H, Tanaka T, Ishizu T, *et al.* The effect of breath termination criterion on breathing patterns and the work of breathing during pressure support ventilation. *Anesth Analg* 2001; 92: 161–165.

38. Aslanian P, El Atrous S, Isabey D, *et al.* Effects of flow triggering on breathing effort during partial ventilatory support. *Am J Respir Crit Care Med* 1998; 157: 135–143.

39. Prinianakis G, Delmastro M, Carlucci A, Ceriana P, Nava S. Effect of varying the pressurisation rate during noninvasive pressure support ventilation. *Eur Respir J* 2004; 23: 314–320.

40. Nava S, Bruschi C, Rubini F, Palo A, Iotti G, Braschi A. Respiratory response and inspiratory effort during pressure support ventilation in COPD patients. *Intensive Care Med* 1995; 21: 871–879.

41. Smith TC, Marini JJ. Impact of PEEP on lung mechanics and work of breathing in severe airflow obstruction. *J Appl Physiol* 1988; 65: 1488–1499.

42. Mancebo J, Albaladejo P, Touchard D, *et al.* Airway occlusion pressure to titrate positive end-expiratory pressure in patients with dynamic hyperinflation. *Anesthesiology* 2000; 93: 81–90.

43. MacIntyre NR, Cheng KC, McConnell R. Applied PEEP during pressure support reduces the inspiratory threshold load of intrinsic PEEP. *Chest* 1997; 111: 188–193.

44. L'Her E, Deye N, Lellouche F, *et al.* Physiologic effects of noninvasive ventilation during acute lung injury. *Am J Respir Crit Care Med* 2005; 172: 1112–1118.

45. Lellouche F, Maggiore SM, Deye N, *et al.* Effect of the humidification device on the work of breathing during noninvasive ventilation. *Intensive Care Med* 2002; 28: 1582–1589.

46. Beck J, Gottfried SB, Navalesi P, *et al.* Electrical activity of the diaphragm during pressure support ventilation in acute respiratory failure. *Am J Respir Crit Care Med* 2001; 164: 419–424.

47. Peter JV, Moran JL, Phillips-Hughes J, Warn D. Noninvasive mechanical ventilation in acute respiratory failure – a meta-analysis update. *Crit Care Med* 2002; 30: 555–562.

48. Meecham Jones DJ, Paul EA, Grahame-Clarke C, Wedzicha JA. Nasal ventilation in acute exacerbations of chronic obstructive pulmonary disease: effect of ventilator mode on arterial blood gas tensions. *Thorax* 1994; 49: 1222–1224.

49. Navalesi P, Fanfulla F, Frigerio P, Gregoretti C, Nava S. Physiologic evaluation of noninvasive mechanical ventilation delivered with three types of masks in patients with chronic hypercapnic respiratory failure. *Crit Care Med* 2000; 28: 1785–1790.

50. Vitacca M, Rubini F, Foglio K, Scalvini S, Nava S, Ambrosino N. Non-invasive modalities of positive pressure ventilation improve the outcome of acute exacerbations in COLD patients. *Intensive Care Med* 1993; 19: 450–455.

51. Girault C, Richard JC, Chevron V, *et al.* Comparative physiologic effects of noninvasive assist-control and pressure support ventilation in acute hypercapnic respiratory failure. *Chest* 1997; 111: 1639–1648.

52. Patrick W, Webster K, Ludwig L, Roberts D, Wiebe P, Younes M. Noninvasive positive-pressure ventilation in acute respiratory distress without prior chronic respiratory failure. *Am J Respir Crit Care Med* 1996; 153: 1005–1011.

53. Younes M. Proportional assist ventilation, a new approach to ventilatory support. Theory. *Am Rev Respir Dis* 1992; 145: 114–120.

54. Younes M. Proportional assist ventilation. *In*: Tobin MJ, ed. Principles and practice of mechanical ventilation. New York, McGraw-Hill, 1994; pp. 349–369.

55. Vitacca M, Clini E, Pagani M, Bianchi L, Rossi A, Ambrosino N. Physiologic effects of early administered mask proportional assist ventilation in patients with chronic obstructive pulmonary disease and acute respiratory failure. *Crit Care Med* 2000; 28: 1791–1797.

56. Gay PC, Hess DR, Hill NS. Noninvasive proportional assist ventilation for acute respiratory insufficiency. Comparison with pressure support ventilation. *Am J Respir Crit Care Med* 2001; 164: 1606–1611.

57. Fernández-Vivas M, Caturla-Such J, González de la Rosa J, Acosta-Escribano J, Alvarez-Sánchez B, Cánovas-Robles J. Noninvasive pressure support *versus* proportional assist ventilation in acute respiratory failure. *Intensive Care Med* 2003; 29: 1126–1133.

58. Rusterholtz T, Bollaert PE, Feissel M, *et al.* Continuous positive airway pressure *vs.* proportional assist ventilation for noninvasive ventilation in acute cardiogenic pulmonary edema. *Intensive Care Med* 2008; 34: 840–846.

59. Farré R, Mancini M, Rotger M, Ferrer M, Roca J, Navajas D. Oscillatory resistance measured during noninvasive proportional assist ventilation. *Am J Respir Crit Care Med* 2001; 164: 790–794.

60. Younes M, Webster K, Kun J, Roberts D, Masiowski B. A method for measuring passive elastance during proportional assist ventilation. *Am J Respir Crit Care Med* 2001; 164: 50–60.

61. Ferrer M, Esquinas A, Leon M, Gonzalez G, Alarcon A, Torres A. Noninvasive ventilation in severe hypoxemic respiratory failure. *Am J Respir Crit Care Med* 2003; 168: 1438–1444.

62. Tobin MJ, Jubran A, Laghi F. Patient–ventilator interaction. *Am J Respir Crit Care Med* 2001; 163: 1059–1063.

63. Kondili E, Prinianakis G, Georgopoulos D. Patient–ventilator interaction. *Br J Anaesth* 2003; 91: 106–119.

64. Conti G, Antonelli M, Navalesi P, *et al.* Noninvasive *vs.* conventional mechanical ventilation in patients with chronic obstructive pulmonary disease after failure of medical treatment in the ward: a randomized trial. *Intensive Care Med* 2002; 28: 1701–1707.

65. Chiumello D, Polli F, Tallarini F, *et al.* Effect of different cycling-off criteria and positive end-expiratory pressure during pressure support ventilation in patients with chronic obstructive pulmonary disease. *Crit Care Med* 2007; 35: 2547–2552.

66. Lourenço RV, Cherniack NS, Malm JR, Fishman AP. Nervous output from the respiratory center during obstructed breathing. *J Appl Physiol* 1966; 21: 527–533.

67. Sinderby CA, Beck JC, Lindström LH, Grassino AE. Enhancement of signal quality in esophageal recordings of diaphragm EMG. *J Appl Physiol* 1997; 82: 1370–1377.

68. Sinderby C, Beck J, Spahija J, Weinberg J, Grassino A. Voluntary activation of the human diaphragm in health and disease. *J Appl Physiol* 1998; 85: 2146–2158.

69. Beck J, Sinderby C, Lindström L, Grassino A. Effects of lung volume on diaphragm EMG signal strength during voluntary contractions. *J Appl Physiol* 1998; 85: 1123–1134.

70. Moerer O, Beck J, Brander L, *et al.* Subject-ventilator synchrony during neural *versus* pneumatically triggered non-invasive helmet ventilation. *Intensive Care Med* 2008; 34: 1615–1623.

71. Beck J, Sinderby C, Lindström L, Grassino A. Influence of bipolar esophageal electrode positioning on measurements of human crural diaphragm electromyogram. *J Appl Physiol* 1996; 81: 1434–1449.

72. Sinderby C, Navalesi P, Beck J, *et al.* Neural control of mechanical ventilation in respiratory failure. *Nat Med* 1999; 5: 1433–1436.

73. Sinderby C, Beck J, Spahija J, *et al.* Inspiratory muscle unloading by neurally adjusted ventilatory assist during maximal inspiratory efforts in healthy subjects. *Chest* 2007; 131: 711–717.

74. Beck J, Brander L, Slutsky AS, Reilly MC, Dunn MS, Sinderby C. Non-invasive neurally adjusted ventilatory assist in rabbits with acute lung injury. *Intensive Care Med* 2008; 34: 316–323.

75. Moritz F, Benichou J, Vanheste M, *et al.* Boussignac continuous positive airway pressure device in the emergency care of acute cardiogenic pulmonary oedema: a randomized pilot study. *Eur J Emerg Med* 2003; 10: 204–208.

76. Moritz F, Brousse B, Gellée B, *et al.* Continuous positive airway pressure *versus* bilevel noninvasive ventilation in acute cardiogenic pulmonary edema: a randomized multicenter trial. *Ann Emerg Med* 2007; 50: 666–675.

77. Takeuchi M, Williams P, Hess D, Kacmarek RM. Continuous positive airway pressure in new-generation mechanical ventilators: a lung model study. *Anesthesiology* 2002; 96: 162–172.

78. Schettino G, Altobelli N, Kacmarek RM. Noninvasive positive-pressure ventilation in acute respiratory failure outside clinical trials: experience at the Massachusetts General Hospital. *Crit Care Med* 2008; 36: 441–447.

79. Miyoshi E, Fujino Y, Uchiyama A, Mashimo T, Nishimura M. Effects of gas leak on triggering function, humidification, and inspiratory oxygen fraction during noninvasive positive airway pressure ventilation. *Chest* 2005; 128: 3691–3698.

80. Battisti A, Tassaux D, Janssens JP, Michotte JB, Jaber S, Jolliet P. Performance characteristics of 10 home mechanical ventilators in pressure-support mode: a comparative bench study. *Chest* 2005; 127: 1784–1792.

81. Bunburaphong T, Imanaka H, Nishimura M, Hess D, Kacmarek RM. Performance characteristics of bilevel pressure ventilators: a lung model study. *Chest* 1997; 111: 1050–1060.

82. Patel RG, Petrini MF. Respiratory muscle performance, pulmonary mechanics, and gas exchange between the BiPAP S/T-D system and the Servo Ventilator 900C with bilevel positive airway pressure ventilation following gradual pressure support weaning. *Chest* 1998; 114: 1390–1396.

83. Tassaux D, Strasser S, Fonseca S, Dalmas E, Jolliet P. Comparative bench study of triggering, pressurization, and cycling between the home ventilator VPAP II and three ICU ventilators. *Intensive Care Med* 2002; 28: 1254–1261.

84. Tassaux D, Dalmas E, Gratadour P, Jolliet P. Patient–ventilator interactions during partial ventilatory support: a preliminary study comparing the effects of adaptive support ventilation with synchronized intermittent mandatory ventilation plus inspiratory pressure support. *Crit Care Med* 2002; 30: 801–807.

85. Richard JC, Carlucci A, Breton L, *et al.* Bench testing of pressure support ventilation with three different generations of ventilators. *Intensive Care Med* 2002; 28: 1049–1057.

86. Vignaux L, Tassaux D, Jolliet P. Performance of noninvasive ventilation modes on ICU ventilators during pressure support: a bench model study. *Intensive Care Med* 2007; 33: 1444–1451.
87. Mancebo J, Amaro P, Mollo JL, Lorino H, Lemaire F, Brochard L. Comparison of the effects of pressure support ventilation delivered by three different ventilators during weaning from mechanical ventilation. *Intensive Care Med* 1995; 21: 913–919.

CHAPTER 12

NIV in the acute setting: technical aspects, initiation, monitoring and choice of interface

S.M. Maggiore, G. Mercurio, C. Volpe

Dept of Anaesthesiology and Intensive Care, Università Cattolica del Sacro Cuore, Policlinico A. Gemelli, Rome, Italy.

Correspondence: S.M. Maggiore, Dept of Anaesthesiology and Intensive Care, Università Cattolica del Sacro Cuore, Policlinico A. Gemelli, Largo Agostino Gemelli, 8, 00168 Rome, Italy. Fax: 39 063013450; E-mail: smmaggiore@rm.unicatt.it

Introduction

Noninvasive ventilation (NIV) is the delivery of mechanical ventilation without the need for an invasive artificial airway [1] and is a safe and effective means to improve gas exchange and reduce the work of breathing in patients with acute respiratory failure (ARF) of various origin [2, 3]. In patients with acute exacerbation of chronic obstructive pulmonary disease (COPD) and hypercapnic respiratory failure, the application of NIV to standard therapy decreases the need for endotracheal intubation, and reduces mortality [2, 4–6]. Similarly, NIV is effective in patients with cardiogenic pulmonary oedema, particularly in those with hypercapnia [7–9]. In patients with acute *de novo* respiratory failure, randomised controlled studies have shown that NIV reduces mortality in selected patients, such as those with immunosuppression [10] or with postoperative complications [11, 12]. However, the success rate of NIV in hypoxaemic ARF is strictly dependent on the ARF aetiology [5, 13], and the application of NIV in these patients is still controversial [14]. Advantages of NIV application include the reduction of the complications associated with endotracheal intubation [15], the improvement of patient comfort and the preservation of airway defence mechanisms, speech and swallowing [16]. NIV, however, is not successful in all patients; due to peculiarities of this ventilatory modality, such as the possibility of leaks and the need for patient compliance, technical aspects are of the utmost importance to improve its efficacy [17].

In order to optimise the success rate, NIV should be used as soon as incipient signs of respiratory failure develop and some technical aspects should be thoroughly taken into account. The correct choice of ventilator type should rely on the patient's conditions and the global performance of the machine. The use of intensive care unit (ICU) ventilators is generally preferable in the acute setting, since they are more powerful and have more adjustable features compared with home ventilators. Additionally, circuits with dual tubes reduce the risk of CO_2-rebreathing in patients with ARF. An important part of recent technical development for NIV application has concerned the interfaces. Nasal masks may be used in cooperative patients, to increase comfort and reduce complications but facial masks are generally preferable for dyspnoeic patients. Recently, an alternative interface, the helmet, has been proposed to decrease complications and improve tolerance. Recent data have also contributed to elucidate the role of gas humidification during NIV. The success rate during NIV will depend on

Eur Respir Mon, 2008, 41, 173–188. Printed in UK - all rights reserved. Copyright ERS Journals Ltd 2008; European Respiratory Monograph; ISSN 1025-448x.

the ability of the treatment to increase alveolar ventilation and reduce the work of breathing. Consequently, monitoring is crucial to assess the quality of assistance, an adequate patient–ventilator interaction and the amount of leaks.

The present chapter discusses the technical aspects of NIV application in the acute setting, with a particular focus on specific equipment and monitoring.

Initiation of NIV treatment: patient selection and preparation

Practical experience with NIV may not achieve success rates as high as those reported in the literature. Differences in patient selection and level of expertise of some practitioners with the application of NIV may account for discrepancies among published studies on NIV.

NIV has been used successfully in patients with hypercapnic respiratory failure due to COPD or restrictive lung diseases, in patients with acute cardiogenic pulmonary oedema, in immunocompromised patients and as a means of weaning from invasive mechanical ventilation in patients with COPD. NIV has also been successfully applied in selected patients with hypoxaemic respiratory failure due to pneumonia, asthma exacerbations and acute lung injury, although the evidence supporting the use of NIV in these conditions is weak [14]. Alert and cooperative patients are appropriate candidates to NIV treatment, although COPD hypercapnic patients with narcosis may represent an exception [18, 19].

In order to improve success rates in awake and cooperative patients, it is essential to reassure the patient and explain the technique in detail. It is also beneficial to gently hold the device on the patient's face before tightening it, in order to improve patient comfort. Finally, it is recommended that physicians do not tighten the device excessively or weakly, since an excessive pressure can cause skin breakdown and reduce patient tolerance, while a weak sealing may facilitate air leakage and patient–ventilator asynchronies.

NIV should be avoided in patients with cardiac or respiratory arrest, facial surgery or trauma, upper-airway obstruction, severe hypotension or life-threatening arrhythmia, and in those who require protection of the airways and who are at high risk of aspiration (coma, impaired swallowing, *etc.*) or have inability to clear secretions, while patients who have severe hypoxaemia (arterial oxygen tension (P_a,O_2)/inspiratory oxygen fraction (F_I,O_2) of ≤ 100), morbid obesity (>200% of ideal body weight) or with unstable angina or acute myocardial infarction, should be closely managed by experienced staff [20]. Criteria for NIV discontinuation and endotracheal intubation are shown in table 1 and must be taken into account in order to avoid dangerous delays of intubation.

Table 1. – Common criteria for discontinuation of noninvasive ventilation and endotracheal intubation

Respiratory arrest
Respiratory pauses with loss of consciousness or gasping
Psychomotor agitation making nursing care impossible and requiring sedation
Failure to improve oxygenation (*i.e.* P_a,O_2 ≤ 65 mmHg with an F_I,O_2 ≤ 0.6)
Inability to decrease P_a,CO_2 and improve academia (*i.e.* pH <7.25 and below the value at baseline)
Inability to correct dyspnoea, with tachypnoea and activation of accessory respiratory muscles
Development of conditions requiring protection of the airways (coma or seizure disorders)
Inability to manage copious tracheal secretions
Haemodynamic instability (*i.e.* systolic arterial tension <70 mmHg despite fluid resuscitation)
Heart rate or electrocardiographic instability
Inability to tolerate the mask or helmet

P_a,O_2: arterial oxygen tension; F_I,O_2: inspiratory oxygen fraction; P_a,CO_2: arterial carbon dioxide tension.

Mechanical ventilators, ventilatory modes and settings

NIV can be performed with either modern ICU ventilators or chronic long-term home ventilators [21]. The choice of ventilator type to deliver NIV should depend on both the patient's conditions and the technical characteristics of the machine, such as: 1) availability of different modes of ventilation; 2) quality of monitoring (detection of asynchronies and quantification of air leaks); 3) mechanisms of compensation for leaks; and 4) performance. These aspects have recently gained a greater interest in the literature, as they have a clinical impact in terms of work of breathing [22] and represent the key factors to improve patient–ventilator interaction during NIV, as well as tolerability of the technique. Despite being large in size and expensive, the modern ICU ventilators are more powerful and have more adjustable features (trigger type and sensitivity, slope of pressurisation, and cycling criteria), compared with home ventilators. The latter are portable, easier to use and less costly but often lack power, fine tuning of settings and monitoring capabilities.

When NIV is applied to treat a patient with a mild COPD exacerbation, the use of home ventilators may be appropriate, particularly if the patient is already using home NIV ventilator and is adapted to the machine. By contrast, patients with severe hypoxaemia and/or hypercarbia have a high risk of intubation and should be treated with more sophisticated machines and monitored in dedicated units. Data from bench and clinical studies have shown that home ventilators are generally less homogenous than ICU ventilators, with regards to the global performance [23]. The ICU ventilators have good monitoring capabilities and may adapt better to patients with ARF who have a high risk of NIV failure. A survey by DEMOULE *et al.* [24], conducted to evaluate the application of NIV in ICUs, showed that an ICU ventilator is used in 79% of cases, a ventilator dedicated to NIV in 12% and a home device in 5%.

In theory, NIV can be delivered with similar modalities used to deliver invasive ventilation through an endotracheal tube or a tracheotomy cannula. In practice, assisted ventilation is the primary mode of ventilation applied during NIV, while controlled modes are rarely used [14]. Among assisted modes of ventilation, pressure support ventilation (PSV) with positive end-expiratory pressure (PEEP) is certainly the most widely used mode during NIV [24]. PSV is usually delivered with swings of pressure above baseline ranging 8–20 cmH$_2$O. The setting depends on the patient's tolerance and the efficacy of the preset support level in terms of the delivered tidal volume and respiratory rate.

With regards to the application of PEEP during NIV, it is specifically used to improve oxygenation and increase lung volume in patients with hypoxaemic respiratory failure and to counteract intrinsic PEEP or to maintain airway patency in patients with COPD and sleep apnoea, respectively. In COPD patients, the level of PEEP should be titrated according to the actual intrinsic PEEP of the patient. Since this value cannot be reliably measured during NIV, the use of low PEEP levels (≤ 5 cmH$_2$O) is recommended for two main reasons: 1) intrinsic PEEP rarely exceeds this value in COPD patients, and 2) the higher is the level of PEEP, the greater is the likelihood of leaks, autocycling and asynchronies [25]. In hypoxaemic patients, the use of higher PEEP levels may be justified in the attempt to improve gas exchange. In a prospective, crossover, physiological study performed in 10 patients with acute lung injury, L'HER *et al.* [26] assessed the short-term effects of NIV with two combinations of PSV and PEEP (10–10 and 15–5 cmH$_2$O, respectively), and with continuous positive airway pressure (CPAP; 10 cmH$_2$O). Those authors found that tidal volume increased with PSV and not with CPAP, while neuromuscular drive and inspiratory muscle effort were significantly lower with the two PSV levels than with CPAP. The application of PEEP (10 cmH$_2$O), alone or in combination with PSV, improved oxygenation, but dyspnoea relief was significantly better with high level of PSV (15–5 cmH$_2$O). Thus, in patients with hypoxaemic respiratory failure, the application of PEEP or CPAP ameliorates gas exchange; however, PSV is needed in order to reduce inspiratory muscle effort and dyspnoea.

One specific problem with PSV during NIV concerns the cycle into expiration in case of leaks. Indeed, in PSV mode, the ventilator recognises the end of inspiration when the decelerating flow has fallen to a preset value. When air leaks occur, the flow threshold required to cycle into expiration cannot be achieved by the ventilator, and the inspiration is prolonged, thus causing patient–ventilator asynchronies and poor tolerance of the technique by the patient. Several strategies can be adopted to solve such a problem [27]. First, a small reduction in peak pressure (by reducing PSV or PEEP level) may be attempted in order to reduce leaks and eliminate asynchronies. Alternatively, the flow threshold can be set above the leak flow rate, by using expiratory flow sensitivity settings >30–40% of the peak-flow rate. Alternatively, a pressure controlled ventilation mode with a fixed inspiratory time (≤ 1 s) can be used [28].

Details on these aspects can be found in a dedicated chapter of this *European Respiratory Monograph* (*ERM*).

Selection of the interface

Apart from the choice of ventilator type, the use of an optimal interface is a crucial issue when NIV treatment is started [17]. Over the last few years, the development of new interfaces has contributed to improving the tolerance and the efficacy of the technique and has favoured the application of NIV in patients with ARF of various origins. A large array of interfaces is now available to deliver NIV (table 2).

The masks

Nasal and facial masks are the most commonly used interfaces during NIV and consist of two parts: a soft inflatable cushion that is directly in contact with the patient's face and a mask holder with two to five attachment points to secure the elastic head-straps. Increasing the number of the attachment points increases the adherence and stability of the mask and allows for a more uniform distribution of pressure on the skin surface. The adequate insufflation of the cushion is essential to improve patient comfort and reduce air leaks during NIV. Indeed, an excessive mask fit pressure causes skin damage at the site of mask contact, while a weak mask sealing may facilitate air leakage. In a bench study, it has been shown that air leaks increase when the difference between the pressure inside the cushion and the airway pressure is <2 cmH$_2$O [29]. Thus, it seems reasonable to keep the mask fit pressure 2–5 cmH$_2$O above airway pressure.

The nasal mask is usually well tolerated because it causes less claustrophobia and discomfort. It allows eating, drinking and expectorating and is commonly used for chronic long-term home ventilation [21, 30]. As an alternative to nasal masks, nasal pillows can be used to reduce the risk of pressure sores. The facial mask is preferable in acute respiratory failure because dyspnoeic patients are often mouth-breathers and mouth opening during nasal mask ventilation may cause air leakage and decrease the efficacy of NIV [21, 31]. In these patients, facial mask greatly improves alveolar ventilation and may prevent the increase in nasal resistances observed with the nasal mask in case of mouth leaks [32]. Different mask sizes are now commercially available and facilitate adaptation to individual facial contour. Total face masks are also available and give the theoretical advantages of reducing the risk of leakage and improving

Table 2. – Main characteristics of commercially available interfaces for noninvasive ventilation

Interface	Disposable (D) or re-usable (R)	Use in the intensive care unit (ICU) or at home	Advantages	Disadvantages
Nasal (simple) Respironics (Comfort classic) ResMed (Ultra mirage II nasal) Fisher-Paykel (Flexy fit nasal) SomnoTech (Somno Plus) Invacare (Twilight II)	R	Home and/or ICU	Comfort	Mouth leaks, nasal discomfort for long-term use
Nasal (moulded) Respironics (Profile lite) Sleepnet (IQ nasal) Circadiance (Sleepweaver) PMI ProBasics (Zzz-mask) DeVilbiss (Flexset)	D	Home only	Comfort	Mouth leaks, cost
Nasal pillows ResMed (Mirage swift) RespCare (Bravo nasal) AEIOMed (Headrest nasal) Respironics (Comfort lite nasal interface) CPAPPro (Nasal pillow interface) Fisher-Paykel (Opus 360) Puritan Bennett (Breeze Sleepgear)	R	Home and/or ICU	Comfort	Mouth leaks, cost
Nasal Prong systems Innomed (Nasal Aire II) Tiara (SNAPP-X)	D	Home	Comfort	Mouth leaks
Mouthpiece Fisher-Paykel (Oracle) ResMed (Liberty) Hybrid (Universal interface)	D	Home and/or ICU	For mouth breathing only, avoid nasal wound	Poor tolerance, leaks
Facial with inflatable cushion (simple) Tyco (KOO)	D	ICU		Basic
Facial with chin rest Hans Rudolph (7600 series V2)	R	Home and/or ICU	Avoid nasal wound	Leaks
Facial with internal flap and forehead support ResMed (Ultra mirage) Respironics (Comfort full 2) Fisher-Paykel (Flexifit HC 432) Tiara (Full Advantage)	R or D	Home and/or ICU	Tolerance	Cost
Total face Inspiraid (Fernez-Bacou/Draeger Medical, Lübeck, Germany) Respironics (Total Face, Performax)	R	ICU only	Tolerance, no pressure over nasal bridge	Dead space (low), claustrophobia
Helmet Rusch (4 vent) StarMed (CaStar) Harol (PN 500)	D	ICU only	Tolerance, long-term use, no pressure over the face	Dead space, asynchronies, claustrophobia, auxiliary support, disconnection

patient tolerance [33, 34]. Few studies [33, 35–38] have compared nasal and facial masks in terms of physiological effects, efficacy and patient comfort (table 3).

In 26 stable hypercapnic patients, NAVALESI *et al.* [35] evaluated the effect of three types of masks (nasal, facial and nasal plugs) and two ventilatory modes (PSV or assist-control volume ventilation) in terms of gas exchange, breathing pattern and tolerance to ventilation. The application of NIV significantly improved gas exchange and minute ventilation, regardless of the ventilatory mode, the underlying pathology or the type of mask. Overall, the nasal mask was better tolerated than the other two interfaces, but P_{a,CO_2} was significantly lower with the face mask or nasal plugs, than with the nasal mask. Minute ventilation was significantly higher with the face mask than with the nasal mask, and mouth air-leaks were likely the cause of the loss of tidal volume with nasal mask. Interestingly, the type of interface affected the NIV outcome more than the ventilatory mode. In another physiological study [36], conducted on 14 patients with stable COPD, to assess the efficacy of and tolerance for nasal and full-face masks during NIV, the authors found that NIV improved arterial blood gases and indices of respiratory effort regardless of the type of mask used; patient tolerance was also similar between interfaces. One randomised controlled trial [37] assessed patient tolerance and clinical outcome of facial *versus* nasal mask ventilation in 70 patients with ARF. Mask intolerance was significantly higher in the nasal than the facial mask group (34 *versus* 11%; p<0.05). Mouth leaks were the most common cause of intolerance during nasal ventilation. Conversely, intolerance of facial mask was due mainly to claustrophobia. Despite these differences, the overall success rate of NIV treatment was similar among the two groups.

In terms of comfort and patient tolerance, differences among models of a given interface can be as important as differences among interfaces. This has been recently shown by GREGORETTI *et al.* [38], who demonstrated improved comfort ratings and reduced skin breakdown among patients with hypercapnic and hypoxaemic ARF using a prototype full face mask. According to the authors, because this prototype mask had six points of attachment and a larger and thinner inflatable air cushion than commercially available masks, it can achieve an adequate air seal using less strap tension and may distribute pressure over a larger surface area on the face, reducing skin pressure at any one point such as the nasal bridge; additionally, the mask had an adapter for a nasogastric tube that eliminated the problems of air leak.

The dead-space volume of masks is a potentially important factor that should be taken into account. Indeed, physiological dead space is increased with any type of mask but the application of PEEP can favour carbon dioxide lavage during the respiratory cycle. Using a spontaneous breathing model, SAATCI *et al.* [39] have recently assessed static and dynamic dead space with 19 face masks, five turbine ventilators and three ventilatory modes. The authors found that total dynamic dead space was increased above physiological dead space from 32 to 42% of tidal volume by the use of face masks. The use of NIV modes with continuous pressure throughout the expiratory phase, such as bilevel and CPAP, reduced total dynamic dead space to approach physiological dead space, even with the total face masks. Pressure assist and pressure support ventilation decreased total dynamic dead space to a lesser degree, from 42 to 39% of tidal volume. Face masks with expiratory ports over the nasal bridge resulted in beneficial flow characteristics within the face mask and nasal cavity, with an increase in carbon dioxide lavage and a decrease in dynamic dead space to less than physiological dead space (from 42 to 28.5% of tidal volume). In another bench study, SCHETTINO *et al.* [40] reported that exhalation port location and mask design can affect carbon dioxide rebreathing; in particular, carbon dioxide rebreathing was less with the smallest mask volume and when the exhalation port was located within the mask rather than in the ventilator circuit.

Mouthpiece

This interface has not been evaluated to date in patients with ARF. The need for patient cooperation and the risk of a decreased NIV efficacy, due to nasal leaks,

Table 3. – Main characteristics of clinical trials comparing facial and nasal masks during noninvasive ventilation (NIV)

First author [ref.]	Study design	Patient population	NIV mode	Interfaces	Endpoints	Results
CRINER [33]	Single centre, prospective, observational	Stable hypercapnic (n=9; 30% COPD)	PSV plus PEEP	TF, F, N	Breathing pattern, tolerance, blood gas analysis	Tolerance: TF>N>F Leaks: TF<F=N V_T: TF>F>N f_R: TF=F=N P_{a,CO_2}: TF<F=N
NAVALESI [35]	Two centres, physiological, randomised, cross-over	Stable hypercapnic (n=26; 50% COPD)	PSV and VAC, without PEEP (30 min)	F, N, NP	Blood gas analysis, tolerance, breathing pattern (compared with SB)	↑ P_{a,O_2}: F=NP=N ↓ P_{a,CO_2}: F=NP>N Tolerance: N>F≥N; ↑ V_T: F>N; ↓ f_R: F=NP=N
GREGORETTI [38]	Multicentre (eight centres), prospective, randomised	Heterogeneous ARF (n=46; 45% hypoxaemic; 55% hypercapnic)	PSV plus PEEP	Fp, Fc	Complications, tolerance, blood gas analysis	Complications: Fp<Fc Tolerance: Fp>Fc ↑ P_{a,O_2}: Fp>Fc ↓ P_{a,CO_2}: Fp≥Fc
ANTON [36]	Single centre, physiological, randomised	Stable hypercapnic (n=14; 100% COPD)	PSV plus PEEP (15 min)	F, N	Blood gas analysis, respiratory effort, tolerance (compared with SB)	↑ P_{a,O_2}: F=N ↓ P_{a,CO_2}: F=N Tolerance: F=N ↓ effort: F=N ↑ f_R: F>N
KWOK [37]	Single centre, prospective, randomised	Heterogeneous ARF (n=70; 46% ACPO; 33% COPD; 17% hypoxaemic)	CPAP (~41%) or PSV plus PEEP (~50%)	F, N	Tolerance, intubation, hospital LOS, mortality, dyspnoea, blood gas analysis	Tolerance: F>N Intubation: F=N Hospital LOS: F=N Mortality: F=N ↓ dyspnoea: F=N ↓ P_{a,CO_2}: F=N ↓ f_R: F=N

Statistically significant differences are presented as < and >, trends towards significance are presented as ≤ and ≥ and no significant difference is presented as =. COPD: chronic obstructive pulmonary disease; PSV: pressuresupport ventilation; PEEP: positive end-expiratory pressure; TF: total face mask; F: facial mask; N: nasal mask; V_T: tidal volume; f_R: respiratory rate; P_{a,CO_2}: arterial carbon dioxide tension; VAC: volume assist-controlled; NP: nasal plugs; ↑: increase; P_{a,O_2}: arterial oxygen tension; ↓: decrease; ARF: acute respiratory failure; Fp: facial mask (prototype); Fc: facial mask (conventional); SB: spontaneous breathing; ACPO: acute cardiogenic pulmonary oedema; CPAP: continuous positive airway pressure; LOS: length of stay.

probably explain this lack of data. Alternatively, positive results have been reported in patients with chronic respiratory failure due to post-traumatic tetraplegia [41] or neuromuscular diseases [42].

The helmet

NIV treatment can fail as a consequence of complications directly or indirectly linked to the mask, such as air leaks, skin lesions, discomfort and intolerance [21, 43].

In attempt to improve tolerability, the helmet has been proposed as a new interface to administer NIV [44]. The helmet contains the head and the neck of the patient and is secured by two armpit braces at a pair of hooks on the plastic ring that joins the helmet to a soft collar; the collar adheres to the neck and ensures a sealed connection, once the helmet is inflated. The helmet is provided with an anti-asphyxia mechanism and two inner inflatable cushions to increase comfort and reduce the internal volume. Unlike the face mask, the helmet is not in touch with the patient's face and so it does not cause any skin breakdown and it improves the patient's comfort allowing longer periods of NIV delivery. The helmet can also be used in particular conditions, such as in edentulous patients and in patients with facial trauma. The ventilator delivers pressure to the patient through the helmet inlet. Patients receive only part of the large volume delivered by the ventilator after inspiratory trigger activation; the rest of the volume is compressed around the head, pressurising the helmet. It is, therefore, impossible to measure patient tidal volume and flow with conventional ventilator monitoring. During expiration, the patient exhales into the helmet, which is connected to the ventilator expiratory line through the helmet outlet.

Few studies on the bench or in healthy subjects have evaluated the physiological effects of NIV delivered through the helmet and have compared the performances of this interface with those of facial mask [45–48]. Two main problems have been discovered when NIV is administered through a helmet: 1) carbon dioxide rebreathing and 2) poor patient–ventilator interaction. These problems have been related to the large inner volume of the helmet and to its high compliance. Both are expected to cause a substantial dissipation of the inspiratory pressure delivered by the ventilator to expand the compliant helmet (in particular the soft collar). It has been demonstrated that the use of the helmet to deliver CPAP with a ventilator may predispose to carbon dioxide rebreathing, unless a continuous high-flow system is used [48]. Using this system, large and small helmets were demonstrated to be as efficient as a face mask in delivering CPAP [45]. In comparison with a standard face mask, RACCA et al. [47] showed that the use of helmet to deliver NIV with PSV increased inspiratory muscle effort and patient–ventilator asynchrony, worsened carbon dioxide clearance and increased dyspnoea when a resistive load was imposed in healthy subjects. Autocycled breaths accounted for 12 and 25% of the total minute ventilation and for 10 and 23% of the total inspiratory muscle effort during mask and helmet PSV, respectively. Only one physiological study has compared the efficacy of the helmet and the conventional facial mask in delivering NIV in COPD patients [49]. In that study, NIV significantly improved gas exchange and inspiratory effort with both interfaces. However, the helmet was less efficient than the mask in reducing inspiratory effort and it worsened the patient–ventilator interaction, as suggested by the longer delays to trigger on and cycle off the mechanical assistance, and by the higher number of ineffective efforts. Patient comfort was no different with the two interfaces.

To date, only one randomised and controlled clinical trial [50] has evaluated the effectiveness of CPAP delivered by helmet as compared with standard treatment in preventing the need for intubation and mechanical ventilation in hypoxaemic patients after elective major abdominal surgery. Patients were randomly assigned to receive oxygen (n=104) or oxygen plus CPAP with the helmet (n=105). Patients who received oxygen plus CPAP had a lower intubation rate (1 *versus* 10%; p=0.005) and a lower incidence of pneumonia (2 *versus* 10%; p=0.02), infection (3 *versus* 10%; p=0.03) and sepsis (2 *versus* 9%; p=0.03) than patients treated with oxygen alone. The duration of ICU stay was shorter in the group treated with CPAP than the control group (1.4 *versus* 2.6 days; p=0.09). Interestingly, the helmet allowed a prolonged application of NIV (19±22 h).

Other authors have suggested that the helmet is a valid alternative to the conventional face mask during CPAP, even in patients with severe respiratory acidosis and hypercapnia [51]. In those patients, the helmet provided long-duration CPAP, without any adverse events or clinical intolerance.

Only a few prospective and uncontrolled studies have assessed the clinical efficacy of noninvasive PSV delivered by helmet [44, 52, 53]. In a prospective, matched case–control study, ANTONELLI *et al.* [44] evaluated the efficacy of noninvasive PSV administered through an helmet as first-line intervention to treat patients with hypoxaemic ARF, in comparison with NIV and standard facial mask. Although the intubation rate was similar (24 *versus* 32% with helmet and facial mask, respectively; p=0.3), patients in the helmet group had a better tolerance of the technique (p=0.047). Complications related to the technique (skin necrosis, gastric distension and eye irritation) were fewer in the helmet group compared with the facial mask group (0 *versus* 21%; p=0.002). Moreover, the helmet allowed the continuous application of NIV for a longer period of time (36±29 *versus* 26±13 h; p=0.05). Similar results have been reported in immunosuppressed patients with hypoxaemic respiratory failure [52]. In another study, ANTONELLI *et al.* [53] showed that NIV by helmet was a feasible treatment for COPD patients with acute exacerbation but was not as efficient as the facial mask in improving carbon dioxide elimination. According to the authors, two possible factors could explain the reduced efficacy of the helmet in reducing hypercapnia: 1) carbon dioxide rebreathing and 2) less reduction of inspiratory effort, likely due to the lower quality of inspiratory assistance.

Interfaces: conclusions

The choice of interface is crucial to improve efficacy and patient tolerance during NIV. The facial mask is usually more effective and is tolerated as well as the nasal mask in acute setting; thus, it should be considered as the first choice interface in this setting. However, nasal mask may be used in cooperative patients to increase comfort and reduce complications. The helmet is an effective and better tolerated interface to deliver CPAP in selected patients with hypoxaemic ARF (post-operative ARF, cardiogenic pulmonary oedema and pneumonia, especially in immunosuppressed patients). Three factors should be taken into account when considering the helmet to deliver noninvasive PSV: 1) selection of patients and aetiology of ARF (hypoxaemic or hypercapnic), 2) quality of patient–ventilator interaction (which is better with the masks) and 3) patient tolerance (which is probably better with the helmet). While hypercapnic ARF is not a good indication for helmet PSV, this interface may be an option in patients with hypoxaemic ARF, especially when NIV is applied for prolonged periods of time and patient tolerance is a concern. Because of the risks of asynchronies and rebreathing and the lack of tidal volume monitoring, the use of the helmet during PSV should be restricted in the ICU and in experienced centres.

The ideal interface should be comfortable, stable, easy and quick to apply, inexpensive, and either disposable or re-usable; it should accommodate as many face sizes and shapes as possible while minimising air leaks, claustrophobic reactions and skin trauma. Due to the fact that it is difficult to conceive that a single interface would combine all these attributes, the most rational approach is to have a variety of interfaces, with different types and sizes, to satisfy individual patient needs (table 2). A strategy incorporating the sequential utilisation of different interfaces may prove useful to improve patient tolerance and the efficacy of NIV.

Airway humidification

Failure of NIV has been reported in 20–50% of patients [54] and attributed to inadequate carbon dioxide removal [55] and poor tolerance of the technique [43]. Gas humidification may be important to improve patient tolerance. Compared with invasive mechanical ventilation, upper airways, the main structure responsible for inspired gas heating and humidification, are not by-passed during NIV. This probably explains why, on the one hand, gas conditioning has been considered not necessary during NIV and, on the other hand, the lack of data until recent years. The importance of gas humidification during noninvasive CPAP has been shown, however, by several studies in patients with sleep apnoea syndrome [32, 56–58]. RICHARDS et al. [32] reported that nasal resistance may increase up to 300% during nasal CPAP without humidification and in case of mouth leaks. This phenomenon could be prevented by using a heated humidifier (HH). Other studies performed during home ventilation with nasal CPAP have shown that the use of an HH resulted in a decrease in nasal and upper airways symptoms (i.e. dryness, obstruction, sneezing and nasal drainage), while increasing the compliance with CPAP treatment [57, 58]. These data suggest that humidification of inspired gases may affect patient tolerance to NIV, particularly in case of prolonged applications. Indeed, when NIV is delivered by ICU ventilators, upper airways receive dry inspiratory gases. The upper airways may be unable to humidify these gases adequately, particularly in mouth breathers and when high inspiratory flows are used. Consequently, the lack of humidification may cause patient distress, as emphasised by the recent consensus conference on NIV [31], and life-threatening inspissated secretions [59].

Two humidifying devices are commonly used with ICU ventilators: HHs and heat and moisture exchangers (HMEs). The latter are generally preferred for their simplicity and low cost but add a significant dead space to the circuit and a marginal resistance to flow. These problems cannot be easily compensated during NIV and are dangerous in patients with ARF, who are likely more sensitive to dead space effects. In a physiological study performed in healthy subjects, LELLOUCHE et al. [60] measured hygrometry and comfort during NIV delivered with different humidification strategies: HH, HME or no humidification. For each strategy, a turbine and an ICU ventilator were used with different FI,O_2 setting, with and without leaks. Without humidification, delivered humidity was very low when an ICU ventilator was used but equivalent to the ambient air hygrometry with a turbine ventilator at minimal FI,O_2. HME and HH had comparable performances, but HME's effectiveness was considerably reduced by leaks. These data suggest that: 1) when using dry gases, as with an ICU ventilator, humidification is needed; 2) without leaks, HH and HME provide gas with comparably high water content; and 3) with leaks, a common situation when NIV is performed in acute setting, HH is the only system assuring an adequate humidification. The same authors have performed a randomised cross-over study to investigate the impact of HH and HME on arterial blood gases and patient effort in patients with moderate-to-severe hypercapnic ARF under NIV treatment [61]. Each device was studied without and with a PEEP of 5 cmH$_2$O. Despite similar Pa,CO_2 levels (60 ± 16 versus 57 ± 16 mmHg), minute ventilation was significantly higher with HME than with HH (15.8 ± 3.7 versus 12.8 ± 3.6 L·min^{-1}, without PEEP). HME was associated with a greater increase in work of breathing and indices of patient effort, with and without PEEP. Compared to baseline (unassisted breathing), NIV with HME failed to decrease the work of breathing, which even tended to increase (p=0.06) without PEEP. These data, corroborated by others [62], confirm that, in patients with hypercapnic ARF, the use of an HME lessens the efficacy of NIV in reducing patient effort compared with an HH.

Only one randomised controlled trial has investigated the effects of the two humidifying devices on clinical outcome during NIV in the acute setting [63]. In that study, 247 patients with hypercapnic or hypoxaemic ARF were included in 15 centres and randomised to receive NIV with an HME (n=128) or with an HH (n=119). The intubation rate was similar between the two groups (30.6 *versus* 37.6% with HME and HH, respectively; p=0.31), with no differences in the subgroup analyses. Duration of NIV, length of stay in ICU and in the hospital, and mortality in ICU and in the hospital were also similar between groups. In spite of strong physiological data favouring HH during NIV, no differences in clinical outcome were found in this study. The physiological effects observed in short term studies may be counterbalanced by other important factors in the clinical settings or may play a role only in marginal cases.

In conclusion, data available on the issue of humidification during NIV in the acute setting suggest that: 1) gas conditioning during NIV is important to improve patient tolerance; 2) humidification of inspired gases can be performed indifferently with one of the two available devices (HH or HME); and 3) in specific cases (less tolerant or more severe patients with hypercapnic ARF), HH may offer an advantage to improve the efficacy of NIV.

Monitoring

Monitoring is essential to verify the efficacy of NIV, which results from the ability of ventilatory assistance to increase alveolar ventilation and to decrease the patient effort to breathe, while assuring adequate patient comfort. In turn, this depends on a good patient–ventilator interaction and the amount of leaks. Monitoring during NIV is performed by a periodical evaluation of the patient's clinical status and arterial blood gases, and analysing the curves upon ventilatory screen.

Clinical evaluation and physiological response

Bedside patient evaluation helps physicians to assess the physiological response to treatment and it is crucial, especially during the initial period of NIV. Clinical monitoring is important to assess patient comfort, intensity of patient's efforts (as evaluated by palpation of sternocleidomastoid muscle to assess the use of accessory respiratory muscles, by the observation of paradoxical abdominal motion or by palpation of transversus abdominis muscle to assess active expiration), and efficacy of ventilatory assistance. Adequate clinical evaluation requires the monitoring of neurological status (especially in patients with hypercapnic ARF) and haemodynamic parameters (heart rate and blood pressure), as well. Improvements within 1 or 2 h of NIV treatment include a decrease in respiratory and cardiac frequencies and a reduction either in the use of accessory respiratory muscles or in paradoxical abdominal motion.

Improvement in gas exchange, as determined by percutaneous oximetry and blood gas analysis, is crucial during NIV treatment in acute setting. A lack of improvement in gas exchange within 1 or 2 h of treatment is suggestive of treatment failure and must be taken into account in order to avoid dangerous delays in intubation [13, 55]. Several studies have reported that the degree of acidosis/acidaemia (pH and Pa,CO_2 at admission and after 1 h of NIV) is the best predictor for NIV outcome in patients with hypercapnic ARF [43, 55, 64, 65]. By contrast, the inability to improve oxygenation after 1 h of NIV was associated with treatment failure in patients with hypoxaemic ARF [13, 66].

Arterial blood gas analysis must be performed every day and in case of modifications of clinical status or after changes of ventilatory settings. Arterial blood gases should be performed both during NIV (to assess the efficacy of treatment) and without NIV (to evaluate patient respiratory status and the possibility of weaning from NIV). Blood gas analysis is particularly important when NIV is delivered through the helmet because of the impossibility to monitor inspired and expired tidal volumes with this interface. Continuous noninvasive monitoring of oxygen saturation is an essential monitoring during NIV, particularly in hypoxaemic patients, while Pa,CO_2 evaluation is more important in hypercapnic patients. Although noninvasive carbon dioxide monitoring might be useful for trending purpose during NIV, abnormalities of lung parenchyma, air leaks and dilution, due to bias flow, with some ventilators make end-tidal carbon dioxide monitoring inaccurate. As such, this monitoring has poor indications in the acute setting.

Detection of air leaks and patient–ventilator asynchronies

Patient tolerance is a major determinant of the success of the technique and can be impaired by patient–ventilator asynchronies, defined as a mismatch between the patient and the ventilator inspiratory and expiratory times (details on this issue can be found in a dedicated chapter of this *ERM*). Asynchronies occur frequently during NIV, facilitated by the presence of leaks [67]. Detection of leaks is at best performed by analysing the curves at ventilatory screen. Although allowing the identification of major leaks around the mask, clinical detection ("hand detection") has a low sensitivity and it does not allow quantification of the amount of air leakage. The difference between inspired and expired tidal volumes, as well as the shape of the flow waveform (area included in the inspiratory flow curve, above zero, greater than the area included in the expiratory flow curve, below zero) and the identification of leak-associated phenomena (*e.g.* ventilator autocycling and prolonged inspirations) allow for an early and accurate detection of leaks [27]. Monitoring of expired tidal volume is particularly important to assure an adequate alveolar ventilation (>6 mL·kg^{-1}). Monitoring of respiratory rate (as measured by the ventilator and by the direct observation of the patient) can also be helpful to detect asynchronies, such as ventilator autotriggering (ventilator's respiratory rate greater than the patient's respiratory rate) and ineffective patient efforts (ventilator's respiratory rate less than the patient's respiratory rate).

Summary

Noninvasive ventilation (NIV) reduces the work of breathing, improves gas exchange and may improve clinical outcome in patients with acute respiratory failure (ARF) of various origin. Failure of NIV occurs, however, in ~20–30% of patients with hypercapnic ARF and in an even higher percentage of patients with hypoxaemic ARF. NIV failure may be due to clinical or technical factors such as the ventilatory mode and settings. Poor adaptation to the interface may also be responsible for some cases of NIV failure. It is therefore important to take into account these technical aspects in order to increase the efficacy of NIV.

Both home and intensive care unit ventilators have been used to delivered NIV but the latter are preferred in the most severe critically ill patients. Three main types of interfaces are currently available in acute situation: facial, nasal and the helmet. The facial mask is generally considered the first choice in terms of efficacy. The helmet is an acceptable alternative to deliver continuous positive airway pressure in selected patients with hypoxaemic ARF. The most rational approach is, however, to adapt the type and the size of the interface on an individual basis. Humidification of inspired gas, often considered of minor relevance, is important to improve patient's comfort. In spite of a theoretical superiority of heated humidifiers over heat and moisture exchangers, particularly in patients with hypercapnic ARF, no study has yet confirmed it to date. Finally, adequate patient selection, preparation and monitoring are crucial in making NIV successful.

Keywords: Heat and moisture exchanger, heated humidifier, helmet, mask, noninvasive ventilation, ventilators.

References

1. Meduri GU. Noninvasive ventilation. *In*: Marini J, Slutsky A, eds. Physiological basis of ventilatory support. New York, Marcel Dekker Inc., 1998; pp. 921–998.

2. Brochard L, Mancebo J, Wysocki M, *et al.* Noninvasive ventilation for acute exacerbations of chronic obstructive pulmonary disease. *N Engl J Med* 1995; 333: 817–822.

3. Antonelli M, Conti G, Rocco M, *et al.* A comparison of noninvasive positive-pressure ventilation and conventional mechanical ventilation in patients with acute respiratory failure. *N Engl J Med* 1998; 339: 429–435.

4. Bott J, Carroll MP, Conway JH, *et al.* Randomised controlled trial of nasal ventilation in acute ventilatory failure due to chronic obstructive airways disease. *Lancet* 1993; 341: 1555–1557.

5. Meduri GU, Turner RE, Abou-Shala N, Wunderink R, Tolley E. Noninvasive positive pressure ventilation *via* face mask. First-line intervention in patients with acute hypercapnic and hypoxemic respiratory failure. *Chest* 1996; 109: 179–193.

6. Lightowler JV, Wedzicha JA, Elliott MW, Ram FS. Non-invasive positive pressure ventilation to treat respiratory failure resulting from exacerbations of chronic obstructive pulmonary disease: Cochrane systematic review and meta-analysis. *BMJ* 2003; 326: 185–187.

7. Rasanen J, Heikkila J, Downs J, Nikki P, Vaisanen I, Viitanen A. Continuous positive airway pressure by face mask in acute cardiogenic pulmonary edema. *Am J Cardiol* 1985; 55: 296–300.

8. Bersten AD, Holt AW, Vedig AE, Skowronski GA, Baggoley CJ. Treatment of severe cardiogenic pulmonary edema with continuous positive airway pressure delivered by face mask. *N Engl J Med* 1991; 325: 1825–1830.

9.   Masip J, Roque M, Sanchez B, Fernandez R, Subirana M, Exposito JA. Noninvasive ventilation in acute cardiogenic pulmonary edema: systematic review and meta-analysis. *JAMA* 2005; 294: 3124–3130.

10. Hilbert G, Gruson D, Vargas F, *et al.* Noninvasive ventilation in immunosuppressed patients with pulmonary infiltrates, fever, and acute respiratory failure. *N Engl J Med* 2001; 344: 481–487.

11. Antonelli M, Conti G, Bufi M, *et al.* Noninvasive ventilation for treatment of acute respiratory failure in patients undergoing solid organ transplantation: a randomized trial. *JAMA* 2000; 283: 235–241.

12. Auriant I, Jallot A, Herve P, *et al.* Noninvasive ventilation reduces mortality in acute respiratory failure following lung resection. *Am J Respir Crit Care Med* 2001; 164: 1231–1235.

13. Antonelli M, Conti G, Moro ML, *et al.* Predictors of failure of noninvasive positive pressure ventilation in patients with acute hypoxemic respiratory failure: a multi-center study. *Intensive Care Med* 2001; 27: 1718–1728.

14. Ambrosino N, Vagheggini G. Noninvasive positive pressure ventilation in the acute care setting: where are we? *Eur Respir J* 2008; 31: 874–886.

15. Girou E, Schortgen F, Delclaux C, *et al.* Association of noninvasive ventilation with nosocomial infections and survival in critically ill patients. *JAMA* 2000; 284: 2361–2367.

16. Hill NS. Noninvasive positive pressure ventilation. *In*: Tobin MJ, ed. Principles and Practice of Mechanical Ventilation. 2nd Edn. New York, McGraw-Hill, 2006; pp. 433–471.

17. Elliott MW. The interface: crucial for successful noninvasive ventilation. *Eur Respir J* 2004; 23: 7–8.

18. Diaz GG, Alcaraz AC, Talavera JC, *et al.* Noninvasive positive-pressure ventilation to treat hypercapnic coma secondary to respiratory failure. *Chest* 2005; 127: 952–960.

19. Scala R, Nava S, Conti G, *et al.* Noninvasive *versus* conventional ventilation to treat hypercapnic encephalopathy in chronic obstructive pulmonary disease. *Intensive Care Med* 2007; 33: 2101–2108.

20. Nava S, Ceriana P. Causes of failure of noninvasive mechanical ventilation. *Respir Care* 2004; 49: 295–303.

21. Mehta S, Hill NS. Noninvasive ventilation. *Am J Respir Crit Care Med* 2001; 163: 540–577.

22. Vitacca M, Barbano L, D'Anna S, Porta R, Bianchi L, Ambrosino N. Comparison of five bilevel pressure ventilators in patients with chronic ventilatory failure: a physiologic study. *Chest* 2002; 122: 2105–2114.

23. Richard JC, Carlucci A, Breton L, *et al.* Bench testing of pressure support ventilation with three different generations of ventilators. *Intensive Care Med* 2002; 28: 1049–1057.

24. Demoule A, Girou E, Richard JC, Taille S, Brochard L. Increased use of noninvasive ventilation in French intensive care units. *Intensive Care Med* 2006; 32: 1747–1755.

25. Navalesi P, Maggiore SM. Positive end expiratory positive pressure. *In*: Tobin MJ, ed. Principles and Practice of Mechanical Ventilation. 2nd Edn. New York, McGraw-Hill, 2006; pp. 273–325.

26. L'Her E, Deye N, Lellouche F, *et al.* Physiologic effects of noninvasive ventilation during acute lung injury. *Am J Respir Crit Care Med* 2005; 172: 1112–1118.

27. Brochard L, Maggiore SM. Noninvasive ventilation: modes of ventilation. *In*: Muir JF, Ambrosino N, Simonds AK, eds. Noninvasive Mechanical Ventilation. *Eur Respir Mon* 2001; 16: 67–75.

28. Calderini E, Confalonieri M, Puccio PG, Francavilla N, Stella L, Gregoretti C. Patient-ventilator asynchrony during noninvasive ventilation: the role of expiratory trigger. *Intensive Care Med* 1999; 25: 662–667.

29. Schettino GP, Tucci MR, Sousa R, Valente Barbas CS, Passos Amato MB, Carvalho CR. Mask mechanics and leak dynamics during noninvasive pressure support ventilation: a bench study. *Intensive Care Med* 2001; 27: 1887–1891.

30. Schonhofer B, Sortor-Leger S. Equipment needs for noninvasive mechanical ventilation. *Eur Respir J* 2002; 20: 1029–1036.

31. International Consensus Conferences in Intensive Care Medicine: noninvasive positive pressure ventilation in acute respiratory failure. *Am J Respir Crit Care Med* 2001; 163: 283–291.

32. Richards GN, Cistulli PA, Ungar RG, Berthon-Jones M, Sullivan CE. Mouth leak with nasal continuous positive airway pressure increases nasal airway resistance. *Am J Respir Crit Care Med* 1996; 154: 182–186.

33. Criner GJ, Travaline JM, Brennan KJ, Kreimer DT. Efficacy of a new full face mask for noninvasive positive pressure ventilation. *Chest* 1994; 106: 1109–1115.

34. Cuvelier A, Pujol W, Molano LC, Muir JF. Efficacy and tolerance of cephalic mask for noninvasive ventilation during acute hypercapnic respiratory failure. A randomized controlled study. *Proc Am Thorac Soc* 2006; 3: A471.

35. Navalesi P, Fanfulla F, Frigerio P, Gregoretti C, Nava S. Physiologic evaluation of noninvasive mechanical ventilation delivered with three types of masks in patients with chronic hypercapnic respiratory failure. *Crit Care Med* 2000; 28: 1785–1790.

36. Anton A, Tarrega J, Giner J, Guell R, Sanchis J. Acute physiologic effects of nasal and full-face masks during noninvasive positive-pressure ventilation in patients with acute exacerbations of chronic obstructive pulmonary disease. *Respir Care* 2003; 48: 922–925.

37. Kwok H, McCormack J, Cece R, Houtchens J, Hill NS. Controlled trial of oronasal versus nasal mask ventilation in the treatment of acute respiratory failure. *Crit Care Med* 2003; 31: 468–473.

38. Gregoretti C, Confalonieri M, Navalesi P, *et al.* Evaluation of patient skin breakdown and comfort with a new face mask for non-invasive ventilation: a multi-center study. *Intensive Care Med* 2002; 28: 278–284.

39. Saatci E, Miller DM, Stell IM, Lee KC, Moxham J. Dynamic dead space in face masks used with noninvasive ventilators: a lung model study. *Eur Respir J* 2004; 23: 129–135.

40. Schettino GP, Chatmongkolchart S, Hess DR, Kacmarek RM. Position of exhalation port and mask design affect CO_2 rebreathing during noninvasive positive pressure ventilation. *Crit Care Med* 2003; 31: 2178–2182.

41. Viroslav J, Rosenblatt R, Tomazevic SM. Respiratory management, survival, and quality of life for high-level traumatic tetraplegics. *Respir Care Clin N Am* 1996; 2: 313–322.

42. Bach JR, Alba AS, Saporito LR. Intermittent positive pressure ventilation *via* the mouth as an alternative to tracheostomy for 257 ventilator users. *Chest* 1993; 103: 174–182.

43. Carlucci A, Richard JC, Wysocki M, Lepage E, Brochard L. Noninvasive *versus* conventional mechanical ventilation. An epidemiologic survey. *Am J Respir Crit Care Med* 2001; 163: 874–880.

44. Antonelli M, Conti G, Pelosi P, *et al.* New treatment of acute hypoxemic respiratory failure: noninvasive pressure support ventilation delivered by helmet – a pilot controlled trial. *Crit Care Med* 2002; 30: 602–608.

45. Chiumello D, Pelosi P, Carlesso E, *et al.* Noninvasive positive pressure ventilation delivered by helmet *vs* standard face mask. *Intensive Care Med* 2003; 29: 1671–1679.

46. Patroniti N, Foti G, Manfio A, Coppo A, Bellani G, Pesenti A. Head helmet *versus* face mask for non-invasive continuous positive airway pressure: a physiological study. *Intensive Care Med* 2003; 29: 1680–1687.

47. Racca F, Appendini L, Gregoretti C, *et al.* Effectiveness of mask and helmet interfaces to deliver noninvasive ventilation in a human model of resistive breathing. *J Appl Physiol* 2005; 99: 1262–1271.

48. Taccone P, Hess D, Caironi P, Bigatello LM. Continuous positive airway pressure delivered with a "helmet": effects on carbon dioxide rebreathing. *Crit Care Med* 2004; 32: 2090–2096.

49. Navalesi P, Costa R, Ceriana P, *et al.* Non-invasive ventilation in chronic obstructive pulmonary disease patients: helmet *versus* facial mask. *Intensive Care Med* 2007; 33: 74–81.

50. Squadrone V, Coha M, Cerutti E, *et al.* Continuous positive airway pressure for treatment of postoperative hypoxemia: a randomized controlled trial. *JAMA* 2005; 293: 589–595.

51. Tonnelier JM, Prat G, Nowak E, *et al.* Noninvasive continuous positive airway pressure ventilation using a new helmet interface: a case-control prospective pilot study. *Intensive Care Med* 2003; 29: 2077–2080.

52. Rocco M, Dell'Utri D, Morelli A, *et al.* Noninvasive ventilation by helmet or face mask in immunocompromised patients: a case-control study. *Chest* 2004; 126: 1508–1515.

53. Antonelli M, Pennisi MA, Pelosi P, *et al.* Noninvasive positive pressure ventilation using a helmet in patients with acute exacerbation of chronic obstructive pulmonary disease: a feasibility study. *Anesthesiology* 2004; 100: 16–24.

54. Keenan SP, Kernerman PD, Cook DJ, Martin CM, McCormack D, Sibbald WJ. Effect of noninvasive positive pressure ventilation on mortality in patients admitted with acute respiratory failure: a meta-analysis. *Crit Care Med* 1997; 25: 1685–1692.

55. Ambrosino N, Foglio K, Rubini F, Clini E, Nava S, Vitacca M. Non-invasive mechanical ventilation in acute respiratory failure due to chronic obstructive pulmonary disease: correlates for success. *Thorax* 1995; 50: 755–757.

56. Martins De Araujo MT, Vieira SB, Vasquez EC, Fleury B. Heated humidification or face mask to prevent upper airway dryness during continuous positive airway pressure therapy. *Chest* 2000; 117: 142–147.

57. Massie CA, Hart RW, Peralez K, Richards GN. Effects of humidification on nasal symptoms and compliance in sleep apnea patients using continuous positive airway pressure. *Chest* 1999; 116: 403–408.

58. Rakotonanahary D, Pelletier-Fleury N, Gagnadoux F, Fleury B. Predictive factors for the need for additional humidification during nasal continuous positive airway pressure therapy. *Chest* 2001; 119: 460–465.

59. Wood KE, Flaten AL, Backes WJ. Inspissated secretions: a life-threatening complication of prolonged noninvasive ventilation. *Respir Care* 2000; 45: 491–493.

60. Lellouche F, Maggiore SM, Fischler M, *et al.* Hygrometry during non invasive ventilation (NIV) with different humidification strategies in healthy subjects. *Am J Respir Crit Care Med* 2001; 163: A680.

61. Lellouche F, Maggiore SM, Deye N, *et al.* Effect of the humidification device on the work of breathing during noninvasive ventilation. *Intensive Care Med* 2002; 28: 1582–1589.

62. Jaber S, Chanques G, Matecki S, *et al.* Comparison of the effects of heat and moisture exchangers and heated humidifiers on ventilation and gas exchange during non-invasive ventilation. *Intensive Care Med* 2002; 28: 1590–1594.

63. Lellouche F, L'Her E, Abrouk F, *et al.* Impact of the humidification device on intubation rate during NIV: results of a multicenter RCT. *Proc Am Thorac Soc* 2006; 3: A471.

64. Anton A, Guell R, Gomez J, *et al.* Predicting the result of noninvasive ventilation in severe acute exacerbations of patients with chronic airflow limitation. *Chest* 2000; 117: 828–833.

65. Plant PK, Owen JL, Elliott MW. Non-invasive ventilation in acute exacerbations of chronic obstructive pulmonary disease: long term survival and predictors of in-hospital outcome. *Thorax* 2001; 56: 708–712.

66. Antonelli M, Conti G, Esquinas A, *et al.* A multiple-center survey on the use in clinical practice of noninvasive ventilation as a first-line intervention for acute respiratory distress syndrome. *Crit Care Med* 2007; 35: 18–25.

67. Lellouche F, L'Her E, Fraticelli A, *et al.* Frequency of patient-ventilator asynchrony during non invasive ventilation. *Intensive Care Med* 2005; 31: S193.

CHAPTER 13

Where to perform NIV

S.D.W. Miller, M. Latham, M.W. Elliott

Dept of Respiratory Medicine, St James's University Hospital, Leeds, UK.

Correspondence: M.W. Elliott, Dept of Respiratory Medicine, St James's University Hospital, Beckett Street, Leeds, LS9 7TF, UK. Fax: 44 113 206 6042; E-mail: mark.elliot@leedsth.nhs.uk

Introduction

Noninvasive positive pressure ventilation (NPPV) has been shown to be an effective treatment for ventilatory failure, particularly resulting from acute exacerbations of chronic obstructive pulmonary disease (COPD) but also resulting from hypoxaemic respiratory failure, community acquired pneumonia, cardiogenic pulmonary oedema and following solid organ transplants in randomised controlled trials (RCTs). There have also been RCTs of NPPV in weaning and for patients with post-extubation respiratory failure. Most strikingly, NPPV reduces the need for intubation and invasive mechanical ventilation (IMV), which, in the larger studies, translates into improved survival [1, 2], reduced complication rates, and length of both intensive care unit (ICU) and hospital stay [1]. Infectious complications, particularly pneumonia are markedly reduced [1, 3–5]. The use of NPPV opens up new opportunities in the management of patients with ventilatory failure, particularly with regard to location and the timing of intervention. Paralysis and sedation are not required with NPPV and ventilation can be performed outside the ICU. Given the considerable pressure on ICU beds in some countries, the high costs associated with ICU care and that for some patients, admission to ICU is a distressing experience [6], this is an attractive option.

Definitions

In any discussion about the location of an NPPV service, it is important to note that the model of hospital care differs from country to country and that ICUs, high dependency units (HDUs) and general wards will have different levels of staffing, facilities for monitoring, *etc*. Care must, therefore, be taken in the extrapolation of results obtained in one study environment to other hospitals and countries. The King's Fund panel [7] define intensive care as: "A service for patients with potentially recoverable diseases who can benefit from more detailed observation and treatment than is generally available in the standard wards and departments". This broad definition does not unfortunately assist in the problem of comparisons of individual ICUs between studies. The definition of HDU is even less clear, with some HDUs allowing invasive monitoring while in others only noninvasive monitoring is performed. A multicentre study [2] of NPPV in general respiratory wards illustrates the large variation in nurse to patient ratios in different centres; the mean nurse to patient ratio was 1:11 with a range of 1:2.6–1:13.

Eur Respir Mon, 2008, 41, 189–199. Printed in UK - all rights reserved. Copyright ERS Journals Ltd 2008; European Respiratory Monograph; ISSN 1025-448x.

For the purpose of the present chapter, the following definitions are used. ICU: implies continuous monitoring of vital signs, facilities for IMV *via* oral or nasal endotracheal tube with high levels of nurse staffing throughout a 24-h period in a specified clinical area. Patients generally require support for more than one failing organ system. HDU: implies continuous monitoring of vital signs with a nurse to patient ratio intermediate between that of the ICU and the general ward in a specified clinical area. These are able to care for tracheostomised patients receiving ventilation but otherwise do not look after invasively ventilated patients. Patients generally have single organ failure. General ward: these take unselected emergency admission and, although most will have a particular speciality interest, it is likely that, because of the unpredictability of demand, patients with a variety of conditions and degrees of severity will be cared for in the same clinical area. Nurse staffing levels will vary but the intensity of nursing input available on HDUs and ICUs will not be possible.

Where to perform NPPV

Most of the RCTs have been in patients with COPD which will, therefore, be the main focus for the discussion about location of an acute NPPV service. The ICU is the usual setting for NPPV although there have been prospective randomised controlled studies of NPPV outside the ICU [2, 8–11].

BOTT *et al.* [8] randomised 60 patients with COPD to either conventional treatment or NPPV. NPPV initiation, by research staff, took an average of 90 min (range 15–240 min) and led to a more rapid correction of pH and arterial carbon dioxide tension (Pa,CO_2). A total of nine out of 30 subjects in the conventional treatment group died compared three out of 30 in the NPPV group. In an intention to treat analysis, these figures were not statistically significant but when those unable to tolerate NPPV were excluded, a significant survival benefit was seen (nine out of 30 *versus* one out of 26; p=0.014). Translating the data from this study into routine practice, on general wards, is difficult given that staff supplementary to the normal ward complement set up NPPV. The high mortality rate (30%) in the control group was surprising considering that the mean pH was only 7.34. Additionally, the low intubation rate, while probably reflecting UK practice, has been criticised.

BARBE *et al.* [9] initiated NPPV in the emergency department in patients presenting with an acute exacerbation of COPD and continued it on a general ward. In order to ease some of the problems of workload and compliance, NPPV was administered for 3 h, twice a day. In this small study (n=24) there were no intubations or deaths in either group and arterial blood gas tensions improved equally in both the NPPV group and in the controls. However, the mean pH at entry in each group was 7.33 and at this level of acidosis, significant mortality is not expected; in other words it was unlikely that such a small study would show an improved outcome when recovery would be expected anyway [12].

WOOD *et al.* [10] randomised 27 patients with acute respiratory distress, due to a variety of different conditions, to conventional treatment or NPPV in the emergency department. Intubation rates were similar (seven out of 16 *versus* five out of 11) but there was a nonsignificant trend towards increased mortality in those given NPPV (four out of 16 *versus* zero out of 11; p=0.123). The authors attributed the excess mortality to delay in intubation as conventional patients requiring IMV were intubated after a mean of 4.8 h compared with 26 h in those on NPPV (p=0.055). It is difficult to draw many conclusions from this study given its small size, the fact that the numbers of patients in each group was different, the patients were not matched for aetiology of respiratory failure and that the level of ventilatory support was very modest (inspiratory positive airway pressure of 8 cmH_2O).

ANGUS et al. [11] compared NPPV and Doxapram in patients with COPD and type II respiratory failure in a small (n=17; nine in the NPPV group and eight in Doxapram group) randomised trial on a general ward. NPPV resulted in a significant improvement in both arterial oxygen tension (Pa,O_2) and Pa,CO_2 at 4 h. Contrastingly, no fall in Pa,CO_2 occurred in those patients treated with Doxapram and an initial improvement in Pa,O_2 was not sustained at 4 h. At both 1 and 4 h, pH was significantly better in the NPPV group compared with the Doxapram group. All the patients in the NPPV group were discharged home, although one required Doxapram in addition to NPPV during their acute illness. A total of three out of eight patients in the Doxapram group died and a further two received NPPV. This small study suggests that NPPV is more effective than Doxapram in the treatment of respiratory failure associated with COPD. However, no comparisons were made of nursing work load, patient tolerance or complication rates between the two groups.

In a multicentre RCT of NPPV in acute exacerbations of COPD (n=236) on general respiratory wards in 13 centres [2] NPPV was applied, by the usual ward staff, using a bilevel device in spontaneous mode according to a simple protocol. "Treatment failure", a surrogate for the need for intubation, defined by a priori criteria was reduced from 27 to 15% by NPPV (p<0.05) and in-hospital mortality was also reduced from 20 to 10% (p<0.05). Subgroup analysis suggested that the outcome in patients with pH <7.30 after initial treatment was inferior to that in the studies performed in the ICU. There was no difference in length of stay between the groups median (length of stay median 10 days; range standard group 2–119 days, NPPV group 4–137 days; p=0.269). Due to a reduction in ICU utilisation, NPPV was highly cost effective, resulting in a saving of GBP 4,114 for each death avoided [13]. This study suggests that, with adequate staff training, NPPV can be applied with benefit outside the ICU by the usual ward staff and that the early introduction of NPPV on a general ward results in a better outcome with cost savings than providing no ventilatory support for acidotic patients outside the ICU. It must, however, be put into an international perspective. In North America and in many European countries, NPPV would not be considered an appropriate treatment for the ward environment. The fact that early intervention has been confirmed as having an advantage, potentially increases the number of patients with an exacerbation of COPD who should receive ventilatory support. In the UK and other countries, in which ICU beds are in short supply, if COPD patients are to receive NPPV, it will usually be in the ward location, where nurses provide global care and can adopt some of the roles of the respiratory therapist. These features of the UK setting may reduce the general application of the mortality data to countries with good ICU provision. The study certainly does not suggest that NPPV should be performed on a general ward in preference to an ICU or a higher dependency setting.

There have been no direct comparisons between outcomes from NPPV in the ICU and on a general ward and it is unlikely that there ever will be such a trial. It should be appreciated that, while there is some overlap, the skills needed for noninvasive ventilation are different to those required for IMV and the outcome from NPPV is likely to be better on a general ward where the staff have a lot of experience of NPPV, than on an ICU with high nurse, therapist and doctor to patient ratios and a high level of monitoring but little experience of NPPV. The patient's perspective is also important; many find their experience of ICU to be unpleasant [6] and the less-intensive atmosphere of a noninvasive unit may be less distressing, although there is no evidence to support this assertion. The best location for a NPPV service will depend critically upon local factors, particularly the skill levels of doctors, nurses and therapists in looking after patients receiving NPPV. Patient throughput is an important factor which impacts upon the development and retention of the particular skills needed for NPPV. A study from the UK suggested that for the average general hospital, serving a population of 250,000 and with a standardised mortality rate for COPD of 100, six patients per month, with an acute exacerbation of COPD, will require NPPV, assuming that ventilation is initiated in patients with a pH <7.35 after initial treatment [14]. This number excludes patients with other conditions requiring NPPV and those who require it later in their hospital stay, *e.g.* for weaning *etc.* With relatively small numbers of patients per month, NPPV is best performed in a single location, in order to facilitate staff training and to maximise throughput and skill retention.

Implications for staffing

Noninvasive ventilation has been reported to be a time-consuming procedure [15] but, as with any new technique, there is a learning curve and the same group have subsequently published more encouraging results [16]. A number of studies on the ICU have shown that, in the initial stages, a significant amount of time is required to establish the patient on NPPV [17, 18]. It is possible, therefore, that NPPV may have a much-greater impact on nursing workload outside the ICU, where nurses have responsibility for a larger number of patients. In the study of BOTT *et al.* [8] there was no difference in nursing workload, assessed by asking the senior nurse to rate, on a visual analogue scale, the amount of care needed in the conventional and NPPV groups. However, this is an insensitive way of measuring nursing needs and, in addition, some of the potential extra work associated with NPPV was performed by supernumerary research staff. In the study of PLANT *et al.* [2] NPPV resulted in a modest increase in nursing workload, assessed using an end-of-bed log in the first 8 h of the admission, equating to 26 min, but no difference was identified thereafter. There are, however, no data regarding the effect NPPV has on either the care other patients on the ward received or whether the outcome would have been better if the nurses had spent more time with the patients receiving NPPV. In other words, although that study showed that NPPV was feasible in the general ward environment, it does not mean that it was the optimal situation. Furthermore, even if good results can be obtained it may be at the expense of the care of other patients. Most of the centres that participated in the study had little or no previous experience of NPPV and, therefore, required training in mask fitting and application of NPPV. The mean ± SD amount of formal training given in the first 3 months of opening a ward by the research doctor and nurse was 7.6±3.6 h; thereafter, each centre received 0.9±0.82 h·month^{-1} in order to maintain the skills. It should be appreciated that there was no need to make subtle adjustments to ventilator settings which was all done according to protocol. Much more training would be needed if more sophisticated ventilators are used. However, it underlines the fact that NPPV, in whatever location, is a question not only of purchasing the necessary equipment but also of staff training. Although a considerable amount of input is likely when a unit first starts to provide a NPPV service, thereafter, as long as a critical mass of nurses and therapists remain, new staff will gain the necessary skills from their colleagues.

Predicting the outcome with NPPV

A proportion of patients will fail with NPPV, requiring intubation and IMV; it is important that personnel and the facility for intubation are rapidly available if needed, if the trend to increased mortality with NPPV, as reported by WOOD *et al.* [10] is to be avoided. The likelihood of success or failure with NPPV is a key factor in deciding the most appropriate location. It could be argued that, for patients with a high likelihood of failing, NPPV should be initiated on the ICU and, once stabilised, the patient could be transferred to the ward normally providing NPPV. It is, therefore, helpful to be aware of when NPPV is likely to fail since this may affect the decision as to the most appropriate location for NPPV in a particular patient. A number of studies have looked at predictors of outcome for NPPV in acute exacerbations of COPD [1, 8, 19, 20–25]. The major limiting factor is that prediction models are only as good as the data entered; data that are not collected, cannot be entered into the model. Furthermore, the chosen outcome may influence the results. For instance if "failure of blood gas tensions to improve within a certain time" is taken as an indication for intubation then this will, by default, become a failure criterion even if, perhaps with persistence and adjustment of ventilator settings, success with NPPV could have been achieved.

Data available at the time NPPV is initiated and after a short period can predict the likelihood of success or failure with a reasonable degree of precision (table 1). Patients with high Acute Physiological and Chronic Health Evaluation (APACHE) II scores, pneumonia, who are underweight or have a greater level of neurological deterioration are more likely to fail on NPPV [19]. A reduction in respiratory rate with NPPV has been shown in a number of studies, with larger falls generally being associated with a successful outcome [1, 19, 20], although this is not always seen [26]. The change in arterial blood gas tensions, particularly pH, after a short period of NPPV, predicts a successful outcome [1, 8, 19, 20, 26, 27]. An improvement in arterial blood pH and/or Pa,CO_2 at 30 mins [22], 1 h [27] or after a longer period [28, 29] predicts successful NPPV. After 4 h of therapy, improvement in acidosis and/or a fall in respiratory rate is associated with success [28, 29]. Although NPPV results in lower rates of nosocomial infections compared with IMV, colonisation with nonfermenting gram-negative bacilli, mainly *Pseudomonas aeruginosa*, is strongly associated with NPPV failure in exacerbations of COPD [30]. The tolerance of NPPV also predicts subsequent outcome. Patients with an inability to minimise the amount of mask leak or an inability to co-ordinate with NPPV are less likely to improve with NPPV [19, 23, 24], and there should be a low threshold for IMV. In addition, NPPV is more likely to fail if there is reduced compliance with ventilation [19]. NPPV is less likely to be successful if there are associated complications or if the patients pre-morbid condition is poor [31, 32]. Late failure after initially successful NPPV is a bad prognostic factor, with over half the patients dying, even with IMV [31].

Although there have been a number of studies to ascertain predictors of outcome for patients with COPD requiring NPPV [19, 22, 24, 28, 29, 33, 34], these studies have a number of limitations. Most have recruited small numbers of patients from a small number of centres, have been retrospective and important variables that have been shown to be predictive in other studies may not have been included. Furthermore, the outcome variable is usually survival to hospital discharge. There are few data about longer term outcome, post discharge health status or the longer term outcome of patients who fail an initial trial of NPPV and either receive no further treatment or receive IMV. The clinician needs to make two decisions; first, the likelihood of success of a particular technique in the short term (most patients who fail with NPPV do so in the first 12–24 h [1]) and secondly, the effect of an intervention upon longer term outcome. It is possible that ready recourse to IMV results in better short-term results but worse long-term survival than NPPV and there is some evidence to support this theory [35]. There is, therefore, a need for a prospective study of predictors of outcome for patients receiving NPPV in a wide variety of different centres. It is important that the predictors be those that are readily available at the time when decisions need to be made. At the time of writing, the European Predictors of Outcome from Ventilation (EPOV) study,

Table 1. – Predictors of failure and success in noninvasive positive pressure ventilation (NPPV)

Predictors of failure
  Patient Factors
    Pneumonia
    Excessive secretions
    Colonisation with nonfermenting gram-negative bacilli (*e.g. Pseudomonas aeruginosa*)
    Low BMI
    Poor premorbid condition
    High APACHE II scores
    Low level of consciousness
    Low pH prior to starting NPPV
    Late failure after initially successful NPPV
  Technical factors
    Inability to minimise leak
    Inability to co-ordinate with NPPV
    Reduced compliance with ventilation
Predictors of success
  Large reduction in respiratory rate
  Improvement in pH and/or carbon dioxide tension at 30 min, 1 h or after a longer period
  Improvement in acidosis and/or a fall in respiratory rate after 4 h of therapy

BMI: body mass index; APACHE: Acute Physiological and Chronic Health Evaluation.

based in Leeds, UK, is recruiting patients to determine more robust predictors of outcome. These factors, in addition to others summarised in table 2, will have a bearing upon the chosen location for NPPV, although it must be stressed again that local factors more than any other will be the key determinants.

Should NPPV be started in the emergency room?

Again the type of treatment that is undertaken in the emergency room and the length of time that patients typically stay there vary from country to country. In some countries, patients remain in the emergency room for a very short period whereas in others they may remain there for a day or more. The two studies in which NPPV was initiated in the emergency room [9, 10] both failed to show any advantage to NPPV over conventional therapy. There are a number of possible explanations for this, which include the fact that patients are usually admitted to ICU when other therapies have failed, whereas most of those presenting to the emergency room have not received any treatment. In addition, a proportion is going to improve after initiation of standard medical therapy. In a 1-yr period prevalence study [14] of patients with acute exacerbations of COPD, of 954 patients admitted through the emergency rooms in Leeds, 25% were acidotic on arrival in the department and of those, 25% had completely corrected their pH by the time of arrival onto the ward. There was a weak relationship between the Pa,O$_2$ on arrival at hospital and the presence of acidosis, suggesting that, in

Table 2. – Factors to be considered in determining where noninvasive positive pressure ventilation should be carried out

Location of staff with training and expertise in noninvasive ventilation
Adequate staff available throughout a 24-h period (will depend upon nursing needs of other patients; for instance, one nurse responsible for two very ill patients may have less time than one nurse responsible for four less-severely ill patients)
Rapid access to endotracheal intubation and invasive mechanical ventilation
Severity of respiratory failure and likelihood of success
Facilities for monitoring

at least some patients, respiratory acidosis had been precipitated by high-flow oxygen therapy administered in the ambulance on the way to the hospital. It is important to note that the Yorkshire Noninvasive Ventilation (YONIV) study [2], the only study to show an unequivocal benefit from NPPV outside the ICU, only recruited patients who remained acidotic and tachypnoeic on arrival to the ward.

A cohort of patients for whom intubation is not considered appropriate because their previous medical history is well known, present to the emergency room *in extremis* and require immediate ventilatory support. In that situation, it would be reasonable to start noninvasive ventilation in the emergency room to stabilise the patient for transfer to the ward, on which NPPV is normally performed. In other patients, the clinical findings suggest that intubation would not be appropriate but the medical notes or a family member are not available to corroborate this. NPPV may be useful in this situation to create time in which to obtain further information or to allow the patient to recover to the point at which they can give a history. However, if there is no improvement, the patient should be intubated and transferred to the ICU.

In summary, most patients presenting to the emergency room with an acute exacerbation of COPD do not need NPPV but particular attention should be paid to controlled oxygen therapy. NPPV may be needed in occasional patients who are *in extremis* and for whom intubation is not considered appropriate. If it is normal policy for patients to receive the first 24 h of treatment in the emergency department, then NPPV should be started there in those who remain acidotic and tachypnoeic, a short time after standard medication has been administered and oxygen therapy optimised.

Conditions other than COPD

There are no RCTs of NPPV outside the ICU in hypoxaemic respiratory failure or weaning and it is, therefore, in patients with exacerbations of COPD only that there is an evidence base for its use outside of the ICU. The study of ANTONELLI *et al.* [4], in which conventional mechanical ventilation and NPPV were compared in patients with acute hypoxic respiratory failure, showed NPPV to be as effective as conventional ventilation in improving gas exchange. Patients receiving NPPV had significantly lower rates of serious complications and those successfully treated with NPPV had shorter ICU stays. *Post hoc* subgroup analysis of patients with simplified acute physiological scores (SAPS) of <16 and those of ≥16, showed that patients in the latter group had similar outcomes irrespective of the type of ventilation. However, NPPV was superior to conventional mechanical ventilation in patients with SAPS <16. CONFALONIERI *et al.* [37] evaluated the early application of NPPV in patients with acute respiratory failure due to severe community-acquired pneumonia, on three intermediate respiratory ICUs. A total of 28 patients were randomly assigned to standard treatment and 28 to NPPV. NPPV resulted in a significant reduction in intubation. Six (21%) patients in the NPPV group and 17 (61%) in the standard treatment group met the pre-selected criteria for intubation (p=0.007). A total of 20 patients were intubated: six in the NPPV group and 14 in the standard treatment group (p=0.03). The three remaining patients in the standard treatment group, who met the pre-selected criteria for intubation but were not intubated, were all successfully treated with NPPV. Patients randomised to NPPV had significantly shorter ICU stays (1.8±07 *versus* 6±2 days; p=0.04) and required similar nursing care intensity to those in the standard treatment group. The two groups did not significantly differ in terms of duration of hospital stay, complications, hospital and 2-month mortality. *Post hoc* analysis of the subgroup of patients without COPD showed that a high APACHE II score was significantly associated with intubation requirement (p=0.004), and hospital (p=0.04) and 2-month mortality (p=0.03) but was not an independent predictor of outcome.

As with acute exacerbations of COPD, it would, therefore, appear that it is possible to manage patients with milder disease successfully with NPPV. Further data are needed but it would be reasonable for patients with milder disease to have a trial of NPPV in an experienced noninvasive unit outside the ICU. Rapid access to intubation and mechanical ventilation must, however, be available.

There have been a large number of studies of the use of NPPV, including CPAP, in patients with cardiogenic pulmonary oedema. If NPPV is to be used, it must be initiated early because of the natural history of the condition and, in practice, this will mean initiation at the point of entry to hospital. Indeed, out of hospital NPPV for cardiogenic pulmonary oedema has been described, although in one RCT was not shown to be of benefit [36].

Starting NPPV on a general ward

Nursing and technical staff should be adequately prepared and the necessary equipment must be available before NPPV is first tried (table 3).

Staff should use the equipment on each other in a nonclinical setting and practise the theoretical knowledge and skills prior to use on real patients. Two or three enthusiastic staff members are a real boon as they will often enthuse the rest of the team. Nurses with previous experience of ICU or NPPV are particularly useful, since they will be confident with ventilators. If such individuals are not available within the existing complement, recruitment of such an individual should be considered. An experienced practitioner should be available 24 h a day in order to help solve problems until staff are able to solve them themselves. As experience is gained, further types of ventilator, new masks, etc. can be added, widening the range of patients who can be successfully ventilated noninvasively.

Table 3. – Staff training requirements and recommended equipment

Staff training requirements
Understanding rationale for assisted ventilation
Mask and headgear fitting techniques
Ventilator circuit assembly
Theory of operation and adjusting ventilation to achieve desired outcome
Cleaning and general maintenance
Problem solving, the ability to recognise serious situations and act accordingly
Above all medical, nursing and technical staff need to be convinced that the technique works

Recommended equipment
A simple ventilator; pressure cycled machines are usually simple, compensate for moderate leaks and are generally better tolerated by patients
A supply of circuits already made up
A range of sizes (at least three) of masks, both nasal, full face and head gear; a minimum of two of each should always be available
Connectors to allow customisation of ventilator circuits e.g. for entrainment of oxygen
Facility for cleaning masks, circuits and headgear to an acceptable standard or a budget to allow single patient use of these items

Conclusion

Staff training and experience are more important than location, and adequate numbers of staff, skilled in NPPV, must be available 24 h a day. Due to the demands of looking after acutely ill patients and to aid training and skill retention, NPPV is usually best carried out in a single location with one nurse responsible for no more than three to four patients in total. Whether this is called an ICU, an HDU or is part of a general ward is largely irrelevant. Further studies are needed to determine the optimal threshold for initiating NPPV, particularly in conditions other than COPD, to assess the feasibility, safety and effectiveness in lower intensity settings and to determine the cost-effectiveness, in both the short and long terms.

Summary

This chapter reviews the evidence base for the use of noninvasive ventilation (NIV) in a variety of locations. Ultimately individual circumstances, different between different countries and indeed within an individual country, will determine the best location for an NIV service. Staff training and expertise, however, are key. The need to have a mechanism for monitoring progress and a clear plan, from the outset, of what to do in case of deterioration is stressed. Although the main focus is upon patients with chronic obstructive pulmonary disease, other conditions are touched on.

Keywords: Chronic obstructive pulmonary disease, high dependency unit, intensive care unit, general ward, noninvasive ventilation.

References

1. Brochard L, Mancebo J, Wysocki M, *et al.* Noninvasive ventilation for acute exacerbations of chronic obstructive pulmonary disease. *N Engl J Med* 1995; 333: 817–822.
2. Plant PK, Owen JL, Elliott MW. Early use of non-invasive ventilation for acute exacerbations of chronic obstructive pulmonary disease on general respiratory wards: a multicentre randomised controlled trial. *Lancet* 2000; 355: 1931–1935.
3. Nava S, Ambrosino N, Clini E, *et al.* Noninvasive mechanical ventilation in the weaning of patients with respiratory failure due to chronic obstructive pulmonary disease. A randomized, controlled trial. *Ann Intern Med* 1998; 128: 721–728.
4. Antonelli M, Conti G, Rocco M, *et al.* A comparison of noninvasive positive-pressure ventilation and conventional mechanical ventilation in patients with acute respiratory failure. *N Engl J Med* 1998; 339: 429–435.
5. Antonelli M, Conti G, Bufi M, *et al.* Noninvasive ventilation for treatment of acute respiratory failure in patients undergoing solid organ transplantation: a randomized trial. *JAMA* 2000; 283: 235–241.
6. Easton C, MacKenzie F. Sensory-perceptual alterations: delirium in the intensive care unit. *Heart Lung* 1988; 17: 229–237.
7. Intensive care in the United Kingdom: report from the King's Fund panel. *Anaesthesia* 1989; 44: 428–431.
8. Bott J, Carroll MP, Conway JH, *et al.* Randomised controlled trial of nasal ventilation in acute ventilatory failure due to chronic obstructive airways disease. *Lancet* 1993; 341: 1555–1557.

9. Barbe F, Togores B, Rubi M, Pons S, Maimo A, Agusti AGN. Noninvasive ventilatory support does not facilitate recovery from acute respiratory failure in chronic obstructive pulmonary disease. *Eur Respir J* 1996; 9: 1240–1245.

10. Wood KA, Lewis L, Von Harz B, Kollef MH. The use of Noninvasive positive pressure ventilation in the Emergency Department. *Chest* 1998; 113: 1339–1346.

11. Angus RM, Ahmed AA, Fenwick LJ, Peacock AJ. Comparison of the acute effects on gas exchange of nasal ventilation and doxapram in exacerbations of chronic obstructive pulmonary disease. *Thorax* 1996; 51: 1048–1050.

12. Jeffrey AA, Warren PM, Flenley DC. Acute hypercapnic respiratory failure in patients with chronic obstructive lung disease: risk factors and use of guidelines for management. *Thorax* 1992; 47: 34–40.

13. Plant PK, Owen J, Elliott MW. A cost effectiveness analysis of non-invasive ventilation (NIV) in acute exacerbations of COPD. *Thorax* 1999; 54: A11.

14. Plant PK, Owen J, Elliott MW. One year period prevalence study of respiratory acidosis in acute exacerbation of COPD; implications for the provision of non- invasive ventilation and oxygen administration. *Thorax* 2000; 55: 550–554.

15. Chevrolet JC, Jolliet P, Abajo B, Toussi A, Louis M. Nasal positive pressure ventilation in patients with acute respiratory failure. *Chest* 1991; 100: 775–782.

16. Chevrolet JC, Jolliet P. : Workload on non-invasive ventilation in Acute respiratory failure. *In*: Vincent JL, ed. Year book of Intensive and Emergency Medicine. Berlin, Springer, 1997; pp. 505–513.

17. Kramer N, Meyer TJ, Meharg J, Cece RD, Hill NS. Randomized, prospective trial of noninvasive positive pressure ventilation in acute respiratory failure. *Am J Respir Crit Care Med* 1995; 151: 1799–1806.

18. Nava S, Evangelisti I, Rampulla C, Compagnoni ML, Fracchia C, Rubini F. Human and financial costs of noninvasive mechanical ventilation in patients affected by COPD and acute respiratory failure. *Chest* 1997; 111: 1631–1638.

19. Ambrosino N, Foglio K, Rubini F, Clini E, Nava S, Vitacca M. Non-invasive mechanical ventilation in acute respiratory failure due to chronic obstructive airways disease: correlates for success. *Thorax* 1995; 50: 755–757.

20. Meduri GU, Abou-Shala N, Fox RC, Jones CB, Leeper KV, Wunderink RG. Noninvasive face mask mechanical ventilation in patients with acute hypercapnic respiratory failure. *Chest* 1991; 100: 445–54.

21. Meduri GU, Turner RE, Abou-Shala N, Wunderink R, Tolley E. Noninvasive Positive Pressure Ventilation Via Face Mask - First line intervention in patients with acute hypercapnic and hypoxemic respiratory failure. *Chest* 1996; 109: 179–93.

22. Poponick JM, Renston JP, Bennett RP, Emerman CL. Use of a ventilatory support system (BiPAP) for acute respiratory failure in the emergency department. *Chest* 1999; 116: 166–671.

23. Benhamou D, Girault C, Faure C, Portier F, Muir JF. Nasal mask ventilation in acute respiratory failure. *Chest* 1992; 102: 912–917.

24. Soo Hoo GW, Santiago S, Williams AJ. Nasal mechanical ventilation for hypercapnic respiratory failure in chronic obstructive pulmonary disease: determinants of success and failure. *Crit Care Med* 1994; 22: 1253–1261.

25. Anton A, Guell R, Gomez J, *et al.* Predicting the result of noninvasive ventilation in severe acute exacerbations of patients with chronic airflow limitation. *Chest* 2000; 117: 828–833.

26. Meduri GU, Turner RE, Abou-Shala N, Wunderink R, Tolley E. Noninvasive positive pressure ventilation via face mask. First- line intervention in patients with acute hypercapnic and hypoxemic respiratory failure. *Chest* 1996; 109: 179–193.

27. Meduri GU, Fox RC, Abou-Shala N, Leeper KV, Wunderink RG, *Noninvasive mechanical ventilation* via *face mask in patients with acute respiratory failure who refused endotracheal intubation. Critical Care Medicine* 1994; 22: 1584–1890.

28. Plant PK, Owen JL, Elliott MW. Non-invasive ventilation in acute exacerbations of chronic obstructive pulmonary disease: long term survival and predictors of in-hospital outcome. *Thorax* 2001; 56: 708–712.

29. Confalonieri M, Garuti G, Cattaruzza MS, *et al.* A chart of failure risk for noninvasive ventilation in patients with COPD exacerbation. *Eur Respir J* 2005; 25: 348–355.

30. Ferrer M, Ioanas M, Arancibia F, Marco MA, De La Bellacasa JP, Torres A. Microbial airway colonization is associated with noninvasive ventilation failure in exacerbation of chronic obstructive pulmonary disease. *Crit Care Med* 2005; 33: 2003–2009.

31. Moretti M, Cilione C, Tampieri A, Fracchia C, Marchioni A, Nava S. Incidence and causes of non-invasive mechanical ventilation failure after initial success. *Thorax* 2000; 55: 819–825.

32. Scala R, Bartolucci S, Naldi M, Rossi M, Elliott MW. Co-morbidity and acute decompensations of COPD requiring non-invasive positive-pressure ventilation. *Intens Care Med* 2004; 30: 1747–1754.

33. Lightowler JV, Elliott MW. Predicting the outcome from NIV for acute exacerbations of COPD. *Thorax* 2000; 55: 815–816.

34. Putinati S, Ballerin L, Piattella M, Panella GL, Potena A. Is it possible to predict the success of non-invasive positive pressure ventilation in acute respiratory failure due to COPD? *Respir Med* 2000; 94: 997–1001.

35. Confalonieri M, Parigi P, Scartabellati A, *et al.* Noninvasive mechanical ventilation improves the immediate and long-term outcome of COPD patients with acute respiratory failure. *Eur.Respir.J* 1996; 9: 422–430.

36. Sharon A, Shpirer I, Kaluski E, *et al.* High-dose intravenous isosorbide-dinitrate is safer and better than Bi-PAP ventilation combined with conventional treatment for severe pulmonary edema. *J Am Coll Cardiol* 2000; 36: 832–837.

37. Confalonieri M, Potena A, Carbone G, Porta RD, Tolley EA, Meduri UG. Acute respiratory failure in patients with severe community-acquired pneumonia. A prospective randomized evaluation of noninvasive ventilation. *Am J Respir Crit Care Med* 1999; 160: 1585–1591.

Part II

Chronic respiratory failure and NIV

CHAPTER 14

NIV and obstructive lung diseases

J-F. Muir, C. Molano, A. Cuvelier

Pneumology and Respiratory Intensive Care Unit, Rouen University Hospital, Rouen, France.

Correspondence: J-F. Muir, Service de Pneumologie et Unité de Soins Intensifs Respiratoires (Hôpital de Bois-Guillaume), CHU de Rouen 76031 Rouen, France. Fax: 33 232889000; E-mail: Jean-Francois.Muir@chu-rouen.fr

Introduction

The standard treatment of severe chronic obstructive pulmonary disease (COPD) with chronic hypoxia and cor pulmonale is long-term oxygen therapy (LTOT), as shown in two previous randomised controlled trials [1–2], to improve survival when used for ≥ 15 h·day^{-1}. In the British Medical Research Council multicentre trial [2], it also appeared that, in spite of the good compliance of the group under LTOT, the most hypercapnic and polycythaemic patients at inclusion were the earliest to die, during the first 500 days of LTOT, confirming, as in other studies [3–7], that the pejorative significance of an elevated level of arterial carbon dioxide tension (Pa,CO_2) before onset of LTOT. If the incidence of an elevated Pa,CO_2 under LTOT, which, itself, also worsens Pa,CO_2 in many patients, remains debated [8–13] then its negative significance on prognosis, when a progressively worsening level of Pa,CO_2 appears during the course of COPD in spite of a maximal medical treatment combined with LTOT, is well established [11,14]. Then, the place of an external respiratory assistance, in order to compensate for night-time hypoventilation and thus correct hypercapnia [14], warranted further evaluation, considering the good results of noninvasive mechanical ventilation (NIV) in hypercapnic patients with chronic respiratory failure (CRF) secondary to restrictive pulmonary diseases [15] and in COPD patients with acute hypercapnic respiratory failure (AHRF) [16–21].

Long-term home mechanical ventilation (LTHMV) is generally considered in patients with COPD and CRF when LTOT fails, with progressive worsening of general and respiratory status, associated with frequent episodes of acute respiratory failure (ARF) leading the patients to intensive care unit [22]. Home mechanical ventilation represents the discharge to home from acute (or chronic) care hospital of ventilator-assisted patients who require long-term use of their ventilator (at least 3 h·day^{-1}) intermittently or continuously, either with a tracheostomy, mouthpiece, facial or nasal mask, or an external device [23, 24]. However, LTHMV in severe COPD patients is still controversial since only limited prospective data have been published to date in this population. This chapter will highlight the present data from the literature concerning noninvasive positive pressure ventilation (NPPV) in acute and chronic care management of COPD patients and will suggest an algorithm for selecting the subpopulation of patients who will beneficiate from NPPV on a long-term basis.

Eur Respir Mon, 2008, 41, 203–223. Printed in UK - all rights reserved. Copyright ERS Journals Ltd 2008; European Respiratory Monograph; ISSN 1025-448x.

History

LTHMV with intermittent positive pressure ventilation was introduced in clinical practice after the iron lung era during the 1950s. LTHMV development was favored by a rapid progress in ventilator technology and a net survival improvement of patients treated by tracheotomy-mediated ventilation, later reported by ROBERT *et al.* [25] in a retrospective study including various aetiologies of CRF. After the poliomyelitis epidemics, LTHMV was further indicated in patients with chronic respiratory insufficiency secondary to many restrictive disorders like muscular dystrophies and tuberculosis sequelae but also to obstructive diseases such as chronic obstructive pulmonary disease (COPD). At the beginning of the 1960s, SADOUL *et al.* [26], documented satisfactory arterial blood gases controls by using volumetric ventilators and facial masks in COPD patients with ARF. However, that technique was abandoned because of the large extent of ventilation with tracheostomy at that period and because convenient masks were not available.

The relative interest of intermittent positive pressure ventilation (IPPV) through mouthpiece or tracheotomy *versus* LTOT for COPD patients was discussed as soon as the early 1970s [27]. At the end of the 1970s, the multicentric study of the British Medical Research Council (BMRC) [2] confirmed the first results from the Denver group [28] and showed a significant improvement of survival among COPD patients receiving LTOT *versus* a control group without LTOT. The simultaneous publication of the American Nocturnal Oxygen Therapy Trial (NOTT) study also demonstrated benefits in the group receiving continuous LTOT *versus* a control group in which only nocturnal oxygen therapy had been given [1]. Oxygen therapy seemed to put an end to the cumbersome and constraining long-term mechanical ventilation techniques for which indications had never been clearly documented in COPD patients. However, within the present decade, general advances in respiratory care and rehabilitation, better home-care services and a new generation of compact, portable ventilators have prompted renewed interest in long-term mechanical ventilation [29]. Improvement of interfaces, such as nasal masks [30, 31] or external prostheses of the 1980s, gave a new interest in noninvasive mechanical ventilation. Thus, many thousands of patients, mainly with a restrictive ventilatory defect, are currently treated by LTHMV all over the world [32]. However, NPPV is not new, if we consider the important results obtained in polio patients in the 1950s with perithoracic ventilation.

In the late 1980s, the publications from MEDURI *et al.* [16] about facial mask ventilation in COPD patients with ARF were confirmed in a controlled fashion successively by BROCHARD *et al.* [19], KRAMER *et al.* [17] and BOTT *et al.* [18]. Such data favoured numerous publications proving benefits of this technique not only in the acute care setting but also in the long-term, similarly reported in neuromuscular patients by BACH and ALBA [33] and by RIDEAU [34] for patients with muscular dystrophy. As a result, NPPV was reconsidered for patients with severe hypoxic and hypercapnic COPD whose condition was unstable and who had poor responsiveness to LTOT [35].

NPPV may be delivered through various ventilatory methods, which are generally divided in two concepts, internal methods using intermittent positive pressure ventilation, and external methods with mainly negative pressure ventilation using perithoracic prostheses.

Negative pressure ventilation

The use of negative intermittent pressure ventilation has been reconsidered in COPD patients at the beginning of the 1980s [36] due to the existence of new devices which were better performing than the classic iron lung. These devices, such as cuirass, external shells and jackets (poncho or wrap), are applied to the thorax and/or the abdomen. Several trials have been conducted to determine whether respiratory muscles can be rested by negative pressure ventilation and if this is beneficial on a long-term basis. Preliminary results showed that there was a real effect on the dyspnoea level, on the capture of diaphragmatic activity and on the respiratory muscle strength [37]. In terms of dyspnoea levels, negative intermittent pressure ventilation seems better tolerated by "type B" COPD patients (*i.e.* hypercapnic) than by "type A" (*i.e.* eucapnic) emphysematous patients. However, randomised trials failed to prove efficiency of this treatment and compliance was poor [38, 39]. A controlled, randomised study [40] showed no beneficial effects on arterial blood gases, walking tests, level of dyspnoea and quality of life in 184 COPD patients treated over 12 weeks with effective negative intermittent pressure ventilation by poncho, compared with a sham ventilation with poncho. Compliance was poor within the 63 patients not using the poncho or it was stopped before the end of the study. These poor results and a low compliance with such a cumbersome technique explain that negative pressure ventilation was supplanted by the rapidly growing nasal ventilation.

Positive pressure ventilation

NPPV may be applied to the nose *via* a mask or pillows as initially proposed by RIDEAU [34] for LTHMV in patients with muscular dystrophy and to the mouth *via* a mask or a mouthpiece [41]. Many patients are nowadays ventilated with facial masks including the nasal and the buccal methods. Survival rates for home positive pressure ventilation are lower for patients with chronic airflow obstruction, with a 10-yr survival of ~10% [42–44], decreased hospitalisation and some improvement in right heart failure and arterial gases, than for those with restrictive chest wall or neuromuscular disease.

Mouth positive pressure ventilation

Intermittent oral positive pressure is generally referred to "intermittent positive pressure breathing" (IPPB) when used for short time periods with pressure-cycled ventilators and to "mouth intermittent positive pressure ventilation" (MIPPV) when used for a longer period of time with a volume-cycled ventilator [41]. MIPPV was very popular in Europe during the 1970s but was rapidly found to be nonbeneficial for patients because of its constraints and the impossibility to provide long-term periods of mechanical ventilation [42–44]. Consequently, compliance and efficiency of the technique were poor. It is more than likely that a number of patients treated by MIPPV during the 1970s for moderate hypercapnia would have been offered simple LTOT in the 1980s. It differed from the IPPB programs studied in the USA during the same period because IPPB does not provide a real respiratory assistance [45, 46]. A prospective study [47] has shown no benefit from IPPB compared with simple nebulisations in a group of less-severe COPD patients.

From home mechanical ventilation with tracheostomy to nasal NPPV

The major potential benefit from mechanical ventilation by tracheostomy is the potential of longer periods of efficient mechanical ventilation sessions, especially during the night. Evaluation of long-term results of home mechanical ventilation with tracheostomy (HMVT) in COPD patients is impaired because of a lack of controlled studies. Different studies [42, 44] have reported the prognosis of COPD with HMVT, which appeared less favorable compared with patients with restrictive chest wall or neuromuscular disorders. In the series by ROBERT et al. [25], the 5-yr survival was 30% and the 10-yr survival was 8%, with stabilisation after the tenth year for a population of 112 COPD patients using HMVT (fig. 1). However, these results must be considered as an attempt at improving patient comfort by reducing the frequency of hospitalisations for ARF [29, 48, 49].

This led the present authors to conduct a similar multicentric retrospective study in a larger population of 259 COPD patients treated by HMVT with the help of ANTADIR (*Association Nationale pour le Traitement a Domicile des Insuffisants Respiratoires*) [50]. Survival curves (fig. 2) were drawn between that of the study by ROBERT et al. [25] and the previous reports of LTOT alone in the BMRC [2] and NOTT [1] trials. The latter reported recruited patients with less-severe COPD: 42% with 5-yr survival and 22% with 8-yr survival. However, survival in the ANTADIR study was better than the survival of treated patients from the BMRC trial until the fourth year of follow-up, where survival curves become identical. In spite of the difficulty to extrapolate from one study to another, comparison of the survival curves from the ANTADIR group to those of the BMRC study seems to favour a more-interventional approach for these patients including a trial of mechanical ventilation. Indeed, the BMRC study showed that early deaths were recruited in the most hypercapnic and the most polyglobulic patients; *i.e.* those with the most severe chronic respiratory failure. Logically, mechanical ventilation should have been beneficial to those patients since LTOT appeared to provide no benefit during the first 500 days after initiation.

Nasal positive pressure ventilation

Since the early 1980s, nasal NPPV has been extensively studied in patients with restrictive chronic respiratory insufficiency as well as in those with acute [19, 32, 51, 52–55]

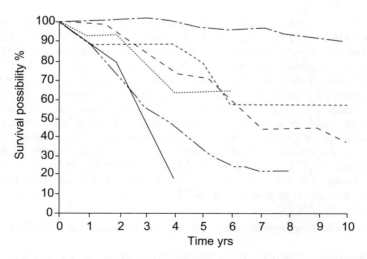

Fig. 1. – Survival of patients treated at home by long-term mechanical ventilation with tracheostomy according to the aetiology of the chronic respiratory failure. — - —: post-polio syndrome; ....: myopathies; - - - - - -: kyphoscoliosis; – – –: damaging sequelae of tuberculosis; — - - —: chronic obstructive pulmonary disease; ———: bronchiectasis. Reproduced from [25] with permission from the publisher.

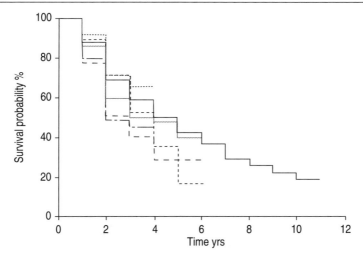

Fig. 2. – Actuarial survival curve of chronic obstructive pulmonary disease (COPD) patients treated by home mechanical ventilation with tracheotomy as compared with long-term oxygen therapy. In this figure are presented the results implying tracheotomised patients from the studies of ROBERT *et al.* [25] (- - - - - (n=50)) and of MUIR *et al.* [50], (——— (n=259)). Survival curves are compared with patients treated by oxygen therapy alone from the American Nocturnal Oxygen Therapy Trial (NOTT) [8] (12 h group: — — (n=101)); 24 h group: .... (n=101)) and the British Medical Research Council (BMRC) [2] (15 h group: ——— (n=42); control group: — - — - (n=45)) studies. Study/NOTT O_2 12 h group, p<0.05 and study/BMRC control group p<0.05.

and chronic conditions [56, 57]. After 1–2 months of nasal IPPV at night, transcutaneous Pa,CO_2 and Sa,O_2 improved.

Important results were obtained in COPD patients with ARF [16, 19, 51–55] whereby nasal NPPV may avoid endotrachal intubation in more than 50% of patients when used as the initial treatment [19]. It was then attractive to perform NPPV on a long-term basis in COPD patients with CRF but this subject remains controversial [52]. In the first uncontrolled studies with COPD patients treated with NPPV for three to nine months, a significant improvement occurred in the diurnal arterial blood gases with an improvement of sleep quality [31, 53], the best results being obtained in the more hypercapnic patients [56, 57] with nevertheless a less satisfactory compliance than in restrictive patients.

However, there is currently only minimal data to assess usefulness of NPPV in COPD patients on a long-term basis [55–57]. In 12 patients, ELLIOTT *et al.* [21] reported an interesting compliance to the nasal ventilation with an improvement of arterial blood gases at the 12th month (fig. 3), with an improvement of sleep quality and of quality of life. In a collective of 276 patients under NPPV (among which, 50 COPD were included), LÉGER *et al.* [58] reported an improvement of Pa,O_2 and Pa,CO_2 after 1 and 2 yrs. After 1 yr, the authors showed a marked reduction of the numbers of days in hospital for ARF, the probability to pursue NPPV was 55% at the 36th month of treatment (fig. 4). A retrospective study in 33 COPD patients followed during 5 yrs [59] showed that the probability of continuing ventilation was lower (∼43%); however, this study concerned patients at the end stage of their disease (fig. 5). In 14 patients with hypercapnic COPD followed during 6 months, PERRIN *et al.* [60] showed that daytime arterial blood gases were improved with NPPV and that the total St George Respiratory Questionnaire score and the impact components of it, were improved (fig. 6).

Some controlled studies are available but remain controversial: STRUMPF *et al.* [61], using NPPV in a randomised crossover study within 23 patients with COPD, failed to

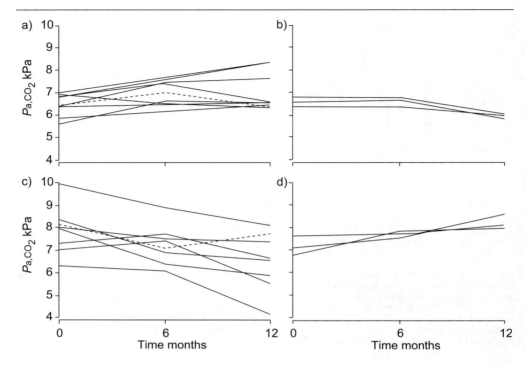

Fig. 3. – Arterial blood gas tensions a and b) arterial oxygen tension (P_{a,O_2}) and c and d) arterial carbon dioxide tension (P_{a,CO_2}) during spontaneous breathing and after 6 months and 1 yr in patients submitted to noninvasive mechanical ventilation (NIMV): seven patients still using NIMV at home and one who discontinued ventilation after 9 months. Three patients who discontinued home mechanical ventilation before 6 months. Reproduced from [21] with permission from the publisher.

note a clear improvement with mechanical ventilation. No modifications were assessed concerning dyspnoea, pulmonary function tests, respiratory muscle strength, arterial blood gases, exercise tests and sleep parameters. The only benefits were noticed on the neuropsychological function. However, only seven patients completed the study; such a poor compliance was linked to the nasal mask interface. Moreover, the authors used bi-level positive pressure ventilation with BiPAP® [61, 62] and the patients, in spite of a frank obstructive defect, had only a moderate alteration of arterial blood gases, some of them being even normocapnic at stable state. In a randomised crossover study, MEECHAM-JONES *et al.* [63] compared the benefit of NPPV plus oxygen therapy *versus* LTOT alone in 18 patients followed during two successive periods of 3 months with each treatment. Significant improvements in daytime arterial blood gases were assessed with a mean P_{a,O_2} increase and a mean P_{a,CO_2} reduction under NPPV (fig. 7) associated with an improvement of nocturnal P_{a,CO_2} and sleep parameters. That study also showed that the improvement of daytime arterial blood gases was correlated with the change in overnight P_{a,CO_2}. Compliance was satisfactory: 14 out of the 18 patients completing the study. This was attributed to the fact that the included patients were in-patients with better education of NPPV and also more-severe patients with more-severe hypercapnia. Because quality of life scores (symptom, impact, and total quality of life scores) were also improved, the authors suggested that such a benefit could be associated with the improvement of arterial blood gases and to the improvement of sleep quality. LIN [64] prospectively compared the benefits of 2-week treatment periods by LTOT alone, NPPV alone and NPPV in COPD patients. No difference was found for pulmonary function

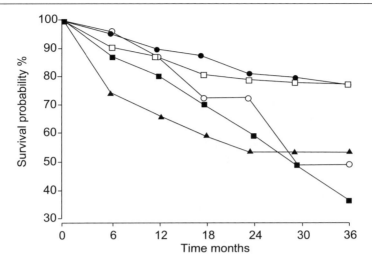

Fig. 4. – Probability to continue noninvasive mechanical ventilation in various aetiologies of chronic respiratory failure. ●: kyphoscolliosis; □: tuberculosis; ○: chronic obstructive pulmonary disease; ▲: bronchiectasis; ■: duchenne. Reproduced from [58] with permission from the publisher.

tests, arterial blood gases, index of respiratory muscle strength or ventilatory drive. Sleep quality was worse under NPPV. This negative study was flawed by the low level of IPAP used (8–15 mmHg), which did not allow to control nocturnal hypoventilation, and also by the duration of each treatment period, which was too short to achieve a satisfactory adaptation to treatment. In the same direction, GAY *et al.* [65] studied 35 severe hypercapnic COPD patients randomised for a 3-month period of either NPPV with BiPAP® at 10 cmH$_2$O IPAP or sham NPPV with IPAP at 0 cmH$_2$O. Only four of the seven patients from the NPPV group completed the study compared with all 6 patients from the sham NPPV group. Only one patient had a substantial reduction of Pa,CO$_2$ under NPPV. Indeed, no significant change and no difference were observed

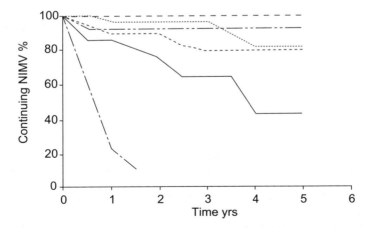

Fig. 5. – Probability of continuing noninvasive mechanical ventilation (NIMV) in UK according to different diagnostic groups. ——: poliomyelitis; — - - —: tuberculosis; ....: neuromuscular; - - -: kyphoscoliosis; ——: chronic obstructive pulmonary disease; — - —: bronchiectasis. Reproduced from [59] with permission from the publisher.

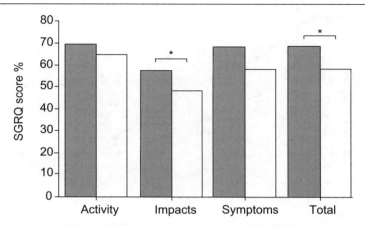

Fig. 6. – Evolution of the St George's Respiratory Questionnaire (SGRQ) scores after 6 months of nasal intermittent positive pressure ventilation. ■: SGRQ before NPPV. □: SGRQ after 6 months of NPPV. *: p<0.05. From PERRIN et al. [60].

between both arms of the study considering Pa,CO_2 decrease, modification of lung function, nocturnal O_2 saturation and sleep efficiency. Again, this study included only a small group of patients for rather short periods of NPPV.

In a more-recent paper, CASANOVA et al. [66] studied 52 patients with severe COPD receiving, in a randomised order, either NPPV plus standard care or standard care alone (93% with LTOT) for 1 yr. Survival was identical at 1 yr (78%) as well as the number of acute exacerbations. The number of hospital admissions fell significantly at 3 months in the NPPV group (5 versus 15%) but remained unchanged after the third month (fig. 8). The only benefits observed in the NPPV arms were a reduction of dyspnoea and an improvement of one of the neuropsychological tests (psychomotor coordination) at 6 months. Again, it was concluded that there was a trend towards a marginal benefit of NPPV in severe COPD patients but on a limited population and during a too short period of follow-up of 1 yr.

The trial conducted by CLINI et al. [67] included 122 patients during 2 yrs, using pressure support ventilators in the NIV arm, and showed a similar rate of mortality between the two groups: 18% with NIV and 17% with LTOT. The design of the study aimed to assess the effect of the treatment on severity of hypercapnia, use of healthcare resources and health related quality of life (HRQL). This trial showed no reduction of hospital admission in the two arms in the study; however, in the NIV group, there were a trend towards a reduction of hospital admission when comparing the follow-up with the follow-back period, as there was a trend towards increment in the LTOT group. Using the MRF-28, use of NPPV and oxygen was associated with an improvement of HRQL versus oxygen alone (fig. 9).

In another study, TUGGEY et al. [68] showed that domiciliary NIV, applied in a highly selected population of COPD patients with recurrent admissions for acidotic exacerbations requiring acute NIV, was effective at reducing admissions and minimising costs from the perspective of the acute hospital. Then NIV could be associated in selected patients with a reduction of the severity of AHRF episodes and perhaps also with a stabilization role on the course of the disease at least during the first year of application of NIV; this initial trend for improvement is not clear, but could be linked to the acute effect of NIV in responders as the final prognosis is recaptured by the spontaneous evolution of the disease.

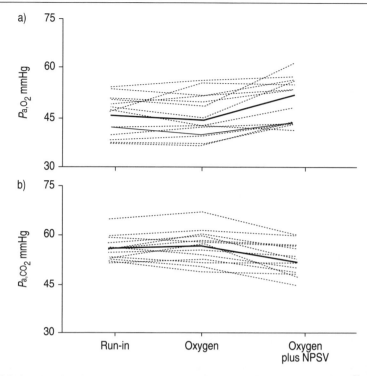

Fig. 7. – Individual (----) and mean (——) values of a) daytime arterial oxygen (Pa,O_2) and b) carbon dioxide (Pa,CO_2) tensions at run-in, after 3 months of oxygen alone and 3 months of oxygen and nasal pressure support (NPSV) in 14 chronic obstructive pulmonary disease patients. Reproduced from [63] with permission from the publisher.

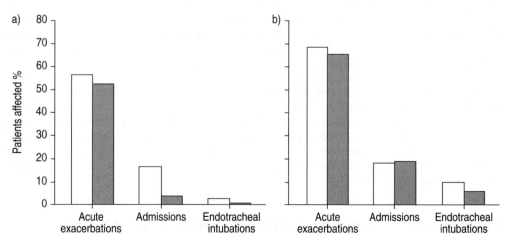

Fig. 8. – Long-term morbidity (acute exacerbations, admissions to the hospital and endotracheal intubation) in patients with severe chronic obstructive pulmonary disease after oxygen treatment alone and oxygen plus noninvasive positive pressure ventilation (NPPV). There were no significant differences in any outcome at either a) 3 or b) 12 months. □: controls; ■: NPPV. Reproduced from [66] with permission from the publisher.

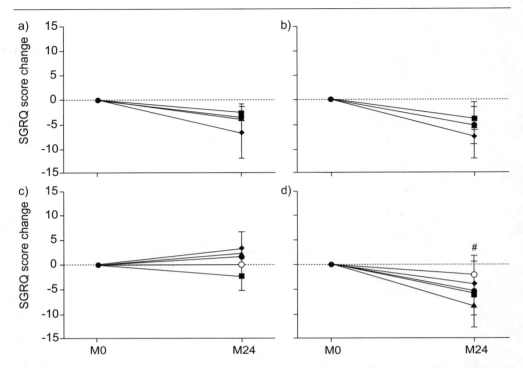

Fig. 9. – Change from baseline in total and dimension scores of St George's Respiratory Questionnaire (SGRQ). a and b) ♦: symptoms; ■: activity; ▲: impact; ●: total and Maugeri Foundation Respiratory Failure Questionnaire (MRF-28). c and d) ○: cognitive behaviour; ♦: activity; ■: disability; : others; ●: total. M0 : discharge; M24: 24 months after discharge. Group comparision for changes from baseline in total SGRQ score was not significant (p=0.554). #: p=0.041, treatment effect 7.100, 95% confidence interval 0.13–4.07. Reproduced from [67] with permission from the publisher.

Even if such studies are difficult to manage, there is clearly a need for prospective studies comparing LTOT and NPPV in the most severe obstructive pulmonary diseases, in a large amount of patients and on a real long-term basis of several years. Many patients with COPD are currently using NPPV at home, as showed in a recent European survey [69]. Two randomised prospective studies have been completed in Europe [70] and in Australia to assess the real role of NPPV in severe hypercapnic patients either under mechanical ventilation with volume preset machines or with pressure preset respirators.

Evaluation of NPPV in diffuse bronchiectasis and cystic fibrosis (CF) brings arguments to the contention that patients with severe airway obstruction and hypercapnia may respond favorably to NPPV. In bronchiectasis patients, BENHAMOU et al. [70, 71] showed a Pa,CO_2 decrease and less frequent hospitalizations during the year after NPPV initiation (compared with the previous year). Other series have reported stabilisation of severe hypercapnic patients with CF under NPPV while they awaited lung transplantation [72–74].

Rationale for chronic mechanical ventilation in COPD

CRF secondary to COPD is a complex situation associating a parenchymal impairment with reduced efficiency of its gas exchange function. Hypoxia is a marker of ventilation/perfusion abnormalities and hypercapnia is a marker of chronic pump failure and alveolar hypoventilation. As low-flow oxygen therapy is commonly able to compensate hypoxia in COPD patients, external mechanical ventilation will compensate for hypoventilation. Thus, improvement of arterial blood gases is one of the main objectives that determines ventilator adjustments.

Several hypotheses have been suggested to explain the beneficial effects of long-term mechanical ventilation in patients with COPD and CRF. NPPV is preferentially indicated during sleep periods, in order to achieve longer duration of ventilation; this is probably necessary to compensate nocturnal hypoventilation and episodes of arterial oxygen desaturation which occur predominantly during rapid eye movement sleep when breathing room air [75]. Indeed, the main beneficial effect of NPPV implies a correction of nocturnal hypoventilation and Pa,CO_2 reduction is the hallmark of improvement in alveolar ventilation under all types of mechanical ventilation. Such an improvement could persist after interruption of the ventilation period because of a temporary improvement in CO_2 sensitivity of the respiratory centers, that is often blunted in COPD patients [76]. However, the same results might be obtained when using NPPV 8 h during the daytime [77].

The improvement of nocturnal Pa,O_2 could also lead to an improvement of the diurnal Pa,O_2 [45, 78]; an effect that can be related to the correction of the alveolar-arterial gradient under NPPV and to the increase in spontaneous breathing pattern following mechanical ventilation. This is the consequence of an improved compliance of the chest wall and the lungs [79], an improved respiratory muscle function, an increased respiratory drive [76] and a decreasing oxygen consumption secondary to a decrease in work of breathing or an increase in efficiency of the respiratory muscle function or perhaps a reduction of chronic respiratory muscle fatigue [80–82]. The relief of chronic respiratory muscle fatigue remains controversial as well as the concept of chronic respiratory muscle fatigue. Indeed, it is difficult to assess whether the modifications of respiratory muscle strength are a cause or a consequence of the arterial blood gases improvement under NPPV [40, 83–85]. Respiratory muscle fatigue is probably not an important contributing factor when evaluating patients during periods of clinical stability. Thus, patients with severe CO_2 retention, particularly those with nocturnal oxygen desaturation, appear to be the best candidates to get a favorable response to nocturnal NPPV.

Alternatively, hypercapnia in COPD patients is not always synonymous with predominant hypoventilation, and may be linked to an increase in physiological dead space secondary to a ventilation/perfusion mismatch in relation with bronchospasm and/or parenchymal destruction, secondary to extension of emphysema. It is always debated as to whether hypercapnia *per se* defines an adaptative mechanism in severe COPD (permissive hypercapnia, *i.e.* sensible to NIV), when the respiratory centres are tuned towards a higher Pa,CO_2, in order to lessen the respiratory work as advocated by DUBOIS *et al.* [12] and COOPER and colleagues [7, 13], and later shown by AIDA *et al.* [11], or is a marker of the terminal phase of the disease (progressive hypercapnia, *i.e.* no more sensible to NIV) with an acceleration of the rise of Pa,CO_2 in the 3 yrs before death [7], or is a mixture of the two mechanisms. An illustration of this hypothesis is represented by the positive results obtained by NIV in severe hypercapnic patients with COPD published by ELLIOTT *et al.* [21] in a highly selected population of COPD patients described as intolerant to LTOT, with worsening of hypercapnia and incomplete correction of hypoxia under nocturnal oxygen therapy, which could be ranged in the responders patients with predominant hypoventilation. Thus, long-term nocturnal mechanical ventilation, which acts *via* a correction of Pa,CO_2 should be most effective only with the first clinical group, *i.e.* COPD with adaptative ventilatory pump failure, but could only be palliative in the second group with terminal parenchymal disease.

Selection of COPD patients to NPPV

In the last ACCP Consensus Conference on NPPV in chronic respiratory failure [74], it was proposed to indicate NPPV in COPD patients presenting with the characteristics detailed in table 1. However, these recommendations do not apply perfectly to patients with COPD [86]. Symptoms of chronic nocturnal hypoventilation are difficult to screen in patients with a poor quality of sleep, frequent morning headaches and chronic fatigue linked to their poor general and respiratory condition. Although the Consensus considered the presence of hypercapnia as mandatory, the presence of chronic hypercapnia by itself is not an indication of NPPV if stable and well tolerated. The presence of nocturnal oxygen desaturation is common in such patients and not always corrected by nocturnal oxygen therapy, as previously showed by DOUGLAS et al. [75]. Conversely, the notion of frequent episodes of decompensation leading to repeated hospitalisations is a good criterion, if the associated LTOT and medical management are optimal.

To indicate NPPV in a patient with COPD and CRF, the present authors prefer to consider the presence of a progressive deterioration of respiratory status based on clinical and biological criteria. Thus, in spite of the controversial results previously reported, they suggest to consider NPPV for patients with severe hypoxic and hypercapnic COPD in the two following practical situations.

COPD patients who present with blue and bloated type associated with chronic hypoxia and hypercapnia and develop an unstable respiratory condition. This may be appreciated on a clinical basis with chronic dependent oedemas and deterioration of respiratory and clinical status in spite of a well-prescribed and well-followed medical treatment, associating physiotherapy and LTOT. Instability may be confirmed by a progressive worsening of arterial blood gas tensions, leading to frequent cardiorespiratory decompensations with ominous ARF episodes [35, 86]. NPPV is a preventive

Table 1. – Clinical indicators for institution of nasal positive pressure ventilation in patients with COPD

Disease documentation	
Establish and document an appropriate diagnosis	History
	Physical examination
	Results of diagnostic tests
The most common obstructive lung diseases would include	Chronic Bronchitis
	Emphysema
	Bronchiectasis
	Cystic fibrosis
Assure optimal management of COPD	Bronchodilators
	Oxygen therapy when indicated
Optimal management of other underlying disorders	Multichannel sleep study to exclude associated OSAS if clinically indicated
Indications for usage	
Symptoms	Fatigue
	Dyspnoea
	Morning headache, *etc.*
Physiological criteria (one of the following)	Pa,CO_2 $\geq$55 mmHg
	Pa,CO_2 between 50 and 54 mmHg with nocturnal desaturation (Sa,O_2 by pulse oximetry $\leq$88% for 5 continuous min while receiving oxygen therapy $\geq$2 L·min^{-1})
	Pa,CO_2 between 50 and 54 mmHg with hospitilisation related to recurrent episodes of hypercapnic respiratory failure ($\geq$2 in a 12-month period)

OSAS: obstructive sleep apnoea syndrome; Pa,CO_2: arterial carbon dioxide tension; Sa,O_2: arterial oxygen saturation. Adapted from [74].

treatment of future dangerous episodes of ARF. Associated obesity is a further argument of indicating NPPV even in the presence of an overlap syndrome associating COPD and obstructive sleep apnoea; in such a case, the setting of expiratory positive airway pressure (EPAP) will be adapted during polysomnographic recordings which are mandatory when obesity is present [87].

NPPV should also be considered after an ARF episode, successfully treated by noninvasive ventilation [88, 89] but with the impossibility to wean the patient from the ventilator [90] or even patients receiving NPPV to be successfully weaned from endotracheal mechanical ventilation [41]. In such acute conditions, NPPV will be maintained beyond the ARF episode and re-evaluated on a long-term basis a few weeks or months later. Consequently, tracheotomy-mediated ventilation has nowadays restricted indications, such as failure of NPPV, often after a further episode of ARF and weaning failure from endotracheal ventilation.

Thus, NPPV could be proposed as a preventative treatment in severe COPD patients with unstable respiratory condition associated with fluctuating hypercapnia before, during and after an ARF episode, avoiding the need for a tracheotomy. An algorithm can be suggested to designate indications for HMVT (table 1), long-term oxygen therapy and IPPV by the nasal route in patients with severe COPD (fig. 10) [41].

Ventilators and interfaces

Ventilators for use in NPPV, devoted to patients with COPD are generally used for long periods of time, and generally overnight. Therefore, ventilators should be simple, reliable and easy to use, which is allowed by regular technological improvements. As COPD patients needing NPPV are generally partially dependent upon their machine, the presence of a battery-operated ventilator is only mandatory if patients need to ventilate more than 12 h·day^{-1}. Ventilators must also be light and portable. Both high- and low-pressure alarms are required to indicate airflow obstruction, disconnection or failure of the ventilator and must be set according to a leaky ventilation. At the present time, available studies are in favor of clinical equivalence of volume-preset and pressure-preset ventilation modes [91–94]. Besides, availability of volume assured pressure support respirators makes this difference in most of the situations academic. However, the actual trend is to use pressure-support ventilators on a first-line basis, especially with pressure-support mode, which is easier to adjust and to synchronise with the patient. Secondly, in case of failure, poor tolerance or inefficiency of pressure-support ventilation, pressure controlled or, more often, flow-preset ventilators may be proposed, as patients may appear to be responder or not to either volumetric or barometric ventilation [95]. By the end of the 1990s, release of dual portable ventilators providing either pressure-support ventilation or volume-preset ventilation opened the way for new potent turbine pressure-support ventilators able to deliver real volume ventilation with the average volume assured pressure-support ventilation mode which represents a flexible way for managing the most difficult patients [96]. The concept of prophylactic intermittent NPPV (i.e. given only one or two nights per week) might be developed in patients with poor adherence to a regular ventilation period during the night.

When pressure support ventilation is used [19, 61, 62, 86, 94] the level of inspiratory aid is progressively raised from 10 to 20 cmH$_2$O with a low level of EPAP around 5 cmH$_2$O in order to optimise CO$_2$ removal and control of auto-positive end-expiratory pressure (PEEP), according to the patient tolerance. Levels of IPAP, which are too low,

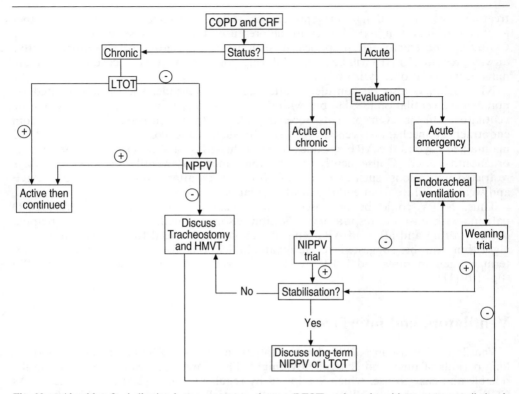

Fig. 10. – Algorithm for indicating long term oxygen therapy (LTOT) and nasal positive pressure ventilation in patients with chronic obstructive pulmonary disease (COPD) and chronic respiratory failure (CRF). HMVT: home mechanical ventilation *via* tracheotomy; -: failure; +: success. Reproduced from [41] with permission from the publisher.

could be associated with long-term failure of NPPV, as showed by WINDISCH *et al.* [97]. A back-up frequency is usually set at 12 breaths·min^{-1} and the inspiratory duration as short as possible. The fraction of inspired oxygen (F_{I,O_2}) is adjusted to correct nocturnal hypoxaemia and controlled by night oximetry. The comfort of the patient remains crucial and conditions the long-term compliance. VITTACCA *et al.* [98] confirmed that ventilatory settings established according to patient tolerance, patient comfort and arterial blood gases controls were as satisfactory as ventilatory settings established more rigorously upon more conventional criteria, mechanics and respiratory muscle function assessments.

When pressure-support ventilation fails, trials of pressure assist-controlled ventilation and/or flow-preset ventilation may be used. With volume-preset ventilation, settings are similar to those of mechanical ventilation in COPD with ARF (tidal volume 10–15 mL·kg^{-1} with nasal mask ventilation; inspiratory/expiratory ratio of 1/3 or less, back up frequency respiratory rate 12 breaths·min^{-1}; inspiratory trigger set for optimal confort of the patient; F_{I,O_2} as needed). Oxygen supplementation of the respirator can be achieved conventionally by cylinders, liquid oxygen or a concentrator.

Nasal or facial masks commonly in use are similar to the devices used to treat sleep apnoea syndrome. Nasal pillows are sometimes preferred for local skin tolerance and/or particular anatomical configuration. Alternate use between different masks or nasal cannulae may be proposed as needed to improve comfort of the patient.

NPPV initiation and follow-up in COPD patients

Initiating NPPV is a very important phase conditioning the future compliance to the treatment. As COPD patients are generally the most difficult patients to adapt to NPPV, the best way is to initiate the ventilatory trial during an in hospital stay of 1 week, in order to familiarise the patient and their family to a treatment which is a part of his rehabilitation programme. Apart from the ventilatory treatment itself, the patient must learn how to use nasal or facial connections which are crucial to the compliance. Nocturnal assessment with clinical scores, monitoring of $Sa_{,}O_2$ and transcutaneous $Ptc_{,}CO_2$ are useful, as well as serial arterial blood gases controls. The suspicion of an overlap syndrome always implies a nocturnal ventilatory polygraphic recording. The development in the most recent respirators of potent softwares allows useful monitoring of the respiratory pattern of the patient treated by mechanical ventilation at home; respiratory assistance must correct the incidence of asynchrony between patient and machine as much as possible [99]. Long-term follow-up implies regular visits at the hospital every 3–6 months. Close technical supervision is achieved by home respiratory care organisations of various compositions and structures according to the different countries and social organisations.

NPPV and rehabilitation

Despite medication and respiratory assistance, many patients with severe COPD suffer from dyspnoea resulting in limitation of physical capacity and even in their activities of daily living. Thus, methods to improve the ability of patients with severe COPD to function in the home and work environment with reduced symptoms (the goals of rehabilitation) have become accepted forms of therapy [100]. That approach, called "pulmonary rehabilitation" has been defined as "an art of medical practice wherein an individually tailored, multidisciplinary programme is formulated which, through accurate diagnosis, therapy, emotional support and education, stabilises or reverses both the physio- and psychopathology of pulmonary diseases and attempts to return the patient to the highest possible functional capacity allowed by their pulmonary handicap and overall life situation" [101]. Adjunction of NPPV to exercise rehabilitation is under evaluation [54, 102–107]. Thus, the key elements which will return the patient back to home with their ventilator are education about their disease and the management of their own therapy (*i.e.* NPPV), including physical therapy, exercise conditioning (adapted to those severely disabled patients), breathing retraining, psychosocial counseling and vocational training.

Conclusion

In conclusion, long-term noninvasive positive pressure ventilation in chronic obstructive pulmonary disease should be considered as a preventative treatment in severe patients with unstable respiratory condition associated with fluctuating hypercapnia before, during and after an acute respiratory failure episode. Instability may be appreciated on a clinical basis and confirmed by a progressive worsening of arterial blood gas tensions, leading to frequent cardiorespiratory decompensations with ominous acute respiratory failure episodes. In this setting, the association of NPPV with pulmonary rehabilitation programmes is promising.

Summary

The key role of noninvasive positive pressure ventilation (NPPV) is well documented in chronic obstructive pulmonary disease (COPD) patients with acute respiratory failure (ARF) since it may avoid endotracheal intubation in >50% of cases when used as the initial treatment. However, there is currently only minimal data to assess usefulness of NPPV in COPD patients on a long-term basis. Even if such studies are difficult to manage, there is clearly a need for prospective studies comparing long-term oxygen therapy and NPPV in the most severe COPD in a large amount of patients and on a real long-term basis of several years. Two randomised, prospective studies are being completed in Europe and the first preliminary results show that NPPV is associated with a reduction of hospitalisation for CRF decompensation.

The main beneficial effect of long-term mechanical ventilation in COPD patients with chronic respiratory failure implies a correction of nocturnal hypoventilation that could persist beyond the ventilation period because of a temporary improvement in CO_2 sensitivity that is often blunted in these patients.

The literature suggests considering NPPV for severe COPD patients who present with chronic hypoxia and hypercapnia and develop an unstable respiratory condition. Instability may be appreciated on a clinical basis and confirmed by a progressive worsening of arterial blood gas tensions, leading to frequent cardiorespiratory decompensations with ominous ARF episodes. NPPV should also be considered after an ARF episode successfully treated by noninvasive ventilation but with the impossibility to wean the patient from the ventilator.

Thus, NPPV could be proposed as a preventative treatment in severe COPD patients with unstable respiratory condition associated with fluctuating hypercapnia before, during and after an ARF episode, avoiding the need for a tracheotomy. Adjunction of NPPV to exercise rehabilitation is under evaluation.

Keywords: Chronic obstructive pulmonary disease, noninvasive ventilation, respiratory failure, short- and long-term outcome.

References

1. Continuous or nocturnal oxygen therapy in hypoxemic chronic obstructive lung disease: a clinical trial. Nocturnal Oxygen Therapy Trial Group. *Ann Intern Med* 1980; 93: 391–398.
2. Long term domiciliary oxygen therapy in chronic hypoxic cor pulmonale complicating chronic bronchitis and emphysema. Report of the Medical Research Council Working Party. *Lancet* 1981; 1: 681–686.
3. Burrows B, Ferle RH. Course and prognosis of chronic obstructive lung disease. A prospective study of 200 patients. *N Engl J Med* 1969; 280: 397–404.
4. Boushy SF, Thompson HK Jr, North LB, Beale AR, Snow TR. Prognosis in chronic obstructive pulmonary disease. *Am Rev Respir Dis* 1973; 108: 1373–1383.
5. Postma DS, Burema J, Gimeno F, *et al.* Prognosis in severe chronic obstructive pulmonary disease. *Am Rev Respir Dis* 1979; 119: 357–367.
6. Kawakami Y, Kishi F, Dohsaka K, Nishiura Y, Suzuki A. Reversibility of airway obstruction in relation to prognosis in chronic obstructive pulmonary disease. *Chest* 1988; 93: 49–53.

7. Cooper CB, Waterhouse J, Howard P. Twelve year clinical study of patients with hypoxic cor pulmonale given long term domiciliary oxygen therapy. *Thorax* 1987; 42: 105–110.
8. Keller R, Ragaz A, Borer P. Predictors for early mortality in patients with longterm oxygen home therapy. *Respiration* 1985; 48: 216–221.
9. Strom K, Boe J. Quality assessment and predictors of survival in long-term domiciliary oxygen therapy. The Swedish Society of Chest Medicine. *Eur Respir J* 1991; 4: 50–58.
10. Chailleux E, Fauroux B, Binet F, Dautzenberg B, Polu JM. Predictors of survival in patients receiving domiciliary oxygen therapy or mechanical ventilation. A 10-year analysis of ANTADIR Observatory. *Chest* 1996; 109: 741–749.
11. Aida A, Miyamoto K, Nishimura M, Aiba M, Kira S, Kawakami Y. Prognostic value of hypercapnia in patients with chronic respiratory failure during long-term oxygen therapy. *Am J Respir Crit Care Med* 1998; 158: 188–193.
12. Dubois P, Jamart J, Machiets J, Smeets F, Lulling J. Prognosis of severely hypoxemic patients receiving long-term oxygen therapy. *Chest* 1994; 105: 469–474.
13. Cooper CB. Life expectancy in severe COPD. *Chest* 1994; 105: 335–337.
14. Hill NS. Noninvasive ventilation in chronic obstructive pulmonary disease. *Clin Chest Med* 2000; 21: 783–797.
15. Simonds AK. Outcomes of long-term mechanical ventilation. *In*: Hill NS, ed. Long-term mechanical ventilation, Lung Biology in Health and Disease. New York, Marcel Dekker; 2001; pp. 471–500.
16. Meduri GU, Conoscenti CC, Menashe P, Nair S. Noninvasive face mask ventilation in patients with acute respiratory failure. *Chest* 1989; 95: 865–870.
17. Kramer N, Meyer TJ, Meharg J, Cece RD, Hill NS. Randomized prospective trial of noninvasive positive pressure ventilation in acute respiratory failure. *Am J Respir Crit Care Med* 1995; 151: 1799–1806.
18. Bott J, Carroll MP, Conway JH, *et al.* Randomised controlled trial of nasal ventilation in acute ventilatory failure due to chronic obstructive airways disease. *Lancet* 1993; 341: 1555–1557.
19. Brochard L, Mancebo J, Wysocki M, *et al.* Noninvasive ventilation for acute exacerbations of chronic obstructive pulmonary disease. *N Engl J Med* 1995; 333: 817–822.
20. Plant PK, Owen JL, Elliott MW. Early use of non-invasive ventilation for acute exacerbations of chronic obstructive pulmonary disease on general respiratory wards: a multicentre randomised controlled trial. *Lancet* 2000; 355: 1931–1935.
21. Elliott MW, Simonds AK, Carroll MP, Wedzicha JA, Branthwaite MA. Domiciliary nocturnal nasal intermittent positive pressure ventilation in hypercapnic respiratory failure due to chronic obstructive lung disease: effects on sleep and quality of life. *Thorax* 1992; 47: 342–348.
22. Hill NS. Noninvasive ventilation. Does it work, for whom and how? *Am Rev Respir Dis* 1993; 147: 1050–1055.
23. O'Donohue WJ, Giovannoni RM, Goldberg AI, *et al.* Long-term mechanical Ventilation. Guidelines for management in the home and at alternate community sites. Report of the Ad Hoc Committee, Respiratory Care Section American College of Chest Physicians. *Chest* 1986; 90:1 Suppl., 1S–37S.
24. Plummer AL, O'Donohue WJ, Petty TL. Consensus conference on problems in home mechanical ventilation. *Am Rev Respir Dis* 1989; 140: 555–560.
25. Robert D, Gérard M, Léger P, *et al.* Ventilation mécanique à domicile des insuffisants respiratoires chroniques. *Rev Fr Mal Resp* 1983; 11: 923–936.
26. Sadoul P, Aug MC, Gay R. Traitement par ventilation instrumentale de 100 cas d'insuffisance respiratoire aigue sévère (Pa,CO_2 supérieure ou égale à 70 mmHg) chez des pulmonaires chroniques. *Bull Eur Physiopathol Respir* 1965; 1: 519–546.
27. Levi-Valensi P. : Traitement ambulatoire des : IRC graves. *In*: Boehringer Ed. Actes du Colloque d'Amiens. 1973.
28. Petty TL. Ed. Intensive and rehabilitative respiratory care. 2nd Edn. Philadelphia, Lea & Febiger. 1974.

29. Pierson DJ, George RB. Mechanical ventilation in the home: possibilities and prerequisites. *Respir Care* 1986; 31: 266–270.

30. Carroll N, Branthwaite MA. Control of nocturnal hypoventilation by Nasal Intermittent Positive Pressure Ventilation. *Thorax* 1988; 43: 349–353.

31. Branthwaite MA. Non invasive and domiciliary ventilation: Positive pressure techniques. *Thorax* 1991; 46: 208–212.

32. Make BJ. Epidemiology of Long-Term Ventilatory Assistance. *In*: Hill NS, Ed. Long-Term Mechanical Ventilation. New York, Dekker, 2000; pp. 1–17.

33. Bach JR, Alba AS. Management of chronic alveolar hypoventilation by nasal ventilation. *Chest* 1990; 97: 52–57.

34. Rideau Y. The Duchenne dystrophy child. International congress on neuromuscular disease. *Muscle Nerve* 1986; 9: 55.

35. Muir JF, Levi-Valensi P. When should patients with COPD be ventilated? *Eur J Respir Dis* 1987; 70: 135–139.

36. Braun NM. Effect of daily intermittent rest on respiratory muscles in patients with CAO. *Chest* 1984; 85: 59S–60S.

37. Dubois F. Negative pressure ventilation improves respiratory muscle strength and dyspnea in patients with severe COPD. *Am Rev Respir Dis* 1990; 141: A37.

38. Celli B, Lee H, Criner G, *et al.* Controlled trial of external negative pressure ventilation in patients with severe chronic airflow obstruction. *Am Rev Respir Dis* 1989; 140: 1251–1256.

39. Zibrak JD, Hill NS, Federman EC, Kwa SL, O'Donnell C. Evaluation of intermittent long-term negative pressure ventilation in patients with severe chronic obstructive pulmonary disease. *Am Rev Respir Dis* 1988; 138: 1515–1518.

40. Shapiro SH, Ernst P, Gray-Donald K, *et al.* Effect of negative pressure ventilation in severe chronic obstructive pulmonary disease. *Lancet* 1992; 340: 1425–1429.

41. Muir JF. Intermittent positive pressure ventilation (IPPV) in patients with chronic obstructive pulmonary disease (COPD). *Eur Respir Rev* 1992; 2: 335–345.

42. Kauffmann F, Drouet D, Brille D, Hatzfeld C, Liot F, Kompalitch M. La prescription en France de la ventilation à domicile dans le traitement des insuffisants respiratoires chroniques. *Rev Fr Mal Resp* 1979; 7: 370–376.

43. Muir JF, Hermant A, Laroche D, Levi-Valensi P, Duwoos H. Résultats à long terme de l'assistance ventilatoire intermittente chez 74 IRCO graves appareillés depuis plus d'un an. *Rev Fr Mal Resp* 1979; 7: 421–423.

44. Kinnear WJ, Shneerson JM. Assisted ventilation at home : is it worth considering ? *Br J Dis Chest* 1985; 79: 313–351.

45. Sukumalchantra Y, Park SS, William MH. The effects of intermittent positive pressure breathing (IPPB) in acute respiratory failure. *Am Rev Respir Dis* 1965; 92: 885–893.

46. Kamat SR, Dulfano MJ, Segal MS. The effects of IPPB with compressed air in patients with severe chronic non-specific obstructive pulmonary disease. *Am Rev Respir Dis* 1962; 86: 360–380.

47. Intermittent positive pressure breathing therapy of chronic obstructive pulmonary disease. A clinical trial. The IPPB Trial Group. *Ann Intern Med* 1983; 99: 612–620.

48. Jones SE, Packham S, Hebden M, Smith AP. Domiciliary nocturnal intermittent positive pressure ventilation in patients with respiratory failure due to severe COPD: long term follow up and effect on survival. *Thorax* 1998; 53: 495–498.

49. Branthwaite MA. Mechanical ventilation at home. *Br Med J* 1989; 298: 1409–1411.

50. Muir JF, Girault C, Cardinaud JP, Polu JM. Survival and long-term follow-up of tracheostomized patients with COPD treated by home mechanical ventilation. A multicenter French study in 259 patients. French Cooperative Study Group. *Chest* 1994; 106: 201–209.

51. Benhamou D, Girault C, Faure C, Portier F, Muir JF. Nasal mask ventilation in elderly patients with ARF. *Chest* 1992; 102: 912–917.

52. Rossi A. Noninvasive ventilation has not been shown to be ineffective in stable COPD. *Am J Respir Crit Care Med* 2000; 161: 688–689.

53. Laier-Groeneveld G, Hutteman U, Criee CP. Non invasive nasal ventilation in acute and chronic ventilatory failure. *Am Rev Respir Dis* 1990; 141: A237.

54. Ambrosino N, Goldstein RS Ed. : Ventilatory support for chronic respiratory failure vol. 1– Informa Healthcare, New York, 2008, p. 595.

55. Leger P, Jennequin J, Gaussorgue D, Robert D. Acute respiratory failure in COPD patients treated by home IPPV via nasal mask. *Eur Respir J* 1989; 3: 683S.

56. Léger P, Hill NS. : Long-term mechanical ventilation for restrictive thoracic disorders. In: Hill NS, Ed. Long-term mechanical ventilation. New York, Dekker, 2000; pp. 105–150.

57. Marino W. Intermittent volume cycled mechanical ventilation via nasal mask in patients with respiratory failure due to COPD. *Chest* 1991; 99: 681–684.

58. Leger P, Bedicam JM, Cornette A, *et al.* Nasal intermittent positive pressure ventilation. Long term follow-up in patients with severe chronic respiratory insufficiency. *Chest* 1994; 105: 100–105.

59. Simonds AK, Elliott MW. Outcome of domiciliary nasal intermittent positive pressure ventilation in restrictive and obstructive disorders. *Thorax* 1995; 50: 604–609.

60. Perrin C, El Far Y, Vandenbos F, *et al.* Domiciliary nasal intermittent positive pressure ventilation in severe COPD: effects on lung function and quality of life. *Eur Respir J* 1997; 10: 2835–2839.

61. Strumpf DA, Millman RP, Carlisle CC, *et al.* Nocturnal positive pressure ventilation via nasal mask in patients with severe COPD. *Am Rev Respir Dis* 1991; 144: 1234–1239.

62. Strumpf DA, Carlisle CC, Millman RP, Smith KW, Hill NS. An evaluation of the Respironics BiPAP bi-level CPAP device for delivery of assisted ventilation. *Respir Care* 1990; 35: 415–422.

63. Meecham-Jones DJ, Paul EA, Jones PW, Wedzicha JA. Nasal pressure support ventilation plus oxygen compared to oxygen therapy alone in hypercapnic COPD. *Am J Respir Crit Care Med* 1995; 152: 538–544.

64. Lin CC. Comparison between nocturnal nasal positive pressure ventilation combined with oxygen therapy and oxygen monotherapy in patients with severe COPD. *Am J Respir Crit Care Med* 1996; 154: 353–358.

65. Gay PC, Hubmayr RD, Stroetz RW. Efficacy of nocturnal nasal ventilation in stable, severe chronic obstructive pulmonary disease during a 3-month controlled trial. *Mayo Clin Proc* 1996; 71: 533–542.

66. Casanova C, Celli BR, Tost L, *et al.* Long-term controlled trial of nocturnal nasal positive pressure ventilation in patients with severe COPD. *Chest* 2000; 118: 1582–1590.

67. Clini E, Sturani C, Rossi A, *et al.* The Italian multicentre study on noninvasive ventilation in chronic obstructive pulmonary disease patients. *Eur Respir J* 2002; 20: 529–538.

68. Tuggey JM, Plant PK, Elliott MW. Domiciliary non-invasive ventilation for recurrent acidotic exacerbations of COPD : an economic analysis. *Thorax* 2003; 58: 867–871.

69. Lloyd-Owen SJ, Donaldson GC, Ambrosino N, *et al.* Patterns of home mechanical ventilation use in Europe: Results of the Eurovent study. *Eur Respir J* 2005; 25: 1025–1031.

70. Muir JF, De la Salmonière P, Cuvelier A, the European Group. Survival of severe hypercapnic COPD under long-term home mechanical ventilation with NIPPV plus Oxygen versus oxygen therapy alone: Results of a European multicenter study. *Am J Respir Crit Care Med* 1999; 159: A295.

71. Benhamou D, Muir JF, Raspaud C, *et al.* Long-term efficiency of home nasal mask ventilation in patients with diffuse bronchiectasis and severe chronic respiratory failure: a case control study. *Chest* 1997; 112: 1259–1266.

72. Piper AI, Parker S, Torzillo PJ, Sullivan CE, Bye PT. Nocturnal nasal IPPV stabilizes patients with cystic fibrosis and hypercapnic respiratory failure. *Chest* 1992; 102: 846–850.

73. Hodson ME, Madden BP, Steven MH, Tsang VT, Yacoub MH. Non-invsive mechanical ventilation for cystic fibrosis patients – a potential bridge to transplantation. *Eur Respir J* 1991; 4: 524–527.

74. ACCP Consensus report. Clinical indications for non invasive positive pressure ventilation in chronic respiratory failure due to restrictive lung disease, COPD, and nocturnal hypoventilation. *Chest* 1999; 116: 521–534.

75. Douglas NJ, Calverley PM, Leggett RJ, Brash HM, Flenley DC, Brezinova V. Transient hypoxaemia during sleep in chronic bronchitis and emphysema. *Lancet* 1979; 1: 1–4.

76. Fleetham JA, Mezon B, West P, Bradley CA, Anthonisen NR, Kryger MH. Chemical control of ventilation and sleep arterial oxygen desaturation in patients with COPD. *Am Rev Respir Dis* 1980; 122: 583–589.

77. Schonhofer B, Geibel M, Sonneborn M, Haidl P, Kohler D. Daytime mechanical ventilation in chronic respiratory insufficiency. *Eur Respir J* 1997; 10: 2840–2846.

78. Elliott MW, Mulvey DA, Moxham J, Green M, Branthwaite MA. Domiciliary nocturnal nasal intermittent positive pressure ventilation in COPD: mechanisms underlying changes in arterial blood gas tensions. *Eur Respir J* 1991; 4: 1044–1052.

79. Grassino AE, Lewinsohn GE, Tyler JM. Effects of hyperinflation of the thorax on the mechanics of breathing. *J Appl Physiol* 1973; 35: 336–342.

80. Ambrosino N, Nava S, Bertone P, Fracchia C, Rampulla C. Physiologic evaluation of pressure support ventilation by nasal mask in patients with stable COPD. *Chest* 1992; 101: 385–391.

81. Nava S, Ambrosino N, Rubini F, *et al.* Effect of nasal pressure support ventilation and external PEEP on diaphragmatic activity in patients with severe stable COPD. *Chest* 1993; 103: 143–150.

82. Macklem PT. The clinical relevance of respiratory muscle research: J Burns Amberson Lecture. *Am Rev Respir Dis* 1986; 134: 812–815.

83. Gutierrez M, Beroiza T, Contreras G, *et al.* Weekly cuirass ventilation improves blood gases and inspiratory muscle strength in patients with chronic air-flow limitation and hypercarbia. *Am Rev Respir Dis* 1988; 138: 617–623.

84. Elliott MW, Mulvey D, Moxham J, Green M, Branthwaite MA. NIPPV reduces respiratory muscle activity. *Am Rev Respir Dis* 1990; 141: A722.

85. Carrey Z, Gottfried SB, Levy RD. Ventilatory muscle support in respiratory failure with NIPPV. *Chest* 1990; 97: 150–158.

86. Elliott MW. Long-term mechanical ventilation in severe COPD. *In*: Hill NS, Ed. Long-term mechanical ventilation. New York, Dekker, 2000; pp. 151–175.

87. Fletcher EC, Luckett RA, Miller T, Costarangos C, Kutka N, Fletcher JG. Pulmonary vascular hemodynamics in chronic lung disease patients with and without oxyhemoglobin desaturation during sleep. *Chest* 1989; 95: 757–764.

88. Udwadia ZF, Santis GK, Steven MH, Simonds AK. Nasal ventilation to facilitate weaning in patients with chronic respiratory insufficiency. *Thorax* 1992; 47: 715–718.

89. Girault C, Daudenthun I, Chevron V, Tamion F, Leroy J, Bonmarchand G. Non invasive ventilation as a systematic extubation and weaning technique in acute on chronic respiratory failure: a prospective randomized controlled study. *Am J Respir Crit Care Med* 1999; 160: 86–92.

90. Cuvelier A, Viacroze C, Bénichou J, *et al.* Dependency on mask ventilation after acute respiratory failure in the intermediate care unit. *Eur Respir J* 2005; 26: 289–297.

91. Meecham-Jones DJ, Wedzicha JA. Comparison of pressure and volume preset nasal ventilator systems in stable chronic respiratory failure. *Eur Respir J* 1993; 6: 1060–1064.

92. Restrick LJ, Fox NC, Braid G, Ward EM, Paul EA, Wedzicha JA. Comparison of nasal pressure support ventilation with nasal intermittent positive pressure ventilation in patients with nocturnal hypoventilation. *Eur Respir J* 1993; 6: 364–370.

93. Smith IE, Shneerson JM. Secondary failure of nasal intermittent positive ven-tilation using the Monnal D: Effects of changing ventilator. *Thorax* 1997; 52: 89–91.

94. Simonds A, Ed. Non invasive respiratory support. A practical handbook. Vol. 1. Hodder Arnold, London, 2007, 3rd Ed, p. 370.

95. Schonhofer B, Sonneborn M, Haidl P, Bohrer H, Kohler D. Comparison of two different modes for noninvasive mechanical ventilation in chronic respiratory failure: volume versus pressure controlled device. *Eur Respir J* 1997; 10: 184–191.

96. Storre JH, Seuthe B, Fiechter R, *et al.* Average volume-assured pressure support in obesity hypoventilation: a randomized crossover trial. *Chest* 2006; 130: 815–821.

97. Windisch W, Kostic S, Dreher M, Virchow JC, Sorichter S. Outcome of patients with stable COPD receiving controlled noninvasive positive pressure ventilation aimed at a maximal reduction of PaC02. *Chest* 2005; 128: 657–662.

98. Vittaca M, Nava S, Confalonieri M, *et al.* The appropriate setting of noninvasive pressure support ventilation in stable COPD patients. *Chest* 2000; 118: 1286–1293.

99. Fanfulla F, Delmastro M, Berardinelli A, D'Artavilla Lupo N, Nava S. Effects of different ventilator settings on sleep and inspiratory effort in patients with neuromuscular disease. *Am J Respir Crit Care Med* 2005; 172: 619–624.

100. Lucas J. Home ventilator care. *In*: O'Ryan JA, Burns DG, Eds. Pulmonary rehabilitation : from hospital to home. Saint Louis, Mosby Publishers, 1984; p. 260.

101. Make BJ. Pulmonary rehabilitation : myth or reality? *Clin Chest Med* 1986; 7: 519–540.

102. Garrod R, Mikelsons C, Paul EA, Wedzicha JA. Randomized controlled trial of domiciliary non invasive positive pressure ventilation and physical training in severe chronic obstructive pulmonary disease. *Am J Respir Crit Care Med* 2000; 162: 1335–1341.

103. Barakat S, Michele G, Nesme P, Nicole V, Guy A. Effect of a noninvasive ventilatory support during exercise of a program in pulmonary rehabilitation in patients with COPD. *Int J Chron Obstruct Pulmon Dis* 2007; 2: 585–591.

104. Van't Hul A, Gosselink R, Hollander P, Postmus P, Kwarkkele G. Training with inspiratory pressure support in patients with severe COPD. *Eur Respir J* 2006; 27: 65–72.

105. Costes F, Agresti A, Court-Fortune I, Rocher F, Vergnon JM, Barthelemy JC. Noninvasive ventilation during exercise training improves exercise tolerance in patients with chronic obstructive pulmonary disease. *J Cardiopulm Rehabil* 2003; 23: 307–313.

106. Dreher M, Storre JH, Windisch W. Noninvasive ventilation during walking in patients with severeee COPD : a randomised cross-over trial. *Eur Respir J* 2007; 29: 930–936.

107. Ambrosino N. Assisted ventilation as an aid to exercise training : a mechanical doping? *Eur Respir J* 2006; 27: 3–5.

CHAPTER 15

NIV and neuromuscular disease

A.K. Simonds

Correspondence: A.K. Simonds, Academic Unit of Sleep & Breathing, Royal Brompton Hospital, London SW3 6NP, UK. Fax: 44 2073518911; E-mail: A.Simonds@rbht.nhs.uk

General considerations

Neuromuscular patients comprise a heterogeneous group, at different stages of the natural history of the disorders and include many uncommon diseases, so it is not surprising that there have been few systematic or randomised studies of noninvasive ventilation (NIV) in neuromuscular disease. In the present chapter, general considerations will be discussed and outcomes presented in relatively stable conditions such as previous poliomyelitis and spinal cord injury, and the progressive disorders Duchenne muscular dystrophy (DMD) and amyotrophic lateral sclerosis (ALS; motor neurone disease (MND)) as these exemplify key principles of therapy.

In addition specific problems in the neuromuscular group may include: ineffective cough and secretion clearance; bulbar weakness and swallowing dysfunction; generalised limb weakness creating difficulty placing and removing interfaces, and operating ventilators; and accompanying cardiomyopathy in some conditions, e.g. DMD, glycogen storage disorders and Emery Dreifuss muscular dystrophy.

Overview of neuromuscular disorders

The probability of respiratory failure in neuromuscular conditions is shown in table 1, although cases always need to be judged on an individual basis. It should be noted that co-pathology (e.g. mild asthma, obesity or left ventricular dysfunction) can significantly add to respiratory muscle load so all pertinent medical factors should be taken into account.

Assessment for respiratory function

The purpose of monitoring patients is to detect symptoms and deterioration in lung function. In broad terms individuals with progressive conditions and those with a vital capacity (VC) <60% should be followed with measurements of spirometry and cough peak flow. RAGETTE et al. [1] showed that in a group with heterogeneous muscle conditions, sleep disordered breathing predominantly in rapid eye movement sleep was first seen when VC fell below 60% predicted. With a VC <40% predicted continuous hypoventilation was seen, and once VC was <25%, predicted daytime ventilatory failure was likely.

Eur Respir Mon, 2008, 41, 224–239. Printed in UK - all rights reserved. Copyright ERS Journals Ltd 2008; European Respiratory Monograph; ISSN 1025-448x.

Table 1. – Likelihood of developing respiratory insufficiency in inherited and acquired neuromuscular disease

Inevitable	Duchenne MD, type I SMA
Frequent	Limb girdle MD 2C,2D,2F,2I
	Nemaline myopathy
	Acid maltase deficiency
	Int SMA
	X-linked myotubular myopathy
	Multicore myopathy
	Congenital myasthenia
	Congenital myotonic dystrophy
	High spinal cord injury
Occasional	Emery Dreifuss MD, Becker MD, Bethlem myopathy, Minicore myopathy
Rare	Facioscapulohumeral MD, Mitochondrial myopathy, Central core disease, Limb girdle MD 1, 2A,B,G,H

MD: muscular dystrophy; SMA: spinal muscular atrophy.

Symptoms of nocturnal hypoventilation should always be sought. These include poor sleep quality, sudden wakenings with a panic sensation, morning headaches, daytime sluggishness and concentration problems [2]. Sleep studies should be carried out yearly and probably at 6-month intervals once early hypoventilation is noted. A general monitoring plan incorporating consensus conference recommendations [3] and algorithm of treatment interventions are shown in table 2 and figure 1, respectively.

Initiation of NIV

Most authorities now advise that NIV is started once symptomatic nocturnal hypoventilation has been identified before the development of diurnal hypercapnia [4]. This allows sensible planning and may prevent episodes of uncontrolled ventilatory decompensation. Outpatient or inpatient initiation may be equally safe and provides patients and families with a choice.

Evolution of NIV in neuromuscular and other restrictive disorders

Following its introduction in the early 1980s, when it was pioneered in DMD by RIDEAU et al. [5], NIV entered mainstream clinical practice in 1986–1987. In a large French multicentre series [6] the 3-yr probability of continuing domiciliary NIV was 75–80% for patients with post-polio respiratory muscle weakness, scoliosis and old tuberculous restrictive disease. Equivalent results were seen in a single-centre UK cohort [7],

Table 2. – Consensus recommendations for respiratory care in neuromuscular disease

Measure VC, peak cough flow, Sa,O_2 yearly
Patients with VC < 1 L or rapid decline should be assessed more frequently *e.g.* every 3–6 months
Arterial blood gases should be analysed if symptoms or signs of nocturnal hypoventilation, daytime Sa,O_2 <93%
A sleep study should be performed annually if VC <60% predicted or if there are symptoms of nocturnal hypoventilation (or wheel chair use)

VC: vital capacity; Sa,O_2: arterial oxygen saturation.

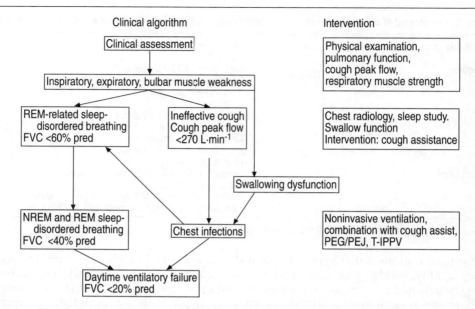

Fig. 1. – Clinical algorithm including timing of interventions. REM: rapid eye movement; FVC: forced vital capacity; % pred: % predicted; NREM: non-REM; PEG/PEJ: percutaneous enteral gastrostomy/percutaneous jejunostomy; T-IPPV: tracheostomy intermittent positive pressure ventilation.

which showed a 5-yr actuarial probability of continuing domiciliary NIV of 100% in post-polio patients, 94% (95% confidence interval (CI) 83–100%) in patients with post tuberculous lung disease, 79% (95% CI 66–92%) for scoliotic patients and 81% (95% CI 61–100%) in those with neuromuscular disorders excluding poliomyelitis. This compared with 5-yr figures of 43% in COPD patients and <20% in bronchiectasis. In that study, the probability of continuing NIV equated almost completely with survival, as the main reason for discontinuing NIV was death. Almost a third of DMD patients in the French study transferred to tracheostomy (T-) intermittent positive pressure ventilation (IPPV) long term.

Effects of NIV on physiological outcomes, morbidity and quality of life

Improvements in symptoms and daytime arterial blood gas tensions are consistently seen in NIV users [6, 7]. Sleep architecture and nocturnal blood gas tensions in children and adults with restrictive disorders also show improvement [8]. While changes in spirometry and respiratory muscles strength are equivocal (see the following section), SCHONHOFER et al. [9] have shown a substantial gain in endurance in three different tests in NIV users with restrictive disorders compared with controls. Endurance time increased by $278 \pm 269\%$ during inspiratory threshold loading, by $176 \pm 159\%$ during cycle ergometry and by $32 \pm 22\%$ during a shuttle-walk test.

LEGER et al. [6] report significant reductions in inpatient days for at least 2 yrs after the initiation of NIV in patients with muscular dystrophy, scoliosis and post-tuberculous lung disease, implying that worthwhile economic savings can be made.

A UK NIV subgroup who received the SF36 health status questionnaire gave comparable results to other groups with chronic disorders such as diabetes mellitus and ischaemic heart disease [7]. Although physical function was reduced in contrast to age-matched population norms, mental health and energy/vitality were similar. Sleep quality is a significant contributor to quality of life scores and, contrary to popular belief, patients using nocturnal NIV rated their sleep quality as average (67%) or very good (27%), with only 5% describing sleep quality as poor.

Mechanisms of action of NIV in restrictive disorders

Several mechanisms have been proposed to explain the physiological effects of long term ventilatory support, particularly the fact that nocturnal application of treatment is translated into improvements in daytime blood gas tensions. These are: relief of chromic respiratory muscle fatigue; improvement in central respiratory drive; improvement in chest wall/lung mechanics; improvement in sleep efficiency and quality; and alteration in cardiopulmonary/renal haemodynamics.

It may be that the relative importance of these mechanisms differs in restrictive neuromuscular disease and chest wall disorders and, of course, the explanations are not mutually exclusive. It has often been assumed that respiratory muscle fatigue is an important factor in the development of ventilatory failure. However, the presence of fatigue is difficult to confirm in practice. In addition, although some uncontrolled studies have demonstrated small improvements in respiratory muscle strength after NIV [6, 10, 11], others have not [12, 13]; it may be that these increases in respiratory muscle strength are due to an improvement in general wellbeing and/or a learning effect. Indeed it should always be remembered that any stabilisation in respiratory muscle strength in a progressive condition may represent improvement but is difficult to confirm without controlled studies.

HILL et al. [14] examined the efficacy of NIV by withdrawing it from restrictive patients who had acclimatised to the technique for at least 2 months. All had demonstrated improvements in symptoms and arterial blood gas tensions following initiation. A week after withdrawal patients experienced an increase in breathlessness, morning headaches and somnolence in the absence of any change in daytime blood gas tensions, pulmonary function or respiratory muscle strength. Moreover, nocturnal monitoring without NIV showed greater desaturation, a larger rise in arterial carbon dioxide tension (Pa,CO_2) and an increase in tachypnoea and tachycardia compared with results when receiving noninvasive IPPV (NIPPV), suggesting that one of the prime mechanisms of action is *via* control of nocturnal hypoventilation.

The impact of withdrawal of NIV after successful implementation have also been analysed by PIPER et al. [12]. In 14 neuromuscular and scoliotic patients treated with nocturnal NIV for at least 6 months, mean $\pm$ SD arterial blood gas tensions measured while breathing spontaneously during the day improved for arterial oxygen tension (Pa,O_2) from 7.5 ± 1.2 to 10.2 ± 1.3 kPa, and for Pa,CO_2 from 8.2 ± 1.6 to 6.4 ± 0.7 kPa and maximum inspiratory mouth pressures rose from 41 to 65 mmHg (p<0.003). During full polysomnography without ventilatory support breathing during sleep was improved compared with a pre-NIV study, but was still abnormal. The REM sleep-related fall in arterial oxygen saturation and rise in transcutaneous carbon dioxide tension were 20% and 1.5 kPa, respectively, compared with values of 41% and 2.8 kPa in the baseline study before NIV. There was no difference in effects between patients with primary neuromuscular disease and those with idiopathic scoliosis and, in both patient groups, there was no correlation between the increase in respiratory muscle strength and improvement in nocturnal gas exchange. As a consequence the authors argue that the improvement in nocturnal gas exchange following NIV is due to a reduction in hypoxic and hypercapnic induced arousals with resulting beneficial effects on sleep quality. Sleep fragmentation and deprivation caused by arousal are known to have a negative effect on ventilatory drive and, therefore, it is postulated that central drive is increased by the enhanced sleep quality.

To add weight to this theory, ANNANE *et al.* [13] have shown that the decrease in Pa,CO_2 that occurs after initiation of NIV in patients with neuromuscular disease and scoliosis is correlated with an increase in the slope of the ventilatory response to carbon dioxide (r= -0.68; p=0.008). This study also showed no improvement in respiratory muscle strength or lung mechanics. An additional mechanism contributing to increased chemosensititvity to carbon dioxide may be the washout of carbon dioxide stores following correction of overnight hypercapnia.

However, SCHONHOFER *et al.* [15] have challenged the belief that correction of nocturnal hypoventilation is of key importance in a study using ventilatory support solely during the day in patients who remained awake. There was no significant difference in improvement in arterial blood gas tensions in patients using daytime and night-time ventilator support, although obviously support during sleep is more convenient for patients.

More recently, the interaction between NIV use and change in chemosensitivity to carbon dioxide has been re-explored [16], this time using a combination of invasive and noninvasive measures of respiratory function, in order to obviate volitional effects, and difficulties using mouth pressure meters. A direct comparison with the results obtained by ANNANE *et al.* [13] is not possible as measurements were made at baseline, after 5 days and 3 months of NIV. However, the overall outcome was similar in that in a group with restrictive disorders (12 subjects with stable neuromuscular disease and eight with scoliosis) as mean $\pm$ SD, hypercapnic ventilatory response increased significantly from 2.8 ± 2.3 to 3.6 ± 2.4 $L \cdot min^{-1} \cdot kPa^{-1}$ at 5 days and further to 4.3 ± 3.3 $L \cdot min^{-1} \cdot kPa^{-1}$ after 3-months nocturnal NIV (p=0.044). There was an interesting "dose response" in that those using NIV for >4 $h \cdot night^{-1}$ showed a significant improvement in hyercapnic ventilatory response and Pa,CO_2 at 3 months, compared with those in whom average use was <4 $h \cdot night^{-1}$ where chemosensitivity and arterial blood gas tensions fell back to baseline levels at 3 months after initial improvement at 5 days. Invasive measurements of respiratory muscle strength and lung/chest wall compliance obtained using oesophageal and gastric balloon pressure catheters showed no significant improvement. Sleep stage distribution was not assessed in that study, so it is not clear whether it played a part, as sleep deprivation has previously been shown to depress chemosenstivity to carbon dioxide.

Overall, however, these results suggest that in stable neuromuscular (and scoliosis) patients, one of the key mechanisms by which NIV affects improvement is by an increase in ventilatory drive.

T-IPPV in restrictive disorders

It is instructive to compare results from NIV and T-IPPV. Outcome information on T-IPPV in restrictive disorders is mainly available from a French multicentre series dating from several decades ago. ROBERT *et al.* [17] have shown 5-yr survival rates of 95% in post-polio patients and 70% in those with tuberculosis sequelae. In a 20-yr experience of T-IPPV in the home from 1962–1983, SPLAINGARD *et al.* [18] report on 40 adults and children with neuromuscular disease, including spinal cord injury or central hypoventilation syndromes. The 3-yr survival was 63% for spinal cord injury patients and 74% for other neuromucular diagnoses combined *i.e.* figures not dissimilar from

NIV results. However, as discussed elsewhere, patients prefer noninvasive modes where these are feasible [19], and certainly the practicalities of implementing NIV are simpler than those of T-IPPV. The possibility of weaning onto NIV should always be considered in any patient using T-IPPV in the long term. Currently the main indications for T-IPPV in neuromuscular disease are: extreme ventilator dependency; upper airway problems *e.g.* tracheomalacia; marked bulbar weakness with swallowing and cough difficulties; inability to use mask; failure to thrive on NIV, inadequate ventilation; and neonatal ventilatory problems.

Quality of life in NIV *versus* T-IPPV users

Direct comparisons of quality of life between NIV and T-IPPV users are problematical as there have been no randomised trials and are unlikely to be any. Furthermore, those who are treated with T-IPPV are likely to have more advanced disease, greater ventilatory dependency and/or bulbar disease. Most comparisons are historical or have been done in ALS. BACH [19] has shown where patients and caregivers have swapped between T-IPPV and NIV (and therefore have experience with both techniques), NIV is preferred in nearly all respects. Clearly, NIV is simpler, less intensive in terms of care package, carer training and risk management. Aspects such as voice control, need to use suction, *etc.* also influence choice where both options are feasible. It has been suggested [20] even 24-h NIV reduces pulmonary morbidity compared with T-IPPV but here, individual choice is important. Although the burden of evidence indicates that NIV has significant quality of life advantages over T-IPPV where feasible, MARKSTROM *et al.* [21] found divergent results in a survey of home ventilator dependent patients in Sweden. In these individuals with post-polio respiratory failure, other neuromuscular disease or scoliosis, Sickness Impact Profile (SIP) and Heath Index scores were higher in T-IPPV recipients than NIV users. Interestingly, daytime fatigue level was higher and sleep quality rated worse in NIV patients, suggesting overnight control of ventilation might have been better in T-IPPV patients. The authors speculate that the fact that the follow-up care plan for T-IPPV users was more intensive and supportive than for NIV users (who were seen once a year) may have played a part. T-IPPV patients also received a highly personalised service with customised tracheostomy tubes which is likely to have reduced tube- and stoma-related complications. In addition, most T-IPPV recipients would probably receive NIV if treatment was initiated according to current guidelines.

DMD

As an X-linked recessive disorder, DMD is the most common muscular dystrophy in childhood with an incidence of around 1:3500 live male births. The gene and gene product (dystrophin) have been identified, paving the way to gene-therapy trials. A lack of dystrophin leads to the most severe forms of DMD. About 20% of cases are diagnosed before the age of 2 yrs, others are identified as "motor milestones" are missed. Previously, most boys lost ambulation by the age of 10–12 yrs, although, since the widespread use of steroid therapy in childhood, wheelchair dependence may now occur several years later. This change may also reduce the severity and impact of scoliosis which tends to become more marked as the child becomes wheelchair bound. Loss of lung volume tends to occur in mid teens with the onset of ventilatory failure in late teens or early 20s. Once daytime hypercapnia is present, death within 1–2 yrs is virtually inevitable unless ventilatory support is provided [22]. Nearly all young men now begin NIV; in some countries they progress to T-IPPV once failure to thrive or bulbar problems intervene. In other countries a noninvasive approach combining NIV and cough assistance is preferred. Pulmonary morbidity has been shown to be reduced in some series using the combined noninvasive approach [20] although once again there have been no true randomised comparisons. A cardiomyopathy is an almost inevitable accompaniment and should be monitored with yearly echocardiography and ECG. Comprehensive treatment of left ventricular insufficiency is recommended with ACE inhibitor and β-blocker. It should be noted that cardiac failure and respiratory insufficiency do not necessarily progress in tandem. For example in Becker muscular dystrophy, cardiac dysfunction may predate respiratory problems and significant heart block and malignant dysrhythmias can be seen in this condition and in Emery Dreifuss muscular dystrophy. A 5-yr survival of $\geq 70\%$ in DMD patients on NIV [23, 24] should be expected with increasing numbers of patients living into their 30s and 40s [25]; most report a satisfactory quality of life [26]. Later complications include chronic constipation/ bowel problems and urinary retention.

ALS/MND

The incidence of ALS is 1 in 50,000 per year, with a mean age at onset of 56 yrs. The most frequent presentation is a mixture of progressive upper and lower motor neurone signs in the spinal and bulbar territory ("classical ALS") although diagnosis may be problematical and up to 40% of patients experience a delayed diagnosis [27]. An acute presentation with overt respiratory failure [28] or features of nocturnal hypoventilation is not uncommon [29] and most units have seen an increasing number of referrals for ventilatory support in the last 5 yrs. Bulbar involvement affects up to 30% of individuals at the onset the disease [30] but is virtually inevitable by the terminal phase. Median survival is ~2.5 yrs but a quarter of affected individuals may live for 5 yrs or more. Prognosis tends to be better in younger patients. The cause of nerve degeneration in MND is unknown but it may be related to the excessive stimulation of glutamate receptors on the motor neurone. The only available pharmacological therapy, Riluzole (Rilutek, Rhone-Poulenc Rorer), was introduced into Europe in 1996 as an anti-excitogenic agent and is known to inhibit glutamate release.

The key respiratory problems in ALS/MND patients are: dypsnoea; aleovolar hypoventilation, morning headaches; sleep disturbance, daytime sleepiness; ineffective cough resulting in chest infections; excessive oral secretions; aspiration and choking episodes secondary to bulbar involvement; and panic attacks.

The American Academy of Neurology Practice parameter guidelines on care of ALS patients [31] lists five main respiratory issues to address: "what are the early indications of respiratory insufficiency?"; "does NIV affect respiratory function or survival?"; "does NIV and invasive ventilation improve quality of life or palliate symptoms?"; "does experience with NIV aid decision-making regarding progression to invasive ventilation?"; and "what is the optimal method or withdrawing NIV and invasive ventilation?"

Additionally one could ask: "what is the best time to initiate NIV?"; "how should one select ventilatory mode or settings?"; "which patients are most likely to benefit from NIV?"; and "who needs a cough assist device?"

Identification of respiratory problem

Dyspnoea is unlikely if VC exceeds 70% predicted, but respiratory muscle function should be closely monitored if the VC falls below this value, as respiratory decompensation commonly ensues within the following 12 months. Respiratory failure is virtually inevitable if VC falls below 30% predicted. Analysis of flow–volume loops will demonstrate abnormalities suggestive of upper airway dysfunction in many patients with ALS. Not surprisingly, these findings occur more often, but not exclusively, in patients with bulbar involvement. Bulbar insufficiency can worsen respiratory function by causing recurrent clinical and subclinical episodes of aspiration pneumonia. Comprehensive evaluation of bulbar and swallowing function can be obtained by videofluoroscopy.

Respiratory failure early in the course of the disease denotes phrenic nerve involvement, often in conjunction with weakness of accessory and other respiratory muscles. Respiratory muscle strength can be accurately measured using tests such as maximal sniff pressure [32, 33] with minimal discomfort to patients. LYALL et al. [32] have shown that, while a fall in VC is a useful predictor of respiratory failure, sniff pressure may be a better prognostic guide. Recently, there has been a renewed interest in expiratory muscle strength, as this is a major determinant of cough efficacy. The subgroup of patients with early respiratory muscle involvement but normal or only mildly impaired bulbar function and preserved limb strength is the group that usually responds best to noninvasive ventilation. Use of cough assist devices in ALS/MND is described in the following section.

Choice of ventilatory technique in ALS

T-IPPV has been used widely in ALS patients in the USA in order to circumvent progressive bulbar problems. For practical purposes, selection of patients is often heavily influenced by the degree of insurance cover, the extent of independent financial resources and the availability of family help/carers. SALAMAND et al. [34] reported a 1-yr survival of 24% in 24 ALS patients receiving home T-IPPV. However, OPPENHEIMER [35] showed an improved outcome with an up to 85% 1-yr survival. In that series, >50% of patients survived for 3 yrs or more using T-IPPV at home. A French cohort of patients using nasal/mouth ventilation or T-IPPV showed a transient improvement in pulmonary function and it was possible to discharge all patients home [36]. Clearly T-IPPV is the only ventilatory option in patients with severe bulbar disease.

On theoretical grounds, NIV should be helpful in patients with ALS and early respiratory muscle involvement as it may help stabilise the upper airway during sleep. PINTO et al. [37] showed a significant increase in survival in patients with respiratory insufficiency using bilevel ventilatory support compared with a nonventilated control group. However, the quality of life measure used in that study showed no improvement. ABOUSSOUAN et al. [38] also found that prognosis was improved in patients who could tolerate NIV.

There has only been one randomised controlled trial of NIV in ALS. BOURKE et al. [39] followed 92 patients and randomly allocated 19 to standard care and 22 to NIV when they developed either orthopnoea, a maximum inspiratory pressure of <60% predicted or symptomatic daytime hypercapnia. Bulbar function was assessed on a 6-point scale, with normal of moderate bulbar function score 4–6 and severe bulbar impairment score 0–3. NIV was supplied using a bilevel pressure support device (ResMed VPAP STII) in spontaneous timed mode via either a nasal, facial, total or mouthpiece interface, according to patient choice. Ventilator settings were adjusted, with the aim of normalising daytime arterial blood gas tensions. Patients were reviewed at 3-month intervals and were assessed for symptoms, lung function and quality of life using the SF36, a sleep related score (SAQLI) and the chronic respiratory disease questionnaire (CRQ). In that trial, cough assist devices were not provided but all patients were given physiotherapy advice. Importantly, the subgroup with better bulbar function on NIV showed a survival advantage of 205 days, with improvement in quality of life scores compared with controls. In the group with poor bulbar function there was no survival advantage to NIV, but some quality of life measures, particular those related to sleep symptoms, improved.

Other research [40] also demonstrated an increase in energy and vitality in patients after starting NIV, and this benefit was sustained even in the face of declining general muscle function. It is crucial to note that, once daytime Pa,CO_2 rises above 6.0 kPa, severe ventilatory decompensation is imminent (this is confirmed by the BOURKE et al. study [39] with very high early mortality in hypercapnic patients in the control group). Bulbar symptoms are not a contraindication to NIV, but may make tolerance of NIV more difficult for the patient [38]. Patients with severe bulbar impairment can be advised that NIV is unlikely to prolong survival but may help symptom control, so there is little to be lost from a trial. Favourable features for successful use of NIV in the home in ALS are shown below.

Clinical features favouring NIV success in MND/ALS are: early respiratory muscle involvement; symptomatic nocturnal hypoventilation; some independent breathing capacity; bulbar involvement not marked; strongly motivated; adequate resources (caregivers, family, ventilatory equipment, aids to daily living); experienced home-care team; good liaison between hospital, general practitioner, carers and hospice; and an agreed plan for supportive care/advance directive planning.

Cough assistance

Weakness of the bulbar, and inspiratory and expiratory muscles contribute to poor cough in ALS and other neuromuscular conditions. The key components of an effective cough are maximum inspiration, glottic closure and efficient recruitment of expiratory muscles. Expiratory muscle strength can be measured using maximum expiratory mouth pressure, whistle peak flow or gastric pressures, although accuracy may be affected by buccal weakness, reducing mouthseal, or pseudobulbar problems making compliance with the measurement difficult. In clinical practice cough peak flow provides a simple assessment with values <270 min^{-1}, indicating reduced cough strength. Asking the patient to cough also allows the efficacy to be graded simply as mildly, moderately or severely reduced. Physiotherapy techniques, such as huffing should be taught to all patients. Patients and their families should also be shown how to perform physiotherapy while receiving NIV. Adjusting the settings by increasing inspiratory positive airway pressure (IPAP) or breath stacking, using a volume preset ventilator can be helpful during chest infections. Manual insufflation using an ambu bag with non-rebreathe valve will augment inspiratory capacity and therefore cough peak flow. Carers can follow manual insufflation with an abdominal thrust to increase cough peak flow further.

The cough in-exsufflator (Emerson, and other manufacturers) has been shown to significantly augment cough in ALS/MND. MUSTFA et al. [41] showed that cough peak flow increased by 28% in nonbulbar patients and 17% in bulbar patients. Those with the weakest muscles benefited most. The present author's practice is to first teach cough assistance with NIV and/or ambu bag. If that is not sufficient, a cough in-exsufflator is added, providing it can be demonstrated to improve cough effectiveness, is well tolerated by the patient and can be applied by carers/family. The addition of cough in-exsufflation to NIV has proved extremely helpful in some patients with a markedly reduced peak cough flow. In individuals with vocal cord dysfunction or pseudobulbar palsy the in-exsufflator may not be well tolerated but nothing is lost from trying this on an individual basis.

Dealing with feeding problems, dysphagia and aspiration in NMD

Percutaneous enteral gastrostomy (PEG) placement should be considered in patients with symptomatic dysphagia and/or loss of >10% baseline weight or aspiration problems. Because of the risks of placement, PEG should ideally be sited before FVC is <50% predicted. A PEG or percutaneous jejunostomy (PEJ) can be placed radiologically or endoscopically under local anaesthetic or general anaesthetic. Respiratory management during these procedures is crucial. It is clearly vital to avoid use of sedation without adequate respiratory support. However, providing close peri- and post-operative monitoring is carried out, it is possible to safely insert a PEG feeding tube in a patient reliant on NIV. It is also often prudent to start NIV prior to PEG insertion to familiarise patient with the technique.

Contraindications to PEG insertion are few but include: the patient is unlikely to survive 3 months; the patient is unable to give informed consent; and the patient is unable to manage feeding tube and no carer available [42].

Symptom control

Most ALS patients are under the care of a multidisciplinary team, and there is evidence that multidisciplinary care patients do better than those under single speciality (neurology) care [43]. Palliative medicine advice is highly valuable and strongly recommended in all cases. Admission may occur under the care of the respiratory team and so familiarisation with palliative strategies is vital [44].

Decision making in ALS including progression to tracheostomy ventilation

Moss et al. [45] have shown that 96% of ALS patients are in favour of making advance directives. A majority are able to place limits on the application of long term mechanical ventilation eg. they would wish ventilatory support to be discontinued is they had cardiac arrest or developed a permanent coma. It is crucial that a decision is made as to whether the patient would like to be intubated in the event of an acute reversible respiratory event at the start of NIV.

Oppenheimer [35] found that <25% of ALS patients decided to use mechanical ventilation in advance of an emergency admission but, having started ventilatory support, nearly all wished to continue this. In a subsequent study [46], 100% of those using NIV were glad that they had chosen this form of support. From the family viewpoint, 42% of families who cared for a ALS/MND patient, requiring ventilatory support at home, felt this to be a major burden [45], but 83% would encourage that individual to choose mechanical ventilation again, although they were less sure about receiving this treatment themselves if the need arose. The situation has changed somewhat with the introduction of NIV, and some patients, for example, choose to limit ventilatory support to noninvasive methods. In a European survey of patients with chronic respiratory diseases, including ALS, admitted to high dependency units, ~30% wished to have NIV as a ceiling of ventilatory support [47].

The usual indications for tracheostomy ventilation in progressive conditions are: severe bulbar impairment resulting in recurrent aspiration or choking episodes; total ventilatory dependency or inability to control ventilatory failure using NIV or a combination of noninvasive techniques.

In practice, it may be possible to maintain patients with even severe bulbar disease with a combination of NIV, cough assistance techniques and PEG/PEJ feeding. As in DMD patients, this approach has long been advocated by BACH [48]. Realistically, there is likely to be a subgroup who may wish to progress to tracheostomy care and have the family and personal resources to cope with this. In the authors' recent experience, this has tended to be individuals who wish to extend life as long as possible for cultural of religious reasons. Our approach has been to facilitate these wishes where possible. An algorithm on progressive ventilatory care is shown in figure 2.

Quadriplegia

Patients with high cervical cord or bulbar lesions with no independent ventilatory capacity and an inability to clear secretions require tracheostomy assisted ventilation. Expertise in managing these patients has been gained in many spinal injuries centres.

Recently, it has been demonstrated that a proportion of quadriplegic patients with minimal respiratory reserve may cope with long-term noninvasive methods and, where this is feasible, the option of noninvasive support should be encouraged as it simplifies care and is preferred by patients and carers [23]. Patients with unrecordable VC may be able to self-ventilate for periods, using glossopharyngeal ("frog") breathing. This

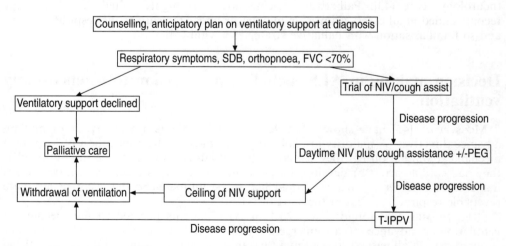

Fig. 2. – Algorithm for ventilatory management of amyotrophic lateral sclerosis. SDB: sleep-disordered breathing; FVC: forced vital capacity; NIV: noninvasive ventilation; PEG: percotaneous enteral gastrostomy; T-IPPV: tracheostomy intermittent positive pressure ventilation.

involves the patient gulping a series of breaths in succession so that breath stacking results.

The aetiology of quadriplegia ranges from traumatic cervical cord injury to stable neurological disorders (*e.g.* spina bifida) to progressive neuromuscular disease. An individual with a cervical cord lesion above C4 is likely to need ventilation immediately. Those with a C4/5 injury may be able to support ventilation independently but will decompensate in the presence of underlying chronic lung disease, spinal shock or the development of a chest infection. Delayed progression to ventilatory failure may occur in others. Critical to the wellbeing of these patients is physiotherapy and assisted coughing. Hyperinflation of the chest may be helpful in reducing the tendency to atelectasis and perhaps improving chest wall and pulmonary compliance, but there are minimal controlled trials in this area.

Assessment should include measurement of lung volumes, mouth pressures and overnight monitoring of respiration when symptoms of nocturnal hypoventilation are present, or VC is <60% predicted. Cough assist devices can be combined with NIV as described.

Anticipatory planning in neuromuscular patients with acute on chronic respiratory failure

Although the use of NIV may reduce the frequency and severity of chest infections in neuromuscular patients, occasional exacerbations are inevitable. Consideration should always be given as to whether an exacerbation represents a simple chest infection, progression of the underlying condition or development of bulbar weakness with aspiration. It is important to appreciate that respiratory muscle strength and swallowing function may temporarily deteriorate at the time of an infection.

Decision making about progression to intubation should ideally be carried out in advance as part of anticipatory care planning [49] and take into account the above considerations. A noninvasive approach is preferred where feasible. If that is insufficient, then intubation and a brief period of invasive ventilation to allow the acute episode to resolve is reasonable in patients with a substantial component of acute reversible pathology. With the advent of NIV it is now rare for individuals to end up "trapped on an ICU ventilator", although this belief is perpetuated by some teams with limited experience of neuromuscular patients. Most patients with reasonable bulbar function can be extubated into NIV. If that fails, the use of a temporary tracheostomy with the aim of stepping down to NIV should be tried. In some individuals with deteriorating overall function, however, it may be entirely appropriate to redirect care to a palliative approach rather than move to invasive ventilation, depending on the patient's wishes and clinical course. A US survey has shown wide variations management of neuromuscular patients with acute respiratory failure, with intensivists less likely to advocate active management plans compared with rehabilitation specialists. Decisions should, of course, be made on an individual basis, rather than by diagnostic label [50]. That includes full assessment of the individual, as even within subgroups of conditions *e.g.* spinal muscular atrophy type 1 there can be substantial variation in functional level and prognosis. Other conditions, *e.g.* nemaline myopathy and limb girdle muscular dystrophy, have hugely variable phenotypic expression. If there is doubt about long-term prognosis, advice should be sought from centres experienced in managing these patients.

Practical tips for managing established NIV users who are admitted with an acute chest infection

Table 3 shows a list of practical tips in the management of these NIV users.

Table 3. – Practical tips for managing established noninvasive ventilation (NIV) users who are admitted with an acute chest infection

Use NIV intensively
Carry out physiotherapy while patient uses NIV as cough enhanced and patient less likely to tire
Add supplemental oxygen therapy to NIV to maintain S_{a,O_2} >93%
May help to increase IPAP by 2–5 cmH$_2$O incrementally according to P_{CO_2} level and EPAP by 1–2 cmH$_2$O to a maximum of 7 cmH$_2$O. Increasing back-up rate to just below spontaneous breathing rate will improve CO$_2$ control
If patient becomes near 24-h NIV dependent during an acute episode consider alternating masks to prevent pressure sores and alternate day and night between two ventilators of the same model, so as not to run ventilator continuously for days
Add humidfication if patient is 24-h NIV dependent
Use nebulised bronchodilator if evidence of wheeze or bronchial hyperreactivity
Add cough in-exsufflator if secretion clearance using NIV inadequate

S_{a,O_2}: arterial oxygen saturation; IPAP: inspiratory positive airway pressure; P_{CO_2}: carbon dioxide tension; EPAP: expiratory positive airway pressure.

Risk management in neuromuscular patients

Neuromuscular patients are often more dependent on ventilatory support than other groups and requirements may progress over time. Careful consideration should be given to regular service of equipment in the home, rapid access to medical advice and attention to equipment breakdowns, and back-up equipment, *e.g.* battery power. This should be supported by a competency training programme provided to the patient, family and carers, and home team input as required. Telemedicine may be relevant in some patient groups to reduce readmissions [51]. Risk management factors are considered in detail elsewhere [52].

Summary

Noninvasive ventilation (NIV) in neuromuscular conditions, associated with respiratory insufficiency, can rapidly improve physiological indices and increase survival. Even in individuals with severe/progressive disorders, NIV may reduce symptom burden and improve quality of life. A combined NIV/cough assist approach may decrease the need for tracheostomy by facilitating sputum clearance, especially at the time of chest infections.

Keywords: Amyotrophic lateral sclerosis, cough assist device, Duchenne muscular dystrophy, nocturnal hypoventilation, spinal muscular atrophy.

References

1. Ragette R, Mellies U, Schwake C, Voit T, Teschler H. Patterns and predictors of sleep disordered breathing in primary myopathies. *Thorax* 2002; 57: 724–728.
2. Simonds AK. Assessment and selection of patients for home ventilation. *In*: Simonds AK, ed. Non-Invasive Respiratory Support: a Practical Handbook. London, Hodder Arnold, 2007; pp. 155–176.
3. American Thoracic Society Consensus Statement. Respiratory care of the patient with Duchenne muscular dystrophy. *Am J Respir Crit Care Med* 2004; 170: 456–465.
4. Ward SA, Chatwin M, Heather S, Simonds AK. Randomised controlled trial of non-invasive ventilation (NIV) for nocturnal hypoventilation in neuromuscular and chest wall disease patients with daytime normocapnia. *Thorax* 2005; 60: 1019–1024.
5. Rideau Y, Gatin G, Bach J, Gines G. Prolongation of life in Duchenne's muscular dystrophy. *Acta Neurol* 1983; 5: 118–124.
6. Leger P, Bedicam JM, Cornette A, *et al.* Nasal intermittent positive pressure ventilation. Long term follow-up in patients with severe chronic respiratory insufficiency. *Chest* 1994; 105: 100–105.
7. Simonds AK, Elliott MW. Outcome of domiciliary nasal intermittent positive pressure ventilation in restrictive and obstructive disorders. *Thorax* 1995; 50: 604–609.
8. Mellies U, Ragette R, Schwake C, Boehm H, Voit T, Teschler H. Long-term noninvasive ventilation in children and adolescents with neuromuscular disorders. *Eur Respir J* 2003; 22: 631–636.
9. Schonhofer B, Wallstein S, Kohler D, Boutellier U. Effect of noninvasive mechanical ventilation on endurance performance in patients with chronic ventilatory insufficiency. *Eur Respir J* 1998; 12: Suppl. 28, 310s.
10. Fauroux B, Boule M, Lofaso F, *et al.* Chest physiotherapy in cystic fibrosis: improved tolerance with nasal pressure support ventilation. *Pediatrics* 1999; 103: E32.
11. Braun NMT, Arora NS, Rochester DF. Respiratory muscle and pulmonary function in polymyositis and other proximal myopathies. *Thorax* 1983; 38: 616–623.
12. Piper AJ, Sullivan CE. Effects of long term nocturnal nasal ventilation on spontaneous breathing during sleep in neuromuscular and chest wall disorders. *Thorax* 1996; 9: 1515–1522.
13. Annane D, Quera-Salva MA, Lofaso F, *et al.* Mechanisms underlying the effects of nocturnal ventilation on daytime blood gases in neuromuscular diseases. *Eur Respir J* 1999; 13: 157–162.
14. Hill NS, Eveloff SE, Carlisle CC, Goff SG. Efficacy of nocturnal nasal ventilation in patients with restrictive thoracic disease. *Am Rev Respir Dis* 1992; 145: 365–371.
15. Schonhofer B, Geibel M, Sonneborn M, Haidl P, Kohler D. Daytime mechanical ventilation in chronic respiratory insufficiency. *Eur Respir J* 1997; 10: 2840–2846.
16. Nickol AN, Hart N, Hopkinson NS, Moxham J, Simonds A, Polkey MI. Mechanisms of improvement of respiratory failure in patients with restrictive thoracic disease treated with non-invasive ventilation. *Thorax* 2005; 754–760.
17. Robert D, Gerard M, Leger P, *et al.* Domiciliary ventilation by tracheostomy for chronic respiratory failure. *Rev Fr Mal Resp* 1983; 11: 923–936.
18. Splaingard ML, Frates FC, Harrison GM, *et al.* Home positive pressure ventilation. Twenty years experience. *Chest* 1983; 84: 376–382.
19. Bach J. A comparison of long-term ventilatory support alternatives from the perspective of the patient and care-giver. *Chest* 1993; 104: 1702–1706.
20. Tzeng AC, Bach JR. Prevention of pulmonary morbidity for patients with neuromuscular disease. *Chest* 2000; 118: 1390–1396.
21. Markstrom A, Sundell K, Lysdahl M, Andersson G, Schedin U, Klang B. Quality of life evaluation of patients with neuromuscular and skeletal diseases treated with noninvasive and invasive home mechanical ventilation. *Chest* 2002; 122: 1695–1700.
22. Vianello A, Bevilacqua M, Salvador V, Cardaioli C, Vincenti E. Long-term nasal intermittent positive pressure ventilation in advanced Duchenne's Muscular Dystrophy. *Chest* 1994; 105: 445–448.

23. Simonds AK, Muntoni F, Heather S, Fielding S. Impact of nasal ventilation on survival in hypercapnic Duchenne muscular dystrophy. *Thorax* 1998; 53: 949–952.

24. Eagle M, Baudouin S, Chandler C, Giddings D, Bullock R, Bushby K. Survival in Duchenne muscular dystrophy: improvements in life expectancy since 1967 and the impact of home nocturnal ventilation. *Neuromusc Disord* 2002; 12: 926–929.

25. Jeppesen J, Green A, Steffensen BF, Rahbek J. The Duchenne muscular dystrophy population in Denmark, 1977–2001: prevalence, incidence and survival in relation to the introduction of ventilator use. *Neuromusc Disord* 2003; 13: 804–812.

26. Kohler M, Clarenbach CF, Boni L, Brack T, Russi EW, Bloch KE. Quality of life, physical disability, and respiratory impairment in Duchenne muscular dystrophy. *Am J Respir Crit Care Med* 2005; 172: 1032–1036.

27. Hardiman O. Pitfalls in the diagnosis of motor neurone disease. *Hosp Med* 2000; 61: 767–771.

28. Al-Shaikh B, Kinnear W, Higenbottam TW, Smith HS, Shneerson JM. Motor neurone disease presenting as respiratory failure. *Br Med J* 1986; 292: 1325–1326.

29. Polkey MI, Lyall RA, Davidson AC, Leigh PN, Moxham J. Ethical and clinical issues in the use of home non-invasive ventilation for the palliation of breathlessness in motor neurone disease. *Thorax* 1999; 54: 367–371.

30. Haverkamp LJ, Appel V, Appel SH. Natural history of amyotrophic lateral sclerosis in a database population. Validation of a scoring system and a model for survival prediction. *Brain* 1995; 118: 707–719.

31. Miller RG, Rosenberg JA, Gelinas H, *et al.* Practice Parameter: the care of the patient with amyotrophic lateral sclerosis (an evidence based review): Report of the quality standards subcommittee of the American Academy of Neurology. *Neurology* 1999; 52: 1311–1331.

32. Lyall, RA, Donaldson N, Polkey MI, Leigh PN, Moxham J. Respiratory muscle strength and ventilatory failure in amyotrophic lateral sclerosis. *Brain* 2001; 124: 2000–2013.

33. Polkey MI, Lyall RA, Green M, Leigh PN, Moxham J. Respiratory muscle function in amyotrophic lateral sclerosis. *Am J Respir Crit Care Med* 1998; 158: 1–8.

34. Salamand J, Robert D, Leger P, Langevin B, Barraud J. Definitive mechanical ventilation via tracheostomy in end-stage amyotrophic lateral sclerosis. 3rd International Conference on Pulmonary Rehabilitation Denver. 1991; 50.

35. Oppenheimer EA. Amyotrophic lateral sclerosis. *Eur Respir Rev* 1992; 10: 323–329.

36. Goulon M, Goulon-Goeau C. Sclerose lateral amyotrophique et assistance respiratoire. [Amyotrophic lateral sclerosis and respiratory assistance]. *Rev Neurol* 1989; 145: 293–298.

37. Pinto AC, Evangelista T, Carvalho M, Alves MA, Sales Luis ML. Respiratory assistance with a non-invasive ventilator (BiPAP) in MND/ALS patients: survival rates in a controlled trial. *J Neurol Sci* 1995; 129: Suppl. 19–26.

38. Aboussouan LS, Khan SU, Meeker DP, Stelmach K, Mitsumoto H. Effect of noninvasive positive-pressure ventilation on survival in amyotrophic lateral sclerosis. *Ann Intern Med* 1997; 127: 450–453.

39. Bourke SC, Tomlinson M, Williams TL, Bullock RE, Shaw PJ, Gibson GJ. Effects of non-invasive ventilation on survival and quality of life in patients with amyotrophic lateral sclerosis: a randomised controlled trial. *Lancet Neurol* 2006; 5: 140–147.

40. Lyall RA, Donaldson N, Fleming T, *et al.* A prospective study of quality of life in ALS patients treated with non-invasive ventilation. *Neurology* 2001; 57: 153–156.

41. Mustfa N, Aiello M, Lyall RA, *et al.* Cough augmentation in amyotrophic lateral sclerosis. *Neurology* 2003; 61: 1285–1287.

42. Leigh PN, Abrahams S, Al-Chalabi A, *et al.* The management on motor neurone disease. *J Neurol Neurosurg Psychiatry* 2003; 74: 32–47.

43. Farrero E, Prats E, Povedano M, Martinez-Matos JA, Manresa F, Escarrabill J. Survival in amyotrophic lateral sclerosis with home mechanical ventilation: the impact of systematic respiratory assessment and bulbar involvement. *Chest* 2005; 127: 2132–2138.

44. Simonds AK. Home ventilation in progressive disorders, quadriplegia and palliative non-invasive ventilation. *In*: Simonds AK, ed. Non-Invasive Respiratory Support: a Practical Handbook. London, Hodder Arnold, 2007; pp. 193–207.

45. Moss AH, Oppenheimer EA, Casey P, *et al.* Patients with amyotrophic lateral sclerosis receiving long-term mechanical ventilation. Advance care planning and outcomes. *Chest* 1996; 110: 249–255.

46. Cazzolli PA, Oppenheimer EA. Home mechanical ventilation for amyotrphic lateral sclerosis: nasal compared to tracheostomy intermittent postive pressure ventilation. *J Neurol Sci* 1996; 139: 123–128.

47. Nava S, Sturani C, Hartl S, *et al.* End of life decision-making in respiratory intermediate care units: A European survey. *Eur Respir J* 2007; 30: 156–164.

48. Bach JR. Amyotrophic lateral sclerosis: Predictors for prolongation of life by noninvasive respiratory aids. *Arch Phys Med Rehabil* 1995; 76: 828–832.

49. Wang CH, Finkel RS, Bertini E, *et al.* Consensus Statement for Standard of Care in Spinal Muscular Atrophy. *J Child Neurol* 2007; 22: 1027–1049.

50. Simonds AK. Respiratory support for the severely handicapped child with neuromuscular disease: ethics and practicality. *Semin Respir Care Med* 2007; 28: 342–354.

51. Vitacca M, Scalvini S, Spanevello A, Balbi B. Telemedicine and home care: controversies and opportunities. *Breathe* 2006; 3: 148–158.

52. Simonds AK. Risk management of the home ventilator dependent patient. *Thorax* 2006; 61: 369–371.

CHAPTER 16

NIV and chronic respiratory failure secondary to restrictive thoracic disorders (obesity excluded)

W. Windisch, M. Dreher

Dept of Pneumology, University Hospital Freiburg, Freiburg, Germany.

Correspondence: M. Dreher, Dept of Pneumology, University Hospital Freiburg, Killianstrasse 5, D-79106 Freiburg, Germany. Fax: 49 7612703704; E-mail: michael.dreher@uniklinik-freiburg.de

Introduction

Noninvasive positive pressure ventilation (NPPV) is widely accepted as a treatment option for patients with chronic hypercapnic respiratory failure (HRF) arising from different aetiologies including chronic obstructive pulmonary disease (COPD), restrictive thoracic disorders (RTDs), neuromuscular disorders and obesity hypoventilation syndrome [1–4]. During the application of NPPV, a face mask serves as an interface between the biological airways of the patient and the artificial airways of the ventilator [1, 2, 5]. Long-term NPPV is applied with the aim of improving physiological parameters, such as blood gases, as well as outcome parameters, such as survival and health-related quality of life (HRQL). NPPV is used intermittently and, most often, during night, in order to preserve the potential for mobility during daytime; however, NPPV application, predominantly during the day, has also been described [6]. The impact of NPPV on both physiological and outcome parameters differs greatly according to the underlying disorder causing chronic HRF. The present article summarises the current knowledge about the impact of long-term NPPV in patients with RTDs. Herein, the different pathophysiological conditions causing chronic HRF in RTD patients are described, with reference to the different underlying diseases. The present article also focuses on the impact of NPPV, on both the physiological parameters and outcome, when used as a treatment for chronic HRF.

Pathophysiology

Different aetiologies, causing deformities of the thoracic rib cage, can lead to RTDs. Irrespective of the underlying disease, RTDs are characterised by reduced chest wall compliance and restrictive lung function pattern [7]. Thus, vital capacity, total lung capacity, functional residual capacity and, to a lesser extent, residual volume are all reduced. Furthermore, if the deformity occurs early in life, particularly before ~4 yrs of age, lung development is impaired [8]. In contrast to parenchymal lung disease, which can also cause a restrictive ventilatory defect, pulmonary gas exchange is not initially impaired. However, rib cage deformity can lead to increased airway resistance following deformity of the airways. Moreover, in patients with RTDs, the respiratory muscles are at a mechanical disadvantage due to their suboptimal contraction length.

Eur Respir Mon, 2008, 41, 240–250. Printed in UK - all rights reserved. Copyright ERS Journals Ltd 2008; European Respiratory Monograph; ISSN 1025-448x.

This causes an ineffective interaction between the respiratory muscles and the thoracic cage. As a consequence, the load imposed on the inspiratory muscles is increased, while the capacities of the inspiratory muscles and especially the diaphragm are reduced [9]. This imbalance, between load and capacity, results in inspiratory muscle insufficiency and can lead to chronic HRF; moreover, this risk of developing chronic HRF increases with advancing age. However, coexisting conditions such as COPD or severe obesity can accelerate the development of chronic HRF. This risk of chronic HRF is known to be high once vital capacity falls below 1–1.5 L, although this can occur earlier [8].

As the disease advances, RTD patients develop a rapid, shallow-breathing pattern in order to overcome the respiratory demand and minimise the work of breathing; thus minimising or even avoiding inspiratory muscle fatigue. However, rapid shallow breathing, where dead space is unchanged but tidal volume is decreased, results in reduced alveolar ventilation, as indicated by increasing arterial carbon dioxide tension (Pa,CO_2). It is, however, unclear if chronically reduced alveolar ventilation reflected by hypercapnia, normal pH and elevated bicarbonate levels already reflect inspiratory muscle fatigue, or whether this scenario represents a physiological mechanism for preventing inspiratory muscle fatigue.

In RTD patients, hypercapnia initially develops during rapid eye movement (REM) sleep, due to increased work of breathing and reduced respiratory muscle activity [10, 11]. As the disease advances, hypercapnia also develops during the deeper stages of non-REM sleep, in the late stages during exercise [12] and, finally, during daytime at rest [8, 13].

Conditions causing restrictive thoracic disorders

In principle, chronic disorders of the sternum, ribs or spine have the potential to result in chronic HRF. However, sternal diseases rarely cause respiratory failure, except in the presence of an unstable chest wall, that is, the coupling of a traumatic sternal fracture with fractures of several ribs that produce a flail segment. In these cases, the affected chest wall moves paradoxically during respiration, often with ineffective ventilation.

Rib cage abnormalities that lead to RTDs are more often responsible for chronic HRF. A still-common rib cage abnormality, with the potential to cause chronic HRF, can occur following thoracoplasty, which was once a treatment for tuberculosis, prior to the availability of specific chemotherapy. Here, a resection or replacement of the ribs was performed in order to promote a reduction in thoracic volume, thus leading to RTDs with the consequences outlined above. The so-called post-tuberculosis syndrome (PTBS) is an RTD characterised by the consequences of thoracoplasty, chest wall deformity from tuberculosis spondylitis and other residuals of tuberculosis. A more-rare condition of RTDs is a cartilaginous disorder of the ribs called asphyxiating thoracic dystrophy ("Jeune's syndrome").

Another common spine abnormality, kyphoscoliosis (KYSC; fig. 1), is a combination of kyphosis and scoliosis that results in severe rib distortion. Although scoliosis is usually combined with kyphosis, the latter can also occur in isolation (*e.g.* as a result of severe osteoporosis). The aetiology of KYSC is heterogeneous. Neuromuscular disorders affecting thoracic muscles, vertebral disease, acquired abnormalities of the thoracic cage, and connective tissue disorders are all well described as conditions that lead to KYSC. Specifically, ankylosing spondylitis is a connective tissue disorder in which chronic inflammation affects the joints of the axial skeleton. This eventually leads to fibrosis and ossification of the ligamentous structures of the spine, sacroiliac joints and rib cage; although diaphragmatic function is usually spared. However, the

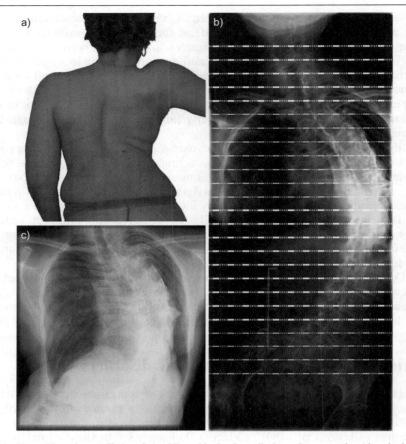

Fig. 1. – A 54-yr-old patient suffering from idiopathic kyphoscoliosis and consecutive chronic hypercapnic respiratory failure with the need for long-term noninvasive positive pressure ventilation: a) physical examination, b) radiograph from the spine and c) chest radiograph.

aetiology, in about 80% of KYSC patients, remains unexplained; the so-called idiopathic KYSC begins in childhood and typically leads to chronic HRF decades later.

Mechanical ventilation for the treatment of patients with restrictive thoracic disorders

In general, both negative- and positive-pressure ventilation can be used to treat chronic HRF. However, negative-pressure ventilation that requires lying on the deformed chest wall is uncomfortable, even painful, for RTD patients. In addition, the use of bulky devices, together with the risk of upper airway obstruction and the fact that triggering is only possible in some modern tank ventilators, has led to a decrease in the use of negative pressure ventilation.

Historically, patients with KYSC and PTBS have been ventilated invasively *via* tracheotomy, but since the late 1980s, NPPV with face masks has become the predominant form of ventilatory support for the treatment of chronic HRF resulting from RTDs [8, 14, 15]. Accordingly, a recent European survey indicated that nasal masks are used in >80% of RTD patients [4]. Only 5% of RTD patients with the need to receive long-term ventilatory support still receive invasive mechanical ventilation *via* tracheotomy [4]. This survey also indicated that nearly one-third of the patients in Europe receiving long-term mechanical ventilation suffered from RTDs, although patients with obesity hypoventilation syndrome were also associated with RTDs [4]. However, a large discrepancy between countries was reported, with Denmark and Poland reporting the lowest, and Spain reporting the highest, relative numbers of patients with RTDs receiving long-term mechanical ventilation [4].

Both pressure- and volume-limited NPPV are being used nowadays to treat chronic HRF [4], although there has been a shift from volume- to pressure-limited NPPV during the last decade [16]. However, randomised controlled cross-over trials, that have included patients with RTDs, have demonstrated that both modes of NPPV are comparably effective on blood gases, sleep quality, physical activity and HRQL [17, 18], although pressure-limited NPPV reportedly causes fewer side effects [17]. Inspiratory positive airway pressures between 20 and 25 cmH$_2$O have been recommended in the past with an inspiratory time of 0.8–1 s, an expiratory time ~2 s and an expiratory positive airway pressure of between 2 and 4 cmH$_2$O [8]. A sensitive trigger system is required to guarantee synchronisation with the ventilator, thus providing maximal comfort and high-quality ventilation.

The difficult decision about when to start long-term NPPV for RTD patients still exists for the clinician [1]. In addition, for neuromuscular patients with various underlying disorders causing chronic HRF, recent data have shown that physiological parameters at NPPV onset were essentially heterogeneous [19]. Therefore, it is also difficult to say if different underlying aetiologies causing RTD require different criteria for NPPV indication. However, the specific complaints of patients with chronic HRF, such as daytime hypersomnolence, excessive fatigue, morning headache, cognitive dysfunction, depression and dyspnoea, are essential for the indication of NPPV. The more-objective parameters, which justify the initiation of NPPV include data on gas exchange, the most important of which is Pa,CO_2; here, a Consensus Conference Report identified two objective parameters for the initiation of NPPV, namely, Pa,CO_2 ≥45 mmHg and nocturnal desaturations (table 1) [1].

Treatment compliance in RTD patients is reportedly high. The total percentage of patients who discontinued treatment is indicatively the lowest in KYSC patients (20%) and PTBS patients (24%), compared with those with COPD and Duchenne muscular dystrophy (both 44%) [14]. This has been confirmed by recent data, which also indicate the highest probability of pursuing NPPV in KYSC patients [16]. However, some RTD patients do not tolerate NPPV for home mechanical ventilation; therefore, a comprehensive follow-up is required in order to overcome problems with NPPV, as well as to ensure optimal patient compliance [20].

Table 1. – Clinical indicators for noninvasive positive pressure ventilation in patients with restrictive thoracic disorders, as outlined by the Consensus Conference Participants in 1999 [1]

Symptoms (fatigue, dyspnoea, morning headache, *etc.*) and one of the following:
Physiological criteria (one of the following):
Pa,CO_2 ≥45 mmHg
Nocturnal oximetry demonstrating an oxygen saturation ≤88% for five consecutive minutes

Pa,CO_2: arterial carbon dioxide tension.

Physiological effects of NPPV

Short- and long-term physiological effects of NPPV in RTD patients are shown in table 2.

Blood gases

Improvements in blood gases following NPPV commencement have been demonstrated by a large number of studies. In particular, there is an increase in arterial oxygen tension (Pa,O_2) and a decrease in Pa,CO_2, once long-term NPPV has been successfully established in RTD patients. Specifically, improvements in blood gases have been achieved during not only NPPV [9, 13, 16], but also subsequent spontaneous breathing following intermittent NPPV, that is applied most often during night [6, 9, 13, 14, 21–24]. Importantly, the improvement in blood gases can be maintained for several years following successful NPPV establishment [14, 25]. Interestingly, daytime NPPV and nocturnal spontaneous breathing, a seemingly reasonable and alternative approach to treating those patients who do not tolerate the nocturnal application of NPPV, have also been shown to effectively improve blood gases to a similar degree as nocturnal NPPV [6].

There are currently three different theories about how NPPV improves alveolar ventilation and gas exchange: 1) by respiratory muscle rest; 2) by resetting the CO_2 sensitivity of the central ventilatory controller; and 3) via changes in pulmonary mechanics [26]. Although the underlying mechanisms of improved gas exchange are still debated [1], recent work suggests that the increased ventilatory response to carbon dioxide is the principal mechanism underlying the long-term improvement in gas exchange following NPPV in RTD patients [9]. This is also supported by the observation that nocturnal NPPV leads to increasing daytime tidal volume, thus providing sustained reductions in Pa,CO_2 during intermittent periods of spontaneous breathing [13].

Lung function

Slight improvements in lung function parameters have been shown in RTD patients following NPPV establishment. Here, improvements were observed in both vital capacity [22–25, 27] and forced expiratory volume in one second [22, 24, 25]. In addition, the increased vital capacity, following NPPV establishment, has been shown to be related to improvements in global inspiratory muscle strength [23]. However, in contrast

Table 2. – Effects of noninvasive positive pressure ventilation in patients with restrictive thoracic disorders

Short-term effects
    Increased ventilation
    Reduced work of breathing
    Improved blood gases
    Increased strength and endurance of respiratory muscles
Long-term effects
    Improved exercise capacity
    Back-formation of cor pulmonale
    Reduced polyglobulia
    Improved sleep duration and quality
    Increased quality of life
    Reduced hospitalisation
    Prolonged survival

to the substantial improvements in blood gases, changes in lung function are only minor, and structural changes of the rib cage, from which substantial improvements in lung function might be expected, do not obviously occur following NPPV establishment. Moreover, lung function reportedly does not improve, despite significant improvements in blood gases [9, 21]. Therefore, improvements of lung function and pulmonary mechanics are unlikely to be the main principles upon which NPPV acts to improve gas exchange.

Respiratory muscle strength

Reduced inspiratory muscle strength is a common finding in RTD patients with chronic HRF [6, 9, 13, 16, 22]. There are several studies which demonstrate an increase in inspiratory muscle strength following successful initiation of NPPV [6, 23, 24, 28, 29]. However, only volitional tests of global inspiratory strength, namely the maximal inspiratory mouth pressure (PI,max), were the sole means of assessment in the above-mentioned studies. This diagnostic test is, however, highly dependent on the subject performing a truly maximal inspiratory effort, and normal values cannot be defined reliably [30, 31]. Therefore, the improvements in PI,max could also be attributed to higher motivation after successful NPPV treatment. Importantly, a recent study conducted more reliable nonvolitional tests on inspiratory muscle strength by using, for the first time, magnetic stimulation techniques [9]. In that study, there was no increase in measures of inspiratory muscle strength, including twitch transdiaphragmatic pressure, following NPPV commencement in RTD patients. However, it was suggested that the hypothesis of improved respiratory muscle function, resulting from NPPV, cannot be completely rejected, since respiratory muscle endurance has not been tested [9].

Quality of sleep

Chronic HRF is associated with nocturnal hypoventilation and a reduction in sleep quality [32]. RTDs exacerbate both the suppressive effects on respiratory centre output and central chemosensitivity, and the increases in upper airway resistance that occur with the onset of sleep [33]. NPPV has the potential to resolve this problem and therefore relieve the symptoms of hypoventilation [28, 33, 34]. It was shown, 20 yrs ago that NPPV is capable of improving sleep architecture in KYSC patients suffering from chronic HRF [29]. In addition, nocturnal ventilation and sleep quality in patients with RTDs have been shown to progressively improve over a 12-month period after NPPV commencement, and this applied to both REM and non-REM sleep [27]. Most interestingly, even after the withdrawal of NPPV for one night, these improvements were still evident during spontaneous breathing; however, the most marked improvements were evident when NPPV was used during the night.

Pulmonary haemodynamics

One study has reported an improvement in pulmonary haemodynamics in RTD patients, whereby decreases both in mean pulmonary arterial pressures and pulmonary vascular resistance were evident after 1 yr of NPPV [21]. Here, the mean pulmonary arterial pressure decreased in RTD patients from 33 ± 10 to 25 ± 6 mmHg after 1 yr of NPPV, whereas no change in mean pulmonary arterial pressure was found in patients with COPD [21].

Impact of NPPV on outcome

A summary of NPPV effects on outcome in RTD patients is shown in table 2.

Survival

Observational studies have provided evidence that 1-yr survival rates reach ~90% in KYSC patients following the commencement of NPPV treatment [14, 15]; moreover, two studies reported that the 5-yr survival rate in these patients was 79% [15, 16]. In addition, 5-yr survival rates in PTBS patients reached 94% in one study [15], but were found to be considerably lower (<50%) in another study [16]. This discrepancy is presumably explained by the different mean baseline ages of patients in those two studies, with PTBS patients being aged 61 ± 8 yrs in the first study [15] and 75 ± 6 yrs in the second study [16]. In addition, patients with chronic HRF, that arose after thoracoplasty for tuberculosis, were reported to have survival rates of 91, 74, 64 and 55% at 1, 3, 5 and 7 yrs, respectively, once long-term NPPV has been started [35]. In addition, uncontrolled trials have clearly shown that KYSC [23] and PTBS patients [36] who receive NPPV have a substantially higher survival rate than those who receive long-term oxygen therapy alone; however, the patients who received NPPV were deemed to be more ill, as estimated from lung function parameters and Pa,CO_2. Therefore, robust data from uncontrolled studies are now available to support the notion that survival is clearly increased when long-term NPPV is used to treat chronic HRF that results from RTD. While no randomised controlled trials have been performed to compare directly the outcome of patients who receive long-term NPPV to those who do not, such trials will, presumably, never be conducted due to ethical concerns.

HRQL

HRQL evaluation is becoming increasingly essential in healthcare practice and research, as it provides an important means of evaluating the human and financial costs and benefits of modern, medical-treatment modalities; this is particularly relevant to patients with chronic and noncurable disorders such as RTD [37–39]. Cross-sectional studies comparing patients with different underlying disorders, who had already received long-term NPPV, revealed that KYSC patients have the overall best HRQL compared with those with PTBS, COPD and neuromuscular disorders [15, 40, 41]. Therefore, it is noteworthy that when using the generic Medical Outcomes Study (MOS) 36-Item Short-Form Health Status Survey (SF-36) [42–44], mental health was shown to be unimpaired, despite a marked reduction in physical health, when compared with a normal reference population [40]. Several studies have also indicated that HRQL effectively improves in KYSC patients upon commencement of NPPV, to treat chronic HRF [45, 46]. Recently, the Severe Respiratory Insufficiency (SRI) Questionnaire was developed for the purpose of specifically measuring HRQL in patients with chronic HRF and the need for long-term NPPV [41]. Using this instrument, a very recent multicentric prospective trial including RTD patients, mainly those with KYSC and PTBS, has indicated a substantial increase in overall HRQL [47]. Importantly, HRQL already showed improvement after 1 month of treatment and remained stable at this elevated level during the subsequent year. Domains showing the strongest improvements included "respiratory complaints", "physical functioning", "attendant symptoms" and "sleep and anxieties".

Exercise ability

Recent work has shown that nocturnal NPPV, applied over a 3-month period, improved exercise capacity in patients with chronic HRF arising from RTD, whereas no change in exercise capacity was found in the control group [22]. Furthermore, the same study also showed that inspiratory muscle endurance improved when nocturnal NPPV was applied for 3 months, whereas no change in respiratory muscle endurance was found in the control group. This provides controlled evidence to suggest that nocturnal NPPV can improve both respiratory and peripheral muscle endurance [22]. NPPV can also be applied during exertion in RTD patients, in order to increase exercise capacity. A recent study demonstrated in severely restrictive patients that NPPV, during exercise, significantly improved exercise duration and tolerance and increased alveolar ventilation [48]. In addition, NPPV applied during exercise has also been investigated in patients with PTBS. Here, NPPV effectively supported ventilation under exertion, with consecutive reductions in breathlessness and improvements in exercise endurance [12]. This is in accord with a previous finding in COPD patients, where NPPV-aided exercise resulted in improved oxygenation, reduced dyspnoea and increased walking distance [49]. Therefore, NPPV-aided exercise is suggested to be a useful adjunct for rehabilitation programmes, which aim to improve exercise capability.

Hospitalisation

Although no controlled studies are available, there is increasing evidence that the need for hospitalisation decreases during the time that follows NPPV commencement. This has been shown for both KYSC and PTBS patients (table 3) [14], as well as for KYSC patients alone, whose days in hospital decreased from 11 to 0 days when comparing the 6-month period preceding and following NPPV establishment [28]. In addition, a recent study, providing long-term follow-up, showed that the mean number of days spent in hospital decreased significantly in RTD and neuromuscular patients following NPPV establishment: 22 ± 2 days in the year before NPPV; 17 ± 4 days in the first year with NPPV; 6 ± 3 days in the second year with NPPV; 6 ± 2 days in the third year with NPPV; 10 ± 4 days in the fourth year with NPPV; and 7 ± 3 days in the fifth year with NPPV [16]. In addition, the hospitalisation rate has been shown to decrease in KYSC patients following NPPV commencement [45, 46]. Therefore, reduced hospitalisation following NPPV establishment, as shown by several studies, indicates an improvement in HRQL, since the number of hospitalisations has been identified as a main variable in predicting HRQL in patients with chronic HRF, who are receiving long-term NPPV [50].

Table 3. – Days in hospital before and after initiation of noninvasive positive pulmonary ventilation (NPPV) in patients with kyphoscoliosis (KYSC) and post-tuberculosis syndrome (PTBS), according to LEGER et al. [14]

	Subjects n	1 yr without NPPV	First year with NPPV	Second year with NPPV
KYSC	56	34 ± 31	6 ± 6	5 ± 9
PTBS	43	31 ± 29	10 ± 17	9 ± 19

Summary

Kyphoscoliosis with different aetiologies and post-tuberculosis syndrome are the most common conditions causing restrictive thoracic disorders that predispose patients to the risk of developing chronic hypercapnic respiratory failure. Noninvasive positive pressure ventilation using face masks has become the standard means of treating chronic hypercapnic respiratory failure that arises from restrictive thoracic disorders. Thereby, noninvasive positive pressure ventilation has been shown to improve physiological parameters, most importantly blood gases, and also pulmonary haemodynamics and sleep architecture. In addition, noninvasive positive pressure ventilation is also strongly suggested to improve important outcome parameters such as long-term survival, health-related quality of life, hospitalisation and exercise ability. Therefore, patients with chronic hypercapnic respiratory failure due to restrictive thoracic disorders should be regularly offered long-term noninvasive positive pressure ventilation.

Keywords: Hypoventilation, intermittent positive pressure ventilation, kyphosis, noninvasive ventilation, respiratory insufficiency, restrictive thoracic disorder.

References

1. Clinical indications for noninvasive positive pressure ventilation in chronic respiratory failure due to restrictive lung disease, COPD, and nocturnal hypoventilation – a consensus conference report. *Chest* 1999; 116: 521–534.
2. Mehta S, Hill NS. Noninvasive ventilation. *Am J Respir Crit Care Med* 2001; 163: 540–577.
3. Simonds AK. Home ventilation. *Eur Respir J* 2003; 22: Suppl. 47, 38s–46s.
4. Lloyd-Owen SJ, Donaldson GC, Ambrosino N, *et al.* Patterns of home mechanical ventilation use in Europe: results from the Eurovent survey. *Eur Respir J* 2005; 25: 1025–1031.
5. Schönhofer B, Sortor-Leger S. Equipment needs for noninvasive mechanical ventilation. *Eur Respir J* 2002; 20: 1029–1036.
6. Schönhofer B, Geibel M, Sonneborn M, Haidl P, Köhler D. Daytime mechanical ventilation in chronic respiratory insufficiency. *Eur Respir J* 1997; 10: 2840–2846.
7. Bergofsky EH. Respiratory failure in disorders of the thoracic cage. *Am Rev Respir Dis* 1979; 119: 643–669.
8. Shneerson JM, Simonds AK. Noninvasive ventilation for chest wall and neuromuscular disorders. *Eur Respir J* 2002; 20: 480–487.
9. Nickol AH, Hart N, Hopkinson NS, Moxham J, Simonds A, Polkey MI. Mechanisms of improvement of respiratory failure in patients with restrictive thoracic disease treated with non-invasive ventilation. *Thorax* 2005; 60: 754–760.
10. Sawicka EH, Branthwaite MA. Respiration during sleep in kyphoscoliosis. *Thorax* 1987; 42: 801–808.
11. Midgren B, Petersson K, Hansson L, Eriksson L, Airikkala P, Elmqvist D. Nocturnal hypoxaemia in severe scoliosis. *Br J Dis Chest* 1988; 82: 226–236.
12. Tsuboi T, Ohi M, Chin K, *et al.* Ventilatory support during exercise in patients with pulmonary tuberculosis sequelae. *Chest* 1997; 112: 1000–1007.
13. Windisch W, Dreher M, Storre JH, Sorichter S. Nocturnal non-invasive positive pressure ventilation: physiological effects on spontaneous breathing. *Respir Physiol Neurobiol* 2006; 150: 251–260.

14. Leger P, Bedicam JM, Cornette A, *et al.* Nasal intermittent positive pressure ventilation. Long-term follow-up in patients with severe chronic respiratory insufficiency. *Chest* 1994; 105: 100–105.

15. Simonds AK, Elliott MW. Outcome of domiciliary nasal intermittent positive pressure ventilation in restrictive and obstructive disorders. *Thorax* 1995; 50: 604–609.

16. Janssens JP, Derivaz S, Breitenstein E, *et al.* Changing patterns in long-term noninvasive ventilation: a 7-year prospective study in the Geneva Lake area. *Chest* 2003; 123: 67–79.

17. Windisch W, Storre JH, Sorichter S, Virchow JC Jr. Comparison of volume- and pressure-limited NPPV at night: a prospective randomized cross-over trial. *Respir Med* 2005; 99: 52–59.

18. Tuggey JM, Elliott MW. Randomised crossover study of pressure and volume non-invasive ventilation in chest wall deformity. *Thorax* 2005; 60: 859–864.

19. Dreher M, Rauter I, Storre JH, Geiseler J, Windisch W. When should home mechanical ventilation be started in patients with different neuromuscular disorders? *Respirology* 2007; 12: 749–753.

20. Criner GJ, Brennan K, Travaline JM, Kreimer D. Efficacy and compliance with noninvasive positive pressure ventilation in patients with chronic respiratory failure. *Chest* 1999; 116: 667–675.

21. Schönhofer B, Barchfeld T, Wenzel M, Köhler D. Long term effects of non-invasive mechanical ventilation on pulmonary haemodynamics in patients with chronic respiratory failure. *Thorax* 2001; 56: 524–528.

22. Schönhofer B, Wallstein S, Wiese C, Kohler D. Noninvasive mechanical ventilation improves endurance performance in patients with chronic respiratory failure due to thoracic restriction. *Chest* 2001; 119: 1371–1378.

23. Buyse B, Meersseman W, Demedts M. Treatment of chronic respiratory failure in kyphoscoliosis: oxygen or ventilation? *Eur Respir J* 2003; 22: 525–528.

24. Budweiser S, Heinemann F, Fischer W, Dobroschke J, Wild PJ, Pfeifer M. Impact of ventilation parameters and duration of ventilator use on non-invasive home ventilation in restrictive thoracic disorders. *Respiration* 2006; 73: 488–494.

25. Duiverman ML, Bladder G, Meinesz AF, Wijkstra PJ. Home mechanical ventilatory support in patients with restrictive ventilatory disorders: a 48-year experience. *Respir Med* 2006; 100: 56–65.

26. Hill NS. Noninvasive ventilation. Does it work, for whom, and how? *Am Rev Respir Dis* 1993; 147: 1050–1055.

27. Schönhofer B, Köhler D. Effect of non-invasive mechanical ventilation on sleep and nocturnal ventilation in patients with chronic respiratory failure. *Thorax* 2000; 55: 308–513.

28. Ferris G, Servera-Pieras E, Vergara P, *et al.* Kyphoscoliosis ventilatory insufficiency: noninvasive management outcomes. *Am J Phys Med Rehabil* 2000; 79: 24–29.

29. Ellis ER, Grunstein RR, Chan S, Bye PT, Sullivan CE. Noninvasive ventilatory support during sleep improves respiratory failure in kyphoscoliosis. *Chest* 1988; 94: 811–815.

30. American Thoracic Society/European Respiratory Society. ATS/ERS Statement on respiratory muscle testing. *Am J Respir Crit Care Med* 2002; 166: 518–624.

31. Windisch W, Hennings E, Sorichter S, Hamm H, Criée CP. Peak or plateau maximal inspiratory mouth pressure: which is best? *Eur Respir J* 2004; 23: 708–13.

32. McNicholas WT. Impact of sleep in respiratory failure. *Eur Respir J* 1997; 10: 920–933.

33. Perrin C, D'Ambrosio C, White A, Hill NS. Sleep in restrictive and neuromuscular respiratory disorders. *Semin Respir Crit Care Med* 2005; 26: 117–130.

34. Hill NS, Eveloff SE, Carlisle CC, Goff SG. Efficacy of nocturnal nasal ventilation in patients with restrictive thoracic disease. *Am Rev Respir Dis* 1992; 145: 365–371.

35. Jackson M, Smith I, King M, Shneerson J. Long term non-invasive domiciliary assisted ventilation for respiratory failure following thoracoplasty. *Thorax* 1994; 49: 915–919.

36. Jäger L, Franklin KA, Midgren B, Löfdahl K, Ström K. Increased survival with mechanical ventilation in posttuberculosis patients with the combination of respiratory failure and chest wall deformity. *Chest* 2008; 133: 156–160.

37. Testa MA, Simonson DC. Assesment of quality-of-life outcomes. *N Engl J Med* 1996; 334: 835–840.

38. Wood-Dauphinee S. Assessing quality of life in clinical research: from where have we come and where are we going? *J Clin Epidemiol* 1999; 52: 355–363.

39. Higginson IJ, Carr AJ. Measuring quality of life: using quality of life measures in the clinical setting. *BMJ* 2001; 322: 1297–1300.

40. Windisch W, Freidel K, Schucher B, *et al.* Evaluation of health-related quality of life using the MOS 36-Item Short-Form Health Status Survey in patients receiving noninvasive positive pressure ventilation. *Intensive Care Med* 2003; 29: 615–621.

41. Windisch W, Freidel K, Schucher B, *et al.* The Severe Respiratory Insufficiency (SRI) Questionnaire: a specific measure of health-related quality of life in patients receiving home mechanical ventilation. *J Clin Epidemiol* 2003; 56: 752–759.

42. Ware JE Jr, Sherbourne CD. The MOS 36-item short-form health survey (SF-36). I. Conceptual framework and item selection. *Med Care* 1992; 30: 473–483.

43. Ware JE Jr, Kosinski M, Bayliss MS, McHorney CA, Rogers WH, Raczek A. Comparison of methods for the scoring and statistical analysis of SF-36 health profile and summary measures: summary of results from the Medical Outcomes Study. *Med Care* 1995; 33: AS264–AS279.

44. Ware JE J. The SF-36 Health Survey. ; 1996. NTA

45. Nauffal D, Doménech R, Martínez García MA, Compte L, Macián V, Perpiñá M. Noninvasive positive pressure home ventilation in restrictive disorders: outcome and impact on health-related quality of life. *Respir Med* 2002; 96: 777–783.

46. Doménech-Clar R, Nauffal-Manzur D, Perpiñá-Tordera M, Compte-Torrero L, Macián-Gisbert V. Home mechanical ventilation for restrictive thoracic diseases: effects on patient quality-of-life and hospitalizations. *Respir Med* 2003; 97: 1320–1327.

47. Windisch W. Impact of home mechanical ventilation on health-related quality of life. *Eur Respir J* 2008; 32: 1328–1336.

48. Borel JC, Wuyam B, Chouri-Pontarollo N, Deschaux C, Levy P, Pépin JL. During exercise noninvasive ventilation in chronic restrictive respiratory failure. *Respir Med* 2008; 102: 711–719.

49. Dreher M, Storre JH, Windisch W. Noninvasive ventilation during walking in patients with severe COPD: a randomised cross-over trial. *Eur Respir J* 2007; 29: 930–936.

50. López-Campos JL, Failde I, Masa JF, *et al.* Factors related to quality of life in patients receiving home mechanical ventilation. *Respir Med* 2008; 102: 605–612.

NIV and chronic respiratory failure secondary to obesity

J-P. Janssens*, J-L. Pépin[#,¶], Y.F. Guo[+]

*Division of Pulmonary Diseases and [#]Sleep Laboratory, Division of Psychiatry, Belle-Idée, Geneva University Hospitals, Geneva, Switzerland, [¶]INSERM ERI 17, HP2 Laboratory, University Hospital, Grenoble, France, and [+]Dept of Pulmonary Diseases, Beijing Hospital, Beijing, China.

Correspondence: J-P. Janssens, Centre antituberculeux, Hôpital cantonal, 1211 Geneva 14, Switzerland. Fax: 41 223729929; E-mail: Jean-Paul.Janssens@hcuge.ch

Introduction

The epidemic of obesity is a growing concern for medical authorities throughout the world, especially in industrialised countries. One of its consequences in these countries is a spectacular increase in the number of patients suffering from obstructive sleep apnoea/hypopnoea syndrome (OSAHS) and obesity–hypoventilation syndrome (OHS); both are associated with the metabolic syndrome and, thus, with a marked increase in cardiovascular and cerebrovascular morbidity. OHS, itself, has a severe prognosis if untreated. In the present chapter, the major consequences of morbid obesity on ventilatory function and ventilatory drive will be analysed, as well as the evidence in favour of noninvasive positive pressure ventilation (NPPV) as an efficient treatment for OHS.

Definition

Originally reported by BICKELMANN et al. [1], OHS is defined by obesity (body mass index (BMI) ≥ 30 kg·m^{-2}) and chronic alveolar hypoventilation leading to daytime hypercapnia (arterial carbon dioxide tension (Pa,CO$_2$) >45 mmHg), after exclusion of all other causes of alveolar hypoventilation (severe obstructive or restrictive diseases, chest wall disorders, neuromuscular diseases) [2]. In ~90% of patients, OHS is associated with OSAHS. The remaining ~10% have nocturnal hypoventilation with a normal apnoea/hypopnoea index (AHI) [3, 4]. If not adequately treated, patients with OHS develop pulmonary hypertension, cor pulmonale and recurrent episodes of hypercapnic respiratory failure. Without ventilatory support, obesity-associated hypoventilation is associated with a high morbidity and mortality [5].

Epidemiology of morbid obesity

The prevalence of obesity has risen three-fold or more in many European countries since the 1980s [6]. According to the World Health Organization, prevalence of obesity in Europe ranges 5–20% in males and up to 30% in females. If the prevalence continues to increase at the same rate as in the 1990s, it is estimated that ~150 million adults in Europe will be obese by 2010. The figures show a clear upward trend, even in countries

Eur Respir Mon, 2008, 41, 251–264. Printed in UK - all rights reserved. Copyright ERS Journals Ltd 2008; European Respiratory Monograph; ISSN 1025-448x.

with traditionally low rates of overweight and obesity such as France, the Netherlands and Norway.

In the United States, the epidemic has taken on much more-severe proportions with a doubling in prevalence of obesity reported over the past 25 yrs; presently 33% of the adult population aged 20–74 yrs has a BMI >30 kg·m^{-2} [7]. US figures could well account for the spectacular rise of OHS patients under NPPV (30% of US adults had class II obesity in 2002, according to the Centers for Disease Control and Prevention); however, prevalence of class II and class III obesity in Europe are not sufficient for explaining this trend. Increasing awareness of obesity-related respiratory disorders by general practitioners and pulmonary physicians is certainly contributive to the increasing use of NPPV in OHS.

Although prevalence of obesity is reaching epidemic proportions in many developed countries, to date, large-scale data regarding the prevalence of OHS are not available. However, prevalence of OHS increases with BMI, averaging $<10\%$ in subjects with a BMI of 30–34 kg·m^{-2} and increasing markedly in subjects with a BMI of 35–39 kg·m^{-2} (10–20%) and >40 kg·m^{-2} (20–25%) [8]. LAABAN and CHAILLEUX [9] studied 1,141 adult patients with OSAHS treated by a nonprofit network for home treatment of chronic respiratory insufficiency (the *Association Nationale pour le Traitment À Domicile de l'Insuffisance Respiratoire chronique*; ANTADIR): prevalence of daytime hypercapnia (Pa,CO$_2$ >45 mmHg) was 7.2% in patients with a BMI <30 kg·m^{-2}, 9.8% for those with a BMI 30–40 kg·m^{-2}, and 23.6% for those with a BMI >40 kg·m^{-2}; 11% of the whole population had daytime hypercapnia before initiating continuous positive airway pressure (CPAP) [9]. Similarly, a Japanese study involving 1,227 patients with OSAHS found that 14% of patients had daytime hypercapnia [10]. In that study, hypercapnia was significantly related to severity of AHI, while BMI was a weak predictor of daytime hypercapnia [10]. NOWBAR et al. [5] noted a similar relationship between prevalence of hypoventilation and increasing BMI among 150 obese patients admitted to a teaching hospital; hypoventilation increased from 35% (in subjects with a BMI of 35–44 kg·m^{-2}) to 71% in subjects with a BMI >45 kg·m^{-2} [5]. That study included hospitalised patients potentially suffering from comorbidities, such as cardiac failure; such unstable conditions can overestimate the prevalence of OHS. Further studies addressing the prevalence of OHS in ambulatory obese subjects in the general population are necessary.

Impact of obesity on respiratory function

Obesity, compliance of the respiratory system and work of breathing

The most important consequence of severe obesity on respiratory mechanics is a decrease in compliance of the respiratory system and an increase in work of breathing (WOB). PELOSI et al. [11] measured lung compliance, resistance and WOB in sedated–paralysed normal subjects (n=10) and morbidly obese patients (n=10; BMI: 49 ± 7 kg·m^{-2}). Respiratory mechanics were markedly altered in obese subjects; functional residual capacity (FRC) was about one-third of normal and compliance of the respiratory system was reduced to ~50% of that of normal subjects due to a decrease in both lung and chest wall compliance. The loss of lung compliance was probably secondary to micro-atelectasis in dependant areas of the lung. The decrease in chest wall compliance was related to structural changes in the chest wall and rib cage (*i.e.* increased adiposity) and to a decreased thoracic volume, bringing the chest wall pressure–volume curve down to its less compliant segment [12]. Total lung resistance was three-fold higher in obese patients compared with normal subjects, resulting from an increase in both airway and lung resistance. Both elastic and resistive WOB were significantly higher in obese subjects [12]. In a similar study, PELOSI et al. [13] demonstrated a highly significant exponential inverse relationship between BMI and compliance. Compliance was further reduced in obese individuals in the supine position [14].

In order to estimate oxygen cost of breathing ($V'O_2$,RESP), KRESS et al. [15] measured baseline oxygen uptake ($V'O_2$) in morbidly obese patients (n=18; BMI 53.4 $\pm$ 14 kg·m^{-2}) prior to gastric bypass surgery and again after intubation, mechanical ventilation and paralysis, and compared change in $V'O_2$ to that obtained in nonobese patients (n=8; BMI 22.2 $\pm$ 4.0 kg·m^{-2}) undergoing abdominal surgery. Changes in $V'O_2$ were highly significant in obese patients (on average, -16%) but not in controls (<1%), obese subjects exhibiting a five-fold increase in $V'O_2$,RESP/$V'O_2$ and a higher baseline $V'O_2$. Thus, obese subjects have a markedly increased WOB, and $V'O_2$,RESP resulting from decreased compliance of the respiratory system and increased total lung and airway resistance.

Obesity, lung volumes and respiratory muscles

As previously mentioned, the most consistent finding in obese subjects is a reduction in FRC , which implies a reduction in expiratory reserve volume, breathing occurring close to residual volume and within closing volume (CV) [16]. A significant inverse relationship between BMI and forced vital capacity (FVC), in subjects aged >40 yrs was noted in the Normative Aging Study (n=507); conversely, increasing BMI was associated with an increase in forced expiratory volume in one second (FEV1)/FVC ratio, and an increase in the maximal mid-expiratory flow (MMEF; probably as a consequence of increased elastic recoil of the respiratory system) [17]. Weight changes are associated with significant changes in pulmonary function tests. In a multicentre study of pulmonary function testing after smoking cessation (Lung Health Study; n=5,346), WISE et al. [18] showed a significant inverse relationship between weight changes and changes in either FEV1 or FVC; in sustained quitters, FVC dropped by 174 $\pm$ 15 mL in males and 106 $\pm$ 17 mL in females, for every 10 kg of weight gain. Severe obesity is, thus, associated with a restrictive defect and impaired ventilation/perfusion relationships resulting from decreased FRC and FRC-CV.

Strength of inspiratory muscles seems to be reduced, to some extent, in OHS [19, 20]. However, values reported in patients with OHS, alone, cannot explain the occurrence of chronic hypoventilation [19]. Individuals with OHS are capable of normalising their daytime Pa,CO_2 levels by voluntarily hyperventilating [21]. Furthermore, although NPPV with a bilevel pressure cycled ventilator has been shown to unload inspiratory muscles, respiratory muscle strength has not been shown to improve after NPPV; thus, respiratory muscle fatigue is an unlikely cause of chronic hypoventilation in OHS [19, 20, 22]. It is probable, however, that an adverse load/capacity ratio occurs in OHS and predisposes to respiratory failure [16]. Acidosis and hypoxaemia encountered in severe OHS can also have a detrimental effect on inspiratory muscle strength.

Leptin, obesity and respiratory drive

Leptin was initially described as an adipose tissue derived hormone implicated in control of body weight and energy expenditure; receptors to leptin have been described in the central nervous system (CNS; e.g. hypothalamus) and in peripheral tissues. Leptin is also a modulator of the respiratory control system. Indeed, leptin-deficient mice (ob/ob strain), which spontaneously develop marked obesity, have a reduced diurnal and, more importantly, nocturnal ventilatory response to inspired carbon dioxide, which is corrected by exogenous administration of leptin [23]. In fact, ventilatory response to carbon dioxide is abolished during rapid eye movement (REM) sleep in ob/ob mice. In humans with OHS, increases in circulating levels of leptin are most-often reported, suggesting leptin resistance rather than leptin deficiency (as in ob/ob mice). SHIMURA *et al.* [24] studied 106 eucapnic (Pa,CO_2 40.9 ± 0.3 mmHg) and 79 hypercapnic (Pa,CO_2 46.6 ± 0.4 mmHg) male patients with OSAHS; circulating leptin levels were higher in the hypercapnic group and serum leptin was the only predictor for the presence of hypercapnia by logistic regression. Levels of leptin increased significantly with BMI, although more in hypercapnic patients (r=0.65) than in normocapnic subjects (r=0.38) [24]. Similar findings were reported by PHIPPS *et al.* [25], who suggest that increased leptin in severe obesity may act, initially, to adapt alveolar ventilation to increased ventilatory load and that failure of this compensatory mechanism may explain hypercapnic respiratory failure. A recent report including 245 obese subjects (BMI ≥ 30 kg·m^{-2}) found a significant and independent inverse relationship between Log of leptin and either mouth occlusion pressure (P0.1) or P0.1/end-tidal carbon dioxide tension (PET,CO_2); in other words, higher leptin levels were associated with a reduced ventilatory drive and reduced response to carbon dioxide [26].

Respiratory disturbances during sleep in OHS

The pathophysiology of OHS results from complex interactions, which involve increased WOB related to obesity, normal or decreased ventilatory drive and various sleep-associated breathing disorders (*i.e.*: OSAHS and REM sleep hypoventilation). Appropriately identifying these different respiratory patterns occurring during sleep may help in selecting the most appropriate ventilatory support in a given patient.

Associated OSAHS (fig. 1) is present in most cases of OHS and may contribute to the occurrence of daytime hypercapnia. The maintenance of eucapnia during sleep in OSAHS patients requires a balance between carbon dioxide loading during apnoea and elimination in the inter-event period. BERGER *et al.* [27] found an inverse relationship between the slope of the post-event ventilatory response and the chronic awake arterial Pa,CO_2, suggesting that this mechanism might be impaired in OHS patients with OSAHS (fig. 2). Similarly, chronic hypercapnia has been shown to be directly related to the apnoea/inter-apnoea duration ratio. With increasing chronic hypercapnia, the inter-apnoea duration shortens, relative to the apnoea duration [28]. There is, therefore, a rationale to an initial trial of nasal CPAP (nCPAP) in OHS patients with OSAHS

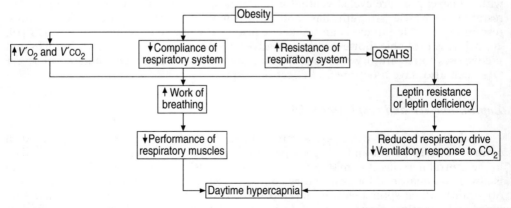

Fig. 1. – Items contributing to chronic hypercapnic respiratory failure in obesity–hypoventilation syndrome. V'O$_2$: oxygen uptake; V'CO$_2$: carbon dioxide production; OSAHS: obstructive sleep apnoea/hypopnoea syndrome.

instead of a more complex bilevel ventilator, although, as discussed in a following section, only a subset of subjects can be successfully managed with nCPAP alone.

The second typical respiratory abnormality taking place during sleep in OHS patients is REM sleep hypoventilation (fig. 3). During REM sleep, rib-cage and accessory breathing muscle activity is suppressed, particularly during bursts of eye movement; breathing is more irregular, rapid and shallow, with a significant decrease in ventilation. REM sleep hypoventilation is central in nature and is related to a reduction in respiratory drive, associated with phasic REM sleep. It has been recently demonstrated that, in OHS, the amount of REM sleep hypoventilation is significantly related with blunted ventilatory responses to carbon dioxide and associated with increased sleepiness [29]. When REM sleep hypoventilation is prominent, CPAP devices are ineffective [30]; the present consensus is for discouraging the use of auto-adjusted CPAP, in this situation, and instead using a bilevel positive pressure ventilator [31].

Morbidity and mortality associated with obesity–hypoventilation

Obesity is a component of the metabolic syndrome (abdominal obesity, insulin resistance, hypertension, low serum high density lipoprotein (HDL) cholesterol, elevated serum triglycerides) and, as such, is associated with a higher risk of hypertension, diabetes mellitus, and associated cardiovascular and cerebrovascular morbidity [3, 32]. OSA is related to glucose intolerance, insulin resistance and diabetes.

There is evidence for an increased cardiovascular morbidity in OHS subjects compared with patients with similar degrees of obesity [3, 8, 33]. OHS patients are much

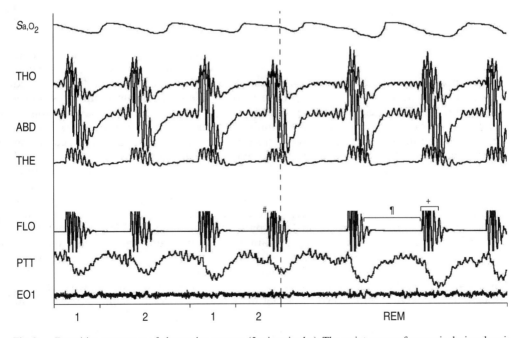

Fig. 2. – Repetitive occurrence of obstructive apnoeas (5-min episodes). The maintenance of eucapnia during sleep is dependent upon the post-event ventilatory response slope ($^{#}$) and the ratio between the inter-apnoea duration ($^{+}$) and the apnoea duration (¶). Sa,O_2: arterial oxygen saturation; THO: thoracic movements; ABD: abdominal movements; THE: buconasal thermistor; FLO: nasal pressure; PTT: pulse transit time; EO1: eye movements.

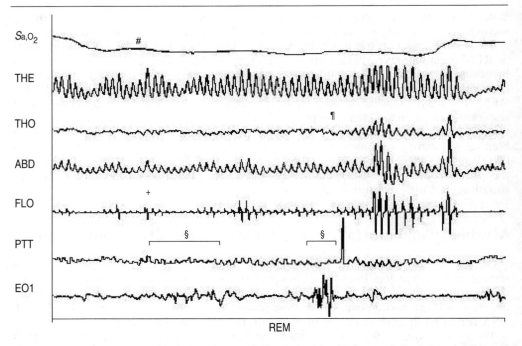

Fig. 3. – Rapid eye movement (REM) sleep hypoventilation (a 5-min epoch is presented). Sa,O_2: arterial oxygen saturation; THE: buconasal thermistor; THO: thoracic movements; ABD: abdominal movements; FLO: nasal pressure; PTT: pulse transit time; EO1: eye movements. [#]: sustained oxygen desaturation; [¶]: predominant reduction of the thoracic contribution to the ventilation during REM sleep; [+]: sustained reduction in flow; [§]: reduction of respiratory effort during phasic REM sleep reflecting reduced respiratory drive. Adapted from [29].

more likely to be diagnosed with systemic hypertension, diabetes mellitus and cardiac failure. Obesity is, apparently, not the only determinant of these cardiovascular consequences. A specific visceral fat inflammation and resistance to leptin demonstrated in these patients could play a role. Leptin-resistant obese subjects may exhibit resistance to the anorectic and weight-reducing effects of leptin while showing preservation of peripheral actions such as increasing renal sympathetic nerve outflow and arterial pressure, subsequently leading to hypertension [34, 35]. In humans, increased serum leptin concentrations are associated with hypertension, myocardial infarction and stroke, independently of obesity status [36]. Elevated plasma leptin levels also contribute to insulin resistance and low-grade inflammation. Leptin has a pro-atherosclerotic effect and leptin deficient mice are resistant to atherosclerosis [36]. Leptin can influence the production of other adipokines involved in fat and systemic inflammation, contributing to a specific inflammatory profile in OHS patients. This high prevalence of metabolic and cardiovascular co-morbidity may explain a higher mortality rate in OHS patients.

PEREZ DE LLANO et al. [37] reported a 40% mortality rate over an average follow-up period of 50 ± 25 months among 15 patients with OHS who did not accept NPPV. Among 4,332 hospital admissions, NOWBAR et al. [5] followed 47 patients with obesity-associated hypoventilation (BMI ≥ 35 kg·m^{-2}) and 103 with "simple obesity"; at 18 months, mortality was 23% in the "obesity-associated hypoventilation" group versus 9% in the "simple obesity" group. Adjusted mortality rate for patients with obesity-associated hypoventilation (corrected for age, sex, BMI, electrolyte disturbances, history of thromboembolism or hypothyroidism) was four times higher than that for subjects with simple obesity.

Use of healthcare resources in OHS

BERG et al. [33] compared use of healthcare resources by patients with OHS (BMI 47 ± 11 kg·m^{-2}) to two control groups (obese without OHS and general population) during the 5 yrs before and the 2 yrs after initiation of positive pressure support; OHS patients had an average of 11 ± 2 physician visits per yr *versus* 5.7 ± 0.8 for obese controls and 4.5 ± 0.4 for the general population. Before treatment, OHS patients had an increased number of hospital admissions; in the year prior to diagnosis, 70% of OHS patients were hospitalised at least once. Risk of being hospitalised prior to treatment was much higher than that of the general population (odds ratio (OR) 8.6, 95% confidence interval (CI) 5.9–12.7) or of obese subjects without hypoventilation (OR 4.9, 95% CI 4.0–10.4). These differences disappeared after treatment. Similar results were reported in Switzerland; in 32 patients treated for OHS, the number of days spent in hospital decreased significantly between the year before NPPV therapy had begun (26 ± 4 days) and the 3 yrs after starting NPPV (year 1: 17 ± 5 days; year 2: mean, 3 ± 1 days; year 3: mean, 9 ± 4 days), then increased slightly [19].

Noninvasive ventilation and OHS

Major factors contributing to respiratory failure and impaired gas exchange in OHS are summarised in tables 1 and 2 and figure 1. Positive pressure support in OHS aims to decrease upper airway resistance during sleep (pneumatic splinting, for OSAHS), decrease nocturnal WOB by improving upper airway patency, increase FRC and thus improve ventilation/perfusion ratio (V'/Q') matching and, when using bilevel positive airway pressure (BiPAP) ventilation, unload the respiratory muscles and increase nocturnal ventilation to improve day- and night-time Pa,CO_2 [38]. Because the strength of respiratory muscles is preserved in most patients with OHS [19], NPPV most probably improves daytime arterial blood gases through a resetting of respiratory centres and target value for Pa,CO_2. Although no NPPV-related improvement of compliance of the respiratory system has been formally documented in OHS, improved VC, reported by some authors, suggests a possible increase in compliance of the respiratory system after several months of treatment [22, 39, 40].

Benefits associated with noninvasive ventilation in OHS

The first report of an alternative treatment to tracheostomy of patients with severe OHS, cardio-respiratory failure and associated OSAHS (Pickwickian syndrome) was published by SULLIVAN et al. in 1983 [41]; low levels of CPAP improved daytime and nocturnal hypoventilation and nocturnal arterial oxygen saturation (Sa,O_2). With the advent of the BiPAP®, SANDERS and KERN [42] established that BiPAP® could be used to treat OSAHS at lower levels of expiratory positive airway pressure (EPAP), improving acceptance to treatment. More-recent reports showed that short term NPPV could successfully treat patients with OHS, OSAHS and hypercapnic respiratory failure, with a persistent correction of daytime hypercapnia. PIPER et al. [43] identified a subset of patients (n=13) with OSAHS, who were "grossly obese" (BMI >35 kg·m^{-2}) and in whom carbon dioxide retention (62 ± 2.5 mmHg) and nocturnal (REM) hypoventilation persisted, despite CPAP therapy; these patients were administered nocturnal NPPV with a volumetric ventilator for 7–18 days. A total of nine of the patients were able to be re-established on a CPAP regimen; one had repeated episodes of daytime hypercapnia and sleepiness and had to be put back onto NPPV; three patients were treated up to

Table 1. – Factors contributing to respiratory failure in severe obesity

Increase in work of breathing and oxygen cost of breathing ($V'O_2$,RESP)
Increase in metabolic demand (increased $V'O_2$ and $V'CO_2$) and in total ventilation for a given effort
Decrease in compliance of the lung (micro-atelectasis)
Decrease in compliance of chest wall (increased adiposity)
Increase in upper airway resistance (when associated with OSAHS)
Increase in airway resistance (Raw)
Decrease in ventilatory drive ($P_{0.1}$, ventilatory response to CO_2)
Changes in ventilatory mode (increased respiratory rate, decreased tidal volume)
Respiratory muscle dysfunction
Mechanical disadvantage (inadequate length–tension relationship, decrease in FRC)
Decrease in respiratory muscle strength?
Increased respiratory load

$V'O_2$,RESP: oxygen cost of breathing; $V'O_2$: oxygen uptake; $V'CO_2$: carbon dioxide production; OSAHS: obstructive sleep apnoea/hypopnoea syndrome; Raw: airway resistance; $P_{0.1}$: mouth occlusion pressure; FRC: functional residual capacity.

3 months before being put back on CPAP. That study clearly showed that, among markedly obese patients with OHS, there were some nonresponders to CPAP therapy who needed long-term NPPV. It also showed that patients with hypercapnic OSAHS, who fail to respond initially to nCPAP, may need transient NPPV as an interim measure [43]. PEREZ DE LLANO et al. [37] described 54 patients with OHS (BMI 44 ± 9 kg·m^{-2}), 87% of whom had OSAHS, followed for a mean period of 50 ± 25 months; 49 patients were treated by BiPAP, and 3 only by nCPAP; all improved their arterial oxygen tension (Pa,O_2), Pa,CO_2 and sleepiness scores (Epworth). Ultimately, NPPV could be withdrawn in 5 patients, and 16 were stabilised with nCPAP. As previously mentioned, for the 15 patients who did not accept NPPV, mortality was high (40%). MASA et al. [20] showed that patients with OHS, treated by NPPV (volume- and pressure-cycled ventilators) for 4 months because of hypercapnic respiratory failure, improved their arterial blood gases in a similar manner to patients with kyphoscoliosis. Symptoms such as morning headache and drowsiness, dyspnoea and leg oedema also improved with NPPV. HEINEMANN et al. [22] reported on 35 stable OHS patients (BMI 45.9 ± 8.8 kg·m^{-2}) treated using BiPAP over 24 months; all patients normalised their daytime Pa,CO_2, and interestingly improved their total lung capacity (TLC), residual volume (RV), VC and FRC. The authors suggest that these improvements result from opening of micro-atelectasis and a decrease in premature closure of dependant airways during expiration. DE LUCAS-RAMOS et al. [40] followed 13 OHS patients (daytime Pa,CO_2 6.6 ± 0.5 kPa, BMI 42.2 ± 7.8 kg·m^{-2}), with an AHI of <10 per h; after 12 months, all patients significantly improved their arterial blood gases, FVC and ventilatory response to

Table 2. – Factors contributing to impaired gas exchange in severe obesity

Ventilation/perfusion mismatch and increase in Δ(A-a)O_2
Decrease in FRC
Increase in CV
Decrease in FRC-CV
Worsening of ventilation/perfusion mismatch when lying supine
Decrease in ventilatory drive ($P_{0.1}$, ventilatory response to CO_2)
Nocturnal and diurnal hypoventilation
Obstructive sleep apnea and hypopnea syndrome
Repeated episodes of nocturnal desaturation
Progressive blunting of ventilatory response to CO_2

Δ(A-a)O_2: Alveolo-arterial gradient; FRC: functional residual capacity; CV: closing volume; FRC-CV: "breathing in closed volume"; $P_{0.1}$: mouth occlusion pressure.

carbon dioxide (change in minute ventilation ($\Delta V'$E)/ΔPa,CO_2 and ΔP0.1/ΔPa,CO_2) [40]. Withdrawal of NPPV after at least 1 yr of treatment was performed in 12 OHS patients (BMI 42.5 ± 7.7 kg·m^{-2}) for 3 months; PFT, arterial blood gases and tests of respiratory drive did not change after 3 months and respiratory polygraphy showed OSAHS in seven out of 12 patients. The authors suggest that among patients on long-term NPPV for OHS in a substantial number of patients, NPPV can either be withdrawn or switched to nCPAP [44]. The follow-up period was short, however, and only 12 patients were included. Whenever measured, subjective or daytime vigilance were also improved by NPPV [20, 29, 37].

nCPAP or BiPAP?

Two short-term studies attempted to distinguish between obese patients who could be treated by nCPAP alone and those who needed BiPAP. RESTA et al. [45] studied 105 OSAHS patients (confirmed by polysomnography), who underwent a first night trial with nCPAP; 81 (77%) patients obtained satisfactory results, monitored by polysomnography, while 24 (23%) required BiPAP. Patients who necessitated BiPAP had a higher BMI (40 ± 6 versus 33 ± 6 kg·m^{-2}), a lower FEV1, FVC and FEV1/FVC than patients who did well on CPAP; they also had a higher daytime Pa,CO_2 (45 ± 6 versus 40 ± 4 mmHg), and a lower Pa,O_2 and lower mean nocturnal Sa,O_2. Among those with OHS, only six (35%) out of 17 could be managed with nCPAP and 65% needed BiPAP therapy. SCHÄFER et al. [46] compared 13 patients with OSAHS who failed to respond to initial CPAP therapy with an AHI-matched control group; nonresponders were significantly more obese (BMI 44 ± 8 versus 31 ± 6 kg·m^{-2}, OR 1.3, 95% CI 1.1–1.6), had a lower Pa,O_2 (OR 0.78, 95% CI 0.6–0.9) and a higher Pa,CO_2 (44.7 versus 38.3 mmHg, OR 1.8, 95% CI 1.1–2.9) and spent more time with a Sa,O_2 <90% on nocturnal pulse oximeter tracings (OR 1.13, 95% CI 1.0–1.26). In a recent randomised study, PIPER et al. [47] found a similar efficacy for CPAP and BiPAP in OHS patients. However, the authors themselves underlined that results were applicable to a subset of patients with OHS only: those without severe persisting hypoventilation during initial CPAP titration. These studies suggest that, in OSAHS patients, increasing BMI, daytime Pa,CO_2 values and REM sleep hypoventilation decrease the probability of clinical response to nCPAP and justify treatment with NPPV.

Leptin, NPPV and chemosensitivity

As previously mentioned, leptin deficiency or, more frequently, resistance to leptin seems to play an important role in OHS-associated decrease in ventilatory drive and blunted response to hypercapnia. Interestingly, NPPV is associated with significant changes in leptin levels. YEE et al. [48] studied 14 patients with OHS (BMI 41 ± 2 kg·m^{-2}, Pa,CO_2 6.7 ± 0.2 kPa, respiratory disturbance index (RDI) 44 ± 35 per h). After a median of 2.3 yrs, NPPV users (n=9) had a significant reduction in leptin levels (p=0.001) with no change in BMI. Improvement in Pa,CO_2 did not reach statistical significance. No change in leptin occurred in nontreated subjects. REDOLFI et al. [49] showed an increase in serum levels of leptin in six cases of OHS after an average of 10.3 months of NPPV. These patients had, prior to treatment, lower levels of serum leptin than obese control patients without OHS. Changes in leptin levels correlated positively and significantly with changes in the ΔP0.1/ΔPET,CO_2 slope. CHOURI-PONTAROLLO et al. [29] studied 15 consecutive patients with OHS (BMI 38.7 ± 6.1 kg·m^{-2}, Pa,CO_2 47 ± 2 mmHg) at baseline and after five nights of NPPV; those with a low baseline carbon dioxide sensitivity (who had the highest proportion of hypoventilation during REM sleep) significantly improved their ventilatory response to carbon dioxide. Those patients were the sleepiest and had the most significant improvements in objective daytime sleepiness after NPPV. The authors hypothesised that improvements in respiratory drive resulted from improving leptin resistance. Thus, NPPV appears to improve respiratory drive, even in short-term studies. These improvements may be related to either a decrease in resistance to leptin or an increase in leptin levels for subjects with low baseline leptin levels.

Survival associated with OHS treated by noninvasive ventilation

In the Geneva lake area study [19], 71 patients (33% of all patients included) were treated for OHS (n=50, BMI 41.9 ± 9 kg·m^{-2}) with or without associated OSAHS. All patients had presented at least one episode of acute hypercapnic respiratory failure and none of the patients included was treated by NPPV solely because of discomfort or intolerance to CPAP. Probability of pursuing NPPV was 76% at 3 yrs and 72% at 5 yrs, the highest among all patients studied, mortality was low (6%), with a 5-yr survival rate of 88%. BUDWEISER et al. [39] performed a retrospective analysis of 126 OHS patients treated by NPPV and followed for 41 ± 27 months, survival was 97% after 1 yr, 92% after 2 yrs and 70% after 5 yrs.

Technical aspects

Choice of ventilator

In patients with a clear diagnosis of OHS, with or without associated OSAHS, BiPAP is clearly the "default" treatment reported in most studies [22, 29, 38–40, 44–46, 48–51]. Earlier reports used either volume-cycled ventilators only [52] or offered BiPAP as a second choice, in case of intolerance to volume-cycled ventilators [20]. Among 71 patients followed in the Geneva Lake area between 1992 and 2000, 58 (82%) used BiPAP, seven (10%) used volume-cycled ventilators and six (8%) used pressure support ventilators such as the Breas PV403® (Breas, Mölnlycke, Sweden) [19]. Average EPAP levels are usually titrated to overcome upper airway obstructive apnoea or hypopnoea (4–12 cmH$_2$O); inspiratory positive airway pressure (IPAP) is adjusted to optimise daytime Pa,CO2 and/or nocturnal transcutaneous carbon dioxide tension (Ptc,CO$_2$). The usual mode used with BiPAP is the "S/T" (spontaneous/timed) mode, allowing triggering by the patient, but with a back-up rate, which can compensate for episodes of central apnoea, hypopnoea or hypoventilation; however, some groups use either the "S" mode (spontaneous) [45] or the "T" (controlled) mode in this indication [46].

A recent bench test study compared performances of 10 bilevel pressure cycled ventilators designed for home care. Variations in pressurisation between ventilators were quite substantial [53]. These observations would tend to favour the use of the ventilators with the highest pressurisation capacities because of the markedly decreased compliance of the respiratory system in OHS. There is to date, however, no clinical study to support this recommendation.

Volume targeting

A limitation of BiPAP is the absence of guarantee as to volume delivered to the patient. Volume targeting is a feature recently made available on certain bilevel ventilators (i.e. Synchrony®; Respironics Inc., Murrysville, PA, USA; VENTIlogic®; VENTImotion®, Weinmann, Hamburg, Germany; VS Ultra® and Elisee®TM 150; ResMed, Sydney,

Australia; Legendair® and Smartair®; Covidien AG, Hamilton, Bermuda), which aims to solve this limitation; the ventilator measures or estimates delivered tidal volume (V_T) through a built-in pneumotachograph and adjusts pressure support within a preset range to provide a V_T as close as possible to a target V_T set by the clinician. Target V_T recommended by Respironics® in obese patients is 8 mL·kg^{-1} (based on a BM1 of 23 kg·m^{-2}). In a randomised cross-over study, STORRE *et al.* [51] showed, in OHS patients (n=10, BMI 41 ± 12 kg·m^{-2}, Pa,CO_2 47 ± 2 mmHg) that BiPAP with volume targeting (7–10 mL·kg^{-1} of ideal body weight) decreased mean nocturnal Ptc,CO_2 and daytime Pa,CO_2 more efficiently than BiPAP alone. The impact of volume targeting on nocturnal Ptc,CO_2 was confirmed in 12 OHS patients, who underwent polysomnography for two consecutive nights with BiPAP with or without volume targeting (7–8 mL·kg^{-1}) in a randomised order, this improvement was however at the expense of a lesser sleep comfort, increased awakenings, wake after sleep onset and a shorter total sleep time [54].

Conclusions

Obesity–hypoventilation has become in many industrialised countries the most frequent indication for home noninvasive positive airway pressure [19]. This phenomenon results from the rapidly progressing epidemic of obesity in industrialised countries and from a greater awareness of physicians as to the respiratory consequences of obesity through the widespread mediatisation of obstructive sleep apnoea and hypopnoea syndrome. Although untreated obesity–hypoventilation syndrome is associated with a high morbidity and mortality, noninvasive positive airway pressure considerably improves survival, physiological parameters, symptoms of chronic hypercapnic respiratory failure, and quality of life, and decreases use of health resources (visits to physicians, hospitalisations). Noninvasive positive airway pressure seems to improve obesity–hypoventilation syndrome mainly through a resetting of respiratory centres and an improvement of respiratory drive. The role of leptin, leptin resistance and impact of noninvasive positive airway pressure on leptin resistance opens interesting perspectives as to a better understanding of hypoventilation and cardiovascular morbidity in obesity and warrants further clinical studies.

Summary

Morbid obesity is associated with an increase in work of breathing and oxygen cost of breathing, a decrease in compliance of the respiratory system, lung volumes, ventilatory drive and respiratory muscle dysfunction. These changes, frequently associated with obstructive apnoea/hypopnoea syndrome, increase the risk of chronic hypercapnic respiratory failure and lead to obesity-hypoventilation syndrome. Untreated obesity-hypoventilation is associated with an increased use of healthcare resources and with a high morbidity and mortality. Although some patients may respond to nocturnal nasal continuous positive airway pressure alone, and correct their daytime hypercapnia, patients with higher body mass index and arterial carbon dioxide tension values will most often require noninvasive positive pressure ventilation. Bilevel positive pressure ventilation is the most frequently chosen option, with high survival rates and a decrease in subsequent hospitalisations for cardiopulmonary failure.

Keywords: Healthcare resources, morbid obesity, noninvasive ventilation, obesity-hypoventilation syndrome, obstructive apnoea/hypopnoea syndrome, respiratory drive.

References

1. Bickelmann AG, Burwell CS, Robin ED, Whaley RD. Extreme obesity associated with alveolar hypoventilation; a Pickwickian syndrome. *Am J Med* 1956; 21: 811–818.

2. Cuvelier A, Muir JF. Acute and chronic respiratory failure in patients with obesity-hypoventilation syndrome: a new challenge for noninvasive ventilation. *Chest* 2005; 128: 483–485.

3. Mokhlesi B, Kryger MH, Grunstein RR. Assessment and management of patients with obesity hypoventilation syndrome. *Proc Am Thorac Soc* 2008; 5: 218–225.

4. Sharp JT, Barrocas M, Chokroverty S. The cardiorespiratory effects of obesity. *Clin Chest Med* 1980; 1: 103–118.

5. Nowbar S, Burkart KM, Gonzales R, *et al.* Obesity-associated hypoventilation in hospitalized patients: prevalence, effects, and outcome. *Am J Med* 2004; 116: 1–7.

6. Seidell JC. Obesity in Europe: scaling an epidemic. *Int J Obes Relat Metab Disord* 1995; 19: Suppl. 3, S1–S4.

7. Flegal KM, Carroll MD, Kuczmarski RJ, Johnson CL. Overweight and obesity in the United States: prevalence and trends, 1960–1994. *Int J Obes Relat Metab Disord* 1998; 22: 39–47.

8. Mokhlesi B, Tulaimat A. Recent advances in obesity hypoventilation syndrome. *Chest* 2007; 132: 1322–1336.

9. Laaban JP, Chailleux E. Daytime hypercapnia in adult patients with obstructive sleep apnea syndrome in France, before initiating nocturnal nasal continuous positive airway pressure therapy. *Chest* 2005; 127: 710–715.

10. Kawata N, Tatsumi K, Terada J, *et al.* Daytime hypercapnia in obstructive sleep apnea syndrome. *Chest* 2007; 132: 1832–1838.

11. Pelosi P, Croci M, Ravagnan I, Vicardi P, Gattinoni L. Total respiratory system, lung, and chest wall mechanics in sedated-paralyzed postoperative morbidly obese patients. *Chest* 1996; 109: 144–151.

12. Harris RS. Pressure-volume curves of the respiratory system. *Respir Care* 2005; 50: 78–98.

13. Pelosi P, Croci M, Ravagnan I, *et al.* The effects of body mass on lung volumes, respiratory mechanics, and gas exchange during general anesthesia. *Anesth Analg* 1998; 87: 654–660.

14. Naimark A, Cherniack RM. Compliance of the respiratory system and its components in health and obesity. *J Appl Physiol* 1960; 15: 377–382.

15. Kress JP, Pohlman AS, Alverdy J, Hall JB. The impact of morbid obesity on oxygen cost of breathing ($V'O_2$,RESP) at rest. *Am J Respir Crit Care Med* 1999; 160: 883–886.

16. Gibson GJ. Obesity, respiratory function and breathlessness. *Thorax* 2000; 55: Suppl. 1, S41–S44.

17. Lazarus R, Sparrow D, Weiss ST. Effects of obesity and fat distribution on ventilatory function: the normative aging study. *Chest* 1997; 111: 891–898.

18. Wise RA, Enright PL, Connett JE, *et al.* Effect of weight gain on pulmonary function after smoking cessation in the Lung Health Study. *Am J Respir Crit Care Med* 1998; 157: 866–872.

19. Janssens JP, Derivaz S, Breitenstein E, *et al.* Changing patterns in long-term noninvasive ventilation: a 7-year prospective study in the Geneva Lake area. *Chest* 2003; 123: 67–79.

20. Masa JF, Celli BR, Riesco JA, Hernandez M, Sanchez De Cos J, Disdier C. The obesity hypoventilation syndrome can be treated with noninvasive mechanical ventilation. *Chest* 2001; 119: 1102–1107.

21. Leech J, Onal E, Aronson R, Lopata M. Voluntary hyperventilation in obesity hypoventilation. *Chest* 1991; 100: 1334–1338.

22. Heinemann F, Budweiser S, Dobroschke J, Pfeifer M. Non-invasive positive pressure ventilation improves lung volumes in the obesity hypoventilation syndrome. *Respir Med* 2007; 101: 1229–1235.

23. O'Donnell C P, Schaub CD, Haines AS, *et al.* Leptin prevents respiratory depression in obesity. *Am J Respir Crit Care Med* 1999; 159: 1477–1484.

24. Shimura R, Tatsumi K, Nakamura A, *et al.* Fat accumulation, leptin, and hypercapnia in obstructive sleep apnea-hypopnea syndrome. *Chest* 2005; 127: 543–549.

25. Phipps PR, Starritt E, Caterson I, Grunstein RR. Association of serum leptin with hypoventilation in human obesity. *Thorax* 2002; 57: 75–76.

26. Campo A, Fruhbeck G, Zulueta JJ, *et al.* Hyperleptinaemia, respiratory drive and hypercapnic response in obese patients. *Eur Respir J* 2007; 30: 223–231.

27. Berger KI, Ayappa I, Sorkin IB, Norman RG, Rapoport DM, Goldring RM. Postevent ventilation as a function of CO_2 load during respiratory events in obstructive sleep apnea. *J Appl Physiol* 2002; 93: 917–924.

28. Ayappa I, Berger KI, Norman RG, Oppenheimer BW, Rapoport DM, Goldring RM. Hypercapnia and ventilatory periodicity in obstructive sleep apnea syndrome. *Am J Respir Crit Care Med* 2002; 166: 1112–1115.

29. Chouri-Pontarollo N, Borel JC, Tamisier R, Wuyam B, Levy P, Pepin JL. Impaired objective daytime vigilance in obesity-hypoventilation syndrome: impact of noninvasive ventilation. *Chest* 2007; 131: 148–155.

30. Banerjee D, Yee BJ, Piper AJ, Zwillich CW, Grunstein RR. Obesity hypoventilation syndrome: hypoxemia during continuous positive airway pressure. *Chest* 2007; 131: 1678–1684.

31. Morgenthaler TI, Aurora RN, Brown T, *et al.* Practice parameters for the use of autotitrating continuous positive airway pressure devices for titrating pressures and treating adult patients with obstructive sleep apnea syndrome: an update for 2007. An American Academy of Sleep Medicine report. *Sleep* 2008; 31: 141–147.

32. Tasali E, Ip MS. Obstructive sleep apnea and metabolic syndrome: alterations in glucose metabolism and inflammation. *Proc Am Thorac Soc* 2008; 5: 207–217.

33. Berg G, Delaive K, Manfreda J, Walld R, Kryger MH. The use of health-care resources in obesity-hypoventilation syndrome. *Chest* 2001; 120: 377–383.

34. Rahmouni K, Fath MA, Seo S, *et al.* Leptin resistance contributes to obesity and hypertension in mouse models of Bardet–Biedl syndrome. *J Clin Invest* 2008; 118: 1458–1467.

35. Rahmouni K, Morgan DA, Morgan GM, Mark AL, Haynes WG. Role of selective leptin resistance in diet-induced obesity hypertension. *Diabetes* 2005; 54: 2012–2018.

36. Gualillo O, Gonzalez-Juanatey JR, Lago F. The emerging role of adipokines as mediators of cardiovascular function: physiologic and clinical perspectives. *Trends Cardiovasc Med* 2007; 17: 275–283.

37. Perez de Llano LA, Golpe R, Ortiz Piquer M, *et al.* Short-term and long-term effects of nasal intermittent positive pressure ventilation in patients with obesity-hypoventilation syndrome. *Chest* 2005; 128: 587–594.

38. Pankow W, Hijjeh N, Schüttler F, *et al.* Influence of noninvasive positive pressure ventilation on inspiratory muscle activity in obese subjects. *Eur Respir J* 1997; 10: 2847–2852.

39. Budweiser S, Riedl SG, Jörres RA, Heinemann F, Pfeifer M. Mortality and prognostic factors in patients with obesity-hypoventilation syndrome undergoing noninvasive ventilation. *J Intern Med* 2007; 261: 375–383.

40. de Lucas-Ramos P, de Miguel-Diez J, Santacruz-Siminiani A, Gonzalez-Moro JM, Buendia-Garcia MJ, Izquierdo-Alonso JL. Benefits at 1 year of nocturnal intermittent positive pressure ventilation in patients with obesity-hypoventilation syndrome. *Respir Med* 2004; 98: 961–967.

41. Sullivan C, Berthon-Jones M, Isswa F. Remission of severe obesity-hypoventilation syndrome after short-term treatment during sleep with nasal continuous positive airway pressure. *Am Rev Respir Dis* 1983; 128: 177–181.

42. Sanders M, Kern N. Obstructive sleep apnea treated by independently adjusted inspiratory and expiratory positive airway pressures *via* nasal mask. Physiological and clinical implications. *Chest* 1990; 98: 317–324.

43. Piper AJ, Sullivan CE. Effects of short-term NIPPV in the treatment of patients with severe obstructive sleep apnea and hypercapnia. *Chest* 1994; 105: 434–440.

44. De Miguel Diez J, De Lucas Ramos P, Perez Parra JJ, Buendia Garcia MJ, Cubillo Marcos JM, Gonzalez-Moro JM. [Analysis of withdrawal from noninvasive mechanical ventilation in patients

with obesity-hypoventilation syndrome. Medium term results]. *Arch Bronconeumol* 2003; 39: 292–297.

45. Resta O, Guido P, Picca V, *et al.* Prescription of nCPAP and nBiPAP in obstructive sleep apnoea syndrome: Italian experience in 105 subjects. A prospective two center study. *Respir Med* 1998; 92: 820–827.

46. Schäfer H, Ewig S, Hasper E, Lüderitz B. Failure of CPAP therapy in obstructive sleep apnoea syndrome: predictive factors and treatment with bi-level positive airway pressure. *Respir Med* 1998; 92: 208–215.

47. Piper AJ, Wang D, Yee BJ, Barnes DJ, Grunstein RR. Randomised trial of CPAP *vs* bilevel support in the treatment of obesity hypoventilation syndrome without severe nocturnal desaturation. *Thorax* 2008; 63: 395–401.

48. Yee BJ, Cheung J, Phipps P, Banerjee D, Piper AJ, Grunstein RR. Treatment of obesity hypoventilation syndrome and serum leptin. *Respiration* 2006; 73: 209–212.

49. Redolfi S, Corda L, La Piana G, Spandrio S, Prometti P, Tantucci C. Long-term non-invasive ventilation increases chemosensitivity and leptin in obesity-hypoventilation syndrome. *Respir Med* 2007; 101: 1191–1195.

50. Guo YF, Sforza E, Janssens JP. Respiratory patterns during sleep in obesity-hypoventilation patients treated with nocturnal pressure support: a preliminary report. *Chest* 2007; 131: 1090–1099.

51. Storre JH, Seuthe B, Fiechter R, *et al.* Average volume-assured pressure support in obesity hypoventilation: A randomized crossover trial. *Chest* 2006; 130: 815–821.

52. Piper A, Sullivan C. Effects of long-term nocturnal nasal ventilation on spontaneous breathing during sleep in neuromuscular and chest wall disorders. *Eur Respir J* 1996; 9: 1515–1522.

53. Battisti A, Tassaux D, Janssens JP, Michotte JB, Jaber S, Jolliet P. Performance characteristics of 10 home mechanical ventilators in pressure-support mode: a comparative bench study. *Chest* 2005; 127: 1784–1792.

54. Janssens JP, Metzger M, Sforza E. Impact of volume targeting on efficacy of bi-level non-invasive ventilation and sleep in obesity-hypoventilation. *Respir Med* 2008; [Epub ahead of print PMID: 18579368].

CHAPTER 18

NIV and pulmonary rehabilitation

N. Ambrosino, N. Carpenè, M. Gherardi

Respiratory Intensive Care and Pulmonary Diseases Unit. Cardio-Thoracic Dept, University Hospital, Pisa and Pulmonary Rehabilitation and Weaning Unit, Auxilium Vitae, Volterra, Italy.

Correspondence: N. Ambrosino, Pulmonary Unit, Cardio-Thoracic Dept, Azienda Ospedaliero- Universitaria Pisana, Via Paradisa 2 Cisanello, 57124, Pisa, Italy. Fax: 39 050996779; E-mail: n.ambrosino@ao-pisa.toscana.it

Progressive worsening of dyspnoea and reduced exercise tolerance are the most common symptoms of patients with chronic obstructive pulmonary disease (COPD). In these patients, dyspnoea leads to inactivity and peripheral muscle deconditioning, resulting in a vicious cycle leading to further inactivity, social isolation, fear of dyspnoea and depression. The patients become less and less mobile and reduce their activities of daily living (ADL). Indeed in a survey of patients with severe COPD on long term oxygen therapy (LTOT), 50% of them, suffering from Medical Research Council (MRC) dyspnoea grade 5, did not leave the house and 78% were breathless walking around at home and performing ADL [1].

Pathophysiology of exercise dyspnoea

Pathophysiological factors contributing to exercise dyspnoea in COPD patients include increased inspiratory muscle dysfunction and work of breathing (WOB) due to hyperinflation and related increased intrinsic mechanical loading *i.e.* the intrinsic positive end-expiratory pressure (PEEPi) [2], increased mechanical restriction of the thorax, increased ventilatory demand relative to capacity, gas exchanges abnormalities, dynamic airway compression, cardiovascular factors and any combination of these symptoms [3]. Peripheral muscle dysfunction is also an important determinant of reduced exercise capacity in COPD [4].

Regular physical activity may reduce lung function decline and risk of developing COPD in active smokers [5] and the risk of hospital admission in COPD patients [6]. Peripheral muscle training counteracts the increased exercise-induced oxidative stress [7] and improves exercise capacity and dyspnoea. Multidisciplinary pulmonary rehabilitation, including exercise training may offer a useful tool to improve these symptoms [8–10]. Nevertheless, in the most compromised patients, extreme breathlessness and/or peripheral muscle fatigue limit training at the highest levels of exercise intensity prescribed in pulmonary rehabilitation programmes.

In the last decade, there has been an increasing interest in the use of noninvasive positive pressure ventilation (NPPV) to increase exercise capacity [11]. Given that intrinsic mechanical loading and inspiratory muscle dysfunction contribute to dyspnoea in COPD, assisted ventilation should provide a symptomatic benefit during exercise, allowing for higher levels of exercise intensity. There is evidence that the WOB needed to sustain heavy intensity exercise is correlated to a reduction in leg blood flow and has a significant influence on the exercise performance of healthy people [12, 13]. In other

Eur Respir Mon, 2008, 41, 265–271. Printed in UK - all rights reserved. Copyright ERS Journals Ltd 2008; European Respiratory Monograph; ISSN 1025-448x.

words, during leg exercise there would be a competition for blood flow between respiratory and limb muscles. Therefore, unloading inspiratory muscles by assisted ventilation would allow for a shift of blood flow to peripheral muscles; therefore, promoting improvement in exercise tolerance. Indeed, proportional assisted ventilation (PAV) [14], prevented exercise-induced diaphragmatic fatigue [15]. Several laboratory studies have examined the acute effects of different modalities of ventilatory assistance on dyspnoea and exercise tolerance in advanced COPD [11, 16, 17].

Continuous positive airway pressure

Theoretically, continuous positive airway pressure (CPAP) should reduce the inspiratory threshold load on the inspiratory muscles of hyperinflated COPD patients and enhance neuromuscular coupling, thus improving dyspnoea and exercise tolerance [18–21] by counterbalancing, at least in part, PEEPi [2]. CPAP reduces the WOB and increases exercise tolerance in patients with cystic fibrosis [22]. For maximal benefit, CPAP should be titrated on an individual basis, in order to optimise comfort. Nevertheless, this, theoretically, implies the measurement of PEEPi, which is rather difficult to perform on a routine basis [23].

Pressure support ventilation

Inspiratory pressure support (IPS) is a pressure-targeted mode of mechanical ventilation, in which each breath is patient triggered and supported, that can effectively assist ventilation when applied noninvasively to patients in acute and chronic respiratory failure [24]. This modality improved dyspnoea and exercise capacity by reducing the excessive load placed upon inspiratory muscles, when COPD patients exercise [25–32]. In fact, patients with severe COPD can sustain exercise-induced lactataemia for longer if assisted with IPS [33].

PAV

PAV is a mode of partial ventilatory assistance endowed with characteristics of proportionality and adaptability to the intensity and timing of spontaneous ventilatory pattern by providing inspiratory flow and pressure in proportion to the patient's effort [12]. Several laboratory studies have shown that PAV can increase exercise capacity of COPD patients [34–37].

Controlled mechanical ventilation

Assist-control ventilation is a combination mode of ventilation in which the ventilator delivers a positive pressure breath, at a preset tidal volume, in response to the patient's inspiratory effort. The ventilator will also deliver breaths at a preset rate if no patient effort occurs within the preselected time period [38]. This modality of assisted ventilation was delivered noninvasively during exercise in patients with restrictive disorders, pulmonary tuberculosis sequelae and kyphoscoliosis, resulting in a significant improvement in breathlessness and increase in exercise endurance [39–41].

Ventilatory assistance and pulmonary rehabilitation

The message of the previously performed physiological studies can be summarised as follows: different modalities of NPPV, during exercise reduce dyspnoea and WOB, and enhance exercise tolerance in COPD patients. Given the established usefulness of NPPV in increasing exercise tolerance and reducing dyspnoea in the acute (*i.e.* laboratory) setting [11], the next step would be to evaluate whether assisted ventilation could be used as an aid, during exercise training sessions. This is an important issue, since the recent development of new therapeutic approaches like lung transplantation and lung volume reduction surgery make most of patients with severe COPD, even with chronic respiratory failure, candidates for rehabilitation programmes [42–46].

Nevertheless, conflicting results have been reported on the application of NPPV in exercise training programmes. A randomised controlled study [47] found no additional benefit of PAV on exercise tolerance, dyspnoea and health status, when compared to training alone. Alternatively, another similar study [48] found that mean training intensity and peak work rate were higher after PAV-assisted than after nonassisted training. Isoworkload lactataemia after training was more reduced in the assisted than in the nonassisted patients. A significant inverse relationship was found between reduction in isoworkload lactataemia after training during the constant work rate test and peak work rate achieved during the last week of training. This was considered as a marker of true physiological training effect [48]. Other authors have confirmed benefits of addition of NPPV to exercise training [49–52]. Furthermore, in chronic hypercapnic COPD under long term ventilatory support, high-intensity NPPV could also be administered during walking, using unchanged ventilator settings compared with settings used at rest, thus resulting in improved oxygenation, decreased dyspnoea and increased walking distance [53].

Problems of ventilatory assistance

Despite promising, although conflicting, results, ventilatory assistance during exercise training programmes is unlikely to have a role in the routine pulmonary rehabilitation setting. Some problems are as follows [54]:

Interfaces. During high intensity exercise, patients may breathe through the mouth rather than the nose, thus requiring a face mask or mouthpiece. Nevertheless, compliance to a face mask may be not as easy.

Comorbidities. Many COPD patients have significant comorbidities [55], including a high proportion of cardiac ischaemic disease [56, 57]. It is of concern that reduction of dyspnoea with this kind of "mechanical doping" [54] might expose an unaware COPD patient to a load greater than his/her coronary ischemic threshold.

Practicalities. In one study [47], a high rate of withdrawal, due to lack of compliance in ventilated group, a mean 17-min spent setting the ventilator and supervising the training session during NPPV, were practical drawbacks of the addition of mask ventilation during a high intensity training programme. Therefore, it might not be worthwhile submitting patients to unpleasant equipment (*e.g.* mask and related troubles) with the need of the constant supervision of an individual operator, to check for leaks and reset the ventilator when needed, and a substantial risk of lack of compliance. Furthermore, there is a need of a one-to-one patient–therapist interaction, which will add to the cost of a rehabilitation programme; especially in the light of the recognised benefits of well conducted standard exercise training programmes, which do not require either complex or sophisticated machinery, or a personalised physiotherapist [9, 10, 54, 58].

Night-time NPPV and day-time exercise

Another way to use NPPV to improve results of exercise training is possible: patients with severe stable COPD, undergoing home nocturnal NPPV and daytime exercise training, showed a significant improvement in exercise capacity and quality of life compared with patients undergoing exercise training alone [59]. The hypothesis, that the observed increase in exercise performance with nocturnal NPPV may be associated with increased quadriceps strength, was not confirmed [60].

In conclusion, noninvasive modalities of mechanical ventilation may be useful in improving exercise tolerance and reducing dyspnoea in patients with ventilatory limitation. The practical role of this modality in pulmonary rehabilitation programmes is still being discussed.

Summary

Dyspnoea is the most common symptom of patients with chronic obstructive pulmonary disease (COPD). Exercise training can improve dyspnoea and exercise tolerance in these patients in whom higher intensity levels may be prevented by extreme breathlessness and/or peripheral muscle fatigue. As mechanical loading and inspiratory muscle dysfunction contribute to dyspnoea in COPD, assisted ventilation should provide a symptomatic benefit by unloading and assisting such overburdened ventilatory muscles.

Continuous positive airway pressure and different modalities of noninvasive positive pressure ventilation (NPPV) applied during exercise resulted in improvement of dyspnoea and exercise tolerance. Inspiratory muscle unloading and reduction in intrinsic positive end-expiratory pressure have been considered among mechanisms underlying these effects in COPD patients. Nevertheless, the role of NPPV in pulmonary rehabilitation, if any, is still controversial. The addition of nocturnal domiciliary NPPV during a day-time exercise programme in patients with severe COPD resulted in an improvement in exercise tolerance and quality of life.

Keywords: Chronic obstructive pulmonary disease, dyspnoea, exercise, fatigue, training.

References

1. Restrick LJ, Paul EA, Braid GM, Cullinan P, Moore-Gillon J, Wedzicha JA. Assessment and follow up of patients prescribed long term oxygen therapy. *Thorax* 1993; 48: 708–713.
2. Rossi A, Polese G, Brandi G, Conti G. Intrinsic positive end-expiratory pressure (PEEPi). *Intensive Care Med* 1995; 21: 522–536.
3. O'Donnell DE. Exertional breathlessness in chronic respiratory disease. *In*: DA Mahler, ed. Dyspnea. New York, Dekker, 1998; pp. 97–147.
4. Skeletal muscle dysfunction in chronic obstructive pulmonary disease. A statement of the American Thoracic Society and European Respiratory Society. *Am J Respir Crit Care Med* 1999; 159: S1–S40.
5. Garcia-Aymerich J, Lange P, Benet M, Schnohr P, Antó JM. Regular physical activity modifies smoking-related lung function decline and reduces risk of chronic obstructive pulmonary disease: a population-based cohort study. *Am J Respir Crit Care Med* 2007; 175: 458–463.

6. Garcia-Aymerich J, Lange P, Benet M, Schnohr P, Antó JM. Regular physical activity reduces hospital admission and mortality in chronic obstructive pulmonary disease: a population based cohort study. *Thorax* 2006; 61: 772–778.

7. Mercken EM, Hageman GJ, Schols AM, Akkermans MA, Bast A, Wouters EF. Rehabilitation decreases exercise-induced oxidative stress in chronic obstructive pulmonary disease. *Am J Respir Crit Care Med* 2005; 172: 994–1001.

8. Lacasse Y, Goldstein R, Lasserson TJ, Martin S. Pulmonary rehabilitation for chronic obstructive pulmonary disease. *Cochrane Database Syst Rev* 2006; 4: CD003793.

9. Nici L, Donner C, Wouters E, *et al.* American Thoracic Society/European Respiratory Society statement on pulmonary rehabilitation. *Am J Respir Crit Care Med* 2006; 173: 1390–1413.

10. Ries AL, Bauldoff GS, Carlin BW, *et al.* Pulmonary rehabilitation: joint ACCP/AACVPR evidence-based clinical practice guidelines. *Chest* 2007; 131: Suppl. 5, 4S–42S.

11. Ambrosino N, Strambi S. New strategies to improve exercise tolerance in chronic obstructive pulmonary disease. *Eur Respir J* 2004; 24: 313–322.

12. Harms CA, Babcock MA, McClaran SR, *et al.* Respiratory muscle work compromises leg blood flow during maximal exercise. *J Appl Physiol* 1997; 82: 1573–1583.

13. Harms CA, Wetter TJ, St Croix CM, Pegelow DF, Dempsey JA. Effects of respiratory muscle work on exercise performance. *J Appl Physiol* 2000; 89: 131–138.

14. Younes M. Proportional assist ventilation. *In*: Tobin MJ, ed. Principles and Practice of Mechanical Ventilation. 2nd Edn. New York, McGraw-Hill Inc., 2006; pp. 335–364.

15. Babcock MA, Pegelow DF, Harms CA, Dempsey JA. Effects of respiratory muscle unloading on exercise-induced diaphragm fatigue. *J Appl Physiol* 2002; 93: 201–206.

16. Ambrosino N. Exercise and noninvasive ventilatory support. *Monaldi Arch Chest Dis* 2000; 55: 242–246.

17. van 't Hul A, Kwakkel G, Gosselink R. The acute effects of noninvasive ventilatory support during exercise on exercise endurance and dyspnea in patients with chronic obstructive pulmonary disease: a systematic review. *J Cardiopulm Rehabil* 2002; 22: 290–297.

18. Lougheed MD, Webb KA, O'Donnell DE. Breathlessness during induced lung hyperinflation in asthma: role of the inspiratory threshold load. *Am J Respir Crit Care Med* 1995; 152: 911–920.

19. O'Donnell DE, Sanii R, Younes M. Improvement in exercise endurance in patients with chronic airflow limitation using continuous positive airway pressure. *Am Rev Respir Dis* 1988; 138: 1510–1514.

20. O'Donnell DE, Sanii R, Giesbrecht G, Younes M. Effect of continuous positive airway pressure on respiratory sensation in patients with chronic obstructive pulmonary disease during submaximal exercise. *Am Rev Respir Dis* 1988; 138: 1185–1191.

21. Petrof BJ, Calderini E, Gottfried SB. Effect of CPAP on respiratory effort and dyspnoea during exercise in severe COPD. *J Appl Physiol* 1990; 69: 179–188.

22. Henke KG, Regnis JA, Bye PT. Benefits of continuous positive airway pressure during exercise in cystic fibrosis and relationship to disease severity. *Am Rev Respir Dis* 1993; 148: 1272–1276.

23. Rossi A, Polese G, Milic-Emili J. Monitoring respiratory mechanics in ventilator depending patients. *In*: Tobin MJ, ed. Principles and Practice of Intensive Care Monitoring. New York, McGraw-Hill Inc., 1998; pp. 553–596.

24. MacIntyre NR. Principles of positive pressure mechanical ventilatory support. *In*: Ambrosino N, Goldstein RS eds. Ventilatory Support for Chronic Respiratory Failure. Informa Healthcare Pub, New York, USA, 2008; pp. 13–27.

25. Wysocki M, Meshaka P, Richard JC, Similowski T. Proportional-assist ventilation compared with pressure-support ventilation during exercise in volunteers with external thoracic restriction. *Crit Care Med* 2004; 32: 409–414.

26. Kyroussis D, Polkey MI, Keilty SE, *et al.* Exhaustive exercise slows inspiratory muscle relaxation rate in chronic obstructive pulmonary disease. *Am J Respir Crit Care Med* 1996; 153: 787–793.

27. Polkey MI, Kyroussis D, Mills GH, *et al.* Inspiratory pressure support reduces slowing of inspiratory muscle relaxation rate during exhaustive treadmill walking in severe COPD. *Am J Respir Crit Care Med* 1996; 154: 1146–1150.

28. Keilty SE, Ponte J, Fleming TA, Moxham J. Effect of inspiratory pressure support on exercise tolerance and breathlessness in patients with severe stable chronic obstructive pulmonary disease. *Thorax* 1994; 49: 990–994.
29. Maltais F, Reissmann H, Gottfried SB. Pressure support reduces inspiratory effort and dyspnea during exercise in chronic airflow obstruction. *Am J Respir Crit Care Med* 1995; 151: 1027–1033.
30. Kyroussis D, Polkey MI, Hamnegård CH, Mills GH, Green M, Moxham J. Respiratory muscle activity in patients with COPD walking to exhaustion with and without pressure support. *Eur Respir J* 2000; 15: 649–655.
31. van 't Hul A, Gosselink R, Hollander P, Postmus P, Kwakkel G. Acute effects of inspiratory pressure support during exercise in patients with COPD. *Eur Respir J* 2004; 23: 34–40.
32. Barakat S, Michele G, Nesme P, Nicole V, Guy A. Effect of a noninvasive ventilatory support during exercise of a program in pulmonary rehabilitation in patients with COPD. *Int J Chron Obstruct Pulmon Dis* 2007; 2: 585–591.
33. Polkey MI, Hawkins P, Kyroussis D, Ellum SG, Sherwood R, Moxham J. Inspiratory pressure support prolongs exercise induced lactataemia in severe COPD. *Thorax* 2000; 55: 547–549.
34. Dolmage TE, Goldstein RS. Proportional assist ventilation and exercise tolerance in subjects with COPD. *Chest* 1997; 111: 948–954.
35. Bianchi L, Foglio K, Pagani M, Vitacca M, Rossi A, Ambrosino N. Effects of proportional assist ventilation on exercise tolerance in COPD patients with chronic hypercapnia. *Eur Resp J* 1998; 11: 422–427.
36. Hernandez P, Maltais F, Gursahaney A, Leblanc P, Gottfried SB. Proportional assist ventilation may improve exercise performance in severe chronic obstructive pulmonary disease. *J Cardiopulm Rehabil* 2001; 21: 135–142.
37. Poggi R, Appendini L, Polese G, Colombo R, Donner CF, Rossi A. Noninvasive proportional assist ventilation and pressure support ventilation during arm elevation in patients with chronic respiratory failure. A preliminary, physiologic study. *Respir Med* 2006; 100: 972–979.
38. Mancebo J. Assist-control ventilation. *In*: Tobin MJ, ed. Principles and Practice of Mechanical Ventilation. 2nd Edn. New York, McGraw-Hill Inc., 2006; pp. 183–200.
39. Tsuboi T, Ohi M, Chin K, *et al.* Ventilatory support during exercise in patients with pulmonary tuberculosis sequelae. *Chest* 1997; 112: 1000–1007.
40. Highcock MP, Smith IE, Shneerson JM. The effect of noninvasive intermittent positive-pressure ventilation during exercise in severe scoliosis. *Chest* 2002; 121: 1555–1560.
41. Borel JC, Wuyam B, Chouri-Pontarollo N, Deschaux C, Levy P, Pépin JL. During exercise non-invasive ventilation in chronic restrictive respiratory failure. *Respir Med* 2008; 102: 711–719.
42. Make B. Pulmonary rehabilitation and lung volume reduction surgery. *In*: Donner CF, Ambrosino N, Goldstein RS, eds. Pulmonary Rehabilitation. London, Arnold Pub, 2005; pp. 297–303.
43. Gay SE, Martinez FJ. Pulmonary rehabilitation and transplantation. *In*: Donner CF, Ambrosino N, Goldstein RS, eds. Pulmonary Rehabilitation. London, Arnold Pub, 2005; pp 304–311.
44. Clini EM, Ambrosino N. Nonpharmacological treatment and relief of symptoms in COPD. *Eur Respir J* 2008; 32: 218–228.
45. Carone M, Patessio A, Ambrosino N, *et al.* Efficacy of pulmonary rehabilitation in chronic respiratory failure (CRF) due to chronic obstructive pulmonary disease (COPD): The Maugeri Study. *Respir Med* 2007; 101: 2447–2453.
46. Ambrosino N, Simonds A. The clinical management in extremely severe COPD. *Respir Med* 2007; 101: 1613–1624.
47. Bianchi L, Foglio K, Porta R, Baiardi R, Vitacca M, Ambrosino N. Lack of additional effect of adjunct of assisted ventilation to pulmonary rehabilitation in mild COPD patients. *Respir Med* 2002; 96: 359–367.
48. Hawkins P, Johnson LC, Nikoletou D, *et al.* Proportional assist ventilation as an aid to exercise training in severe chronic obstructive pulmonary disease. *Thorax* 2002; 57: 853–859.

49. van 't Hul A, Gosselink R, Hollander P, Postmus P, Kwakkel G. Training with inspiratory pressure support in patients with severe COPD. *Eur Respir J* 2006; 27: 65–72.

50. Johnson JE, Gavin DJ, Adams-Dramiga S. Effects of training with Heliox and noninvasive positive pressure ventilation on exercise ability in patients with severe COPD. *Chest* 2002; 122: 464–472.

51. Costes F, Agresti A, Court-Fortune I, Roche F, Vergnon JM, Barthélémy JC. Noninvasive ventilation during exercise training improves exercise tolerance in patients with chronic obstructive pulmonary disease. *J Cardiopulm Rehabil* 2003; 23: 307–313.

52. Toledo A, Borghi-Silva A, Sampaio LM, Ribeiro KP, Baldissera V, Costa D. The impact of noninvasive ventilation during the physical training in patients with moderate-to-severe chronic obstructive pulmonary disease (COPD). *Clinics* 2007; 62: 113–120.

53. Dreher M, Storre JH, Windisch W. Noninvasive ventilation during walking in patients with severe COPD: a randomised cross-over trial. *Eur Respir J* 2007; 29: 930–936.

54. Ambrosino N. Assisted ventilation as an aid to exercise training: a mechanical doping? *Eur Respir J* 2006; 27: 3–5.

55. Fabbri LM, Luppi F, Beghé B, Rabe KF. Complex chronic comorbidities of COPD. *Eur Respir J* 2008; 31: 204–212.

56. Le Jemtel TH, Padeletti M, Jelic S. Diagnostic and therapeutic challenges in patients with coexistent chronic obstructive pulmonary disease and chronic heart failure. *J Am Coll Cardiol* 2007; 49: 171–180.

57. Crisafulli E, Costi S, Luppi F, *et al.* Role of comorbidities in a cohort of COPD patients undergoing pulmonary rehabilitation. *Thorax* 2008; 63: 487–492.

58. Ambrosino N, Palmiero G, Strambi SK. New approaches in pulmonary rehabilitation. *Clin Chest Med* 2007; 28: 629–638.

59. Garrod R, Mikelsons C, Paul EA, Wedzicha JA. Randomized controlled trial of domiciliary noninvasive positive pressure ventilation and physical training in severe chronic obstructive pulmonary disease. *Am J Respir Crit Care Med* 2000; 162: 1335–1341.

60. Schönhofer B, Zimmermann C, Abramek P, Suchi S, Köhler D, Polkey MI. Non-invasive mechanical ventilation improves walking distance but not quadriceps strength in chronic respiratory failure. *Respir Med* 2003; 97: 818–824.

CHAPTER 19

NIV and chronic respiratory failure in children

B. Fauroux*, G. Aubertin*, F. Lofaso[#]

*Paediatric Pulmonary Dept, Armand Trousseau Hospital, Paris, and [#]Physiology Dept, Raymond Poincaré Hospital, Garches, France.

Correspondence: B. Fauroux, AP-HP, Hopital Armand Trousseau, Paediatric Pulmonary Dept, Research Unit INSERM UMR S-893 Equipe 12, Université Pierre et Marie Curie-Paris 6, 28 Avenue du Docteur Arnold Netter, Paris, F-75012 France. Fax: 33 144736174; E-mail: brigitte.fauroux@trs.aphp.fr

Introduction

A growing population of children have chronic respiratory failure, due to conditions, such as muscle disease, abnormalities of the airways, the chest wall and/or the lungs, or disorders of ventilatory control. Two factors explain the important development of noninvasive positive pressure ventilation (NPPV) in this population group. First, most of these disorders are fundamentally hypoventilation disorders. As such, oxygen therapy alone is not only usually ineffective in relieving symptoms, but also has been shown to be dangerous and may lead to a marked acceleration of carbon dioxide retention [1, 2]. Secondly, by definition, NPPV is a noninvasive technique that can be applied on demand and preferentially at night, causing much less morbidity, discomfort and social life and family disruption than a tracheostomy. But NPPV is not applicable to all children. Noninvasive forms of mechanical ventilation are technically more difficult to apply in infants and young children. Usually, NPPV is applied during the night and during the daytime nap in young children. A minimal respiratory autonomy is thus an absolute prerequisite for NPPV, even if the beneficial effects of NPPV can extend, after a certain period, during periods of spontaneous breathing. NPPV is often used on an empirical basis in children, with a gap between the expanding use and the lack of precise knowledge on physiological effects. This makes it difficult to establish both the appropriate timing of initiation of NPPV and the most pertinent therapeutic goals.

The present chapter focuses on long-term noninvasive ventilator management of infants and children. The first section examines the diagnoses requiring ventilatory assistance for infants and children. The second section deals with the (potential) physiological benefits of long term NPPV in children. The third section focuses on special considerations for infants and children concerning ventilation techniques, equipment and practical use.

Disorders that may justify NPPV

The ability to sustain spontaneous ventilation can be viewed as a balance between neurological mechanisms controlling ventilation, together with ventilatory muscle power, on one side, and the respiratory load, determined by lung, thoracic and airway mechanics, on the other (fig. 1). Significant dysfunction of any of these components of

Eur Respir Mon, 2008, 41, 272–286. Printed in UK - all rights reserved. Copyright ERS Journals Ltd 2008; European Respiratory Monograph; ISSN 1025-448x.

the respiratory system may impair the ability to spontaneously generate efficacious breaths. In normal individuals, central respiratory drive and ventilatory muscle power exceed the respiratory load and are, thus, able to sustain adequate spontaneous ventilation. However, if the respiratory load is too high and/or ventilatory muscle power or central respiratory drive is too low, ventilation may be inadequate, resulting in hypercapnia. Chronic ventilatory failure, then, is the result of an imbalance in the respiratory system, in which ventilatory muscle power and central respiratory drive are inadequate to overcome the respiratory load. If this imbalance cannot be corrected with medical treatment, the patient may benefit from long-term ventilatory support. Thus, infants and children may require noninvasive long-term ventilatory support due to three categories of respiratory system dysfunction: increased respiratory load (due to intrinsic cardiopulmonary disorders, upper airway abnormalities, or skeletal deformities), ventilatory muscle weakness (due to neuromuscular diseases or spinal cord injury) or failure of neurological control of ventilation (with central hypoventilation syndrome being the most common presentation; fig. 1).

Increase in respiratory load

Upper or lower airway obstruction or chest wall deformity are characterised by an increase in respiratory load.

Obstructive sleep apnoea (OSA) is less common in children than in adults. The pathophysiology is also different with the predominant role of enlarged tonsils and adenoids [3]. If tonsillectomy and adenoidectomy are not able to relieve upper airway obstruction, then noninvasive continuous positive airway pressure (CPAP) ventilation is proposed as the first therapeutic option [4–6]. Indeed, the maintenance of airway patency by means of a continuous positive pressure reduces the respiratory muscle

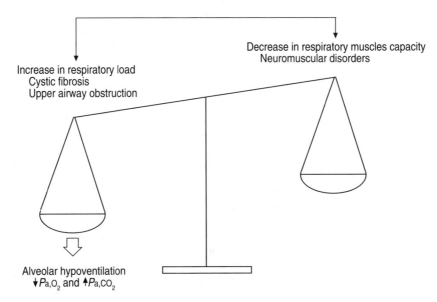

Fig. 1. – Spontaneous ventilation is the result of a balance between neurological mechanisms controlling ventilation together with ventilatory muscle power on one side, and the respiratory load, determined by lung, thoracic and airway mechanics, on the other. If the respiratory load is too high and/or ventilatory muscle power or central respiratory drive is too low, ventilation may be inadequate, resulting in alveolar hypoventilation with hypercapnia and hypoxaemia.

output, which translates into an improvement in alveolar ventilation. Young children are more exposed to these problems; their small lung volumes and the progressive maturation of sleep stages may render them particularly susceptible to the cardiovascular consequences of increased upper airway resistance during sleep.

In children and young adults with advanced pulmonary cystic fibrosis (CF), as lung disease progresses, with a progressive fall in the forced expiratory volume in one second (FEV1), there is an increase in the respiratory muscle load [7]. Indeed, as FEV1 falls, indices reflecting the respiratory muscle output, such as the pressure/time product of the oesophagus (PTPoes) and diaphragm (PTPdi) and the elastic work of breathing increase. Indeed, in a group of children with CF, having a FEV1 of 30–50% of predicted value, PTPoes and PTPdi were increased 3–5-fold [7]. As a result, the patients develop a compensatory mechanism of a rapid, shallow breathing pattern in an attempt to reduce the increase in load. Although this breathing strategy maintains the level of ventilation, arterial carbon dioxide tension (Pa,CO$_2$) rises. Thus, in CF, an imbalance between the load imposed on the respiratory system and the capacity of the respiratory muscles, explains the inability of the respiratory muscle pump to clear carbon dioxide. Short-term physiological studies, during waking and sleep, have demonstrated that NPPV reduces respiratory muscle load and work of breathing [8–10], increases minute ventilation [8, 10] and, thus, improves alveolar ventilation and gas exchange.

Restrictive parenchymal lung diseases are difficult to manage with long-term NPPV. Experience of NPPV in this group of patients is poor. Infants with hypoplastic lungs may be candidates for long-term mechanical ventilation but because of their age and the poor prognosis, they are most-often ventilated with a tracheostomy.

Chest wall abnormalities such as severe scoliosis, kyphosis or thoracic dystrophy are among the chest wall abnormalities that may cause restrictive disease, severe enough to require long-term NPPV. The prognosis of these children depends upon the severity, type and evolution of the disease. In some children, the chest wall abnormalities will cause progressive restrictive pulmonary disease, ultimately resulting in death, even with mechanical ventilation. Other children appear to improve clinically, even in the absence of changes in the chest wall anomaly, due to certain degree of catch-up caused by the physiological growth.

Respiratory muscle weakness

Respiratory muscles are rarely spared in neuromuscular diseases [11]. In general, respiratory muscle weakness is associated with inspiratory muscle weakness, which limits inspiration, resulting in atelectasis and expiratory muscle weakness, causing inability to cough, predisposing to pulmonary infection and hypoventilation, resulting in inadequate gas exchange. Respiratory muscle weakness, dysfunction, or paralysis can occur because of neuromuscular disease, or as a result of spinal cord injury.

The most common neuromuscular diseases requiring NPPV during childhood are Duchenne muscular dystrophy and spinal muscular atrophy. Duchenne muscular dystrophy is a progressive disorder and ventilatory failure is inevitable in the course of the disease, although the time course of progression to it varies between individuals. Home NPPV counteracts the hypoventilation and can improve survival [12–14]. Respiratory failure is also common in children with spinal muscular atrophy (SMA). The SMAs are inherited as autosomal recessive disorders. Severity is inversely proportional to the amount of survival motor-neuron protein in the anterior horn cell. SMAs range from total paralysis and need for ventilatory support from birth, to the relatively mild muscle weakness presenting in the young adult. Diaphragmatic strength is generally preserved and respiratory muscle weakness predominates on the other inspiratory muscles and the expiratory muscles [11]. Respiratory failure is less frequent in other muscular dystrophies, such as Becker, limb-girdle and facioscapulohumeral dystrophies. Congenital myopathies are often static [11]; however, the condition of children may deteriorate functionally with growth because weakened muscles are unable to cope with increasing body mass.

The importance of respiratory failure associated with spinal cord injury depends on the level of the injury. High spinal cord injury, above C-3, causes diaphragm paralysis. This almost always causes respiratory failure in infants and young children. NPPV can be attempted in older children, who have a sufficient respiratory autonomy for at least 8–10 h·day^{-1}. In patients with lower cervical cord injury, expiratory muscle function is severely compromised, impairing cough and the clearance of bronchial secretions. As a result, retention of secretions, leading to atelectasis and bronchopneumonia, frequently occurs in such patients and may require short periods of NPPV during episodes of acute respiratory failure. However, these children, with respiratory muscle weakness, often do not have severe intrinsic or parenchymal lung disease, thus making them good candidates for home NPPV.

Failure of the neurological control of ventilation

Disorders of neurological control of breathing, that are severe enough to cause chronic respiratory failure, are uncommon to rare. Congenital central hypoventilation syndrome ("Ondine's curse") is the most common presentation in childhood and is characterised by the failure of autonomic control of breathing [15]. Hypoxia and hypercapnia worsen during sleep. A tracheostomy is nearly always mandatory in infants and young children but NPPV may be successful in older children, who sustain adequate ventilation during waking but require ventilatory assistance during sleep [16, 17].

Benefits of NPPV

The benefits of NPPV vary according to the underlying disease. Some beneficial effects, such as the correction of nocturnal alveolar hypoventilation are common to the different diagnostic groups, whereas other effects, such as the increase in survival, may be specific for a group of disorders (table 1).

Correction of nocturnal hypoventilation and gas exchange

The most obvious effect, in the paediatric population, is the correction of nocturnal hypoventilation. Sleep is associated with changes in respiratory mechanics, such as an increase in ventilation–perfusion mismatch, an increase in airflow resistance and a fall in functional residual capacity (fig. 2). Although the activity of the diaphragm is preserved, those of the intercostal and upper airway muscles are decreased significantly. Finally, central drive and chemoreceptor sensitivity are less efficient during sleep than during waking. All of these abnormalities explain a physiological degree of nocturnal hypoventilation, even in normal subjects, causing a rise in Pa,CO_2 of up 3 mmHg (0.4 kPa) in adults [18]. This decrease in alveolar ventilation predominates during rapid eye movement (REM) sleep and explains why patients with chronic respiratory failure are vulnerable during this sleep stage. Nocturnal hypoventilation will also predominate during REM sleep in children with OSA because of the physiological relaxation of the upper airway muscles.

Table 1. – Potential benefits of long term noninvasive positive pressure ventilation in children according to the underlying disease.

	Neuromuscular disorders	Obstructive sleep apnoea	Cystic fibrosis
Improvement in nocturnal hypoventilation and gas exchange	Yes	Yes	Yes
Increase in survival	Yes (in patients with Duchenne muscular dystrophy)	Not applicable (tracheostomy is an alternative)	Not proven
Improvement in lung function	Not proven	Not applicable	Limited data
Improvement in respiratory muscle performance	Not proven	Not applicable	Limited data
Improvement in exercise tolerance	Not proven	Not applicable	Yes
Preservation of normal pulmonary mechanics and lung growth	Not proven	Not applicable	Not applicable
Improvement of quality of life	Yes	Yes (as an alternative to tracheostomy)	Not proven

The efficacy of NPPV in relieving nocturnal hypoventilation in children with OSA has been demonstrated in several studies. Nasal CPAP has been used by some experienced teams for several decades [4–6]. Therapy with nasal CPAP eliminated the signs of OSA in 90% (of 80) children in whom this treatment was tried due to the persistence of the symptoms after adenotonsillectomy [4].

Several studies have shown the efficacy of NPPV to correct or improve nocturnal hypoventilation in patients with CF. These patients may experience periods of oxyhaemoglobin desaturation, during sleep, that are most marked during REM sleep [19, 20]. A study including seven adults with CF showed that, compared with a control night without CPAP, nasal CPAP resulted in a significant improvement in arterial oxygen saturation (Sa,O_2) during both REM and non-REM sleep [19]. However, transcutaneous carbon dioxide tension (Ptc,CO_2) measurements were not significantly different between the control and CPAP nights. Another interesting study compared gas exchange and quality of sleep in adults with CF during three nights: a control night, a night with oxygen and a night with NPPV [21]. Similar significant improvements of Sa,O_2 and time spent in REM sleep, were observed during the nights with oxygen and NPPV. Most interestingly, the night with oxygen was associated with a significant increase in Ptc,CO_2, whereas NPPV resulted in a significant decrease in Ptc,CO_2.

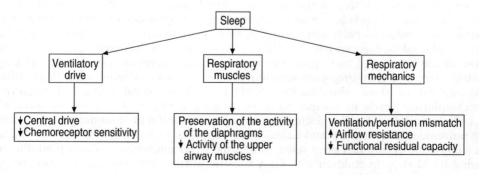

Fig. 2. – Physiological alterations during sleep explaining the worsening of respiratory failure during sleep.

Sleep-related respiratory disturbances are frequent in teenagers and adults with Duchenne muscular dystrophy patients, especially when diurnal arterial hypoxaemia is present [22]. NPPV has been shown to be associated with a substantial improvement in alveolar hypoventilation during both night and day, in children with various neuromuscular diseases [23]. The benefits of NPPV may be due to combined effects of several interrelated processes. The increase in respiratory drive is probably due to a reduction in cerebrospinal fluid bicarbonate concentration which resets the ventilatory response to carbon dioxide, and to an improvement in sleep quality which influences the ventilatory response to carbon dioxide and respiratory muscle endurance [24]. In addition, NPPV may decrease the work of breathing during spontaneous ventilation as a result of an increase in chest wall and lung compliance due to the increase in respiratory movements during NPPV.

Increase in survival

The improvement in survival represents a major expectation of NPPV in patients with progressive neuromuscular or lung disease. But this benefit has only been demonstrated in patients with neuromuscular diseases in a case series [13] and in one nation-wide study. Indeed, the benefit of NPPV on the survival of patients with Duchenne muscular dystrophy in Denmark was evaluated between 1977 and 2001 [14]. While overall incidence remained stable at 2.0 per 100,000 people, prevalence rose from 3.1 to 5.5 per 100,000 people, mortality fell from 4.7 to 2.6 per 100 yrs at risk and the prevalence of ventilator users rose from 0.9 to 43.4 per 100. Ventilator use is probably the main reason of this dramatic increase in survival.

An increase in survival has not been demonstrated in patients with CF. In other diseases, such as OSA, survival is not an issue, because a tracheostomy may constitute an alternative to NPPV.

Improvement in lung function, respiratory muscle performance and exercise tolerance

The stabilisation or slowing of the decline in lung function, by NPPV, in patients whose disease course is characterised by a decline in lung function, such as patients with neuromuscular disease or CF, represents a major expectation of long-term NPPV. No data are presently available to support this hypothesis for patients with neuromuscular disease. Recent data from the French Cystic Fibrosis Observatory have shown that NPPV was associated with a stabilisation of the decline in lung function in patients with advanced lung disease [25]. Indeed, 44 patients (NPPV group) were compared with matched controls (control group), 1 yr prior to the initiation of NPPV, during the year of NPPV initiation, and after 1 yr of NPPV treatment. Each patient of the NPPV group was matched for a control patient for sex, *CFTR* genotype, age $\pm$ 1 yr, weight $\pm$ 2 kg, $FEV_1 \pm 10\%$ predicted and follow up at the same centre. During the year prior to initiation of NPPV, the two groups were comparable but at the year of initiation, the NPPV group had a significantly greater decline in vital capacity (VC) and FEV_1. After 1 yr, the decline in VC and FEV_1 was similar in the two groups, demonstrating a stabilisation of lung function decline in the NPPV group.

NPPV has been associated with an improvement in respiratory muscle performance in patients with CF. PIPER et al. [26] reported an increase in maximal expiratory ($P_{E,max}$) and inspiratory pressure ($P_{I,max}$) in four adults with CF after 1 month of NPPV. However, improvement due to a learning effect or better motivation could not be excluded because of the volitional nature of these tests. Significant decreases have been observed in $P_{E,max}$ and $P_{I,max}$, in 19 children with CF, after a 20-min physiotherapy session [27]. When the physiotherapy session was performed with pressure-support ventilation (PSV) administered by a nasal mask, a significant increase of these parameters was observed. The improvement of $P_{I,max}$ after the PSV session suggests that pressure support may "rest" the inspiratory muscles during chest physiotherapy. The improvement of $P_{E,max}$ after the PSV session could be explained by the increase in tidal volume (V_T) during PSV. During PSV, the V_T tends to the total lung capacity. This allows a larger amount of energy to accumulate, thereby facilitating expiration and decreasing the work of the expiratory muscles.

Noninvasive CPAP ventilation has been associated with an improvement in exercise tolerance in 33 patients with CF [28]. Indeed, 5 cmH_2O CPAP ventilation resulted in a decrease in oxygen consumption, respiratory effort, assessed by the transdiaphragmatic pressure (P_{di}) and dyspnoea score. These beneficial effects during exercise were the most important in the patients with severe lung disease in whom the presence of intrinsic positive end-expiratory pressure (PEEP) may be favourably counteracted by CPAP.

Preservation of normal pulmonary mechanics and lung growth

The physiological changes in the compliance of the lungs and the chest wall play a crucial role in the normal development of the lung. In infancy, the chest wall is nearly three times as compliant as the lung [29]. By the end of the second year of life, chest wall stiffness increases to the point that the chest wall and lung are nearly equally compliant, as in adulthood. Stiffening of the chest wall plays a major role in developmental changes in respiratory system function such as the ability to passively maintain resting lung volume and improved ventilatory efficiency afforded by reduced rib cage distorsion. An important point would be to know if long-term NPPV in infants and young children can preserve a near to normal chest wall compliance, in both children with a too stiff chest, due to chest deformity for example, or those with neuromuscular disease, exposed to ankylosis in the costosternal and costovertebral joints and to gradual stiffening of the rib cage because of a breathing at smaller V_T and greater respiratory frequency.

Chronic hypoventilation can alter the dynamic or static compliance of the lung. The majority of observations in patients with neuromuscular disease have shown a significant reduction in pulmonary compliance [11]. The measurements of these patients were of dynamic compliance reflecting abnormalities in airways rather than a true change in the elastic properties of the lungs. Specific compliance, relating static expiratory compliance to total lung capacity, is normal in patients with respiratory muscle weakness. Atelectasis could explain the hypoxaemia, due to the ventilation–perfusion mismatching.

A major concern in paediatric patients is the effect of chronic hypoventilation on lung growth, and, as a logical consequence, the effect of NPPV in promoting or preserving physiological lung and chest wall growth in the developing child. To the present authors' knowledge, this has not been studied in children; however, animal models have shown that the congenital absence of the diaphragm or the intercostals muscles is associated with both lung hypoplasia and a lack of lung differentiation [30, 31].

Improvement of quality of life

Studies are scarce, but NPPV has not been shown to be associated with deterioration in quality of life in children with neuromuscular disease. In a small group of children with SMA and other neuromuscular diseases, NPPV was associated in an improvement in symptoms of nocturnal hypoventilation, and the maintenance of the different modules of quality of life measures, except the physical module, which reflects the progression of the underlying neuromuscular disease [32]. NPPV was also associated with an improvement in quality of life in boys with Duchenne muscular dystrophy [13]. Such a benefit has not been demonstrated in patients with CF. In patients with OSA, the alternative for NPPV is tracheostomy, which clearly puts the balance in favour of NPPV.

Criteria to initiate NPPV

Validated criteria for beginning long term NPPV are lacking in children [33]. Several consensus conferences agree on the value of daytime hypercapnia and an acute exacerbation to initiate NPPV because these criteria are the signature of established ventilatory failure [34–36]. But these two classical criteria are preceded by a variable period of nocturnal hypoventilation, during which, treatable symptoms, such as frequent arousals, severe orthopnea, daytime fatigue and alterations in cognitive function, may deteriorate the daily life of the patient. There is also a wide agreement to consider that clinical symptoms attributable to nocturnal hypoventilation are most important for the decision of NPPV. Initiation of NPPV before overt daytime hypercapnia may thus be beneficial, not only on quality of sleep but also, according to the underlying disease, on survival, lung growth and lung function and respiratory muscle performance.

A major problem is thus to optimally schedule a polysomnographic sleep study in order to document nocturnal hypoventilation. A polysomnography should be realised without delay when the patient recognises symptoms related to sleep disordered breathing but patients with neuromuscular disorders tend to underestimate symptoms, such as fatigue, before using mechanical ventilation. Sleep disordered breathing may be difficult to establish in children because of reliance on parents and second-hand caregivers, who have a different perception of the child's disease. Lung function parameters are poor indicators of nocturnal hypoventilation. Thus, further studies are mandatory to establish, for every diagnostic group, first, the most pertinent criteria which should ask for a sleep study, and second, those which may require the initiation of NPPV.

A recent study showed that the initiation of NPPV at the stage of nocturnal hypercapnia without daytime hypercapnia in children and adults with neuromuscular disorders and chest wall disease was associated with an improvement in nocturnal gas exchange [37]. Larger prospective studies, in homogeneous groups of patients, are warranted in order to confirm the benefit of this "early" initiation of NPPV.

Ventilation techniques, ventilation equipment and use in children

Ventilation techniques

The type of equipment and the specific ventilator settings that should be chosen remain a matter of debate. The specific equipment available for therapy evolves more rapidly with industry capability rather than with clear indications available from scientific trials.

Nasal CPAP is the treatment of choice for obstructive events during sleep [6, 38]. Upper airway patency is maintained with nasal CPAP by a pneumatic splinting effect. In addition, it has been demonstrated that CPAP reduces the work of breathing in patients with flow limitation [39, 40]. In such patients, CPAP overcomes the inspiratory threshold imposed by auto-PEEP, and pneumatically splints the airways to prevent dynamic collapse during exhalation. Thus, if the main indication of CPAP is OSA, it is also advocated in obstructive lung disease, when intrinsic PEEP increases the work of breathing; however, because upper airway loading with complete or partial obstruction and intrinsic PEEP are not the sole mechanisms of hypoventilation, CPAP should be insufficient in patients with respiratory function abnormalities.

Volume-targeted ventilation is characterised by the delivery of a fixed, predetermined VT. The main advantage of this mode is that a guaranteed minimal VT is delivered, but this can result in detrimentally high inspiratory airway pressures causing discomfort and poor tolerability. Despite many of the volume-targeted ventilators having no leak compensation mechanisms, this mode is suited to patients with neuromuscular diseases, where the ventilator acts as a substitute for the weakened respiratory muscles, which are unable to trigger the ventilator. However, a relatively high back up rate (2–3 breaths lower than the spontaneous respiratory rate of the patient) is required to avoid nocturnal desaturations, and, as a consequence, many patients adopt a controlled mode without triggering the ventilator. Also, the inspiratory triggers of these ventilators are not very sensitive, which is another factor justifying the use of a relatively high back up rate [9, 41]. Initial studies with long term NPPV in children with neuromuscular disease and CF have used volume-targeted devices [42, 43]. These ventilators designed for home use are relatively portable. They are not as technologically sophisticated as hospital ventilators. Furthermore, few of them are capable to operate within certain limits (*i.e.* VT <50–100 mL).

PSV is pressure-targeted, during which each breath is triggered and terminated by the patient and supported by the ventilator; the patient can control their respiratory rate, inspiratory duration and VT [44]. This explains the relative ease in adapting to, and the greater comfort and synchrony of this mode. In contrast to volume-targeted ventilation, VT is not predetermined but depends on the level of PSV, the inspiratory effort of the patient and the mechanical properties of the patient's respiratory system. During this mode, since there are no mandatory breaths present, an in-built low-frequency back-up rate is used to prevent episodes of apnoea. Furthermore, because the breaths are triggered by the patient, the sensitivity of the trigger is crucial. The sensitivity of the inspiratory triggers of the different ventilators designed for the home is variable but some are as sensitive as those of intensive care devices [41, 45]. Because, during PSV, inspiratory muscle activity may influence respiratory frequency and VT, this ventilatory mode is generally proposed in patients who can breathe spontaneously for substantial periods of time and require mainly nocturnal ventilation.

Bi-level PPV is the combination of PSV and PEEP, permitting an independent adjustment of expiratory positive airway pressure (EPAP) and inspiratory positive airway pressure (IPAP). In this condition upper airway obstruction and/or work of breathing induced by intrinsic PEEP are prevented by EPAP and thus PS can be triggered easily by the patient. This ventilatory mode has been used in children with OSA, CF [46, 47] and neuromuscular disease [46, 48, 49].

For all ventilatory modes, alarms must be correctly set. When positive pressure ventilators are used, low pressure or disconnect alarms are classically present. Alarms for high pressure, incorrect timing and power failure are also frequently present. The alarm of a minimal VT is very useful in children. A back-up frequency is generally set on the ventilator. All these alarms must be carefully checked before the discharge of the patient.

Interfaces

The necessity of interfaces, specifically designed for children, represents an important technical limitation of NPPV in paediatric patients. In adults, four different types of interfaces are used: full face masks (enclose mouth and nose); nasal masks; nasal pillows or plugs (insert directly into the nostrils); and mouthpieces. Nasal pillows and plugs are too large for children and mouthpieces require a good co-operation and are difficult to use in neuromuscular patients. In young children, nasal masks are preferred because they have less static dead space, are less claustrophobic and allow communication and expectoration more easily than full face masks. Nasal masks allow also the use of a pacifier in infants, which contributes to the better acceptance of NPPV and the reduction of mouth leaks; however, few industrial masks are available for children. This shortcoming is even more important for infants. Most often, NPPV is thus restrained to some highly specialised paediatric centres which have the possibility of manufacturing custom-made masks for infants and children who can not use industrial masks [50].

The nasal interface represents a crucial determinant of the success of NPPV. The patient will be unable to tolerate and accept NPPV in case of facial discomfort, skin injury or significant air leaks. The evaluation of the short term tolerance of the nasal mask is thus an essential component of NPPV [50]. NPPV is generally used during sleep, which can represent the major part of the day in young infants. In these young patients, there is a potential risk of skin injury and facial deformity, such as facial flattening and maxilla retrusion, caused by the pressure applied by the mask on growing facial structures. These potential side effects justify the systematic follow up of children receiving NPPV by a paediatric maxillo-facial specialist.

Additional therapies

Oxygen therapy at home must be justified on the basis of an individual-based medical necessity, as determined by appropriate physiologic monitoring, such as Sa,O_2 during periods of sleep, wakefulness, feeding and physical activity and arterial blood gases. CO_2 should be minimised first by ventilator use before considering oxygen therapy, especially for patients with neuromuscular disorders and OSA. It is important to remember that supplemental oxygen is not a replacement for assisted ventilation in patients who hypoventilate.

Systematic humidification of the ventilator gas is not necessary for NPPV because of the respect of the upper airway. However, nasal intolerance, due to excessive dryness can resolve after humidification of the ventilator gas.

The maintenance of an optimal nutritional status is of major importance. Chronic respiratory insufficiency is associated with an increased energy demand, feeding difficulties and poor caloric intake. Swallowing problems may occur in patients with neuromuscular disease [51]. In some patients, gastrostomy may be a useful adjunct therapy to NPPV and contribute to postponing the time of a tracheostomy [51, 52].

It is essential that the child, if the age permits it, and the parents should have the opportunity to discuss NPPV therapy in advance. Discussion should start long enough before the anticipated need, to allow the child and the family to evaluate options thoroughly and to discuss their feelings. NPPV, here, has an essential first place as a noninvasive therapy but still represents an objective element reflecting a further step in the severity of a disease. It is crucial to determine short- and intermediate-term goals of NPPV with the child and the family and to explain the principles of NPPV. A wide range of ventilators and masks are available and great care will be taken to choose the most appropriate equipment and settings. The final objective is that NPPV translates into well-being and a better quality of life with a total adherence of the child and their family.

Contraindications, side effects and limits of NPPV

The general point-of-view is that NPPV is preferred over invasive mechanical ventilation as the first therapy of chronic respiratory failure. However NPPV is contraindicated in some circumstances (table 2) [53]. NPPV is also contraindicated in case of recent pneumothorax, which can occur in patients with advanced CF lung disease. Pneumothorax can also occur as a side effect of NPPV in patients with neuromuscular disorders [54]. In patients with CF, nasal polyps are common and should be treated before the initiating of NPPV.

Side effects are common; they are caused by the interface and the delivery of a positive pressure. In the present authors' experience, skin injury, from transient erythema to permanent skin necrosis, due to the nasal mask, has been observed in 53% of the 40 patients during their routine 6-months follow-up [50]. In young children, there is also a potential risk of facial deformity, such as facial flattening and maxilla retrusion, caused by the pressure applied by the mask on growing facial structures. These potential side effects justify the systematic evaluation before the initiation and during the follow up of children receiving NPPV by a paediatric maxillo-facial specialist. Abdominal distension is an uncommon problem which can be lessened by switching to a PSV or decreasing the V_T on a volume-targeted ventilator [53].

NPPV is not always successful in adequately relieving hypoventilation. Air leaks have been shown to be an important cause of persistent hypercapnia in both invasively and noninvasively ventilated neuromuscular patients [55]. In these patients, simple practical measures such as changing the mask, using a chin strap, increasing minute ventilation and changing the type of the ventilator, were able to reduce the volume of air leaks and improve the efficacy of ventilation [55].

In patients with neuromuscular disease, cough assisted techniques are useful when ventilatory dependence is increasing. Several techniques are available such as manual physiotherapy, intermittent positive pressure breathing, and mechanical insufflation-exsufflation [56-59]. These techniques, associated with daytime ventilation by means of a mouthpiece [60], extend the use of NPPV in patients having increasing ventilatory dependency. However, despite these measures, in progressive diseases such as some neuromuscular diseases, a tracheotomy will become necessary at a certain moment. Close monitoring of the patient's physiological status and disease progression, together with clear information of the family are essential. Technical problems, especially with regards to the nasal mask and the ventilator equipment, frequently limit the use of NPPV in infants. Because noninvasive ventilation leaves airway protection, those with copious secretions or severe swallowing dysfunction may respond poorly, requiring the discussion of a tracheostomy with the patient and their family.

Table 2. – Contraindications for noninvasive positive pressure ventilation (NPPV). Adapted from [53]

Relative contraindications
  Severe swallowing impairment
  Inadequate family/caregiver support
  Need for full-time ventilatory assistance
Absolute contraindications
  Complete persistent upper airway obstruction during NPPV
  Uncontrollable secretion retention
  Inability to co-operate
  Inability to achieve adequate peak cough flow, even with assistance
  Inadequate financial resource
  Inability to fit an interface

In conclusion, noninvasive positive pressure ventilation is increasingly used in children and infants. Unfortunately, in this age group, this therapy is generally initiated on an empirical basis. Further studies are urgently needed to determine the most pertinent criteria to initiate noninvasive positive pressure ventilation according to the disease and the age of the patient; to evaluate the long term benefits, with regard to the increase in survival, stabilisation in the decline in lung function and respiratory muscle performance; to promote lung growth and respiratory mechanics; and, most importantly, to improve the quality of life of the child and their family.

Summary

Domiciliary noninvasive positive pressure ventilation (NPPV) is increasingly used in children. Three categories of respiratory system dysfunction can justify long term NPPV: an increase in respiratory load (due to intrinsic cardiopulmonary disorders or skeletal deformities); respiratory muscle weakness (due to neuromuscular diseases or spinal cord injury); or failure of neurologic control of ventilation (such as the central hypoventilation syndrome). In these different diseases, the role of NPPV will be to respectively unload the respiratory muscles, to replace the respiratory muscles or to replace central drive, in order to correct alveolar hypoventilation. The benefit of NPPV on nocturnal and daytime gas exchange has been demonstrated in children. Other effects, such as an improvement of lung function, respiratory muscle performance or respiratory mechanics, are less well documented. The effect of NPPV on lung growth is an important point that needs to be investigated. The type of equipment and the specific ventilator settings that should be chosen remain a matter of debate and evolve more rapidly with industry capability than with clear indications available from scientific trials. The major advantage of NPPV is that it can be applied at home, combining greater potential for psychosocial development and family function, at a lesser cost. The use of home NPPV requires appropriate diagnostic procedures, appropriate titration of the ventilator, co-operative and educated families and a careful, well-organised follow up. NPPV represents a challenge for the future whose objective is to improve the well-being of a child with chronic respiratory insufficiency and his or her family.

Keywords: Alveolar hypoventilation, children, chronic respiratory insufficiency, home care, noninvasive mechanical ventilation.

References

1.   Gay PC, Edmonds LC. Severe hypercapnia after low-flow oxygen therapy in patients with neuromuscular disease and diaphragmatic dysfunction. *Mayo Clin Proc* 1995; 70: 327–330.
2.   Masa JF, Celli BR, Riesco JA, Sánchez de Cos J, Disdier C, Sojo A. Noninvasive positive pressure ventilation and not oxygen may prevent overt ventilatory failure in patients with chest wall disease. *Chest* 1997; 112: 207–213.
3.   Croft CB, Brockbank MJ, Wright A, Swanston AR. Obstructive sleep apnoea in children undergoing routine tonsillectomy and adenoidectomy. *Clin Otolaryngol Allied Sci* 1990; 15: 307–314.
4.   Waters KA, Everett FM, Bruderer JW, Sullivan CE. Obstructive sleep apnea: the use of nasal CPAP in 80 children. *Am J Respir Crit Care Med* 1995; 152: 780–785.

5. Guilleminault C, Nino-Murcia G, Heldt G, Baldwin R, Hutchinson D. Alternative treatment to tracheostomy in obstructive sleep apnea syndrome: nasal continuous positive airway pressure in young children. *Pediatrics* 1986; 78: 797–802.

6. Guilleminault C, Pelayo R, Clerk A, Leger D, Bocian RC. Home nasal continuous positive airway pressure in infants with sleep-disordered breathing. *J Pediatr* 1995; 127: 905–912.

7. Hart N, Polkey MI, Clément A, *et al.* Changes in pulmonary mechanics with increasing disease severity in children and young adults with cystic fibrosis. *Am J Respir Crit Care Med* 2002; 166: 61–66.

8. Fauroux B, Pigeot J, Polkey MI, Isabey D, Clément A, Lofaso F. *In vivo* physiologic comparison of two ventilators used for domiciliary ventilation in children with cystic fibrosis. *Crit Care Med* 2001; 29: 2097–2105.

9. Fauroux B, Louis B, Hart N, *et al.* The effect of back-up rate during non-invasive ventilation in young patients with cystic fibrosis. *Intensive Care Med* 2004; 30: 673–681.

10. Fauroux B, Nicot F, Essouri S, *et al.* Setting of pressure support in young patients with cystic fibrosis. *Eur Respir J* 2004; 24: 624–630.

11. Nicot F, Hart N, Forin V, *et al.* Respiratory muscle testing: a valuable tool for children with neuromuscular disorders. *Am J Respir Crit Care Med* 2006; 174: 67–74.

12. Vianello A, Bevilacqua M, Salvador V, Cardaioli C, Vincenti E. Long-term nasal intermittent positive pressure ventilation in advanced Duchenne's muscular dystrophy. *Chest* 1994; 105: 445–448.

13. Simonds AK, Muntoni F, Heather S, Fielding S. Impact of nasal ventilation on survival in hypercapnic Duchenne muscular dystrophy. *Thorax* 1998; 53: 949–952.

14. Jeppesen J, Green A, Steffensen BF, Rahbek J. The Duchenne muscular dystrophy population in Denmark, 1977–2001: prevalence, incidence and survival in relation to the introduction of ventilator use. *Neuromuscul Disord* 2003; 13: 804–812.

15. Gozal D. Congenital central hypoventilation syndrome: an update. *Pediatr Pulmonol* 1998; 26: 273–282.

16. Nielson DW, Black PG. Mask ventilation in congenital central alveolar hypoventilation syndrome. *Pediatr Pulmonol* 1990; 9: 44–45.

17. Zaccaria S, Braghiroli A, Sacco C, Donner CF. Central hypoventilation in a seven year old boy. Long-term treatment by nasal mask ventilation. *Monaldi Arch Chest Dis* 1993; 48: 37–38.

18. Gothe B, Altose MD, Goldman MD, Cherniak NS. Effect of quiet sleep on resting and CO_2-stimulated breathing in humans. *J Appl Physiol* 1981; 50: 724–730.

19. Regnis JA, Piper AJ, Henke KG, Parker S, Bye PT, Sullivan CE. Benefits of nocturnal nasal CPAP in patients with cystic fibrosis. *Chest* 1994; 106: 1717–1724.

20. Milross MA, Piper AJ, Norman M, *et al.* Low-flow oxygen and bilevel ventilatory support: effects on ventilation during sleep in cystic fibrosis. *Am J Respir Crit Care Med* 2001; 163: 129–134.

21. Gozal D. Nocturnal ventilatory support in patients with cystic fibrosis: comparison with supplemental oxygen. *Eur Respir J* 1997; 10: 1999–2003.

22. Barbé F, Quera-Salva MA, McCann C, *et al.* Sleep-related respiratory disturbances in patients with Duchenne muscular dystrophy. *Eur Respir J* 1994; 7: 1403–1408.

23. Barbé F, Quera-Salva MA, de Lattre J, Gajdos P, Agustí AG. Long-term effects of nasal intermittent positive-pressure ventilation on pulmonary function and sleep architecture in patients with neuromuscular disease. *Chest* 1996; 110: 1179–1183.

24. White DP, Douglas NJ, Pickett CK, Zwillich CW, Weil JV. Sleep deprivation and the control of ventilation. *Am Rev Respir Dis* 1983; 128: 984–986.

25. Fauroux B, Le Roux E, Ravilly S, Bellis G, Clément A. Long-term noninvasive ventilation in patients with cystic fibrosis. *Respiration* 2008; 76: 168–174.

26. Piper AJ, Parker S, Torzillo PJ, Sullivan CE, Bye PT. Nocturnal nasal IPPV stabilizes patients with cystic fibrosis and hypercapnic respiratory failure. *Chest* 1992; 102: 846–850.

27. Fauroux B, Boulé M, Lofaso F, *et al.* Chest physiotherapy in cystic fibrosis: improved tolerance with nasal pressure support ventilation. *Pediatrics* 1999; 103: E32.

28. Henke KG, Regnis JA, Bye PT. Benefits of continuous positive airway pressure during exercise in cystic fibrosis and relationship to disease severity. *Am Rev Respir Dis* 1993; 148: 1272–1276.

29. Papastamelos C, Panitch HB, England SE, Allen JL. Developmental changes in chest wall compliance in infancy and early childhood. *J Appl Physiol* 1995; 78: 179–184.

30. Inanlou MR, Kablar B. Abnormal development of the diaphragm in *mdx:MyoD*$^{-/-}$(9th) embryos leads to pulmonary hypoplasia. *Int J Dev Biol* 2003; 47: 363–371.

31. Inanlou MR, Kablar B. Abnormal development of the intercostal muscles and the rib cage in *Myf5*$^{-/-}$ embryos leads to pulmonary hypoplasia. *Dev Dyn* 2005; 232: 43–54.

32. Young HK, Lowe A, Fitzgerald DA, *et al.* Outcome of noninvasive ventilation in children with neuromuscular disease. *Neurology* 2007; 68: 198–201.

33. Fauroux B, Lofaso F. Non-invasive mechanical ventilation: when to start for what benefit? *Thorax* 2005; 60: 979–980.

34. Robert D, Willig TN, Leger P, Paulus J. Long-term nasal ventilation in neuromuscular disorders: report of a consensus conference. *Eur Respir J* 1993; 6: 599–606.

35. Rutgers M, Lucassen H, Kesteren RV, Leger P. Respiratory insufficiency and ventilatory support. 39th ENMC International Workshop, Naarden, The Netherlands, 26-28 January 1996. European Consortium on Chronic Respiratory Insufficiency. *Neuromuscul Disord* 1996; 6: 431–435.

36. Clinical indications for noninvasive positive pressure ventilation in chronic respiratory failure due to restrictive lung disease, COPD, and nocturnal hypoventilation – a consensus conference report. *Chest* 1999; 116: 521–534.

37. Ward S, Chatwin M, Heather S, Simonds AK. Randomised controlled trial of non-invasive ventilation (NIV) for nocturnal hypoventilation in neuromuscular and chest wall disease patients with daytime normocapnia. *Thorax* 2005; 60: 1019–1024.

38. Waters KA, Everett F, Sillence DO, Fagan ER, Sullivan CE. Treatment of obstructive sleep apnea in achondroplasia: evaluation of sleep, breathing, and somatosensory-evoked potentials. *Am J Med Genet* 1995; 59: 460–466.

39. Fauroux B, Pigeot J, Polkey MI, *et al.* Chronic stridor caused by laryngomalacia in children: work of breathing and effects of noninvasive ventilatory assistance. *Am J Respir Crit Care Med* 2001; 164: 1874–1878.

40. Essouri S, Nicot F, Clement A, *et al.* Noninvasive positive pressure ventilation in infants with upper airway obstruction: comparison of continuous and bilevel positive pressure. *Intensive Care Med* 2005; 31: 574–580.

41. Fauroux B, Leroux K, Desmarais G, *et al.* Performance of ventilators for noninvasive positive-pressure ventilation in children. *Eur Respir J* 2008; 31: 1300–1307.

42. Hodson ME, Madden BP, Steven MH, Tsang VT, Yacoub MH. Non-invasive mechanical ventilation for cystic fibrosis patients – a potential bridge to transplantation. *Eur Respir J* 1991; 4: 524–527.

43. Bellon G, Mounier M, Guidicelli J, Gerard M, Alkurdi M. Nasal intermittent positive ventilation in cystic fibrosis. *Eur Resp J* 1992; 2: 357–359.

44. Brochard L, Pluskwa F, Lemaire F. Improved efficacy of spontaneous breathing with inspiratory pressure support. *Am Rev Resp Dis* 1987; 136: 411–415.

45. Lofaso F, Brochard L, Hang T, Lorino H, Harf A, Isabey D. Home *versus* intensive care pressure support devices. Experimental and clinical comparison. *Am J Respir Crit Care Med* 1996; 153: 1591–1599.

46. Padman R, Lawless S, Von Nessen S. Use of BiPAP by nasal mask in the treatment of respiratory insufficiency in pediatric patients: preliminary investigation. *Pediatr Pulmonol* 1994; 17: 119–123.

47. Caronia CG, Silver P, Nimkoff L, Gorvoy J, Quinn C, Sagy M. Use of bilevel positive airway pressure (BIPAP) in end-stage patients with cystic fibrosis awaiting lung transplantation. *Clin Pediatr (Phila)* 1998; 37: 555–559.

48. Robertson PL, Roloff DW. Chronic respiratory failure in limb-girdle muscular dystrophy: successful long-term therapy with nasal bilevel positive airway pressure. *Pediatr Neurol* 1994; 10: 328–331.

49. Guilleminault C, Philip P, Robinson A. Sleep and neuromuscular disease: bilevel positive airway pressure by nasal mask as a treatment for sleep disordered breathing in patients with neuromuscular disease. *J Neurol Neurosurg Psychiatry* 1998; 65: 225–232.

50. Fauroux B, Lavis JF, Nicot F, *et al.* Facial side effects during noninvasive positive pressure ventilation in children. *Intensive Care Med* 2005; 31: 965–969.

51. Güell MR, Avendano M, Fraser J, Goldstein R. [Pulmonary and nonpulmonary alterations in Duchenne muscular dystrophy]. *Arch Bronconeumol* 2007; 43: 557–561.

52. Yuan N, Wang CH, Trela A, Albanese CT. Laparoscopic Nissen fundoplication during gastrostomy tube placement and noninvasive ventilation may improve survival in type I and severe type II spinal muscular atrophy. *J Child Neurol* 2007; 22: 727–731.

53. Hill NS. Ventilator management for neuromuscular disease. *Semin Respir Crit Care Med* 2002; 23: 293–305.

54. Simonds AK. Pneumothorax: an important complication of non-invasive ventilation in neuromuscular disease. *Neuromuscul Disord* 2004; 14: 351–352.

55. Gonzalez J, Sharshar T, Hart N, Chadda K, Raphaël JC, Lofaso F. Air leaks during mechanical ventilation as a cause of persistent hypercapnia in neuromuscular disorders. *Intensive Care Med* 2003; 29: 596–602.

56. Chatwin M, Ross E, Hart N, Nickol AH, Polkey MI, Simonds AK. Cough augmentation with mechanical insufflation/exsufflation in patients with neuromuscular weakness. *Eur Respir J* 2003; 21: 502–508.

57. Miske LJ, Hickey EM, Kolb SM, Weiner DJ, Panitch HB. Use of the mechanical in-exsufflator in pediatric patients with neuromuscular disease and impaired cough. *Chest* 2004; 125: 1406–1412.

58. Winck JC, Gonçalves MR, Lourenço C, Viana P, Almeida J, Bach JR. Effects of mechanical insufflation-exsufflation on respiratory parameters for patients with chronic airway secretion encumbrance. *Chest* 2004; 126: 774–780.

59. Fauroux B, Guillemot N, Aubertin G, *et al.* Physiologic benefits of mechanical insufflation-exsufflation in children with neuromuscular diseases. *Chest* 2008; 133: 161–168.

60. Toussaint M, Steens M, Wasteels G, Soudon P. Diurnal ventilation *via* mouthpiece: survival in end-stage Duchenne patients. *Eur Respir J* 2006; 28: 549–555.

CHAPTER 20

NIV and palliative care

R. Scala*, S. Nava[#]

*Respiratory Unit, Ospedale San Donato di Arezzo, Arezzo, and [#]Respiratory Intensive Care Unit, Fondazione Salvatore Maugeri, IRCCS, Istituto Scientifico di Pavia, Pavia, Italy.

Correspondence: S. Nava, Respiratory Intensive Care Unit, Fondazione Salvatore Maugeri, Via Maugeri n.10, 27100 Pavia, Italy. Fax: 39 0382592075; E-mail: stefano.nava@fsm.it

Introduction

Thanks to modern pharmacological and nonpharmacological approachs (*i.e.* long-term oxygen therapy and home mechanical ventilation), pulmonologists are able to prolong the survival of patients with chronic respiratory diseases until very advanced stages of their natural course [1]. However, the increase in the survival rate is not always associated with a satisfactory quality of life since an impaired lung function is often associated with a limitation in the patients' activities of daily living (ADLs) and with discomfort and distress (*i.e.* dyspnoea, weakness, depressive symptoms) [2, 3].

It is known that, with the technological innovations in both the diagnosis and the multidisciplinary treatment, the mortality rate, at least for selected types of both solid cancers and haematological malignancies, has been reduced. However, patients with malignant neoplasms may often develop respiratory complications related to the underlying disorder and/or the aggressive treatment strategy; this may adversely affect their outcome even if intensive care measures are adopted [4].

For both clinical scenarios (*i.e.* end-stage non-neoplastic respiratory diseases and respiratory complications in malignancies), prolonging survival is not always a desirable goal to achieve for both the physician and the patient according to the modern vision of patient-centred management of diseases [3]. Conversely, palliation of symptoms and shared end-of-life decisions are the main target of the care in order to maintain human dignity in death [5].

With the introduction of noninvasive ventilation (NIV) to treat acute respiratory failure (ARF) of different aetiologies ~20 yrs ago, classical outcome measures, such as hospital mortality, need for endotracheal intubation, complications of invasive ventilation and length of hospital stay, have been drastically improved [6]. The feasibility and usefulness of NIV in the palliative care of patients with ARF near the end of their lives is still not well demonstrated [5, 7]. In the present chapter, the rationale and the little available literature about this nonconventional use of NIV in end-stage non-neoplastic chronic respiratory diseases and in malignancy will be widely discussed.

Eur Respir Mon, 2008, 41, 287–306. Printed in UK - all rights reserved. Copyright ERS Journals Ltd 2008; European Respiratory Monograph; ISSN 1025-448x.

End-stage non-neoplastic respiratory diseases

Clinical and ethical scenario of end-of-life decisions

Although advances in medicine have greatly improved the ability to treat seriously ill patients and prolong life, there is increasing recognition that extension of life might not always be an appropriate goal. This is particularly true for patients with end-stage chronic respiratory failure for whom palliative care plays a crucial role within the complex ethical and medical burden of end of life. As a matter of a fact, in that subset of patients with poor life expectancy, who are commonly admitted to general and respiratory intensive-care settings for the management of what could be the "terminal" episode of ARF, the palliation of symptoms (*e.g.* dyspnoea) should be one of the more important "musts" for physicians who have to face the dilemma of end-of-life decisions [2, 3, 8, 9].

Pulmonary physicians, especially those dealing with mechanical ventilation, are facing the problem of end-of-life decisions in critically ill patients affected by acute or chronic respiratory disorder everyday. End-of-life decisions include several kinds of practice, which show substantial differences among each other despite a potential overlap between some of them (table 1) [8–11].

The overall incidence of these practices in Europe and the rest of the World is only partially known and, even more importantly, it has been shown that there are important differences between countries or regions, reflecting the absence of a common strategy even within the European Community [10–17].

A very recent survey performed on behalf of the European Respiratory Society to assess end-of-life practices in >6,000 patients with chronic respiratory diseases admitted to European respiratory intermediate care units (RICUs) and high-dependency units over a 6-month period, reported that an end-of-life decision was taken in 21.5% of cases with significant differences in some practices (*i.e.* "do not intubate" (DNI)/"do not resuscitate" (DNR)) between northern and southern countries [11].

In everyday clinical practice it is often difficult to identify the "ideal" candidate for this dramatic end-of-life decision. In fact, it is almost impossible to always determine the preference of individual patients; indeed patient preference may change over time with changing circumstances [3, 18]. The decision to withhold or withdraw life-sustaining treatment is often hindered by prognostic uncertainly, since it is usually difficult to identify at an early stage and without reasonable doubts, those patients who will inevitably die. Typically the prognosis only becomes obvious late in the evolution of the acute illness and not, for example, when the patient is admitted to the hospital.

Table 1. – End-of-life decisions in patients with acute or chronic respiratory failure

Withholding	A planned decision not to institute therapies that were otherwise warranted (*i.e.* intubation, renal replacement therapy, increased doses of vasopressor infusions, surgery, transfusion, nutrition and hydration).
Withdrawal	Discontinuation of treatments that had been started (*i.e.* decreasing fraction of inspired oxygen to 21%, extubation, turning off the ventilator, suspend the vasopressors *etc.*).
Palliative sedation	Consists of pain and symptom treatment with the possible side effect of shortening life.
Euthanasia	From the Greek words ευ θανατοσ meaning "good death". It means that a doctor is intentionally killing a person who is suffering unbearably and hopelessly at the latter's voluntary, explicit, repeated, well-considered and informed request.
Physician-assisted suicide	It means that a doctor is intentionally helping/assisting/co-operating in the suicide of a person who is suffering unbearably and hopelessly at the latter's voluntary, explicit, repeated, well-considered and informed request. These acts do not include withholding or withdrawing treatments although these latter may occur prior to physician-assisted suicide.

Unfortunately the available severity scoring systems such as the Acute Physiologic and Chronic Health Evaluation (APACHE) and Simplified Acute Physiologic (SAPS) scores, do not predict outcome in individual patients with sufficient accuracy to be useful in end-of-life decision making [15].

In a prospective survey conducted in French ICUs, FERRAND et al. [16] showed that, among the patients with chronic illness prior to ICU admission (i.e. cirrhosis, malignant diseases, AIDS, chronic heart failure, chronic respiratory failure, chronic neurological and psychiatric diseases), the proportions of patients with cirrhosis, severe cardiac or respiratory insufficiency and solid cancer were significantly higher in the group with decisions to withdraw or withhold therapy, than in the group without decisions.

Recently, COOK et al. [17] demonstrated that the strongest determinants of the withdrawal of ventilation were the physician's perception that the patient preferred not to use life support, the physician's predictions of a low likelihood of survival in ICU and poor cognitive function.

Similarly, the recent European pulmonologist survey confirmed that the indications given for withdrawing and withholding treatment, as well DNI/DNR decisions, were highly related to the judgement of the involved physician [11].

The results of these surveys highlighted the idea that a reduced life expectancy may influence the end-of-life decision of the physician and this may hold particularly true for the subset of patients affected by end-stage chronic respiratory failure (i.e. chronic obstructive pulmonary disease (COPD), amyotrophic lateral sclerosis, other neuromuscular diseases, and pulmonary fibrosis). Additionally, the way in which end-of-life decisions were handled is likely to be influenced by other factors, such as age, religion, skill and experience of the attending physician [18]. Last, but not least, the existing local legislation and guidelines concerning the end-of-life decision may vary dramatically among the different European countries [11]: in the Netherlands, withholding, withdrawal and euthanasia are legally covered in the law on contracts for medical treatment [19]; in Belgium, despite there being no law covering end-of-life care in the ICU, it is no longer a criminal offence to commit euthanasia if several strict conditions are fulfilled [20]; conversely, in Italy, the legal context of end-of-life decision is very confused due to the lack of specific laws, and the decision must be made on the basis of civil and penal codes of law that date from the 1940s [21].

Mechanical ventilation near the end of life

Mechanical ventilation is one of the life-sustaining measures which is much more involved in the end-of-life decision and, therefore, raises controversial ethical issues for what withholding and withdrawing concern, especially in end-stage chronic lung diseases [8, 11]. With any life-sustaining interventions, the decision of the institution, or for discontinuation of mechanical ventilation, should be based on the analysis of the balance between beneficence and maleficence, which needs an up to date understanding of what mechanical ventilation could achieve for the patient and the burden that it will impose (table 2) [9].

A good communication between physician and patient is essential to reach a shared end-of-life decision about mechanical ventilation in end-stage respiratory patients. Physicians should target their chronic respiratory patients for efforts to improve patients' education about diagnosis and disease process, treatment, prognosis, what dying might be like and advance care planning. In order to address these issues, DALES et al. [18] developed and tested an aid to assist COPD patients with making decisions concerning mechanical ventilation. From that study, it can be concluded that, with the help of an informative aid (i.e. an audiocassette and a booklet describing intubation and

Table 2. – Use of noninvasive ventilation near end of life

Pro	Con
May prolong survival	May unduly delay the process of dying
May improve quality of life	May increase depression and anxiety
May improve quality of dying	May increase suffering
May improve communication	May increase hospital costs
May give time to say good bye and solve "open" personal problems	Withdrawing may be difficult
May improve dyspnoea and discomfort	Discharge at home may be impossible without a ventilator

mechanical ventilation and its possible outcomes), a firm decision may be made easier by patients with satisfaction and confidence.

Unfortunately, several studies [9–14, 22] have shown that inadequate and insufficient communication between the medical staff and the members of the family is a key issue. For example, it has been reported that, in some countries (*i.e.* Sweden and Italy), in >50% of patients (competent and incompetent) undergoing end-of-life decisions, these issues were discussed with neither the patient nor relatives [14]. Similarly, in a recent European survey performed specifically on advanced chronic respiratory disorders, only a relatively small percentage of the patients (<40%) participated in end-of-life decision making [11].

Even when it was performed, the outcome of mechanical ventilation is often discussed without the correct emphasis on its burden. FRIED *et al.* [23] have assessed how treatment preferences are affected by the burden of treatment (*i.e.* length of stay in hospital, extent of tests, invasiveness of interventions), as well as the outcome, in a groups of patients with COPD, cardiogenic pulmonary oedema (CPO) or cancer. The authors showed that the burden of treatment had a significant impact on decision making, as 98.7% of participants would accept a low-burden treatment if it restored current level of health while only 11.2% of them would refuse high-burden treatment that produced a similar outcome. Alternatively, >70% of the patients would reject a low-burden treatment that resulted in a severe functional or cognitive impairment. Interestingly, for the three age-matched categories of patients, although there was no difference in treatment preferences, subjects with COPD had the worst perceived health and functional levels.

Finally, it should not be forgotten that the awareness of the prognosis of end-stage respiratory patients, such as those with COPD, could be strongly influenced by mass media (*i.e.* educational television programmes) [24].

NIV in end-stage lung diseases

Patients with end-stage chronic respiratory diseases may be the "ideal" candidate for the limitation of life support treatment [25]. However, a nihilistic behaviour of physicians towards such kind of respiratory patients may not be always appropriate, since "alternative" methods of life support (*i.e.* NIV) may be successfully employed in the case of severe acute or chronic respiratory failure in patients with end-stage respiratory disease, not judged to be appropriate for intubation [5, 7]. In the European survey [11], the use of NIV as the treatment ceiling together with withholding of mechanical ventilation and DNR orders accounted for >80% of end-of-life decisions. Moreover, withdrawing was rarely used in European RICUs, mainly because NIV was used as the ceiling of ventilatory care in almost a third of the patients. Indeed, NIV has increasingly been used as an alternative to invasive ventilation in patients with a DNI order [26–31]. It is clear that the availability of a noninvasive tool to sustain ventilation in end-stage respiratory patients has changed in recent years and is likely to greatly modify the behaviour of physicians and patients towards the possibilities of end-of-life decision making.

This option of using NIV in end-of-life decisions is particularly emerging in RICUs where a European epidemiological survey has clearly shown that a large majority of patients with end-stage chronic respiratory disorders are treated by pulmonologists [32]. This is not surprising, as RICUs differ substantially from classical ICUs in terms of patient population, staffing, monitoring systems and the use of NIV as the preferred ventilatory approach, where applicable. Furthermore, a very recent American survey showed that the stated use of NIV and the confidence on its utility in end-of-life patients was greater for pulmonologists than for intensivists [7]. This discrepancy could be due to the belief that NIV relieves dyspnoea is greater in pulmonologists than in intensivists. A pulmonologist's point of view may be also influenced by caring for end-stage respiratory patients over the entire spectrum of their illness compared with the greater focus on acute care among intensivists.

The overlap existing between some definitions of end-of-life decision practices may be a cause of confusion for both physicians and patients. For example, the use of NIV as the treatment ceiling may be considered similar to a DNR/DNI order and, alternatively, in some instances as a "full" form of ventilatory support. Perhaps the time has come to add the term "do not noninvasively ventilate order" to the DNI/DNR orders.

Goals of NIV for palliative care

Although NIV is a widely accepted treatment for selected patients with ARF who desire maximum life-prolonging treatment without preset limits on advanced life support measures, the palliative use of NIV in patients, who have decided to forego endotracheal intubation, and in those with end-stage respiratory disease is still controversial, according to several clinical studies and two position papers [5–8].

Some authors have proposed the palliative use of NIV in this scenario to alleviate respiratory distress, to allow the communication and/or to provide additional time to finalise personal affairs and to come to terms with death [33]. Conversely, other authors consider this use to be inappropriate because NIV is still a form of life support even if delivered noninvasively by a mask, which may itself cause discomfort and may unnecessarily prolong the dying process, while diverting critical care resources away from other patients more likely to survive [34].

Clinicians themselves may be unclear about the goals of NIV when applied in end-of-life conditions, with adverse consequences, including unmet or conflicting patient/family expectations, inappropriate use of medical resources, inadvertent prolongation of dying process, intensification of patient/family anxiety and psycho–physical stress [5]. Specific concerns have been raised about whether patients and their families have an adequate discussion and a clear understanding about the goals of care when NIV is used in the end-of-life context: DNI/DNR and/or "comfort measures only" (CMO) [35]. Physicians should be aware and should clearly understand that when NIV is applied with palliative aims, the aim is not patient survival but symptom control.

It must be kept in mind that, compared with other fields of medicine, evidence-based guidelines or recommendations are difficult to establish for what end-of-life care concerns. This is particularly true for NIV indications in end-stage respiratory patients due to their complex and dynamic ethics and medical connotations. However, an attempt to clarify the rationale of the application of NIV in patients with end-of-life decisions is helpful for both physicians and patients/families to better understand the expected benefits and the potential disadvantages of NIV and to stimulate an active and dynamic communications between patient and caregiver.

Very recently, a Task Force on the "Palliation Use of NIV" from the Society of Critical Care Medicine [5] suggested classifying the use of NIV, for patients with ARF, into three categories: 1) NIV as life support with no preset limitations on life-sustaining treatments; 2) NIV as life support when patients and families have decided to forego endotracheal intubation; and 3) NIV as a palliative measure when patients and families have chosen to forego all life support, receiving CMO. The Task Force suggested an approach to the use of NIV for patients and families who choose to forego endotracheal intubation. NIV should be applied after careful discussion of the goals of care, with explicit parameters for likelihood of success and failure, by experienced personnel, and in appropriate healthcare settings. It is important to acknowledge that individual patients may transition from one category to another as the goals of the care or the risk/benefit balance of NIV dynamically change [5].

The difference in goals of NIV, when applied for palliative purpose compared with "conventional" use, must be stressed. In the first category of patients, without preset limits on the provision of and advance life support (*i.e.* endotracheal intubation) NIV must be considered successful only if it improves gas exchanges, is reasonably tolerated and provides an efficient support to buy time to treat the precipitating cause of ARF. In this scenario, even though it is important for the patient to be comfortable on NIV, they may be encouraged to tolerate some discomfort for a short time if NIV is improving oxygenation and ventilation and is likely to avoid endotracheal intubation and to survive. NIV will be discontinued in case of successful ability of the patient to breath spontaneously without mechanical support or in case of either NIV failure or poor mask tolerance, with the need for invasive ventilation [6, 36]. Moreover, a reduced level of consciousness is not an absolute contraindication for NIV, in this subset of patients, provided that NIV is used in only a close monitored setting with a skill and experienced clinical team ready to intubate the patient if their sensorium does not improve quickly [37].

The goals and the time for discontinuation of NIV are similar for those patients who decline endotracheal intubation and invasive mechanical ventilation, with the difference that NIV will be withdrawn if not successful and/or tolerated any longer, and CMO will be intensified. From the ethical point of view, before the application of NIV to DNI patients, it is crucial to have their informed consent [5, 9].

Additionally, patients belonging to a third category, such as those at the end stage of a chronically progressive disease (*i.e.* COPD, neuromuscular disorders and chronic heart failure) or those with terminal malignancy, do not want any form of life-prolonging therapy as their baseline quality of life is found unacceptable despite a maximal therapy. In this subset of patients, who choose CMO to palliate their symptoms, NIV will be considered successful only if it improves dyspnoea, without having negative consequences, and improves the ability to communicate with the family [38]. In contrast to the other categories, patients in this category should not be encouraged to tolerate the discomfort associated with NIV because the goal of the chosen therapy is only the palliation of the symptoms and not the improvement of physiological parameters. Consequently, NIV should be discontinued if patients feel that NIV is not making them more comfortable. In this scenario, there is no sense in providing NIV to patients who are unable to communicate (*i.e.* have a decreased level of consciousness) as they could not feel the potential impact of NIV on their symptoms [5]. This palliative use of NIV may also allow CMO patients to be transferred home in order to spend the end of their lives in their own beds [30].

An ambivalent behaviour towards life-sustaining treatments may be found in at least some patients or some families who choose CMO, as they may still maintain a desire or hope for a cure or a miracle [39]. A patient who has chosen not to undergo endotracheal intubation and is using NIV, hoping it will, if only briefly, prolong their life should be considered as the second category rather than the third. It may also be that some patients who do not want prolonged life-sustaining therapy may choose to undergo a short-term trial of NIV in order to achieve the goal of surviving either until they get their personal affairs in order or until the arrival of family members or friends [7]. Although these patients may have a terminal illness and may be actively dying, the use of NIV in this scenario would be an example of the second category's rationale. It is important to acknowledge that the boundaries between the two categories of NIV use in patients refusing intubation have not yet been exactly defined. As a matter of a fact, the Critical Care Medicine Task Force advises that the goals of the care should be continually reassessed, because risks, benefits and treatment preferences change over time and, therefore, the goals of the care and the category of NIV also change in the same patient [5].

Evidence and behaviour for NIV use at the end of life

Data from the European survey [11] showed that in 40% of patients undergoing NIV, it was used solely as a palliative treatment. This finding was confirmed by a more recent multicentre self-administered survey performed in North America [7] to determine the attitudes of clinicians (*i.e.* physicians and respiratory therapists (RTs)) towards the use of NIV for patients with ARF who have a DNR/DNI order or have chosen CMO, aiming to understand if NIV helped those patients to achieve important health or personal goals, or whether it merely prolonged the dying process. According to that study, 62% of physicians and 87% of RTs included the potential use of NIV during life support discussions with their DNR patients at least sometimes. For patients choosing CMO, 49% of physicians and 41% of RTs reported including NIV sometimes as an option in their discussions [7].

The application of NIV to treat ARF in DNI/DNR patients and to palliate symptoms in CMO patients is based more on personal clinical experience and patient shared decisions than on any clear scientific data. This is mostly due to the fact that most of the randomised controlled trials (RCTs) on the use of NIV in ARF, systematically excluded DNI patients [36]. The recent American Academy of Critical Care Medicine recommendations for end-of-life care in the ICU, which included palliative use of NIV, did not use an evidence grading system because most of the reported suggestions were based on ethical and legal principles and not derived from empirically based evidence [8].

As far as the evidence supporting NIV use in the Critical Care Medicine Task Force second category is concerned, three UK RCTs [40–42], which showed reduced rates of mortality and endotracheal intubation in COPD exacerbations with NIV compared with the standard medical therapy, did not exclude DNI patients. However, as these studies did not conduct an *a priori* or *post hoc* subgroup analysis, specifically on patients from the second caegory, conclusions about the benefits of NIV in those patients could not be drawn.

Observational studies have examined the potential usefulness of NIV in ARF patients who have a DNI order. In a single-centre study of 17 patients who were considered DNI because endotracheal intubation was contraindicated, NIV was initially successful in 10 (59%) patients with a hospital mortality of 47% (9 out of 17) [26]. MEDURI *et al.* [27] reported a 64% hospital discharge in a series of 11 DNI patients, all with hypercapnic ARF.

In a recent multicentre study [28], NIV was applied to treat episodes of ARF in 114 patients with DNI orders. A total of 43% survived and were discharged from the ICU; with ~50% of those patients with COPD and 70% with CPO surviving at hospital discharge. The authors found that a higher level of baseline hypercapnia, the diagnosis of COPD or CPO, the presence of strong cough and of wakefulness were associated with a better hospital survival.

Similar results have recently been obtained by SCHETTINO et al. [30], in a single-centre prospective observational study investigating the use of NIV in 131 consecutive DNI patients with ARF. The authors reported an overall hospital mortality of 65%, with a much poorer prognosis of patients with advanced cancer showing a hospital mortality of 85%; those with COPD and CPO showed a hospital survival rate of 63 and 60%, respectively. It is not clear whether these predictors are specific to DNI patients because in neither of the latter two studies, were patients in category 2 distinguishable from those in category 3; however, it is possible that the majority of the enrolled patients belonged to category 2 because most of them were discharged alive.

A further uncontrolled study compared the long-term outcome of 80 consecutive patients with COPD exacerbations treated with NIV independent of whether they had a DNI order; the former showed a shorter 1-yr survival compared with the latter (30 and 65%, respectively). Patients in the DNI group were significantly older, had a worse dyspnoea and APACHE II scores, and were more limited in their ADLs [29].

Similar findings were observed in another recent retrospective study [31] performed on 233 patients submitted to NIV: hospital survival was lower in 34 DNI patients than in 199 non-DNI patients (25 versus 74%, respectively; p<0.001) and DNI was the strongest independent predictor of both in-hospital and 6-month mortality. However, while hospital survival was better for COPD versus non-COPD patients with and without DNI order, at 6 months, the outcome was not different for COPD versus non-COPD.

These clinical data are in agreement with the findings of the recent American survey about near end of life showing that most physicians (>80%) use NIV and most RTs (>80%) are asked to initiate NIV for DNR patients with COPD or CPO. Conversely, according to this survey fewer clinicians reported using NIV for DNR patients with underlying malignancy (59% of physicians, 69% of RTs) or for patients choosing CMO (40% of physicians, 51% of RTs; p<0.001) [7].

Another potential field of application of NIV in terms of palliative care is as a treatment ceiling in end-stage patients already receiving home NIV, but no data concerning this issue were available.

To date, no studies have fully assessed the effectiveness and the safety of NIV specifically applied in patients who choose to undergo CMO (i.e. category 3), even though NIV has been shown to be effective in reducing dyspnoea in COPD exacerbations [27, 40] and in advanced solid cancer with ARF [43].

The more controversial point is whether the benefit of NIV to palliate dyspnoea may be outweighed by the discomfort and the limited communication induced by a tight-fitting mask. Additionally, the physician should not forget to consider and to let the patient/family be aware of the other possible complications of NIV, such as gastrodistension, eye irritation, pneumothorax, agitation, patient–ventilator asynchrony and haemodynamic instability that may further deteriorate the poor quality of life of CMO/DNI patients [30, 44]. It is important to emphasise that, presently, there is no convincing evidence that NIV will relieve symptoms in CMO patients. However, understanding the attitudes of physicians towards the goals of NIV and the length and the modality of its application in patients at the end of their life may be helpful.

In order to further understand the reasons for the palliative short-term use of NIV in patients with dyspnoea at the end of life, SINUFF et al. [7] reported that about half of the physicians aimed at providing time for patients and their families to come to terms with the patient's death, as well as allowing patients to get their personal affairs in order. Moreover, following an initial successful application of NIV for the acute management of ARF, two-thirds of physicians decided to continue NIV as long as the patient is comfortable, while almost three-quarters withdraw NIV without restarting if patients deteriorate and less than one-quarter did not discharge to home, NIV patients if they were unable to be weaned.

Another unexplored question is whether NIV is more effective than pharmacological therapies, such as opiates, in palliating symptoms. It is imperative that the patient can and must keep control over the decision to continue NIV. If discomfort related to the use of the mask exceeds the benefit, the patient may simply choose to discontinue NIV and their comfort should be achieved with drugs. The use of anticipated doses of opiates before withdrawing NIV at the end of life may be an option to achieve the higher level of patient comfort, similar to what was already reported with invasive mechanical ventilation [8]. The transition from mechanical support to an oxygen mask seems much simpler both ethically and technically with NIV than with invasive ventilation.

However, studies assessing patient comfort, and/or satisfaction of patients and their families, with NIV near or at the end of life are lacking. According to the SINUFF et al. [7], almost 60% of the physicians believed that NIV can provide two benefits in DNR patients: 1) an additive effect to analgesic and/or anxiolytics for the relief of dyspnoea; and 2) a facilitation of verbal communication with families and clinicians due to avoidance of intubation. Less than half of physicians agreed that NIV may provide these benefits in CMO patients.

Underlying respiratory diseases

The great amount of data is still limited to the use of NIV in the palliative care of end-stage respiratory patients with COPD. In addition to the epidemiological weight of this disease, this is due to the fact that NIV has become the first-line therapy in patients with severe exacerbation of COPD and decompensated respiratory acidosis [5].

Another area where ethical and decisional issues frequently arise for respiratory physicians is the management of patients with neuromuscular disease or neurological disorders which impair respiratory function [9, 45]. This is especially the case in Duchenne muscular dystrophy, motor neuron disease/amyotrophic lateral sclerosis and children with severe spinal atrophy, where respiratory complications produce the burdensome of symptoms and are the most common cause of death. Presently, a permanent restoration of health is not possible in these incurable and degenerative conditions but the general principle of beneficence suggests the physician should do all they can to palliate symptoms and maintain or even prolong a quality of life that is considered acceptable to the patient. Long-term home mechanical ventilation, included NIV in the early phases of neuromuscular diseases, has dramatically changed the prognosis of these patients by improving their survival and quality of life [46].

Despite the home ventilatory support, progressive neuromuscular diseases lead to a full dependence on mechanical ventilation and increased disability. Nearly all neuromuscular patients treated with home NIV choose to continue treatment even in the terminal phase of the disease [9, 45]. Although the noninvasive long term management of very advanced neuromuscular disorders has been successfully reported by very specialised teams in patients needing NIV 24 h·day^{-1} [47], the indication for tracheostomy and home invasive ventilation is almost unavoidable, especially in case of severe bulbar involvement and difficult removal of secretions.

A still unexplored and emerging clinical problem is the management of end-stage idiopathic pulmonary fibrosis and other progressive interstitial lung diseases, for which it is known that ARF occurs commonly, often as a terminal event after a prolonged course of illness and the outcome is really disappointing despite the use of invasive and noninvasive mechanical ventilation [48–52]. The potential role of NIV used for CMO in interstitial lung disease patients with ARF has yet to be fully investigated compared with standard medical and oxygen therapy, always presenting the balance between burden and usefulness for the patients.

Neoplastic diseases

The dilemma of the care in cancer patients with ARF

ARF is common in cancer patients. New types and modalities of chemotherapy and radiotherapy, circulating pluripotent haematopoietic cell grafts and bone marrow transplantation have contributed to the increase in successful treatment of solid and haematological malignancies. However, these regimens may predispose patients to various life-threatening complications, such as infection, haemorrhage, capillary leak syndrome, radiation toxicity or drug-related toxicity [53–55]. The lung is the target organ most frequently involved in these complications; BLOT et al. [56] showed that an episode of ARF is by far the most common reason for admitting a cancer patient to the ICU. The reasons leading to referral for intensive care appear quite familiar: pneumonia, followed by exacerbated COPD, pulmonary oedema and haemoptysis. Short-term mortality is mainly related to the severity of organ dysfunction and not to the characteristics of the malignancy [57]. The occurrence of ARF is often seen by oncologists as a terminal phase of the disease, based on studies reporting limited survival at considerable cost [58–64]. Alternatively, a large proportion of cancer patients with severe respiratory failure are denied admission to an ICU because the intensive care specialists are aware that intubation and mechanical ventilation are both strong predictors of mortality in critically ill cancer patients [54, 63, 65, 66]. Despite these problems, the ICU mortality rate of cancer patients has decreased dramatically in the last 20 yrs, and this is particularly true for those patients requiring mechanical ventilation [57].

Mechanical ventilation and prognosis of advanced cancer patients

The overall survival of cancer patients, admitted to the ICU, is still very disappointing, despite the fact that more recent studies have shown that mortality has now decreased below the threshold of 50%. Mortality in the subgroup of patients requiring mechanical ventilation is particularly high and, until the middle of the 1990s, averaged above 90% [58–64]; more recently there seems to have been a turning point, so that mortality in this subgroup is now ∼75–80% [54, 65, 66]. The overall decrease in ICU mortality in the last 5 yrs does, therefore, seem to be related to the improved prognosis of the patients requiring mechanical ventilation. Thus could be attributed to the following factors: 1) patients with poor functional status or patients with no life-prolonging treatment may be denied admission to the ICU; 2) earlier referral of cancer patients to the ICU for noninvasive diagnostic and therapeutic strategies, provided that these strategies do not delay intubation and optimal management; and 3) a better knowledge of certain complications that develop in critically ill patients with malignancies [4, 57]. In fact, among the variables recorded at ICU admission, only two have been shown to be independently associated with mortality and, quite surprisingly, they are not related to the type of cancer (i.e. solid or haematological malignancy) [56, 69].

The first independent predictor of mortality is, obviously, the severity of the patient's clinical condition on admission to the ICU which is recorded by various scores, such as SAPS I and SAPS II [67], APACHE II and APACHE III [68]. The second and "stronger" independent predictive factor of mortality is the need for mechanical ventilation. Despite the efforts made to prevent bacterial contamination of the patient/ventilator circuit, ventilator-associated pneumonia (VAP) and worsening of a pre-existing infection are still the major challenges in intubated patients [70]. The mortality risk may vary from 30 to 76% and is strictly dependent on the bacteria isolated; mortality among patients infected with aerobic Gram-negative bacteria being significantly higher than that among patients with Gram-positive bacteria.

Gram-positive and Gram-negative bacteria are evenly distributed among immuno-compromised cancer patients with pulmonary infiltrates, but fungal pathogens and viral agents are also well represented [53, 64]. The prognosis of these infected patients worsens significantly when respiratory failure occurs and mechanical ventilation is instituted. Despite adequate diagnostic evaluation and treatment in the ICU, the mortality remains so high that the benefit of mechanical ventilation has been seriously questioned; the ethics have also been questioned. This is especially true for bone-marrow transplant recipients [63]. In those patients who do survive, nosocomial pneumonia is responsible for a longer stay in hospital. An endotracheal tube can predispose to the development of pneumonia by impairing cough and mucociliary clearance; furthermore, contaminated secretions can accumulate above the cuff and leak around it and bacterial binding to the surface of bronchial epithelium is increased [70, 71]. Invasive ventilatory support also increases the risk of feeding aspiration. ELPERN et al. [72] showed that ~50% of tracheotomised patients receiving prolonged ventilation had feeding aspiration.

The role of NIV in cancer patients

Since the act of intubation and the institution of invasive mechanical ventilation have been shown to be among the two major determinants of survival in critically ill cancer patients [63, 65, 66, 69], it is important to understand what has changed in the field of mechanical ventilation in the last 5–10 yrs to explain the improvement in short-term survival in these patients.

It is entirely possible that new therapies, in particular for the treatment of infections (e.g. new antibiotics and anti-viral agents), new diagnostic procedures (e.g. diffusion of protected bronchoalveolar lavage), preventive measures (e.g. oro-tracheal intubation instead of naso-tracheal intubation, use of the semirecumbent position to avoid aspiration pneumonia), new ventilatory modes (e.g. low tidal volumes with protective hypercapnia), the development of clinical guidelines and, finally, better monitoring systems, may have led to a better outcome [57]. It is, however, unlikely that these factors alone have increased ICU survival three-fold in the last few years (from 10 to 30%).

AZOULAY et al. [69] retrospectively studied a cohort of patients with solid or haematological cancer admitted to the ICU for ARF. The first group of 132 patients was admitted in the period 1990–1995 and the second group, composed of 105 patients, was admitted in 1996–1998. The types of cancer were equally distributed among the two groups and were acute leukaemia and lymphoma (51%), myeloma (21%), and solid tumours (28%). The survival rate in the period 1996–1998 was significantly higher than that in the previous period (39 versus 18%, respectively; p=0.0003). Univariate analyses of the patients' characteristics, comorbidity and type of malignancy did not show that any of them (including neutropenia and bone-marrow transplant) were significantly associated with 30-day mortality. However, in the multivariate analysis two variables were found to predict ICU outcome: higher SAPS II score at admission was associated with an increased mortality rate, whereas the use of NIV during the 1996–1998 period was associated with a marked improvement in survival. In order to define the impact of NIV on better outcome, a pairwise-matched exposed–unexposed analysis was performed. A total of 48 patients, who received NIV as the first ventilation method, and 48 patients, who did not, were matched for SAPS II score, type of malignancy and period of ICU admission. Crude ICU mortality rates from those exposed to NIV and from the controls were 44 and 71%, respectively. NIV still had a protective effect against mortality after adjustment for matching variables. According to the risk of death attributable to mechanical ventilation, approximately four patients needed to receive NIV in order for one death is prevented.

The use of NIV to treat a severe episode of respiratory failure in acutely ill cancer patients is a new field of application, which is expanding very quickly given the very promising results obtained, particularly in the patients with haematological malignancies.

Between 30–40% of the patients with neutropenia may develop severe pulmonary infections and these are frequently fatal. Indeed, during the window period of immunodepression, patients may also be prone to developing other respiratory complications such as alveolar haemorrhage, capillary leak syndrome, radiation toxicity or drug-related toxicity [53–55].

Endotracheal intubation increases the mortality risk because of the greater possibility of developing new or superimposed infections, such as sinusitis and VAP [73]. The endotracheal tube bypasses the mechanical defenses of the upper airways and causes local damage. In addition, the portion of the trachea between the cuff and the vocal cords becomes a reservoir of secretions colonised by bacteria originating from the sinuses, the nasal passages, pharynx, oral cavity and the stomach. These infected secretions can be introduced into the lung with nursing manoeuvres [37], such as bronchoaspiration [74]. In this situation, NIV seems to be an interesting alternative due to the lower risk of complication [75]. The first attempts to apply NIV in immunocompromised patients, although not in those with haematological disorders, were made in the early 1990s by GREGG et al. [76] and later by GACHOT et al. [77] in patients with ARF due to Pneumocystis carinii infection. Both studies, although uncontrolled, concluded that continuous positive airway pressure (CPAP) delivered via a face mask was an effective supportive therapy in these acutely ill patients.

In 1992 TOGNET et al. [78] reported the first attempt to ventilate patients with haematological malignancies with NIV delivered via a face mask. They found that, for similar severity of disease and arterial oxygen tension (Pa,O_2)/inspired oxygen fraction (FI,O_2), the ICU mortality was significantly higher in the group of patients ventilated invasively than in those managed with NIV (100 and 55%, respectively).

In 1994, the first pioneering study performed in cancer patients was by MEDURI et al. [27]. In that observational investigation the authors applied NIV in a group of 15 patients in the terminal phase of their disease after these patients had refused consent to be intubated or had signed a DNI order. Two of these patients had ARF due to a haematological disorder and one due to lung cancer. Gas exchange and respiratory rate improved very rapidly after the application of NIV, and two of the three were discharged from the ICU a few days later. This highlighted, for the first time, that NIV may be used even in patients in whom endotracheal intubation is clinically or ethically questionable.

The first pilot, prospective study on the use of NIV in immunocompromised patients with haematological malignancies was performed in 1998. CONTI et al. [79] enrolled 16 consecutive patients with severe ARF (mean $Pa,O_2/FI,O_2$ of 87 ± 22) treated with pressure support ventilation (PSV) through a nasal mask. The criteria for intubation were predetermined. A total of 15 out of these 16 patients showed a significant improvement in arterial blood gases and respiratory rate within the first 24 h. In particular, Pa,O_2 increased in the first hour of ventilation from 43 ± 10 to 88 ± 37 mmHg. Five patients died in the ICU following complications independent of the respiratory failure (three septic shock, one gastrointestinal bleeding and one acute myocardial infarction) and 11 were discharged from the ICU in a stable condition after a mean stay of 4.3 ± 2.4 days. The authors concluded that NIV is feasible and may be a good choice for the treatment of a selected population of critically ill patients, who would otherwise have had a high probability of needing intubation.

HILBERT et al. [80], 2 yrs later, expanded the previous observation in a larger group of patients, using noninvasive CPAP. Over a 5-yr period the authors enrolled 64 patients presenting with febrile acute hypoxaemic ($Pa,O_2/FI,O_2$ of <200) respiratory failure and haematological malignancy. CPAP was administered for 6 h·day^{-1} in the first week of ICU admission. The respiratory rate decreased to <25 breaths·min^{-1} in the majority of the patients, while $Pa,O_2/FI,O_2$ increased from 128 ± 32 to 218 ± 28. Despite these favorable results, CPAP successfully avoided intubation in "only" 16 out of the 64 patients. Interestingly, all the responders survived the hospital stay whereas only four nonresponders did so. In the multivariate analysis, two variables were predictive of the failure of CPAP: the SAPS II score and liver failure at entry to the study.

The studies by CONTI et al. [79] and HILBERT et al. [80] gave, apparently, quite different success rates but the discrepancies in the results can be explained. First, the ventilatory techniques used were different, since CONTI et al. [79] employed PSV in combination with CPAP whereas HILBERT et al. [80] used CPAP alone. This latter strategy has been shown to be no more effective than oxygen therapy alone in treating an episode of hypoxaemic ARF [81], while in the same context PSV with CPAP was associated with a better clinical outcome than that produced by oxygen therapy [82]. Secondly, although the authors used different scores to assess the severity of their patients' conditions on admission (SAPS I and SAPS II, respectively), it is possible to extrapolate that, on average, the patients enrolled into the study by HILBERT et al. [80] were more severely ill.

A later study by HILBERT et al. [83] gave scientific dignity to NIV, partly because it was published in one of the most authoritative medical journals, the *New England Journal of Medicine*, and partly because of the very impressive clinical results. The authors conducted a prospective, randomised trial of intermittent NIV compared with standard treatment with supplemental oxygen and no ventilatory support, in 52 immunosuppressed patients with pulmonary infiltrates, fever and an early stage of hypoxaemic ARF ($Pa,O_2/FI,O_2$ ratio of <200). The large majority of the patients had a haematological malignancy and neutropenia or drug-induced immunosuppression. Periods of NIV delivered through a face mask were alternated every 3 h with periods of spontaneous breathing with supplemental oxygen. The decision to intubate was made according to standard, predetermined criteria. The main results of the study were that fewer patients in the NIV group than in the standard-treatment group required endotracheal intubation (12 *versus* 20, respectively; p=0.03), had serious complications (13 *versus* 21, respectively; p=0.02), died in the ICU (10 *versus* 18, respectively; p=0.03) or died in the hospital (13 *versus* 21, respectively; p=0.02). Overall, that study clearly showed that early implementation of NIV was associated with significant reduction in the rate of intubation, serious complications and death, in both the ICU and hospital.

A case–control study (34 patients) was performed to assess the efficacy of early administration of noninvasive CPAP delivered by face mask *versus* the newly developed interface, the helmet, in patients with haematological malignancies and fever, pulmonary infiltrates, and hypoxaemic ARF ($Pa,O_2/FI,O_2$ ratio of <200) [84]. Each patient was treated with CPAP outside the ICU in the haematology ward. The authors described the highest possible rates of success in the patients ventilated with the helmet. As a matter of fact, oxygenation improved in all patients after CPAP but, while no patient failed helmet CPAP because of intolerance, eight patients in the mask group did. Indeed, NIV could be applied continuously for a longer period of time in the helmet group (28.44 ± 0.20 *versus* 7.5 ± 0.45 h in the mask group). The most important conclusions from this study are that NIV can also be applied outside the ICU, at least in the early stage of ARF and only in selected population of patients [85]. Indeed, the helmet may be a feasible alternative to a face mask in case of intolerance. Great caution should be taken however in using a helmet in hypercapnic patients, since the risk of potential CO_2 rebreathing has not yet been completely elucidated [86].

Finally, a few comments should also be made on the use of NIV in cancer patients in the terminal phase of their disease or in those who expressly state that they do no want to be intubated under any circumstances. The large majority of studies in cancer patients are limited to patients affected by haematological cancers, while scant data are available from cases with solid tumours. This may be a field of great potential interest, since a subgroup of these patients may also be affected by comorbid conditions and, at some point, may develop acute failure of a specific organ, not necessarily related to the site of cancer. For example, a substantial number of cancer patients are, or were, smokers, frequently affected by chronic pulmonary or cardiac disease; thus, acute exacerbation of COPD or CPO, leading to ARF, are relatively common. Despite the fact that most of these episodes are promptly reversible if adequately treated, patients do not always receive ventilatory support, just because they "have cancer". For instance in most of the studies performed on NIV, malignancy is an exclusion criterion.

The present authors prospectively recruited 23 patients needing NIV with a pre-existing diagnosis of solid cancer. NIV was delivered with PSV plus CPAP [43]. The application of NIV was associated with a significant improvement in arterial blood gases and dyspnoea score after only 1 h of ventilation. The survival at 6 and 12 months was low, as expected. From this pilot study, it can be suggested that the use of NIV is feasible and associated with a reduction of dyspnoea in patients with ARF and a pre-existing solid tumour [43]. A very appealing goal of NIV in this kind of patients is to achieve a good control of the dyspnoea in addition to the traditional pharmacological therapy. The preliminary results of a recent multicentre RCT [87] performed in advanced solid cancer patients showed that, compared with only oxygen and medical therapy, the adjunct of NIV may reduce the amount of the needed doses of opiates and, therefore, their side effects, such as the depressed level of sensorium. This may mean a better capability of communication for the patient at the end of their life, with a good control of symptoms.

The location for the palliative use of NIV

The choice of the setting in which to perform NIV should be made carefully in order to balance the severity of ARF and the intensity of care needed together with the optimisation of the limited economical resources of health national systems [88].

Whatever environment is established to apply NIV, the experience of the team (medical doctors, RTs, nurses) needs to be adequate to the severity of the acute illness. The more the team is experienced in NIV, the greater the severity of the ARF that can be managed [89], provided that the switch from noninvasive to invasive ventilation may be done very quickly in patients who do not refuse advanced life-sustaining measures. Last but not least, ethical and palliative issues should be taken in account in the assignment of an acute patient to a specific setting [5, 7].

While the use of NIV in ARF patients, without preset limitation on life sustaining treatment, should be reserved for intensive care units, respiratory high-dependency units or the step-down setting with well-trained staff and adequate monitoring, where the transition to invasive ventilation is available if noninvasive ventilation fails; the ideal palliative care of patients belonging to category 2 and 3 is likely to be more appropriate outside the intensive care unit. In fact, for these categories, the failure of noninvasive ventilation requires rapid intensification of comfort measures only, which could be more adequately performed in totally or partially "open" environments, such as respiratory high-dependency units or respiratory/general wards, with the help of the member of the family [5]. However, the same monitoring and alarm system required for category 1 patients should also be in place for patients from categories 2 and 3, to be sure that they are comfortable and at the same time to quickly identify patients for whom NIV is no longer helpful. The hospice setting may be an appropriate setting for category 3 patients provided that the staff and the family are well trained even if it has not been proved. It must be underlined that in a setting in which clinicians are unfamiliar with NIV the chance of benefit is low and there is the risk of increasing discomfort and stress at the end of life [7].

Summary

As pulmonary physicians, especially those dealing with mechanical ventilation, we are facing the problem of withholding and withdrawing life support in terminally ill patients affected by acute or chronic respiratory disorders every day.

The overall incidence of these practices in Europe is only partially known and, even more importantly, it has been shown that there are important differences between countries or regions, reflecting the absence of a common strategy even within the European Community.

The "shared decision" taken together by physicians, nurses and the patient's family may be the best approach to these decisions. There is good evidence that noninvasive ventilation (NIV) may be used in terminally ill patients with different objectives, such as: 1) life support with no preset limitations on life-sustaining treatment; 2) life support when the patients decided to forego intubation (DNI); and 3) a "pure" palliative measure. Up to 30% of end-stage chronic respiratory patients are receiving NIV in the last days of life, solely to relieve dyspnoea, and this "ceiling" practice has also been applied to end-stage cancer patients. About 50% of DNI patients with acute respiratory failure may also be successfully treated and discharged from the hospital, mainly if affected by chronic obstructive pulmonary disease or chronic heart failure. The success of NIV is strictly dependent on the experience of the staff involved, and the patients should be allowed to withdraw from the treatment in every instance.

Keywords: Acute respiratory failure, cancer, chronic obstructive pulmonary disease, dyspnoea, intubation, noninvasive ventilation.

References

1. Wilt TJ, Niewoehner D, MacDonald R, Kane RL. Management of stable chronic obstructive pulmonary disease: a systematic review for a clinical practice guideline. *Ann Intern Med* 2007; 147: 639–653.
2. Lynn J, Ely EW, Zhong Z, *et al.* Living and dying with chronic obstructive pulmonary disease. *J Am Geriatr Soc* 2000; 48: Suppl. 5, S91–S100.
3. Claessens MT, Lynn J, Zhong Z, *et al.* Dying with lung cancer or chronic obstructive pulmonary disease: insights from SUPPORT. Study to Understand Prognoses and Preferences for Outcomes and Risks of Treatments. *J Am Geriatr Soc* 2000; 48: Suppl. 5, S146–S153.
4. Adam AK, Soubani AO. Outcome and prognostic factors of lung cancer patients admitted to the medical intensive care unit. *Eur Respir J* 2008; 31: 47–53.
5. Curtis JR, Cook DJ, Sinuff T, *et al.* Noninvasive positive pressure ventilation in critical and palliative care settings: understanding the goals of therapy. *Crit Care Med* 2007; 35: 932–939.
6. Hill NS, Brennan J, Garpestad E, Nava S. Noninvasive ventilation in acute respiratory failure. *Crit Care Med* 2007; 35: 2402–2407.
7. Sinuff T, Cook DJ, Keenan SP, *et al.* Noninvasive ventilation for acute respiratory failure near the end of life. *Crit Care Med* 2008; 36: 789–794.
8. Truog RD, Campbell ML, Curtis JR, *et al.* Recommendations for end-of-life care in the intensive care unit: A consensus statement by the American Academy of Critical Care Medicine. *Crit Care Med* 2008; 36: 953–963.
9. Simonds AK. Ethics and decision making in end stage lung disease. *Thorax* 2003; 58: 272–277.
10. Sprung CL, Cohen SL, Sjokvist P, *et al.* End-of-life practices in European intensive care units: the Ethicus Study. *JAMA* 2003; 290: 790–797.
11. Nava S, Sturani C, Hartl S, *et al.* End-of-life decision-making in respiratory intermediate care units: a European survey. *Eur Respir J* 2007; 30: 156–164.
12. Prendergast TJ, Claessens MT, Luce JM. A national survey of end-of-life care for critically ill patients. *Am J Respir Crit Care Med* 1998; 158: 1163–1167.
13. Yaguchi A, Truog RD, Curtis JR, *et al.* International differences in end-of-life attitudes in the intensive care unit: results of a survey. *Arch Intern Med* 2005; 165: 1970–1975.
14. van der Heide A, Deliens L, Faisst K, *et al.* End-of-life decision-making in six European countries: descriptive study. *Lancet* 2003; 362: 435–440.
15. Foley KM. How much palliative care do we need? *Eur J Palliat Care* 2003; 10: Suppl., 5–6.
16. Ferrand E, Robert R, Ingrand P, Lemaire F, French LATAREA Group. Withholding and withdrawal of life support in intensive-care units in France: a prospective survey. French LATAREA Group. *Lancet* 2001; 357: 9–14.
17. Cook D, Rocker G, Marshall J, *et al.* Withdrawal of mechanical ventilation in anticipation of death in the intensive care unit. *N Engl J Med* 2003; 349: 1123–1132.
18. Dales RE, O'Connor A, Hebert P, Sullivan K, McKim D, Llewellyn-Thomas H. Intubation and mechanical ventilation for COPD: development of an instrument to elicit patient preferences. *Chest* 1999; 116: 792–800.
19. Kompanje EJO. Care for the dying in intensive care in the Netherlands. *Intensive Care Med* 2006; 32: 2067–2069.
20. Vincent JL. End-of-life practice in Belgium and the new euthanasia law. *Intensive Care Med* 2006; 32: 1908–1911.
21. Zamperetti N, Proietti R. End of life in the ICU: laws, rules and practices: the situation in Italy. *Intensive Care Med* 2006; 32: 1620–1622.
22. Abbott KH, Sago JG, Breen CM, Abernethy AP, Tulsky JA. Families looking back: one year after discussion of withdrawal or withholding of life-sustaining support. *Crit Care Med* 2001; 29: 197–201.

23. Fried TR, Bradley EH, Towle VR, Allore H. Understanding the treatment preferences of seriously ill patients. *N Engl J Med* 2002; 346: 1061–1066.

24. Nava S, Santoro C, Grassi M, Hill N. The influence of the media on patients' knowledge regarding cardiopulmonary resuscitation. *Int J Chron Obstruct Pulmon Dis* 2008; 3: 295–300.

25. Wildman MJ, Sanderson C, Groves J, *et al.* Implications of prognostic pessimism in patients with chronic obstructive pulmonary disease or asthma admitted to intensive care in the UK within the COPD and asthma outcome study: multicentre observational cohort study. *BMJ* 2007; 335: 1132–1135.

26. Benhamou D, Girault C, Faure C, Portier F, Muir JF. Nasal mask ventilation in acute respiratory failure. Experience in elderly patients. *Chest* 1992; 102: 912–917.

27. Meduri GU, Fox RC, Abou-Shala N, Leeper KV, Wunderink RG. Noninvasive mechanical ventilation *via* face mask in patients with acute respiratory failure who refused endotracheal intubation. *Crit Care Med* 1994; 22: 1584–1590.

28. Levy M, Tanios MA, Nelson D, *et al.* Outcomes of patients with do-not-intubate orders treated with noninvasive ventilation. *Crit Care Med* 2004; 32: 2002–2007.

29. Chu CM, Chan VL, Wong IW, Leung WS, Lin AW, Cheung KF. Noninvasive ventilation in patients with acute hypercapnic exacerbation of chronic obstructive pulmonary disease who refused endotracheal intubation. *Crit Care Med* 2004; 32: 372–377.

30. Schettino G, Altobelli N, Kacmarek RM. Noninvasive positive pressure ventilation reverses acute respiratory failure in select "do-not-intubate" patients. *Crit Care Med* 2005; 33: 1976–1982.

31. Fernandez R, Baigorri F, Artigas A. Noninvasive ventilation in patients with "do-not-intubate" orders: medium-term efficacy depends critically on patient selection. *Intensive Care Med* 2007; 33: 350–354.

32. Corrado A, Roussos C, Ambrosino N, *et al.* Respiratory intermediate care units: a European survey. *Eur Respir J* 2002; 20: 1343–1350.

33. Freichels T. Palliative ventilatory support: use of noninvasive pressure support ventilation in terminal respiratory insufficiency. *Am J Crit Care* 1994; 3: 6–10.

34. Clarke DE, Vaughan L, Raffin TA. Noninvasive positive pressure ventilation for patients with terminal respiratory failure: the ethical and economic costs of delaying the inevitable are too great. *Am J Crit Care* 1994; 3: 4–5.

35. Crausman RS. Patient-centered ventilation. *Chest* 1998; 113: 844–845.

36. International Consensus Conferences in Intensive Care Medicine: noninvasive positive pressure ventilation in acute respiratory failure. *Am J Respir Crit Care Med* 2001; 163: 283–291.

37. Scala R, Nava S, Conti G, *et al.* Noninvasive versus conventional ventilation to treat hypercapnic encephalopathy in chronic obstructive pulmonary disease. *Intensive Care Med* 2007; 33: 2101–2108.

38. Steinhauser KE, Christakis NA, Clipp EC, McNeilly M, McIntyre L, Tulsky JA. Factors considered important at the end of life by patients, family, physicians, and other care providers. *JAMA* 2000; 284: 2476–2482.

39. Back AL, Arnold RM, Quill TE. Hope for the best, and prepare for the worst. *Ann Int Med* 2003; 138: 439–443.

40. Bott J, Carroll MP, Conway JH, *et al.* Randomized controlled trial of nasal ventilation in acute ventilatory failure due to chronic obstructive airways disease. *Lancet* 1993; 341: 1555–1557.

41. Plant PK, Owen JL, Elliott MW. Early use of non-invasive ventilation for acute exacerbations of chronic obstructive pulmonary disease on general respiratory wards: a multicentre randomised controlled trial. *Lancet* 2000; 355: 1931–1935.

42. Angus RM, Ahmed AA, Fenwick LJ, Peacock AJ. Comparison of the acute effects on gas exchange of nasal ventilation and doxapram in exacerbations of chronic obstructive pulmonary disease. *Thorax* 1996; 51: 1048–1050.

43. Cuomo A, Delmastro M, Ceriana P, *et al.* Noninvasive mechanical ventilation as a palliative treatment of acute respiratory failure in patients with end-stage solid cancer. *Palliat Med* 2004; 18: 602–610.

44. Mehta S, Hill NS. Noninvasive ventilation. *Am J Respir Crit Care Med* 2001; 163: 540–577.

45. Polkey MI, Lyall RA, Davidson AC, Leigh PN, Moxham J. Ethical and clinical issues in the use of home non-invasive mechanical ventilation for the palliation of breathlessness in motor neurone disease. *Thorax* 1999; 54: 367–371.

46. Hess DR. Noninvasive ventilation in neuromuscular disease: equipment and application. *Respir Care* 2006; 51: 896–911.

47. Bach JR. Continuous noninvasive ventilation for patients with neuromuscular disease and spinal cord injury. *Semin Respir Crit Care Med* 2002; 23: 283–92.

48. Stern JB, Mal H, Groussard O, *et al.* Prognosis of patients with advanced idiopathic pulmonary fibrosis requiring mechanical ventilation for acute respiratory failure. *Chest* 2001; 120: 213–219.

49. Blivet S, Philit F, Sab JM, *et al.* Outcome of patients with idiopathic pulmonary fibrosis admitted to the ICU for respiratory failure. *Chest* 2001; 120: 209–212.

50. Fumeaux T, Rothmeier C, Jolliet P. Outcome of mechanical ventilation for acute respiratory failure in patients with pulmonary fibrosis. *Intensive Care Med* 2001; 27: 1868–1874.

51. Saydain G, Islam A, Afessa B, Ryu JH, Scott JP, Peters SG. Outcome of patients with idiopathic pulmonary fibrosis admitted to the intensive care unit. *Am J Respir Crit Care Med* 2002; 166: 839–842.

52. Collard HR, Moore BB, Flaherty KR, *et al.* Acute exacerbations of idiopathic pulmonary fibrosis. *Am J Respir Crit Care Med* 2007; 176: 636–643.

53. Ewig S, Torres A, Riquelme R, *et al.* Pulmonary complications in patients with haematological malignancies treated at a respiratory ICU. *Eur Respir J* 1988; 12: 116–122.

54. Kress JP, Christenson J, Pohlman AS, Linkin DR, Hall JB. Outcomes of critically ill cancer patients in a university hospital setting. *Am J Respir Crit Care Med* 1999; 160: 1957–1961.

55. Chaflin DB, Carlon GC. Age and utilization of ICU resources of critically ill cancer patients. *Crit Care Med* 1990; 18: 694–698.

56. Blot F, Guiget M, Nitenberg G, Laeclercq B, Gachot B, Escudier B. Prognostic factors for neutropenic patients in an ICU: respective roles of underlying malignancies and acute organ failure. *Eur J Cancer* 1997; 33: 1031–1037.

57. Schönfeld N, Timsit JF. Overcoming a stigma: the lung cancer patient in the intensive care unit. *Eur Respir J* 2008; 31: 3–5.

58. Torrecilla C, Cortes JL, Chamorro C. Prognosis assessment of the acute complications of bone marrow transplantation requiring intensive therapy. *Intensive Care Med* 1988; 14: 393–398.

59. Crawford SW, Schartz DA, Petersen FB, Clark JC. Mechanical ventilation after marrow transplanatation. Risk factors and clinical outcome. *Am Rev Respir Dis* 1988; 137: 682–687.

60. Afessa B, Tefferi A, Hoagland HC, Letendre L, Peters SG. Outcome of recipients of bone marrow transplant who require intensive-care unit support. *Mayo Clinic Proc* 1992; 67: 117–122.

61. Crawford SW, Petersen FB. Long-term survival from respiratory failure after marrow transplantation for malignancy. *Am Rev Respir Dis* 1992; 145: 510–514.

62. Faber-Langendoen K, Kaplan AL, McGlave PB. Survival of adult bone marrow transplant patients receiving mechanical ventilation: a case for restricted use. *Bone Marrow Transplant* 1993; 12: 501–507.

63. Rubenfeld GD, Crawford SW. Withdrawing life support from mechanically ventilated recipients of bone marrow transplant: a case for evidence-based guidelines. *Ann Intern Med* 1996; 125: 625–633.

64. Ewig S, Glasmacher A, Ulrich B, Wilhelm K, Schafer H, Nachtsheim KH. Pulmonary infiltrates in neutropenic patients with acute leukaemia during chemotherapy. Outcome and prognostic factors. *Chest* 1998; 114: 444–451.

65. Groeger JS, Lomeshow S, Price K, *et al.* Multicenter outcome study of cancer patients admitted to the ICU: a probability of mortality model. *J Clinic Oncol* 1998; 17: 991–997.

66. Kroschinsky F, Weise M, Illmer T, *et al.* Outcome and prognostic features of ICU treatment in patients with haematological malignancies. *Intensive Care Med* 2002; 28: 1294–1300.

67. Le Gall JR, Lemeshow S, Saulnier F. A new Simplified Acute Physiology Score (SAPS II) based on a European/North American multicenter study. *JAMA* 1993; 270: 2957–2963.

68. Johnson MH, Gordon PW, Fitzerald FT. Stratification of prognosis in granulocytopenic patients with haematological malignancies using APACHE II severity of illness score. *Crit Care Med* 1986; 14: 693–697.

69. Azoulay E, Alberti C, Bornstain C, *et al.* Improved survival in cancer patients requiring mechanical ventilatory support: impact of noninvasive mechanical ventilatory support. *Crit Care Med* 2001; 29: 519–552.

70. American Thoracic Society; Infectious Diseases Society of America. Guidelines for the management of adults with hospital-acquired, ventilator-associated, and healthcare-associated pneumonia. *Am J Respir Crit Care Med* 2005; 171: 388–416.

71. Craven DE, Steger KA. Nosocomial pneumonia in intubated patients: new concepts on pathogenesis and prevention. *Surg Clin North Am* 1989; 3: 843–866.

72. Elpern EH, Scott MG, Petro L, Ries MH. Pulmonary aspiration in mechanically ventilated patients with tracheostomies. *Chest* 1994; 105: 563–566.

73. Fagon JY, Chastre J, Domart Y, *et al.* Nosocomial pneumonia in patients receiving continuous mechanical ventilation. Prospective analysis of 52 episodes with use of protected specimen brush and quantitative culture techniques. *Am Rev Respir Dis* 1989; 139: 877–884.

74. Elpern EH, Scott MG, Petro L, Ries MH. Pulmonary aspiration in mechanically ventilated patients with tracheostomies. *Chest* 1994; 105: 563–566.

75. Hess DR. The evidence for noninvasive positive-pressure ventilation in the care of patients in acute respiratory failure: a systematic review of the literature. *Respir Care* 2004; 49: 810–829.

76. Gregg RW, Friedman BC, Williams JF, McGrath BJ, Zimmerman JE. Continuous positive airway pressure by face mask in *Pneumocystis carinii* pneumonia. *Crit Care Med* 1990; 18: 21–24.

77. Gachot B, Clair B, Wolff M, Reigner B, Vachon F. Continuous positive airway pressure administered by face mask or mechanical ventilation in patients with immunodeficiency virus infection and severe *Pneumocystis carinii* pneumonia. *Intensive Care Med* 1992; 18: 155–159.

78. Tognet E, Mercatello A, Polo P, *et al.* Treatment of acute respiratory failure with non-invasive intermittent positive pressure ventilation in haematological patients. *Clin Intensive Care* 1994; 5: 282–288.

79. Conti G, Marino P, Cogliati A, *et al.* Noninvasive ventilation for treatment of acute respiratory failure in patients with haematological malignancies: a pilot study. *Intensive Care Med* 1998; 24: 1283–1288.

80. Hilbert G, Gruson D, Vargas F, *et al.* Noninvasive continuous positive airway pressure in neutropenic patients with acute respiratory failure requiring ICU admission. *Crit Care Med* 2000; 28: 3185–3190.

81. Delclaux C, L'Her E, Alberti C, *et al.* Treatment of acute hypoxemic nonhypercapnic respiratory insufficiency with continuous positive airway pressure delivered by a face mask. A randomized controlled trial. *JAMA* 2002; 284: 2352–2360.

82. Ferrer M, Esquinas A, Leon M, Gonzalez G, Alarcon A, Torres A. Non-invasive ventilation in severe hypoxemic respiratory failure: a randomized clinical trial. *Am J Respir Crit Care Med* 2003; 168: 1438–1444.

83. Hilbert G, Gruson D, Vargas F, *et al.* Noninvasive ventilation in immunodepressed patients with pulmonary infiltrates, fever and acute respiratory failure. *N Engl J Med* 2001; 344: 481–487.

84. Principi T, Pantanetti S, Catani F, *et al.* Noninvasive continuous positive airway pressure delivered by helmet in hematological malignancy patients with hypoxemic acute respiratory failure. *Intensive Care Med* 2004; 30: 147–150.

85. Hill NS. Noninvasive ventilation for immunocompromised patients. *N Engl J Med* 2001; 344: 522–524.

86. Navalesi P, Costa R, Ceriana P, *et al.* Non-invasive ventilation in chronic obstructive pulmonary disease patients: helmet *versus* facial mask. *Intensive Care Med* 2007; 33: 74–81.

87. Nava S, Esquinas A, Ferrer M, *et al.* Multicenter, randomised study of the use of non-invasive ventilation (NIV) vs oxygen therapy (O_2) in reducing dyspnea in end-stage solid cancer patients with respiratory failure and distress. *Eur Respir J* 2007; 30: Suppl. 51, 204s.

88. Elliott MW, Confalonieri M, Nava S. Where to perform noninvasive ventilation? *Eur Respir J* 2002; 19: 1159–1166.

89. Carlucci A, Delmastro M, Rubini F, Fracchia C, Nava S. Changes in the practice of non-invasive ventilation in treating COPD patients over 8 years. *Intensive Care Med* 2003; 29: 419–425.

CHAPTER 21

Domiciliary ventilators: from bench to bedside

L. Vignaux*, J-P. Janssens#, P. Jolliet*

*Service des soins intensifs and #Service de Pneumologie, Hôpitaux Universitaires de Genève, Geneva, Switzerland.

Correspondence: P. Jolliet, Service des soins intensifs, Hôpital Cantonal Universitaire, 1211 Geneva 14, Switzerland. Fax: 41 223729105; E-mail: jolliet@medecine.unige.ch

Introduction

The number of patients receiving long-term home ventilation for a variety of diseases causing chronic respiratory insufficiency is steadily increasing [1, 2]. In part, this has been made possible by the major technological developments resulting in the availability of compact, quiet, high-performance home ventilators [3, 4], as well as the creation of a robust technical-support infrastructure [5, 6]. Over the last decade, domiciliary ventilators have gained in power, sophistication and available options. However, the wide spectrum of this offer does not necessarily make choosing a machine easier for clinicians, especially given the cost constraints that are nowadays ubiquitous in healthcare systems. Furthermore, sophistication can lead to the user interface being very complex, making rapid setting changes difficult.

Bench testing can provide useful insights into this problem, by confronting the machines to various abnormal respiratory mechanics and intensity of inspiratory effort, thereby comparing their performances [3, 4, 7] and testing their user friendliness [8]. Nonetheless, the results of bench testing cannot be directly extrapolated to patients, as the clinical relevance of bench test results must be evaluated in the clinical setting. Therefore, clinical and pathophysiological studies must also be conducted to verify bench findings.

In the present chapter, the available data from various bench model studies of domiciliary ventilators is reviewed and the data in discussed in the context of the results of relevant clinical trials.

Domiciliary ventilators: lessons from the bench

Bench testing of ventilators pursues two goals. First, to evaluate the performance of a machine by simulating various situations that it is likely to face in the clinical setting, such as abnormal respiratory mechanics, severe leaks and high ventilatory demand. Secondly, in order to compare these performances with those of other ventilators available on the market, thereby helping the clinician in choosing the most appropriate machine for a given patient's ventilatory support needs. Naturally, bench models can only provide a partial model of the complex situation of real-life patients and their results should always be interpreted with this caveat in mind.

Eur Respir Mon, 2008, 41, 307–318. Printed in UK - all rights reserved. Copyright ERS Journals Ltd 2008; European Respiratory Monograph; ISSN 1025-448x.

Testing performance: the ventilatory cycle

The most logical approach to bench testing is to evaluate the different phases of a typical positive-pressure ventilatory cycle in terms of patient–ventilator interaction [9], given that optimal synchrony is essential in obtaining proper tolerance to noninvasive ventilation (NIV). Each ventilatory cycle comprises four key phases (fig. 1): triggering, pressurisation, cycling and expiration, which will now be examined in the light of the presently available data.

Triggering. The inspiratory trigger should be sensitive enough to allow easy triggering by the patient, without autotriggering, and have a short delay between the onset of patient inspiratory effort and pressurisation by the ventilator (known as "trigger delay"). Ideally, trigger delay should be <100 ms, since higher values can be perceived by the patient and lead to discomfort [10].

Regarding sensitivity, although differences exist among machines, all bilevel devices generally require very little triggering effort [3]. The inspiratory trigger level is adjustable most of the time, but the adjustment is most often done with arbitrary units. During NIV, leaks lead to autotriggering because they generate a flow which mimics that which is generated by the patient's inspiratory effort.

Bench test performances are heterogeneous among domiciliary ventilators. Although some machines rapidly trigger into inspiration (<100 ms), others take considerably longer, sometimes up to 500 ms [3, 11, 12]. In general, ventilators based on pressure triggering have higher trigger delays. Ventilators based on the flow waveform method of triggering (BiPAP® Vision, Synchrony® and Harmony® BPPV ventilators; Respironics, Murrysville, PA, USA) have the shortest trigger delays [12]. However, this approach sometimes leads to a greater occurrence of autotriggering [13]. Leaks can also increase the trigger delay [14].

Trigger delay also increases with obstructive conditions, although not to a great extent [12]. Finally, in a recent study evaluating performances of 17 ventilators available for home ventilation in France with the most common "paediatric profiles" (neuromuscular disease, upper airway obstruction and cystic fibrosis), triggering performances showed a great variability and depended on the type of trigger (flow or pressure), the type of circuit (simple or double), the patient profile and the presence of leaks [15]. No single ventilator was able to ventilate all the profiles. A total of 12

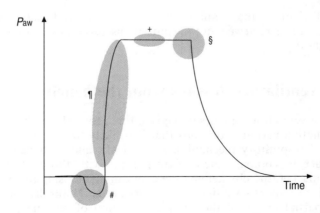

Fig. 1. – Key phases of a typical pressure support cycle. *P*aw: airway pressure. #: trigger; ¶: pressurisation; +: level of pressure support; §: cycling.

ventilators had a trigger delay <150 ms for less than two profiles and only one ventilator for three profiles. In all other cases, the trigger was "inappropriate", meaning that ineffective efforts or autotriggering were present.

Pressurisation. During this phase, inspiratory flow should be sufficient to match inspiratory demand. The matching depends on ventilator performance, pressure support level, pressurisation slope and inspiratory effort level. Leaks, unavoidable during NIV, and high inspiratory effort can impair pressurisation [11, 16, 17].

In a study by BATTISTI *et al.* [3], major differences were found between bilevel devices in terms of pressurisation performance, especially when a high inspiratory demand was present (fig. 2). During pressure-target ventilation, delivered tidal volume (VT) differs substantially between ventilators despite similar adjustments, even in the absence of leaks [18]. These differences are related to variability in inspiratory flow rates, actual pressure delivered and inspiratory duration. The possibility of increasing inspiratory time ("timed (T) mode") on bilevel devices allows insufflation of a higher VT, despite the presence of leaks [17, 18].

Ventilators using volume-target modes deliver the expected volumes fairly accurately; however, in the presence of leaks, airway pressure decreases and delivered volume is reduced. A fall of 50% of the VT has been observed in such ventilators [18]. However, leak compensation differs considerably between the volume-target modes, according to the machine's ability to increase the inspiratory flow rate [18]. With a small or large leak, VT was better maintained by the pressure target modes. This was shown in a study by HIGHCOCK *et al.* [11], testing four bilevel devices in the presence of leaks; the fall in delivered VT was <10%.

Cycling. During ventilatory cycles triggered by the patient ("spontaneous (S) mode" or "spontaneous/timed (S/T) mode" in bilevel pressure support) cycling occurs as the inspiratory flow decreases to a pre-adjusted percentage of the peak inspiratory flow. This cycling criterion is termed "expiratory trigger" (ET) [19]. Ideally, cycling should coincide with the end of the patient's inspiratory effort. However, synchronisation between the latter and the ventilator's ET is mainly determined by respiratory mechanics [20]. Obstructive respiratory mechanics lead to a late cycling [21] and restrictive

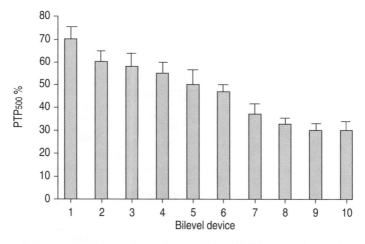

Fig. 2. – Bench model evaluation of the pressurisation capacity of 10 bilevel ventilators. Data are presented as mean±SD % of ideal pressurisation measured 500 ms after onset of ventilator cycle (PTP500 %). Modified from [3].

respiratory mechanics to a premature one [20]. Equally, if not more importantly, during NIV, leaks delay the decrease of the inspiratory flow, leading to a late cycling [22].

Cycling varies markedly among devices, being strongly influenced by the ET used (fig. 3). In the absence of leaks, bilevel devices with "default" ET tend to cycle prematurely with normal and restrictive respiratory mechanics and to exhibit delayed cycling in obstructive respiratory mechanics conditions [3]. As expected, leaks increase in the magnitude of delayed cycling on most machines [3]. Modifying the ET, if possible, allows improvements in both premature and delayed cycling.

The automatic cycling based on the flow waveform method of triggering implemented on an intensive care unit (ICU) ventilator allows for a better cycling despite the presence of leaks than the traditional default 25% of peak flow [14]. Another possible solution is the adjustment of the inspiratory time (T mode).

Expiration. On domiciliary ventilators a single limb circuit is often used, entailing the risk of carbon dioxide rebreathing, which in turn increases work of breathing. A solution to avoid carbon dioxide rebreathing is the fitting of a calibrated leak valve [23] and the maintenance of a minimum mandatory end-expiratory pressure level, known as expiratory positive airway pressure (EPAP; usually 4 cmH$_2$O). The continuous high-level flow which generates EPAP thereby maintains a leak through the calibrated valve, allowing improved carbon dioxide washout [23]. The use of specific valves has been shown to add to the total expiratory resistance of the circuit, although the clinical relevance of this finding remains uncertain [23]. LOFASO *et al.* [24] showed that considerable differences existed between available models, potentially leading to worsening dynamic hyperinflation.

User-friendliness

Over the years, research on the interaction between caregivers and the machines they use has shown that more attention should be given to this topic [25, 26]. Indeed, in order

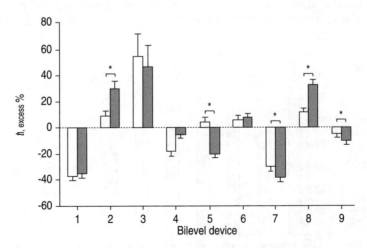

Fig. 3. – Bench model measurement of cycling of nine bilevel ventilators. Data are presented as excess inspiratory time (*t*I,excess) expressed as mean ± SD percentage of patient inspiratory time. Positive values indicate delayed cycling, negative values indicate premature cycling. □: baseline conditions, with the standard leak of the calibrated expiratory valve. ■: presence of a major added leak designed to mimic leaks at the patient–ventilator interface. *: p<0.05 *versus* baseline.

to properly set a ventilator, especially if major asynchrony develops, patient safety depends on a rapid and efficient intervention by the caregiver. Such an intervention not only depends on whether or not that person is familiar with the device but also on the ease with which alarms can be understood, problems identified and settings changed. Therefore, the ergonomics of domiciliary ventilators should be part of their global bench testing, as the benefits derived from good performance can sometimes be outweighed by a confusing, error-prone and time-consuming user interface. So far, only one such study has been performed on these devices. GONZALEZ-BERMEJO et al. [8] evaluated the user-friendliness of 11 home ventilators. The authors asked ICU physicians, experienced in mechanical ventilation but not with the tested devices, to perform a series of standardised tasks (e.g. switching on, unlocking, mode recognition and change). Any action taking longer than 3 min was considered to have failed. Overall, their results showed that major differences between machines existed, with long and potentially dangerous delays necessary to accomplish even the most-simple tasks. Some of the tasks could not even be accomplished in the 3-min allocated time [8]. These findings underline the need for better standardisation of machine–user interfaces and more in-depth research of the ergonomics of user–ventilator interaction. This type of research and development should involve end users early in the development of domiciliary ventilators.

From bench to bedside

Although bench tests can provide valuable data on the performance of domiciliary ventilators, the clinical relevance of these findings is not always obvious. Indeed, the main challenge for the clinician is not necessarily to choose the most powerful machine in terms of pressurisation, but the one which best fits a given patient's needs. Further complicating the issue is the increasing sophistication of home care ventilators, with numerous options and settings that clearly warrant independent clinical and physiological validation. In this section, data from the bench will be discussed in the context of those from clinical trials.

As a preliminary comment, one should note that, although wide differences exist between available options (inspiratory and expiratory trigger adjustment, pressurisation rate or rise time, volume targeting) and performances of ventilators designed for home care [3], there are, to date, no formal recommendations as to the choice of ventilators in national or international guidelines (i.e. volume- or pressure-cycled) or the use of specific options (i.e. volume targeting). Optimal ventilator settings in chronic respiratory failure are also poorly defined and left to the appreciation of the clinician and patient.

Volume- or pressure-cycled ventilator type: the situation in Europe

Customs and practices in relation to home mechanical ventilation (HMV) in Europe have been recently reported on the basis of a large survey performed in 16 European countries [2]: 329 centres reported data on 21,526 patients. Almost all HMV users had positive pressure ventilators. Volume-cycled ventilators were used most frequently for neurological problems (airway diseases: 15%; chest wall deformities and obesity-hypoventilation: 28%; and neuromuscular diseases: 41%). The percentage of pressure-cycled ventilators varied widely from one country to another, ranging from ~50% (Belgium, Spain, the Netherlands) to >90% (Portugal, UK, Ireland) [2]. A Swiss survey performed in the Geneva lake area [1] showed that there was a clear trend over a 7-yr observation period (1992–2000) for an increasing use of bilevel positive pressure ventilation (BPPV) and an increasingly marginal use of volume-cycled ventilators in all indications. As in the Eurovent survey, volume-cycled ventilators were used more frequently in patients with neuromuscular or chest wall disorders, while BPPV was almost exclusively used in chronic obstructive pulmonary disease (COPD) and obesity-hypoventilation syndrome (OHS).

Volume- or pressure-cycled ventilators: clinical trials

Up to the end of the 1980s, noninvasive positive pressure ventilation (NPPV) was delivered through volumetric ventilators only. The first studies of the BiPAP®, were published in 1990 [27, 28]. In the early 1990s, several short-term studies demonstrated the efficacy of the BiPAP® as a mode of positive pressure ventilation: the BiPAP® was capable of markedly decreasing the electromyographic activity of the diaphragm, thereby reducing respiratory muscle workload [29–31]. Reports of the long-term use of either barometric and volumetric ventilators, or barometric ventilators alone appeared as of 1995 [28, 32–36]. When mentioned, the choice of a volumetric versus barometric ventilator by the investigators was determined mainly by the patients' degree of comfort with each ventilator [32–34].

There are a few clinical comparative studies comparing volumetric and barometric ventilators in chronic respiratory failure. In a short-term study, MEECHAM-JONES and WEDZICHA [35] compared the efficacy and the acceptability of two barometric ventilators (BiPAP®; Respironics, Murrysville, PA, USA; and NIPPY®; B&D Electromedical, Strafford upon Avon, UK), and two volumetric ventilators (BromptonPac®; PnevmoPac Ltd, Luton, UK, and Monnal D®; AirLiquide Santé, Paris, France) in patients with stable chronic respiratory failure, who had all previously used NPPV; there were significant changes in arterial blood gases after 2 h with each ventilator with no significant difference between volumetric and barometric ventilators; all ventilators proved equally acceptable to patients studied. LEGER et al. [37] studied 11 patients with restrictive pulmonary disorders, treated by home NPPV. These patients were submitted to two consecutive periods of NPPV, first with a BiPAP® (mean inspiratory positive airway pressure (IPAP) 18.6 ± 2 cmH$_2$O, EPAP 2 cmH$_2$O) and then with a Monnal D® volumetric ventilator; the major endpoint of the study was sleep architecture (i.e. total sleep time, sleep efficiency, % of rapid eye movement (REM) time, mean arterial oxygen saturation (Sa,O$_2$) during REM, number of arousals and desaturation index did not differ between both types of ventilators). RESTRICK et al. [38] compared volume-cycled with BPPV in 12 stable patients already treated with domiciliary ventilatory support. Patients underwent, in a randomised order, three consecutive nocturnal polysomnographic recordings with BPPV (S mode), volume-cycled ventilation (S/T mode with a back-up frequency of 10 breaths·min^{-1}) or without ventilatory support. There were no significant differences between ventilators in terms of correction of arterial blood gases, improvement of mean nocturnal Sa,O$_2$, time spent with a Sa,O$_2$ <90% or mean nocturnal transcutaneous carbon dioxide tension (Ptc,CO$_2$). Visual analogue scale ratings of comfort and quality of sleep were also similar with both types of ventilator. SCHÖNHOFER et al. [39] compared volumetric NPPV with BiPAP® in 30 consecutive patients with chronic respiratory failure due to obstructive or restrictive pulmonary disorders; patients were initially treated by volumetric NPPV for 1 month (Lifecare PLV100®; Respironics, or Drägger EV800®; Drägerwerk AG, Lübech, Germany, in "controlled" mode), then switched to BPPV for 1 month (BiPAP®, Respironics, in the T mode), and classified as "responders" or "nonresponders" to barometric ventilation on the basis of correction of arterial blood gases and nocturnal hypoventilation. Of the 30 patients included, 18 (60%) were classified as "responders" and were equally improved by both ventilatory modes; two did not tolerate volumetric NPPV and were successfully managed with the BiPAP. Ten (33%) patients were considered "nonresponders", *i.e.* had worsening arterial blood gases and symptom scores with barometric ventilation. The likelihood of being a "nonresponder" was not related to the underlying diagnosis. The conclusions of that study are subject to debate because of the "controlled" mode chosen with both ventilators and used in all patients, irrespective of underlying diagnosis, which may have increased patient–ventilator asynchrony [39]. Another short-term study (two 1-h periods of NIV) included 11 patients, all under long-term NIV for at least 1 yr and in a stable clinical condition, comparing BPPV (O'NYX plus®; Puritan Bennett, Boulder, CO, USA, S/T mode) and volumetric NPPV (Eole IINA®; SAIME, Savigny le Temple, France, assisted-controlled mode); the authors found no significant difference in terms of correction of arterial blood gases or increase in VT [40]. More recently, TUGGEY and ELLIOTT [41] compared pressure support and volume ventilation (Breas PV403®, Molyycke, Sweden) in 13 patients with chest wall deformities, over a 4-week randomised cross-over trial. Impact on arterial blood gases, quality of sleep (assessed by polysomnography) and health status (SF-36 and HAD scores) was identical in both modes. Data from the Geneva lake study, comparing patients with volumetric to barometric ventilators, showed no difference in probability of pursuing NPPV, suggesting a similar acceptance by patients and a similar benefit on survival [1]. Thus, except for in the study by SCHÖNHOFER et al. [39], all available reports fail to find any significant differences between volume-cycled and pressure-cycled ventilation, either in short- or long-term studies. Costs of pressure-cycled ventilators are far below that of volume-cycled machines. Furthermore, BPPV ventilators are much less cumbersome, lighter and often perceived as more comfortable [42], which explains their present use as "default" ventilators in most indications for domiciliary NPPV.

S, S/T or T modes: clinical trials

One of the conclusions of the review of the literature regarding volume-cycled *versus* pressure-cycled ventilators is that the choice of the S, S/T or T mode is highly variable from one group to another and does not seem to follow a clear physiological reasoning. In the Geneva lake study, 51% of the patients under BPPV used S mode. RESTRICK et al. [38] compared the efficacy of a BiPAP® in the S mode *versus* S/T mode (with a minimal respiratory rate of 10 breaths·min^{-1}) and found no significant difference between both modes in terms of correction of mean nocturnal Sa,O$_2$ and mean Ptc,CO$_2$, in 12 patients with either chronic airflow limitation or restrictive disorders (chest wall or neuromuscular diseases), suggesting that the BiPAP in S mode (much cheaper than the S/T apparatus) might be sufficient to control these parameters. Conversely, PARREIRA et al. [43] compared effective ventilation during wakefulness and sleep using a BiPAP either in T mode (at 17 and 25 breaths·min^{-1}) or in a spontaneous S mode in eight normal subjects; BiPAP was more effective in the controlled mode (*i.e.* induced a higher minute ventilation (V'E)) at lower IPAP pressures, than in the S mode, mainly because of the frequent occurrence, even in normal subjects, of nocturnal respiratory rhythm instability (*i.e.* periodic breathing and central apnoeas) and associated desaturations. The authors suggest using a back-up respiratory rate of at least 20 min^{-1}. FAUROUX et al. [44] found similar results in 10 patients with cystic fibrosis, aged 9–20 yrs (mean 15±4), naïve to NPPV but fulfilling criteria for home NPPV. Patients underwent consecutive periods of spontaneous breathing, then 20-min trials of either pressure support or volume-cycled ventilation at spontaneous breathing (SB), maximum tolerated ventilation frequency fv,max (individually determined), and fv,max–5 and $f_{V,max}$–10 (5 and 10 breaths below $f_{V,max}$, respectively). No patient–ventilator asynchrony was observed in any of the studied modes. Tidal volume, $V'E$ and Sa,O_2 increased in all modes *versus* SB. However, end-tidal carbon dioxide decreased significantly only at $f_{V,max}$. All indices of respiratory effort were decreased at all frequencies, but these indices were lower during $f_{V,max}$ than during $f_{V,max}$–5. As expected, percentage of assisted breaths decreased at $f_{V,max}$ *versus* $f_{V,max}$–5 or $f_{V,max}$–10. In this specific group of patients, pressure support at $f_{V,max}$ had a maximal impact in decreasing inspiratory effort, expressed as the pressure/time product (PTP). Conversely, lower back-up rates were either poorly tolerated or associated with a significant increase in PTP [44].

Inspiratory triggering

Inspiratory triggering is an option presently available on most home ventilators, except for those with complex synchronisation algorithms ("flow waveform method of triggering": Synchrony® and Harmony® BPPV ventilators, Respironics). Home volumetric ventilators (*i.e.* Lifecare PLV 100®, Breas PV 501®) most often rely on pressure-triggering while barometric ventilators commercialised for home care rely on flow-triggering systems which are more sensitive and may contribute to a lower work of breathing for triggering. NAVA *et al.* [45] compared the effect of flow *versus* pressure triggering on inspiratory effort during pressure support ventilation (PSV) and volumetric assisted controlled (A/C) mode delivered noninvasively in patients with COPD recovering from an acute exacerbation: flow triggering reduced the inspiratory effort by ~15% (oesophageal PTP (PTPoes) and change in airway pressure ΔPaw) during both PSV and A/C modes compared with pressure triggering.

The flow waveform method of triggering (BiPAP® Vision, Synchrony® and Harmony® BPPV ventilators, Respironics) has been compared with the Evita 4 (Drägerwerk) in pressure support mode, in 12 intubated and sedated patients treated for acute respiratory failure (ARF) [13]; the flow waveform method of triggering was more sensitive to patient effort than conventional flow triggering but led to more autotriggerings, and cycling with the flow waveform method of triggering was similar to the use of 25% of peak inspiratory flow criteria.

Time to peak inspiratory pressure

The possibility of adjusting time to peak IPAP pressure (Breas PV 102, VPAP II S and S/T, and Breas PV 401) has been shown to decrease the work of breathing in patients with restrictive disorders [46, 47]; it is also an important factor for patient comfort.

Expiratory trigger setting (cycling)

Recent bilevel pressure cycled ventilators and pressure support ventilators such as the Breas PV430 ventilator, have adjustable expiratory triggers. Commonly, arbitrary units correspond to different percentages of peak inspiratory flow; in some ventilators, percentage of peak inspiratory flow of cycling can be defined.

The relevance of adjusting expiratory trigger was demonstrated by TASSAUX *et al.* [21] in 10 intubated patients with COPD; increasing expiratory trigger from 10 to 70% of peak inspiratory flow was associated with a marked reduction in delayed cycling, intrinsic positive end-expiratory pressure (PEEPi), unrewarded inspiratory efforts and triggering effort. Whether the same would hold true in patients receiving long-term NIV remains to be determined. Indeed, during NIV, even though obstructive mechanics are likely to promote delayed cycling, leaks at the patient–mask interface have been shown to be a major contributor to this problem [22]. When this is the case, reducing the magnitude of leaks and/or adding an upper limit to inspiratory time can improve the situation.

Comparison of different BPPV ventilators in vivo

Very few clinical trials comparing ventilators *in vivo* are available to date. Using five widely used home BPPV ventilators, VITACCA *et al.* [48] studied 28 patients, 11 of whom were on long-term home ventilation; patients were equipped with an oesophageal balloon, and then NPPV was applied, in random order, for 20-min trials. Tubing and nasal mask were the same for all trials. Mean values of comfort reported by the patients varied considerably; however, effort to trigger the ventilators, improvement of $V'E$ and inspiratory muscle unloading was similar between ventilators. HIGHCOCK *et al.* [49] compared, *in vivo*, two BPPV home ventilators, which had showed important differences on bench testing. A total of 10 subjects with chest wall diseases were recruited and underwent polysomnography on two consecutive nights with either ventilator, in a randomised order; sleep quality, sleep architecture, mean Sa,O_2 and Ptc,CO_2 well all unchanged between ventilators, raising the issue of the clinical relevance of in depth bench testing for clinical practice.

Volume targeting

A limitation of BPPV is the absence of guarantee as to the minute-volume delivered to the patient. Volume targeting is a feature recently made available on some bilevel ventilators (*i.e.* Synchrony®, Respironics; VENTIlogic®, VENTImotion®, Weinmann, Hamburg, Germany; VS Ultra® and Elisee®TM 150, ResMed, Sydney, Australia; Legendair® and Smartair®, Covidien AG, Hamilton, Bermuda) which aims to solve this limitation: the ventilator measures or estimates delivered tidal volume (VT) through a built-in pneumotachograph, and adjusts pressure support within a preset range to provide a VT as close as possible to a target VT set by the clinician. Target volume recommended by Respironics® in obese patients is 7–8 $mL \cdot kg^{-1}$ (or 8–12 $mL \cdot kg^{-1}$ of ideal body weight). In a randomised cross-over study, STORRE *et al.* [50] recently showed, in patients with OHS, (n=10, BMI 41 ± 12 $kg \cdot m^{-2}$, Pa,CO_2 47 ± 2 mmHg) that BPPV with volume targeting (7–10 $mL \cdot kg^{-1}$ of ideal body weight) decreased mean nocturnal Ptc,CO_2 and daytime Pa,CO_2 more efficiently than BPPV alone. The impact of volume targeting on nocturnal Ptc,CO_2 was confirmed in 12 OHS patients, who underwent polysomnography during two consecutive nights while receiving BPPV with or without volume targeting (7–8 $mL \cdot kg^{-1}$) in a randomised order; however, this improvement was at the expense of a lesser sleep comfort, increased awakenings and wake after sleep onset, as well as a shorter total sleep time [51].

Conclusion

The steady increase in the number of patients receiving long-term home ventilation and the continuous technical improvements which have made possible the development of compact and sophisticated ventilators has resulted in a wide range of available ventilators on the domiciliary market. Paradoxically, the choice has become more arduous for the clinician in the face of this abundant offer when attempting to equip a given patient with the appropriate ventilator, while attempting to contain costs. Bench tests provide useful data on the performance of ventilators, as well as on their comparative benefits and drawbacks, but their results must be confronted to those of clinical trials in order to determine their relevance on patient care. The ergonomics of ventilators are an area which needs further exploration, as available results indicate that there is a need to improve their user-friendliness.

Summary

The increasing number of patients receiving long-term home ventilation over the years has fuelled demand for the development of reliable, compact, powerful and quiet home ventilators. Manufacturers have been quick to respond and there is now an abundant offer of such machines on the market. However, this large range can sometimes make choosing the appropriate device difficult for physicians. Bench testing can provide valuable data to assist in that decision and several such studies have been published in recent years. However, the clinical relevance of these tests must also be determined through pathophysiological and clinical studies. The combined data stemming from these two complementary approaches should help clinicians in making the right decision when choosing a ventilator for an individual patient in need of chronic home ventilation.

Keywords: Bilevel devices, home ventilation, mechanical ventilation, noninvasive ventilation.

References

1. Janssens JP, Derivaz S, Breitenstein E, *et al.* Changing patterns in long-term noninvasive ventilation: a 7-year prospective study in the Geneva Lake area. *Chest* 2003; 123: 67–79.
2. Lloyd-Owen SJ, Donaldson GC, Ambrosino N, *et al.* Patterns of home mechanical ventilation use in Europe: results from the Eurovent survey. *Eur Respir J* 2005; 25: 1025–1031.
3. Battisti A, Tassaux D, Janssens JP, Michotte JB, Jaber S, Jolliet P. Performance characteristics of 10 home mechanical ventilators in pressure-support mode: a comparative bench study. *Chest* 2005; 127: 1784–1792.
4. Tassaux D, Strasser S, Fonseca S, Dalmas E, Jolliet P. Comparative bench study of triggering, pressurization and cycling between the home ventilator VPAPII® and three ICU ventilators. *Intensive Care Med* 2002; 28: 1254–1261.
5. Farre R, Lloyd-Owen SJ, Ambrosino N, *et al.* Quality control of equipment in home mechanical ventilation: a European survey. *Eur Respir J* 2005; 26: 86–94.
6. Farre R, Navajas D, Prats E, *et al.* Performance of mechanical ventilators at the patient's home: a multicentre quality control study. *Thorax* 2006; 61: 400–404.
7. Bunburaphong T, Imanaka H, Nishimura M, Hess D, Kacmarek RM. Performance characteristics of bilevel pressure ventilators: a lung model study. *Chest* 1997; 111: 1050–1060.
8. Gonzalez-Bermejo J, Laplanche V, Husseini FE, Duguet A, Derenne JP, Similowski T. Evaluation of the user-friendliness of 11 home mechanical ventilators. *Eur Respir J* 2006; 27: 1236–1243.
9. Kondili E, Prinianakis G, Georgopoulos D. Patient-ventilator interaction. *Br J Anaesth* 2003; 91: 106–119.

10. Whitelaw WA, Derenne JP, Milic-Emili J. Occlusion pressure as a measure of respiratory center output in conscious man. *Respir Physiol* 1975; 23: 181–199.

11. Highcock MP, Shneerson JM, Smith IE. Functional differences in bi-level pressure preset ventilators. *Eur Respir J* 2001; 17: 268–273.

12. Stell IM, Paul G, Lee KC, Ponte J, Moxham J. Noninvasive ventilator triggering in chronic obstructive pulmonary disease. A test lung comparison. *Am J Respir Crit Care Med* 2001; 164: 2092–2097.

13. Prinianakis G, Kondili E, Georgopoulos D. Effects of the flow waveform method of triggering and cycling on patient-ventilator interaction during pressure support. *Intensive Care Med* 2003; 29: 1950–1959.

14. Vignaux L, Tassaux D, Jolliet P. Performance of noninvasive ventilation modes on ICU ventilators during pressure support: a bench model study. *Intensive Care Med* 2007; 33: 1444–1451.

15. Fauroux B, Leroux K, Desmarais G, *et al.* Performance of ventilators for noninvasive positive-pressure ventilation in children. *Eur Respir J* 2008; 31: 1300–1307.

16. Schettino GP, Tucci MR, Sousa R, Valente Barbas CS, Passos Amato MB, Carvalho CR. Mask mechanics and leak dynamics during noninvasive pressure support ventilation: a bench study. *Intensive Care Med* 2001; 27: 1887–1891.

17. Smith IE, Shneerson JM. A laboratory comparison of four positive pressure ventilators used in the home. *Eur Respir J* 1996; 9: 2410–2415.

18. Mehta S, McCool FD, Hill NS. Leak compensation in positive pressure ventilators: a lung model study. *Eur Respir J* 2001; 17: 259–267.

19. Brochard L. Inspiratory pressure support. *Eur J Anaesthesiol* 1994; 11: 29–36.

20. Tassaux D, Michotte JB, Gainnier M, Gratadour P, Fonseca S, Jolliet P. Expiratory trigger setting in pressure support ventilation: from mathematical model to bedside. *Crit Care Med* 2004; 32: 1844–1850.

21. Tassaux D, Gainnier M, Battisti A, Jolliet P. Impact of expiratory trigger setting on delayed cycling and inspiratory muscle workload. *Am J Respir Crit Care Med* 2005; 172: 1283–1289.

22. Calderini E, Confalonieri M, Puccio PG, Francavilla N, Stella L, Gregoretti C. Patient-ventilator asynchrony during noninvasive ventilation: the role of expiratory trigger. *Intensive Care Med* 1999; 25: 662–667.

23. Lofaso F, Brochard L, Touchard D, Hang T, Harf A, Isabey D. Evaluation of carbon dioxide rebreathing during pressure support ventilation with airway management system (BiPAP) devices. *Chest* 1995; 108: 772–778.

24. Lofaso F, Aslanian P, Richard JC, *et al.* Expiratory valves used for home devices: experimental and clinical comparison. *Eur Respir J* 1998; 11: 1382–1388.

25. Buckle P, Clarkson PJ, Coleman R, Ward J, Anderson J. Patient safety, systems design and ergonomics. *Appl Ergon* 2006; 37: 491–500.

26. Martin J, Norris B, Murphy E, Crowe J. Medical device development: the challenge for ergonomics. *Appl Ergon* 2008; 39: 271–283.

27. Sanders M, Kern N. Obstructive sleep apnea treated by independantly adjusted inspiratory and expiratory positive airway pressures *via* nasal mask. Physiological and clinical implications. *Chest* 1990; 98: 317–324.

28. Strumpf D, Carlisle C, Millman R, Smith K, Hill N. An evaluation of the Respironics BiPAP bi-level CPAP device for delivery of assisted ventilation. *Respir Care* 1990; 35: 415–422.

29. Ambrosino N, Nava S, Bertone P, Fracchia C, Rampulla C. Physiologic evaluation of pressure support ventilation by nasal mask in patients with stable COPD. *Chest* 1992; 101: 385–391.

30. Lien T, Wang J, Chang M, Kuo C. Comparison of BiPAP nasal ventilation and ventilation *via* iron lung in stable severe COPD. *Chest* 1993; 104: 460–466.

31. Renston J, DiMarco A, Supinski G. Respiratory muscle rest using nasal BiPAP ventilation in patients with stable severe COPD. *Chest* 1994; 105: 1053–1060.

32. Criner G, Brennan K, Travaline J, Kreimer D. Efficacy and compliance with noninvasive positive pressure ventilation in patients with chronic respiratory failure. *Chest* 1999; 116: 667–675.

33. Janssens JP, Cicotti E, Fitting JW, Rochat T. Non-invasive home ventilation in patients over 75 years of age: tolerance, compliance, and impact on quality of life. *Respir Med* 1998; 92: 1311–1320.

34. Janssens JP, Kehrer P, Chevrolet JC, Rochat T. [Non-invasive home ventilation (NIHV): long-term survival of 32 cases]. *Rev Mal Respir* 1999; 16: 511–520.

35. Meecham-Jones D, Wedzicha J. Comparison of pressure and volume preset nasal ventilator systems in stable chronic respiratory failure. *Eur Respir J* 1993; 6: 1060–1064.

36. Simonds AK, Elliott MW. Outcome of domiciliary nasal intermittent positive pressure ventilation in restrictive and obstructive disorders. *Thorax* 1995; 50: 604–609.

37. Leger P, Langevin B, Robert D. Comparative prospective study: 3 months on nasal BiPAP (NIBIPAP) versus 3 months on nasal IPPV (NIPPV) for chronic respirartory insufficiency. *Am Rev Respir Dis* 1993; 147: A883.

38. Restrick LJ, Fox NC, Braid G, Ward EM, Paul EA, Wedzicha JA. Comparison of nasal pressure support ventilation with nasal intermittent positive pressure ventilation in patients with nocturnal hypoventilation. *Eur Respir J* 1993; 6: 364–370.

39. Schönhofer B, Sonneborn M, Haidl P, Böhrer H, Köhler D. Comparison of two different modes for noninvasive mechanical ventilation in chronic respiratory failure: volume *versus* pressure controlled device. *Eur Respir J* 1997; 10: 184–191.

40. Perrin C, Wolter P, Berthier F, *et al.* [Comparison of volume preset and pressure preset ventilators during daytime nasal ventilation in chronic respiratory failure]. *Rev Mal Respir* 2001; 18: 41–48.

41. Tuggey JM, Elliott MW. Randomised crossover study of pressure and volume non-invasive ventilation in chest wall deformity. *Thorax* 2005; 60: 859–864.

42. Mehta S, Hill NS. Noninvasive ventilation. *Am J Respir Crit Care Med* 2001; 163: 540–577.

43. Parreira VF, Delguste P, Jounieaux V, Aubert G, Dury M, Rodenstein DO. Effectiveness of controlled and spontaneous modes in nasal two-level positive pressure ventilation in awake and asleep normal subjects. *Chest* 1997; 112: 1267–1277.

44. Fauroux B, Louis B, Hart N, *et al.* The effect of back-up rate during non-invasive ventilation in young patients with cystic fibrosis. *Intensive Care Med* 2004; 30: 673–681.

45. Nava S, Ambrosino N, Bruschi C, Confalonieri M, Rampulla C. Physiological effects of flow and pressure triggering during non-invasive mechanical ventilation in patients with chronic obstructive pulmonary disease. *Thorax* 1997; 52: 249–254.

46. Bonmarchand G, Chevron V, Menard J, *et al.* Effects of pressure ramp slope values on the work of breathing during pressure support ventilation in restrictive patients. *Crit Care Med* 1999; 27: 715–722.

47. MacIntyre N, Nishimura M, Usada Y, Tokioka H, Takezawa J, Shimada Y. The Nagoya conference on system design and patient-ventilator interactions during pressure support ventilation. *Chest* 1990; 97: 1463–1466.

48. Vitacca M, Barbano L, D'Anna S, Porta R, Bianchi L, Ambrosino N. Comparison of five bilevel pressure ventilators in patients with chronic ventilatory failure: a physiologic study. *Chest* 2002; 122: 2105–2114.

49. Highcock MP, Morrish E, Jamieson S, Shneerson JM, Smith IE. An overnight comparison of two ventilators used in the treatment of chronic respiratory failure. *Eur Respir J* 2002; 20: 942–945.

50. Storre JH, Seuthe B, Fiechter R, *et al.* Average volume-assured pressure support in obesity hypoventilation: A randomized crossover trial. *Chest* 2006; 130: 815–821.

51. Janssens JP, Metzger M, Sforza E. Impact of volume targeting on efficacy of bi-level non-invasive ventilation and sleep in obesity-hypoventilation. *Respir Med* 2008; [Epub ahead of print PMID: 18579368].

CHAPTER 22

Noninvasive mechanical ventilation in chronic respiratory failure: ventilators and interfaces

J.H. Storre*, B. Schönhofer#

*Dept of Pneumology, University Hospital Freiburg, Freiburg im Breisgau, and #Dept of Pneumology and Intensive Care Medicine, Krankenhaus Oststadt-Heidehaus, Hanover, Germany.

Correspondence: J.H. Storre, Abteilung Pneumologie der Medizinischen Klinik, Klinikum der Albert-Ludwigs-Universität, Killianstrasse 5, D-79106 Freiburg in Breisgau, Germany. Fax: 49 7612703704; E-mail: Jan.Storre@uniklinik-freiburg.de; B. Schönhofer, Abteilung für Pneumologie und Internistische Intensivmedizin, Krankenhaus Oststadt-Heidehaus, Klinikum Region Hanover, Podbielskistraße 380, D-30659 Hanover, Germany. Fax: 49 5113779; E-mail: Bernd.Schoenhofer@t-online.de

The present chapter deals with the technical aspects of ventilators and interfaces used in noninvasive ventilation (NIV) of patients with chronic respiratory failure (CRF). Before going into details, it might be helpful to highlight one important clinical issue: patients with CRF are more or less in a respiratory stable condition and are not dependent on ventilatory support 24 hours a day; however, patients with CRF have limited ventilatory capacities, thus the use of NIV as an intermittent treatment should be clinically beneficial and lead to stabilisation of the ventilatory failure. Therefore, in contrast to invasive mechanical ventilation (IMV), cessation of NIV does not cause an immediate life-threatening risk. Complications of IMV, such as failure of the ventilator, changes in ventilator settings, accidental disconnection from ventilator or accidental decannulation, may lead to acute deterioration of clinical status, acute hospitalisation or even death. Therefore, to minimise these complications, ventilators in IMV are equipped with many surveillance devices and alarms [1]. In contrast, such a surveillance system is not necessary when NIV is used to treat CRF, thus avoiding unnecessary irritation to the patient. Accordingly, a recently published study investigated the technical performance of nine portable pressure ventilators (which are also used as NIV ventilators in the home) and found that most of the portable pressure ventilators evaluated were able to respond to high ventilatory demands, even outperforming the intensive care unit (ICU) device [2].

The objective of the first section of the present chapter is to discuss the principal characteristics of ventilators that have been designed for use in patients with CRF requiring NIV. In the second section, the interfaces of NIV are discussed.

Ventilators

Historical development

From an historical point of view, negative pressure ventilation (NPV) was the first mode of NIV to be widely applied to CRF patients (*i.e.* during the 1950s poliomyelitis epidemic). NPV takes place by exposing the chest to subatmospheric pressure during inspiration. During expiration the pressure around the chest wall changes to atmospheric pressure in order to allow passive exhalation [3]. In the past, body ventilation was provided with different models, *e.g.* tank respirator or cuirass type device driven by a negative pressure cycled machine.

Apart from some specialised centres that have maintained the tradition of using NPV as a treatment for CRF, this mode of ventilation has steadily lost its former impact over the last decades and has been almost completely substituted by positive pressure ventilation (PPV) modes. The main reasons for this trend were the large, cumbersome NPV-devices, the lack of accessibility by the patient, the need for considerable experience to operate the device and, finally, the danger of inducing upper airway obstruction [4]. These shortcomings were emphasised by a monocentre retrospective study which investigated, over a 46-yr period, long-term NIV of patients with neuromuscular disorders [5]. It was shown that, compared with NPV, a greater number of patients with PPV (67%) reported positive outcomes (*i.e.* improved sense of wellbeing, independence and perform daily activity). However, there were still patients with CRF who did not tolerate PPV but did well with NPV; therefore, NPV should be considered as an alternative means of ventilation in case of PPV intolerance.

Terminology and classification of modes

The existing set of terminology describing the modes of NIV can sometimes be confusing. The most frequently used modes and abbreviations are shown in table 1. The answers to the following basic questions may facilitate communication and simplify the terminology dealing with NIV. 1) Is the NIV mode pressure-targeted ventilation (PTV) or volume-targeted ventilation (VTV; the frequently used term "volume control" may be inaccurate, since the volume leaving the ventilator is not really controlled; this is due to leakage that can occur during the delivery of air to the patient)? 2) Should positive pressure be applied during inspiration, expiration or both? 3) Does NIV work in the assist (triggering), assist-control (triggering with back-up rate) or cycled (control) mode with a fixed breathing frequency?

Before going into details about the two main types of NIV modes (volume and pressure target-ventilation), it should be noted that the drive of breathing by the patient and ventilators can be set up in the following ways.

Table 1. – Modes of ventilation

Abbreviation	Meaning
ASB	Assisted spontaneous breathing
ASV	Adaptive servo ventilation
ASSPCV	Assisted-pressure controlled ventilation
BiPAP	Biphasic positive airway pressure
CPAP	Continuous positive airway pressure
IPPV	Intermittent positive pressure ventilation
NIV	Noninvasive ventilation
NPPV	Noninvasive positive pressure ventilation
PAV	Proportional assist ventilation
PCV	Pressure controlled ventilation
PEEP	Positive end-expiratory pressure
PSV	Pressure support ventilation
SIMV	Synchronised intermittent mandatory ventilation
VCV	Volume controlled ventilation

Assist mode. When the ventilator detects and supports the patient's spontaneous breath, this process is called "triggering". When NIV is set to assist mode (*e.g.* pressure support ventilation (PSV), proportional assist ventilation (PAV) or assist VTV), it is possible to achieve both a patient-adapted breathing pattern and a high synchrony of ventilation between the patient and the ventilator. However, triggering requires considerable inspiratory work of breathing, which does not end abruptly with the ensuing mechanical pressure support of the inspiration cycle. FLICK *et al.* [6] showed through electromyogram (EMG) recordings that inspiratory work of breathing persisted after triggering diaphragmatic activity. Moreover, it could be demonstrated that the oxygen consumption of the respiratory muscles were clearly higher in the assisted mode of intermittent positive pressure ventilation (IPPV) than in the controlled mode [7].

Control mode. In control mode, there is a preset automatic cycle based on either volumetric ventilation (*i.e.* volume controlled ventilation (VCV)) or barometric ventilation (*i.e.* pressure controlled ventilation (PCV)). In PCV, fixed inspiratory and expiratory pressure levels, breathing frequency and inspiratory and expiratory times are preset. Ventilators for VCV are characterised by the presetting of fixed inspiratory volume, fixed breathing frequency and inspiratory and expiratory times. In pure control mode, the breathing frequency of the ventilator is generally set to a high level in order to avoid the patient's spontaneous efforts. Only this procedure enables actual passive ventilation. In general, preset-controlled volume and pressure modes are preferable in patients with an unreliable respiratory effort, massively overloaded respiratory muscles, apnoea and hypopnoeas, and failure of PSV.

Assist-control mode. This mode is a combination of assisted and controlled modes. Depending on the spontaneous breathing frequency, the patient may either trigger to receive inspiratory support (*i.e.* pressure or volume targeted), or be passively ventilated with the chosen back-up frequency.

Concerning pressure ventilators, this mode is often called "spontaneous/timed", whereas in volumetric ventilators, the mode is called "assist-control ventilation". In principle, the synchronised intermittent mandatory ventilation (SIMV) mode also belongs to this category.

The two main types of NIV-ventilator in CRF: VTV and PTV

Most of the initial studies in the 1990s used VTV as the preferred mode of NIV in CRF [8, 9]. In line with these findings, a study by SIMONDS *et al.* [10] reported that the broad majority of patients (n=170) used VTV, while only ten patients used PTV. Furthermore, a group study by LEGER *et al.* [11] revealed the exclusive use of VTV among the 276 patients studied.

However, due to various reasons, PTV has been increasingly prescribed in recent years and its usage surpassed that of volume respirators by the end of the 1990s [12–14]. This trend is shown in figure 1 [15]. Here, during the observation period from 1990–1999, the entire group of 530 CRF patients were adapted to NIV in the Kloster Grafschaft hospital (Schmallenberg, Germany). The number of new NIV patients per year continuously increased from 13 in 1990 to >100 patients in 1998 and 1999. Apart from in 1990, when NIV was exclusively started with VTV, PTV dominated the years that followed. Within the PTV users, the application of PTV in the assist mode decreased, while PTV in the control or assist-control mode increased (fig. 1).

In general, PTV and VTV are still characterised by some typical advantages and disadvantages which are listed in table 2. In two prospective randomised cross-over

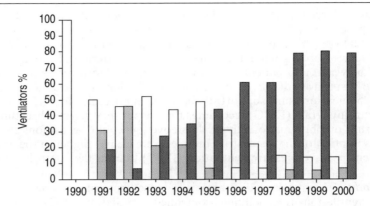

Fig. 1. – Development and distribution of applied noninvasive ventilators from 1990–1999 in the Kloster Grafschaft hospital (Schmallenberg, Germany) [15]. □: volume-targeted ventilators; ▨: pressure-targeted ventilators (assist mode); ■: pressure-targeted ventilators (control or assist-control mode).

studies, no advantages in sleep quality, gas exchange or quality of life over a 4-month period were reported when comparing VTV with PTV in the treatment of CRF [16, 17]. However, reduced patient comfort and increased gastrointestinal side-effects were reported with VTV application [16] while leak compensation is superior in PTV [18, 19]. This trend is particularly obvious in the case of chronic obstructive pulmonary disease (COPD)-induced CRF, where the high airway pressures that arise from the high airway resistance in VTV may partly underlie the development of gastrointestinal side-effects and reduced comfort. In Europe today, PTV is the more commonly used mode in the treatment of CRF, with two-thirds of the 21,526 patients on home mechanical ventilation using this mode of ventilation (fig. 2) [14]. University hospitals are increasingly using PTV, since the percentage of VTV is higher both in non-university hospitals and the long-established centres using NIV [14, 20].

VTV. Most VTV ventilators in NIV have a one-line circuit with an integrated demand valve; therefore, CO_2-rebreathing is not a problem. Furthermore, most VTV ventilators on the market deliver the inspiratory volumes *via* a piston or bellow without integrated PEEP; however, newer devices are blower-driven and capable of internal PEEP adjustment.

VTV ventilators deliver a fixed tidal volume, while the associated airway pressures result from airway resistance, lung and thoracic compliance, flow rate and inspiratory cycle. Although the method of triggering is not consistently specified, VTV is mostly applied in the assist-controlled mode. As mentioned, the use of VTV as a mode of NIV is currently decreasing compared with PCV.

However, VTV as an NIV-mode is still used frequently in CRF due to neuromuscular diseases [14, 21], and in some countries VTV is still used as often as PTV [14]. Volume ventilation may be preferred by some patients with neuromuscular diseases who sometimes need high tidal volumes for ventilation, coughing and increasing the volume of their voice during NIV. According to the need to attain maximal lung insufflations for assisted coughing, adolescent and adult patients with respiratory muscle dysfunction used portable volume-cycled ventilators, rather than pressure-cycled ventilators. This former disadvantage of PTV is now redeemable, since the currently available generation of PTV ventilators deliver higher maximum inspiratory pressures (*i.e.* 40 cm H_2O). VTV with a high flow capacity and pressure limitation may cope adequately with leaks;

Table 2. – Advantages and disadvantages of pressure-targeted ventilators (PTV) and volume-targeted ventilators (VTV)

Aspect	PTV	VTV
Constant inspiratory volume	-	++
Constant inspiratory pressure	++	-
Improvement in sleep quality	+	+
Improvement in gas exchange	+	+
Improvement of quality of life	+	+
Leak compensation	++	-
Gastrointestinal side-effects	+	-
Comfort	+	-

Advantages range from + to ++ and disadvantages are shown as -.

however, in general, PTV still provides better compensation for such leaks. Finally, it should be mentioned that SIMV, a subtype of volume-cycled ventilators, is also available as an NIV mode. However, this is not recommended, since SIMV is associated with increased work of breathing [22].

PTV. In contrast to VTV, all of the currently available PTV ventilators are compressor/blower driven. One-line circuit models with or without an integrated demand valve are available.

PTV ventilators cycle between preset inspiratory positive airway pressure (IPAP) and expiratory positive airway pressure (EPAP), thus providing PSV [23]. This allows the patient to control inspiratory and expiratory times while providing a preset pressure, which, along with patient's effort, determines the inspiratory flow and tidal volume. IPAP and EPAP can be adjusted independently in order to augment alveolar ventilation and maintain upper airway patency during sleep. PSV may facilitate an acceptable patient–ventilator synchrony, while the addition of external PEEP reduces dynamic hyperinflation by offsetting intrinsic PEEP [24]. Therefore, PSV may help the patient to

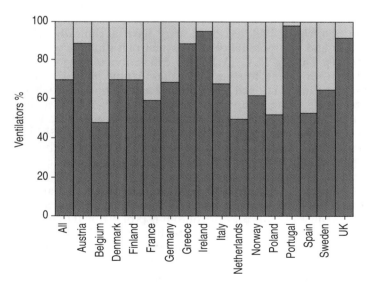

Fig. 2. – Percentage per country of pressure- (■) and volume- (▦) targeted positive pressure ventilators used for home mechanical ventilation (n=21,526) [14].

feel more comfortable. A further advantage of portable PTV devices is the absence of unnecessary alarms (depending on the product) in clinically stable patients. In addition, the PSV equipment is generally lighter and less expensive.

An important advantage of PSV and PCV is the compensation for mild-to-moderate mask or mouth leaks [18, 19]. In the presence of leak the pressure in the patient–ventilator-circle drops and PTV increases inspiratory flow to compensate for the drop in pressure.

CO_2-rebreathing has been documented in PSV, and the risk of CO_2-rebreathing is greater with a single delivery circuit that lacks an active exhalation valve [25, 26]. A recent study from SCHETTINO et al. [27] dealt with CO_2-rebreathing and the influences of the exhalation port position and mask design in the PSV-mode. In that bench study, a lung model with a single-limb circuit was used. In that setting, the full mask with the exhalation port positioned within the mask, demonstrated less CO_2-rebreathing than either the closed full-face mask, with a whisper swivel, or the total face mask [27]. Furthermore, the high respiratory rates and low external PEEP increased the risk of CO_2-rebreathing caused by the shorter expiratory time and lower CO_2 washout of the circuit. A minimal EPAP (>2–4 cmH_2O) is therefore necessary to avoid CO_2-rebreathing in a single tube circuit without valves, in order to wash out CO_2. However, to the best of the present authors' knowledge, no study has shown that CO_2-rebreathing is clinically significant.

A further critical issue of PSV is the detection of the patient's inspiration. There are ventilators fitted with both a fixed and variable trigger. In the past, ventilators were often pressure-triggered. More-recent studies have found that flow-triggered devices appeared to be more sensitive than pressure-triggered devices [28]. Another technical challenge is "pressurisation", in other words, the ability of the ventilator to meet the flow demand of the patient. Flow demand mainly depends on the underlying pathophysiology (e.g. resistance and compliance), the given level of pressure support and inspiratory pressure rise time; the shorter the rise time, the lower the level of work of breathing [29]. Depending on the type of ventilator, the pressure rise time is either adjustable or fixed. It may be possible that in an individual case (e.g. an obese patient with severe airway obstruction) a ventilator does not have enough power to yield adequate pressure.

Both expiratory trigger and resistance may have a clinically relevant impact on expiratory effort and the possibility of desynchronisation between the patient and ventilator [30, 31]. During PSV, cycling to exhalation is triggered by a decrease in inspiratory flow from a peak to threshold value. A time limit of inspiration is usually added because the aforementioned technique becomes inoperative when mask leaks are present. Furthermore, systems using active exhalation valves have shown significant variation in their valve resistance to exhalation. Increased resistance associated with difficulties in exhalation can significantly increase the work of breathing.

Compared with PSV, the aforementioned issues (i.e. CO_2-rebreathing, inspiratory and expiratory triggering) are less critical in the PTV assist-controlled and controlled modes, since they are dominated by automatic cycling.

Compliance might also be improved by allowing the patient to maintain control of the breathing pattern. PAV has been proposed as a mode of synchronised partial ventilatory support, in which the ventilator pressure output is proportional to instantaneous patient effort, thus unloading the resistive and elastic burden [32, 33]. Studies in patients with acute respiratory failure (ARF) have shown that PAV is well-tolerated and just as effective as PSV [34, 35]; however, PAV currently remains as an experimental mode of ventilation. The majority of studies, investigating the short-term application of PAV in patients with CRF, has revealed some interesting pathophysiological insights [36, 37]. PAV has been shown, especially during physical activity, to be more efficient than PSV in assisting the diaphragm and in increasing minute ventilation [37]. Since NIV has been postulated as a promising therapy option for rehabilitation programs in CRF [38–40], PAV could be, in this case, one of the preferred modes of ventilation; however, further studies are needed to investigate this suggestion. Long-term studies, investigating the application of PAV as an NIV mode in sleep or the effect of long-term application in CRF, are yet to be performed.

Finally, it should be mentioned that in both intensive care medicine and anaesthesiology, the biphasic positive airway pressure (BiPAP) mode is associated with a different mode of the Evita ventilator (Draeger, Lübeck, Germany). This mode consists of a phasic change between two preset demand-valve CPAP values ("P-low" and "P-high") during which spontaneous breathing remains unrestricted at each CPAP value. The mechanical support is defined by: 1) the difference between the two pressure levels and 2) the variable duration of both pressure levels.

To conclude this section, it should be added that some manufacturers of home ventilators have recently focused on providing a combination of both PTV and VTV in the same machine. The role of these hybrid modes of ventilation have not yet been sufficiently explored to warrant their use in NIV but a pilot study has indeed shown promising results [41]; in that study, patients with obesity-hypoventilation syndrome were randomised in a cross-over design to either the BiPAP spontaneous/timed or the hybrid combination of BiPAP spontaneous/timed with average volume-assured pressure support (AVAPS). Each mode was applied for 6 weeks of home mechanical ventilation. The authors reported that with the addition of the AVAPS mode there was a significantly greater reduction of transcutaneous carbon dioxide tension (Ptc,CO_2) during the night; however, sleep quality and quality of life did not benefit from the addition of the AVAPS mode when compared with BiPAP spontaneous/timed alone [41]. Similar findings were reported by JANSSENS et al. [42], who reported that the AVAPS mode led to a slight improvement in alveolar ventilation but did not significantly affect the objective indices of sleep structure; however, this new mode was associated with a subjective feeling of reduced sleep quality, increased leaks and increased ventilator pressures. Since these were the first studies to investigate the hybrid mode of ventilation in CRF, it remains unknown as to whether these new modes do actually offer any long-term advantages over the modes in current use.

Choice of ventilator and setting

Regarding the choice of ventilator and ventilator setting, an individualised approach to each patient appears, in general, to be a useful practice [43, 44]. From a practical point of view this means that the ventilator type and its setting should be determined by each patient's degree of comfort, coupled with the patient's ability to increase minute ventilation, improve gas exchange and diminish the work of breathing. Indeed, this constitutes the ideal aim of every specialist in the field of respiratory medicine. However, data that deal with these topics are virtually non-existent in literature, while evidence-based recommendations are also lacking.

Furthermore, despite the described differences between the NIV modes, it still remains open as to whether these differences are of clinical importance. In view of this, HILL [45] stated 15 yrs ago that, based upon the data available at the time, considerations such as leak compensation and reliably delivered volumes, did not appear to be major determinants of NIV success; this statement remains valid to the present day.

Accordingly, data regarding the validity of PTV versus VTV in NIV are available. These data generally emerged from physiological studies, which were conducted mainly over short time periods in small groups of patients [46–48]. A disadvantage of these previous studies was the introduction of additional variables such as assist-control VTV *versus* PSV [47, 48], thus making the comparison between the two ventilation modes more unreliable.

Several studies have compared the long-term efficacy of different NIV modes in CRF [12, 16, 17, 49, 50]. CRINER *et al.* [12] investigated the efficacy and compliance of long-term NIV in 40 patients with CRF; here, the aforementioned trend from VTV to PTV was demonstrated. After initial evaluation, 34 patients received NIV *via* PTV (*i.e.* BiPAP) while only six patients required NIV *via* VTV. During the 6-month follow-up, 14 patients ceased NIV due to incompliance; in the compliant patients, blood gases and functional status improved on a chronic basis. Also, on a long-term basis, SCHÖNHOFER *et al.* [49] conducted a prospective study of the effect of volume- and pressure-cycled ventilation modes of NIV in patients suffering from CRF. After 4 weeks of treatment with VTV in the time-cycled mode, the effect was compared with that of PTV, which was also performed in the same mode over a 4-week period. From these results, the authors concluded that VTV proved superior to PTV in one-third (10 out of 30) of their patients, since this subgroup deteriorated during the PTV period and had to return to VTV. However, the majority of patients (20 out of 30) remained stable during the subsequent PTV period. Subjective scores and carbon dioxide tension values provided a distinction between long-term responders and nonresponders to PTV. It could be speculated that the amount of reduced work of breathing accounted for the discrepancies between the two modes. In contrast to the study of SCHÖNHOFER *et al.* [49], SMITH *et al.* [50] reported that in a mixed collective of 10 CRF patients who deteriorated under VTV, the exchange of the ventilator to PTV led to a reversal of the deterioration observed under VTV.

More recently, PTV and VTV were compared in two prospective randomised cross-over studies [16, 17]. In one of the studies, 12 CRF patients with chest wall deformities underwent a four-week single-blinded randomised cross-over study in either VTV or PTV. In conclusion, the authors suggested that pressure- and volume-ventilation are equivalent in terms of the effects on nocturnal and daytime physiology, resulting daytime function and health status [17]. In line with these findings, WINDISCH *et al.* [16] investigated, in a similar prospective randomised cross-over study, PTV and VTV in 10 patients with obstructive (n=5) and restrictive (n=5) CRF. After 6 weeks of home mechanical ventilation in the assist-controlled mode, an equivalent improvement in gas exchange and sleep quality was seen overnight. However, PTV was better tolerated by the patients, whereas more gastrointestinal side effects were associated with VTV; these findings therefore contribute to the trend towards the use of PTV over the last 15 yrs [16].

Finally, it should be mentioned that the glottis function plays an important role in NIV, since the glottis is known to narrow substantially or even close completely, in response to NIV. This may induce deterioration in the quality of both NIV and sleep [51, 52]. Furthermore, it has been shown that a substantial increase in glottis resistance can occur with the use of different modes of NIV [53, 54], leading to narrowing of the glottis reflex and inducing (amongst others) mouth leaks. It was found that, by altering the delivery of tidal volume, inspiratory flow and ventilatory frequency or positive inspiratory pressure (as well as manipulating the ventilatory mode), the glottis response can be regulated, thus improving ventilatory efficacy. This warrants further trials with CRF patients, since glottis function may act as a practical determinant of ventilator mode and setting, respectively.

General issues concerning technical equipment

The major advantage of NIV is its applicability outside the hospital, *e.g.* in the patient's home. Compared with long-term invasive mechanical ventilation at home [1], which often needs accessory equipment, the technical equipment and design of NIV ventilators should remain simple and be easy to handle. Therefore, NIV ventilators would not need the following technical details in general: a second, back-up ventilator; humidification; external battery; non-rebreathing valve; PEEP; supplemental O_2; pressure and volume monitoring; and alarms for high and low pressure and failure of the battery.

Routine care for patients receiving NIV at home should include the following: patients and caregivers should be properly trained by technicians, specialised nurses or respiratory therapists from the home care company, in the use of the ventilatory equipment prior to hospital discharge. Once assigned to NIV for home mechanical ventilation, patients should be visited at home at least during the first week; subsequent visits would then be dependent on the patient's needs. During these visits, the ventilator should be checked for proper function. Preventative maintenance is performed according to the manufacturer's specifications. The home-care company must guarantee a 24 h technical service, in order to answer emergency calls and repair technical dysfunctions of the ventilatory equipment. After a certain period of usage (e.g. every 5,000 h), the ventilators are to be removed from the home for complete preventative maintenance at the factory. Additional services which are organised by the healthcare providers (such as mask consultation) offer further support for the patient.

A thorough investigation into the frequency of home ventilator failure revealed that such failures were relatively uncommon, with nearly all suspected failures being resolved at home [55]. Caregivers' misuse, tampering or damage led to half of the reported failure. True mechanical failures occurred in only 40% of the reports. No patient suffered any adverse clinical effects, resulting from the failure. However, in a more recent, European survey [56], the quality control of equipment in home mechanical ventilation showed some interesting facts that should be considered: 1) ventilator service was mainly carried out by external companies (62% of centres), with a service occurring every 3–12 months; 2) interaction between servicing companies and prescribers was limited (only 61% of centres were consistently informed of major incidents); 3) participation of centres in equipment quality control was poor; and 4) only 23% of centres were sufficiently aware of the vigilance systems [56]. In line with previous findings, that report revealed that regular assessment of actual ventilator performance at the patient's home is an important quality-control procedure for detecting any malfunctions which could otherwise compromise both the compliance and outcome of home mechanical ventilation [57].

Interfaces

The interface between the patient and ventilator is crucial for the success of NIV; a patient may refuse NIV on the grounds of an uncomfortable mask, or a poorly fitting interface may reduce the efficacy of NIV. Custom sizing and fitting of the mask may require several attempts in order to accommodate the facial architecture. Despite the clinical impact, the choice of different interfaces has received little scientific attention; hence, no general consensus exists in regard to the management of interfaces.

Spectrum of interfaces

As seen historically, the quality of interfaces has markedly improved over the past 25 yrs. In the early 1990s, the percentage of custom-made nasal and facial masks in use was high, due to a lack of sufficient fitting and comfortable commercial masks [15].

Today, a variety of commercial masks are available and more frequently used than custom-made masks (figs 3 and 4). Commercial manufacturers continue to improve mask design and develop gauging tools in order to help the clinician choose the correct mask and size for the patient.

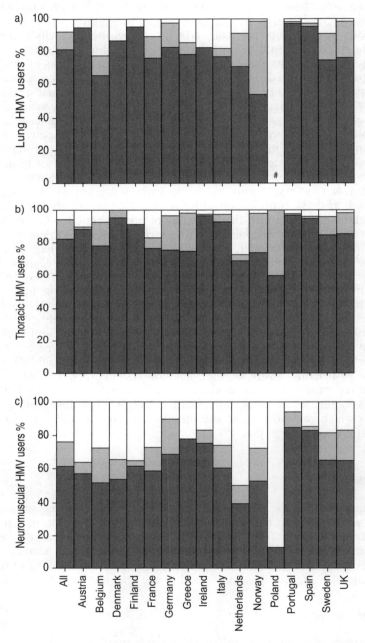

Fig. 3. – Proportion of interfaces for different diseases categorised by country for a) lung, b) thoracic and c) neuromuscular home mechanical ventilation (HMV) users (n=21,526) [14]. ■: nasal masks; ▨: facial masks; □: tracheostomy. #: no data were available for Polish lung users.

In the aforementioned European survey of home mechanical ventilator users, the majority of interfaces are represented by nasal and facial masks, with the majority of patients using nasal masks (fig. 3) [14]. However, as shown in figure 3, there are still patients on home mechanical ventilators who are tracheostomised. The use of this invasive interface is dependent on the underlying disease, whereby the highest rate of the tracheostomised patients suffer from neuromuscular diseases (24%). Fewer patients with lung diseases, like COPD (8%) or restrictive thoracic disorders (5%), require tracheostomy [14]. This distribution also depends on the country of the patient. For example, the respective proportions of tracheostomised patients with neuromuscular diseases in Poland (90%) and the Netherlands (50%) are much higher compared with other countries (fig. 3).

The varieties of interfaces that are currently in frequent use are given in figure 4; approximately 20–30 types of both nasal and face masks are on the market, each being characterised by their own advantages and disadvantages. A comparison of these most-frequently used interfaces is described in table 3. In special indications, total face masks, nasal pillows and mouthpieces are also used (fig. 4).

Commercial interfaces

There are only a few reports which directly compare the success rate of nasal masks, facial masks and other devices. In a study by NAVALESI et al. [58], patients with chronic hypercapnic respiratory failure showed an overall better tolerance of the commercially available nasal masks compared with both the facial masks and nasal pillows (p<0.005). However, the full-face masks were associated with the most favourable reduction in arterial carbon dioxide tension (Pa,CO_2). A recently published study reported that nasal masks are just as effective as full-face masks in terms of sleep quality and gas exchange in CRF patients. Here, the nasal masks were often attached with a chin strap in order to compensate for oral leaks [59]. In line with these findings, the nasal mask was considered to be more comfortable than the face mask during CPAP therapy for sleep apnoea [60]. However, nasal masks dominate as the type of interface used in CRF [14, 61]. In

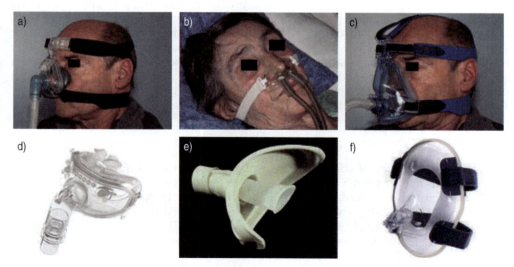

Fig. 4. – Variety of interfaces. a) Commercial nasal mask, b) custom-made nasal mask, c) commercial full-face mask, d) full-face mask with nasal pillows, e) mouthpiece and f) total face mask.

Table 3. – Comparison of oronasal and nasal masks

Aspect	Oronasal mask	Nasal mask
Mouth leak	No	Yes
Mouth breathing	Possible	Decreases NIV quality
Dental status	Independent	Dependent
Application of airway pressure	Higher	Lower
Dead space	High	Low
Dynamic of ABG improvement	Quicker	Slower
Communication	Reduced	Possible
Eating and drinking	No	Possible
Expectoration	No	Possible
Risk of aspiration	Elevated	Reduced
Risk of aerophagia	Elevated	Reduced
Claustrophobia	Elevated	Reduced
Comfort	Lower	Higher

ABG: arterial blood gas; NIV: noninvasive ventilation.

contrast, due to various reasons, oronasal masks are used more often in the treatment of ARF [61, 62].

In order to avoid leaks, masks are often fitted tightly; however, this can induce pressure sores which, in turn, may lead to reduced tolerance. Pressure sores mostly appear on the nasal bridge and different dressings have therefore been evaluated to prevent nasal bridge abrasion. The proper fit of the nose mask can be improved by applying mask cushions or by padding the bridge of the nose. Variations include the bubble type- or gel-masks.

Patients with an intolerance of such nasal interfaces (*i.e.* masks or nasal pillows) might be more willing to try masks that cover both the nose and mouth. Accordingly, CRINER *et al.* [63] found that the total face mask was likely to improve comfort, minimise air leakage and improve ventilation in patients who were previously unable to tolerate NIV *via* nasal or oronasal masks.

Recently, helmets were introduced as a new interface in NIV. In two studies by ANTONELLI *et al.* [64, 65], the helmet was a promising tool in the treatment of acute hypoxemic respiratory failure [64]; however, in patients with CRF, the reduction of Pa,CO_2 with the helmet was not as favourable as that achieved with treatment by the full-face mask [65]. Recently, a study by NAVALESI *et al.* [66] showed, in patients with COPD and CRF, that the helmet and facial mask were equally tolerated and that both were effective in ameliorating gas exchange and decreasing inspiratory effort. However, the helmet was less efficient in decreasing inspiratory effort and worsened the patient–ventilator interaction. Currently, the helmet cannot be recommended as an interface for long-term NIV.

Customised interfaces

Despite the wide use of commercially available masks there are some potential side effects such as a large mask volume, nasal bridge pressure sores or significant leakages. In this case, custom-made nasal or facial masks may be an alternative (fig. 4). In a short-term physiological study, a volumetric ventilator was used to compare commercially available and custom-made nasal masks during NIV [67]; the nasal mask showed a higher effectiveness of NIV, most probably since it has a smaller dead space and reduced air leakage compared with the custom-made mask. In a French population study, masks were constructed by modelling a mixture of silicone and catalyst to the patient's face. The entire mask-making procedure took approximately 30 min and the masks were then usable for around 6 months [11]. The most-recent trend involves the use of semi-customised masks consisting of a prefabricated frame in which quick-drying filler is injected and then moulded to the unique facial contours of each patient.

Mouthpieces

BACH et al. [68] reported on the use of mouthpieces as an interface that precludes the necessity of tracheotomy in patients with neuromuscular disease. A commercially available mouthpiece interface covers the lips and is held in place by straps. Here the mouthpiece, like the nasal mask, facilitates both communication and secretion clearance. A simple mouthpiece may be kept adjacent to the mouth for easy accessibility during the day, with a lip seal added for nocturnal use; the addition of a bite plate may also facilitate the use of an oral interface. However, this type of interface has been associated with adverse effects, e.g. air leakage, dry mouth, risk of aspiration, altered dental occlusion and temporomandibular joint problems.

A recently published study by TOUSSAINT et al. [69] recommends NIV with a mouthpiece as the interface of choice for additional daytime NIV in end-stage Duchenne patients. Here, patients who underwent NIV with a nasal mask and were normocapnic during the night, but developed end-diurnal hypercapnia, were additionally ventilated with a diurnal mouthpiece. A 7-yr follow-up of 42 patients has been performed and revealed NIV with a mouthpiece as a safe means of improving daytime gas exchange, prolonging survival and stabilising vital capacity. The authors also recommended the addition of a self-supporting harness to aid NIV with a mouthpiece.

Dead space

The increase in dead space, as well as the inherent CO_2-rebreathing associated with mask use, is a crucial aspect. CRINER et al. [63] found the following values for dead spaces: total face mask, 1,500 mL; oronasal mask, 250 mL; and nasal mask, 105 mL. Studies in this field are quite rare, but one study of SCHETTINO et al. [27] dealt with CO_2-rebreathing, the position of exhalation port and the design of the mask. In that bench study, a lung model with a single-limb circuit was used. Within this setting, the full-face mask, with its exhalation port fitted in the mask, demonstrated less CO_2-rebreathing compared with either the closed full-face mask with a whisper swivel or the total face mask. A further study investigated the dynamic dead space in 19 commercially available face masks in a lung model; here, with the use of a face mask, the total dynamic dead space during spontaneous ventilation was increased above physiological dead space from 32 to 42% of tidal volume [70]. NIV in either bilevel or CPAP mode that exerts continuous pressure throughout the expiratory phase led to a reduction in total dynamic dead space to approach physiological dead space with most face masks, whereas NIV in PSV mode led to less of a reduction, namely from 42 to 39%. Face masks using expiratory ports over the nasal bridge resulted in beneficial flow characteristics within the face mask and nasal cavity. Here, a decrease in total dynamic dead space to less than physiological dead space from 42 to 28.5% of tidal volume was demonstrated [70]. In conclusion, more studies on this subject are needed to verify the above findings.

Air leakage

The two major sites of air leakage are: 1) between the skin and the mask and 2) through the mouth. Leaks, especially mouth leaks, play a major role in the ineffectiveness of NIV.

Leaks should be monitored and quantified and, for the multiple reasons that have been already mentioned, the potential for leaks should also influence the choice of mask (nasal or oronasal). The effect of a high rate of leakage on the efficiency of ventilation during sleep should be monitored, in addition to the potential effect on arousal and the role of nasal airway resistance.

Leaks may decrease the quality of both ventilation and sleep. BACH et al. demonstrated, through the use of volume ventilators for NIV, that severe leakage (i.e. a loss of 33% of the tidal volume) occurred for a median of 55% of sleep time and was associated with significant hypoventilation. In line with these findings, MEYER et al. [72] found severe mouth leak during sleep. In that study, a single limb bilevel device was used to allow for the possible compensation of leaks. In contrast to the study by BACH et al. [71], oxygenation was well maintained, despite prevalent leaking. Based on polysomnographic studies, it was found that leaks >24 L·min^{-1} were associated with frequent arousals during sleep stages 1, 2 and rapid eye movement (REM) and this contributed to sleep fragmentation; arousals were infrequent during slow-wave sleep.

Indeed, leak-induced deterioration of sleep and ventilation may be compensated by adequate interfaces. For example, CRF patients who wore mouth tape during NIV demonstrated a marked reduction in leakage, improved ventilation (i.e. decrease of PCO$_2$) and improved sleep quality (i.e. reduction of arousal index and increase of REM sleep), when, compared to patients without mouth taping [73]. In order to prevent mouth leaks that are associated with wearing a nose mask, the addition of chin straps can be helpful, and this combination has been shown to be just as effective, in terms of gas exchange and sleep quality, as the full-face mask in patients with CRF [59].

Although several mechanisms may be potentially involved in the development of nasal discomfort during NIV, mouth leaks are particularly important because they cause unidirectional inspiratory nasal airflow and progressive drying of the nasal mucosa. This mechanism is also known to promote the release of inflammatory mediators and increase nasal airway resistance [74, 75], which increase mouth breathing and promote further leakage, respectively.

Furthermore, RICHARDS et al. [74] found that increased nasal resistance can be prevented by the addition of humidification. Their findings showed that, because of the high flows, a cold burst of humidification only increased the relative humidity by 6–9% and thus had no effect on improving airway resistance. However, a hot water bath humidifier increased the relative humidity to >97%, and changes in nasal resistance were either greatly attenuated or abolished. Although no consensus has been found concerning the optimal level of air humidification, it is an issue that deserves much more attention in NIV.

Due to the lack of trials dealing with air humidification during NIV of CRF patients, it seems to be feasible to apply to NIV in CRF the central findings of studies of air humidification during CPAP treating sleep apnoea. Both physiological and long-term clinical trials support the impact of air humidification.

Thus, in physiological studies it has been clearly shown that even during mouth leak, heated humidification can significantly increase relative humidity in the airways [76]. Furthermore CPAP treatment in sleep apnoea was associated with the highest rate of compliance (i.e. hours of CPAP usage) and optimal degree of satisfaction when supplemented with heated humidification, compared to both non-heated humidification and no humidification [77].

Finally, the question of when a face mask should be used instead of a nasal mask could be answered by considering the degree of leak monitoring. Compared to patients with CRF, those with ARF are more closely monitored for ineffective ventilation and mouth leaks. This may account for the reason why oronasal masks are preferred in ARF [61, 62]. Nevertheless, mouth leaks can also be a major problem in CRF. Hence, monitoring the presence of mouth leaks, especially during sleep, should help to optimise mask management.

Conclusions

Although there is an immense variety of both ventilators and interfaces for NIV currently available, this form of therapy is a life-changing treatment in which patients may still feel uncomfortable during ventilation. Therefore, further dedication to this matter is needed to ensure the ongoing improvement of ventilators and interfaces.

Many specialists (*i.e.* physicians, respiratory therapists and skilled nurses), working in hospitals, specialised centres or home-care companies are well-qualified to adapt patients to NIV. However, the choice of the ventilator, the interface and the ventilator are usually based on intuition rather than evidence. Finally, monitoring the patient–ventilator interaction or air leaks during sleep is rarely performed and the knowledge about these phenomena, therefore, remains low.

Even though almost 15 years have passed since MEYER and HILL [8] published their review article, the concluding sentence "...several issues relating to the use of NIV are unresolved. The optimal interface and ventilator design have not been determined, and these may differ among patients" remains true.

Summary

Negative pressure ventilation (NPV) was the first reported form of noninvasive ventilation (NIV) to be widely applied to chronic respiratory failure (CRF). However, during the past decades, NPV has gradually lost its former impact and, apart from in a few centres, has been almost completely replaced by positive pressure ventilation (PPV) modes.

The existing plethora of terminology describing NIV modes can sometimes be confusing, especially with respect to ventilators. Pressure-targeted ventilation (PTV) and volume-targeted ventilation (VTV) are the main modes of NIV; Both types can be used in an assisted or controlled setting.

PTV has surpassed VTV in recent years as the treatment option for CRF. Both modes have been successfully applied to NIV in CRF. However, PTV has become the preferred mode due to the higher comfort level for the patient, as well as the lower costs and the compensation it provides for mild-to-moderate mask or mouth leaks. Recently, hybrid modes of PTV and VTV were introduced.

The choice of ventilator and its setting should address different pathophysiological aspects of the underlying disease, of which is variable amongst CRF patients; in patients with COPD, the expiration time should be set at a higher level to avoid air trapping, while higher pressures may be useful to achieve a sufficient tidal volume. Furthermore, the addition of an positive end-expiratory pressure (PEEP) may be helpful to offset intrinsic PEEP in these patients. Various studies have shown that a controlled mode of ventilation is useful and well tolerated by all patients, irrespective of the underlying disease. When a controlled mode of ventilation is favoured, an assist-controlled mode is suggested to increase the patients' subjective tolerance. However, an individualised approach to each patient is beneficial and further studies investigating ventilator settings are needed to continually improve recommendations. The interface between patient and ventilator is crucial for the success of NIV. In various studies, different interfaces have been used with success. However, despite its high clinical impact, the choice of different interfaces has received little scientific attention. A variety of masks are now available, and manufacturers continue to improve mask design. The majority of interfaces is represented by commercial or custom-made nasal masks and oronasal masks. In special indications, nasal pillows or mouthpieces are used. It is suggested that nasal masks should be used prior to oronasal masks in CRF, since there are fewer limitations and communication with the patients is more convenient. In contrast, if patients are mouth breathers, an oronasal mask is favoured. In patients using nasal masks, leaks can occur through an open mouth, especially during night; these leaks can lead to NIV insufficiency, where both the quality of ventilation and sleep may be reduced. In this case, changing the interface to an oronasal mask should be considered. In general, mechanical ventilation can lead to dryness of the upper airway. Therefore, nasal resistance may be an important reason for reduced compliance, which may be compensated by additional humidification.

Keywords: Chronic respiratory insufficiency, hypoventilation, interfaces, mechanical ventilators, noninvasive positive-pressure ventilation.

Acknowledgements. The authors would like to thank S. Dieni for proofreading the manuscript.

References

1. AARC; Respiratory Home Care Focus Group. AARC clinical practice guideline. Long-term invasive mechanical ventilation in the home 2007 revision & update. *Respir Care* 2007; 52: 1056–1062.
2. Bunburaphong T, Imanaka H, Nishimura M, Hess D, Kacmarek RM. Performance characteristics of bilevel pressure ventilators: a lung model study. *Chest* 1997; 111: 1050–1060.
3. Drinker P, Shaw LA. An apparatus for the prolonged administration of artificial respiration: I. A design for adults and children. *J Clin Invest* 1929; 7: 229–247.
4. Levy RD, Bradley TD, Newman SL, Macklem PT, Martin JG. Negative pressure ventilation. Effects on ventilation during sleep in normal subjects. *Chest* 1989; 95: 95–99.
5. Baydur A, Layne E, Aral H, *et al.* Long term non-invasive ventilation in the community for patients with musculoskeletal disorders: 46 year experience and review. *Thorax* 2000; 55: 4–11.
6. Flick GR, Bellamy PE, Simmons DH. Diaphragmatic contraction during assisted mechanical ventilation. *Chest* 1989; 96: 130–135.
7. Laier-Groeneveld G, Rasche K, Weyland W, Braun U, Hüttemann U, Criée CP. The oxygen cost of breathing in patients with chronic ventilatory failure. *Am Rev Respir Dis* 1992; 145: A155.
8. Meyer TJ, Hill NS. Noninvasive positive pressure ventilation to treat respiratory failure. *Ann Intern Med* 1994; 120: 760–770.
9. Mehta S, Hill NS. Noninvasive ventilation. *Am J Respir Crit Care Med* 2001; 163: 540–577.
10. Simonds AK, Elliott MW. Outcome of domiciliary nasal intermittent positive pressure ventilation in restrictive and obstructive disorders. *Thorax* 1995; 50: 604–609.
11. Leger P, Bedicam JM, Cornette A, *et al.* Nasal intermittent positive pressure ventilation. Long-term follow-up in patients with severe chronic respiratory insufficiency. *Chest* 1994; 105: 100–105.
12. Criner GJ, Brennan K, Travaline JM, Kreimer D. Efficacy and compliance with noninvasive positive pressure ventilation in patients with chronic respiratory failure. *Chest* 1999; 116: 667–675.
13. Claman DM, Piper A, Sanders MH, Stiller RA, Votteri BA. Nocturnal noninvasive positive pressure ventilatory assistance. *Chest* 1996; 110: 1581–1588.
14. Lloyd-Owen SJ, Donaldson GC, Ambrosino N, *et al.* Patterns of home mechanical ventilation use in Europe: results from the Eurovent survey. *Eur Respir J* 2005; 25: 1025–1031.

15. Schönhofer B. Noninvasive mechanical ventilation in chronic respiratory failure: ventilators and interfaces. *In*: Muir JF, Ambrosoin N, Simonds AK, eds. Noninvasive Mechanical Ventilation. *Eur Respir Mon* 2001; 16: 259–273.

16. Windisch W, Storre JH, Sorichter S, Virchow JC Jr. Comparison of volume- and pressure-limited NPPV at night: a prospective randomized cross-over trial. *Respir Med* 2005; 99: 52–59.

17. Tuggey JM, Elliott MW. Randomised crossover study of pressure and volume non-invasive ventilation in chest wall deformity. *Thorax* 2005; 60: 859–864.

18. Mehta S, McCool FD, Hill NS. Leak compensation in positive pressure ventilators: a lung model study. *Eur Respir J* 2001; 17: 259–267.

19. Storre JH, Bohm P, Dreher M, Windisch W. Leak compensation during non-invasive ventilation in COPD. *Eur Respir J* 2006; 28: Suppl. 50, P1117.

20. Janssens JP, Derivaz S, Breitenstein E, *et al.* Changing patterns in long-term noninvasive ventilation. *Chest* 2003; 123: 67–79.

21. Bach JR, Alba AS, Saporito LR. Intermittent positive pressure ventilation *via* the mouth as an alternative to tracheostomy for 257 ventilator users. *Chest* 1993; 103: 174–182.

22. Kacmarek RM. Methods of providing mechanical ventilatory support. *In*: Pierson DJ, Kacmarek RM, eds. Foundation Respiratory Care. New York, Edinburgh, London, Melbourne, Tokyo, Churchill Livingstone, 1992; pp. 953–972.

23. Waldhorn RE. Nocturnal nasal intermittent positive pressure ventilation with bi-level positive airway pressure (BiPAP) in respiratory failure. *Chest* 1992; 101: 516–521.

24. Appendini L, Patessio A, Zanaboni S, *et al.* Physiologic effects of positive end-expiratory pressure and mask pressure support during exacerbations of chronic obstructive pulmonary disease. *Am J Respir Crit Care Med* 1994; 149: 1069–1076.

25. Ferguson GT, Gilmartin M. CO_2 rebreathing during BiPAP ventilatory assistance. *Am J Respir Crit Care Med* 1995; 151: 1126–1135.

26. Lofaso F, Brochard L, Hang T, Lorino H, Harf A, Isabey D. Home *versus* intensive care pressure support devices. Experimental and clinical comparison. *Am J Respir Crit Care Med* 1996; 153: 1591–1599.

27. Schettino GP, Chatmongkolchart S, Hess DR, Kacmarek RM. Position of exhalation port and mask design affect CO_2 rebreathing during noninvasive positive pressure ventilation. *Crit Care Med* 2003; 31: 2178–2182.

28. Aslanian P, El Atrous S, Isabey D, *et al.* Effects of flow triggering on breathing effort during partial ventilatory support. *Am J Respir Crit Care Med* 1998; 157: 135–143.

29. Bonmarchand G, Chevron V, Chopin C, *et al.* Increased initial flow rate reduces inspiratory work of breathing during pressure support ventilation in patients with exacerbation of chronic obstructive pulmonary disease. *Intensive Care Med* 1996; 22: 1147–1154.

30. Fabry B, Guttmann J, Eberhard L, Bauer T, Haberthür C, Wolff G. An analysis of desynchronization between the spontaneously breathing patient and ventilator during inspiratory pressure support. *Chest* 1995; 107: 1387–1394.

31. Lofaso F, Aslanian P, Richard JC, *et al.* Expiratory valves used for home devices: experimental and clinical comparison. *Eur Respir J* 1998; 11: 1382–1388.

32. Younes M, Puddy A, Roberts D, *et al.* Proportional assist ventilation. Results of an initial clinical trial. *Am Rev Respir Dis* 1992; 145: 121–129.

33. Younes M. Proportional assist ventilation, a new approach to ventilatory support. Theory. *Am Rev Respir Dis* 1992; 145: 114–120.

34. Gay PC, Hess DR, Hill NS. Noninvasive proportional assist ventilation for acute respiratory insufficiency. Comparison with pressure support ventilation. *Am J Respir Crit Care Med* 2001; 164: 1606–1611.

35. Wysocki M, Richard JC, Meshaka P. Noninvasive proportional assist ventilation compared with noninvasive pressure support ventilation in hypercapnic acute respiratory failure. *Crit Care Med* 2002; 30: 323–329.

36. Serra A, Polese G, Braggion C, Rossi A. Non-invasive proportional assist and pressure support ventilation in patients with cystic fibrosis and chronic respiratory failure. *Thorax* 2002; 57: 50–54.

37. Poggi R, Appendini L, Polese G, Colombo R, Donner CF, Rossi A. Noninvasive proportional assist ventilation and pressure support ventilation during arm elevation in patients with chronic respiratory failure. A preliminary, physiologic study. *Respir Med* 2006; 100: 972–979.

38. Schönhofer B, Zimmermann C, Abramek P, Suchi S, Köhler D, Polkey MI. Non-invasive mechanical ventilation improves walking distance but not quadriceps strength in chronic respiratory failure. *Respir Med* 2003; 97: 818–824.

39. Dreher M, Storre JH, Windisch W. Noninvasive ventilation during walking in patients with severe COPD: a randomised cross-over trial. *Eur Respir J* 2007; 29: 930–936.

40. Schönhofer B, Dellweg D, Suchi S, Köhler D. Exercise endurance before and after long-term noninvasive ventilation in patients with chronic respiratory failure. *Respiration* 2008; 75: 296–303.

41. Storre JH, Seuthe B, Fiechter R, *et al.* Average volume-assured pressure support in obesity hypoventilation: A randomized crossover trial. *Chest* 2006; 130: 815–821.

42. Janssens JP, Sforza E, Metzger M, Rochat T. Impact of average volume assured pressure support (AVAPS) on sleep structure and efficacy of nocturnal bi-level ventilation in patients with chronic hypercapnic respiratory failure (CRF) : a preliminary study. *Eur Respir J* 2007; 30: Suppl. 51, 4263.

43. Schönhofer B, Sortor-Leger S. Equipment needs for noninvasive mechanical ventilation. *Eur Respir J* 2002; 20: 1029–1036.

44. Schönhofer B. Choice of ventilator types, modes, and settings for long-term ventilation. *Respir Care Clin N Am* 2002; 8: 419–445.

45. Hill NS. Noninvasive ventilation. Does it work, for whom, and how? *Am Rev Respir Dis* 1993; 147: 1050–1055.

46. Hill NS, Eveloff SE, Carlisle CC, Goff SG. Efficacy of nocturnal nasal ventilation in patients with restrictive thoracic disease. *Am Rev Respir Dis* 1992; 145: 365–371.

47. Restrick LJ, Fox NC, Braid G, Ward EM, Paul EA, Wedzicha JA. Comparison of nasal pressure support ventilation with nasal intermittent positive pressure ventilation in patients with nocturnal hypoventilation. *Eur Respir J* 1993; 6: 364–370.

48. Meecham Jones DJ, Wedzicha JA. Comparison of pressure and volume preset nasal ventilator systems in stable chronic respiratory failure. *Eur Respir J* 1993; 6: 1060–1064.

49. Schönhofer B, Sonneborn M, Haidl P, Böhrer H, Köhler D. Comparison of two different modes for noninvasive mechanical ventilation in chronic respiratory failure: volume *versus* pressure controlled device. *Eur Respir J* 1997; 10: 184–191.

50. Smith IE, Shneerson JM. Secondary failure of nasal intermittent positive pressure ventilation using the Monnal D: effects of changing ventilator. *Thorax* 1997; 52: 89–91.

51. Jounieaux V, Aubert G, Dury M, Delguste P, Rodenstein DO. Effects of nasal positive-pressure hyperventilation on the glottis in normal awake subjects. *J Appl Physiol* 1995; 79: 176–185.

52. Jounieaux V, Aubert G, Dury M, Delguste P, Rodenstein DO. Effects of nasal positive-pressure hyperventilation on the glottis in normal sleeping subjects. *J Appl Physiol* 1995; 79: 186–193.

53. Parreira VF, Jounieaux V, Aubert G, Dury M, Delguste PE, Rodenstein DO. Nasal two-level positive-pressure ventilation in normal subjects. Effects of the glottis and ventilation. *Am J Respir Crit Care Med* 1996; 153: 1616–1623.

54. Parreira VF, Delguste P, Jounieaux V, Aubert G, Dury M, Rodenstein DO. Effectiveness of controlled and spontaneous modes in nasal two-level positive pressure ventilation in awake and asleep normal subjects. *Chest* 1997; 112: 1267–1277.

55. Srinivasan S, Doty SM, White TR, *et al.* Frequency, causes, and outcome of home ventilator failure. *Chest* 1998; 114: 1363–1367.

56. Farre R, Lloyd-Owen SJ, Ambrosino N, *et al.* Quality control of equipment in home mechanical ventilation: a European survey. *Eur Respir J* 2005; 26: 86–94.

57. Farré R, Giró E, Casolivé V, Navajas D, Escarrabill J. Quality control of mechanical ventilation at the patient's home. *Intensive Care Med* 2003; 29: 484–486.

58. Navalesi P, Fanfulla F, Frigerio P, Gregoretti C, Nava S. Physiologic evaluation of noninvasive mechanical ventilation delivered with three types of masks in patients with chronic hypercapnic respiratory failure. *Crit Care Med* 2000; 28: 1785–1790.

59. Willson GN, Piper AJ, Norman M, *et al.* Nasal *versus* full face mask for noninvasive ventilation in chronic respiratory failure. *Eur Respir J* 2004; 23: 605–609.

60. Mortimore IL, Whittle AT, Douglas NJ. Comparison of nose and face mask CPAP therapy for sleep apnoea. *Thorax* 1998; 53: 290–292.

61. Elliott MW. The interface: crucial for successful noninvasive ventilation. *Eur Respir J* 2004; 23: 7–8.

62. Meduri GU, Cook TR, Turner RE, Cohen M, Leeper KV. Noninvasive positive pressure ventilation in status asthmaticus. *Chest* 1996; 110: 767–774.

63. Criner GJ, Travaline JM, Brennan KJ, Kreimer DT. Efficacy of a new full face mask for noninvasive positive pressure ventilation. *Chest* 1994; 106: 1109–1115.

64. Antonelli M, Conti G, Pelosi P, *et al.* New treatment of acute hypoxemic respiratory failure: noninvasive pressure support ventilation delivered by helmet – a pilot controlled trial. *Crit Care Med* 2002; 30: 602–608.

65. Antonelli M, Pennisi MA, Pelosi P, *et al.* Noninvasive positive pressure ventilation using a helmet in patients with acute exacerbation of chronic obstructive pulmonary disease: a feasibility study. *Anesthesiology* 2004; 100: 16–24.

66. Navalesi P, Costa R, Ceriana P, *et al.* Non-invasive ventilation in chronic obstructive pulmonary disease patients: helmet *versus* facial mask. *Intensive Care Med* 2007; 33: 74–81.

67. Tsuboi T, Ohi M, Kita H, *et al.* The efficacy of a custom-fabricated nasal mask on gas exchange during nasal intermittent positive pressure ventilation. *Eur Respir J* 1999; 13: 152–156.

68. Bach JR, Alba AS, Bohatiuk G, Saporito L, Lee M. Mouth intermittent positive pressure ventilation in the management of postpolio respiratory insufficiency. *Chest* 1987; 91: 859–864.

69. Toussaint M, Steens M, Wasteels G, Soudon P. Diurnal ventilation *via* mouthpiece: survival in end-stage Duchenne patients. *Eur Respir J* 2006; 28: 549–555.

70. Saatci E, Miller DM, Stell IM, Lee KC, Moxham J. Dynamic dead space in face masks used with noninvasive ventilators: a lung model study. *Eur Respir J* 2004; 23: 129–135.

71. Bach JR, Robert D, Leger P, Langevin B. Sleep fragmentation in kyphoscoliotic individuals with alveolar hypoventilation treated by NIPPV. *Chest* 1995; 107: 1552–1558.

72. Meyer TJ, Pressman MR, Benditt J, *et al.* Air leaking through the mouth during nocturnal nasal ventilation: effect on sleep quality. *Sleep* 1997; 20: 561–569.

73. Teschler H, Stampa J, Ragette R, Konietzko N, Berthon-Jones M. Effect of mouth leak on effectiveness of nasal bilevel ventilatory assistance and sleep architecture. *Eur Respir J* 1999; 14: 1251–1257.

74. Richards GN, Cistulli PA, Ungar RG, Berthon-Jones M, Sullivan CE. Mouth leak with nasal continuous positive airway pressure increases nasal airway resistance. *Am J Respir Crit Care Med* 1996; 154: 182–186.

75. Togias AG, Naclerio RM, Proud D, *et al.* Nasal challenge with cold, dry air results in release of inflammatory mediators. Possible mast cell involvement. *J Clin Invest* 1985; 76: 1375–1381.

76. Martins De Araújo MT, Vieira SB, Vasquez EC, Fleury B. Heated humidification or face mask to prevent upper airway dryness during continuous positive airway pressure therapy. *Chest* 2000; 117: 142–147.

77. Massie CA, Hart RW, Peralez K, Richards GN. Effects of humidification on nasal symptoms and compliance in sleep apnea patients using continuous positive airway pressure. *Chest* 1999; 116: 403–408.

CHAPTER 23

Interfaces and humidification in the home setting

P. Navalesi*, P. Frigerio#, C. Gregoretti¶

*Anesthesia and Intensive Care, Eastern Piedmont University "A. Avogadro", Maggiore della Carità Hospital, Novara, #Spinal Cord Unit, 'Niguarda Ca' Granda Hospital, Milan, and ¶Emergency Dept, CTO-M.Adelaide Hospital, Turin, Italy.

Correspondence: P. Navalesi, SCDU Anestesia, Terapia Intensiva e Rianimazione Generale, Azienda Ospedaliero-Universitaria 'Maggiore della Carità', Corso Mazzini 18, 28100 Novara, Italy. Fax: 39 3213733406; E-mail: paulo.navalesi@fastwebnet.it

Introduction

Noninvasive ventilation (NIV), currently, plays a key role in the treatment of patients with acute respiratory failure [1–7]. NIV is also used for long-term treatment of patients with chronic hypercapnic respiratory failure due to thoracic deformities, neuromuscular diseases, sleep-disordered breathing and chronic obstructive pulmonary disease (COPD) [8–10].

The patient's comfort is crucial for NIV success in both the acute [11, 12] and chronic [13] setting. Because a poorly-fitting interface decreases clinical effectiveness and patient adherence to NIV, the choice of the interface has been recognised as one major determinant of the success of this form of treatment [14, 15]. The patient's comfort may be affected by the interface with respect to many aspects, such as air-leaks, claustrophobia, facial skin erythema, acneiform rash, eye irritation and skin breakdown [14].

The lack of heating and humidification is a less-recognised cause of discomfort for the patient receiving NIV. In patients undergoing overnight nasal continuous positive airway pressure (CPAP) for treatment of obstructive sleep apnoeas (OSAs), in presence of mouth leaks, cold dry air increases nasal resistance [16], which causes nasal symptoms [16] and reduces the patient's compliance to CPAP [17]. Recent work suggests that the same problems could affect nasal NIV and that heated humidification has the potential to reduce these adverse effects and improve NIV comfort [18].

Interfaces

General characteristics

Although the availability of interfaces has greatly increased in the recent years and new products are continuously arriving on the market, the "perfect interface", best for all patients in all situations, does not exist and will likely never exist. When choosing the interface for a patient, one has to compromise between different aims, such as leak minimisation, ease of use and best comfort. The ideal characteristics of the interface for NIV are presented in table 1.

A large variety of masks, both disposable and reusable, are available in different sizes from a number of manufacturers. Ready-to-use masks are usually composed of two parts: a stiff

Eur Respir Mon, 2008, 41, 338–349. Printed in UK - all rights reserved. Copyright ERS Journals Ltd 2008; European Respiratory Monograph; ISSN 1025-448x.

Table 1. – Ideal characteristics of the interface for noninvasive ventilation

Characteristics of the ideal interface
Leak-free
Good stability
Nontraumatic
Light-weight
Long-lasting and nondeformable
Range of sizes
Made of nonallergenic material
Low resistance to airflow
Reduced dead space
Inexpensive
Easy to secure
Easy to clean
Transparent[#]
Quickly removable[#]
Anti-asphyxia valve[#]

[#]: desirable characteristics for oro-nasal mask.

shell and a soft cushioned or flailed surface in direct contact with the patient. These two parts can be either glued in a single block or hooked to one another, in a manner to be easily attached and detached. In this latter case, the same shell is applicable to soft surfaces of different size, so that one single shell can fit a wide range of users. A few masks are composed by a single piece. The shell, commonly transparent, can be made of rigid polyvinyl chloride (PVC), polycarbonate or Orfit®. The piece directly in contact with patient's skin can be made of soft PVC, polypropylene, silicon, silicon elastomer, gel or hygrogel [19].

In the past, especially for long-term home ventilation, custom masks were often moulded directly on the patient or from a previously obtained impression of their face contour [20]. Fabrication time and quality are largely operator-dependent; with respect to the model used, the time required to prepare a mask varies 5–30 mins for a skilled operator [21]. Recently, one manufacturer has proposed a ready-to-use nasal mask that can be customised to the patient's face contour; once removed from the packaging, the mask is put in boiled water and then cooled and pressed against the patient's face.

The body mask includes the prongs to anchor the headgear. In principle, more points of attachment increase the chance of obtaining a good fit and vary the site of maximal pressure application. Prongs sited more peripherally may result in a more uniform distribution of pressure on the face [22].

In some masks the upper part is secured on the forehead rather than at the bridge of the nose. One important feature of these masks is the forehead spacer, made of foam or gel, that, filling the gap between the forehead and the mask, reduces the pressure exerted on the bridge of the nose. In order to further decrease the pressure on the nose, the forehead can be mounted on an adjustable arm.

Masks are connected to the ventilator circuit through connectors, swivels and adapters that can be externally applied or built into the shell. In some models of nasal masks, flexible tubing is mounted between the shell and the connector. This approach improves the comfort, by allowing the patient to move without affecting mask stability but causes an increase in dead space, which may be relevant at low tidal volumes.

Classification of interfaces

Interfaces can be classified according to the manner in which they are connected to the patient as: 1) oral interfaces; 2) nasal interfaces; or 3) oro-nasal interfaces. While the studies performed on acute patients used an oro-nasal mask preferentially, the nasal mask was preferred in more than 75% of the studies evaluating long-term domicilary NIV, followed by nasal pillows (11%), facial mask (6%) and mouthpiece (5%) [15].

The continuous development of new products by the manufacturers has definitely increased the availability of interfaces and the chance of meeting different requirements. In patients necessitating several daily hours of NIV, however, the rotation of different interfaces remains, in the present authors' opinion, the best strategy to avoid or to reduce to a large extent, the risk of skin breakdown, by alternating the distribution of pressure upon the skin and varying the site of maximal friction [23].

Oral interfaces. Mouthpieces are commercially available in different types and sizes in order to meet patient comfort and improve NIV compliance. They can be divided into: 1) standard narrow mouthpieces with different degrees of flexion in order to be grabbed by patient's teeth and/or lips; and 2) custom moulded bite-plates. table 2 summarises advantages and disadvantages of this interface.

Mouthpieces are simple and not expensive. One of their major limitations relies on the large amount of air leaking, which may compromise NIV efficacy and cause unwanted alarming of the ventilator. In order to limit air leaks, mouthpieces configured with a lip seal can be used; some suggest that air leaks can be managed by occluding the nostrils with nose plugs [14]. Mouthpieces may stimulate salivation, elicit gag reflex and, ultimately, cause vomiting. Vomit aspiration is potentially a severe complication but it seems to be more hypothetical than real [14, 24]. Standard mouthpieces may produce orthodontic deformities over time.

Nasal interfaces. Nasal interfaces can be divided into: 1) full nasal masks; 2) external nostril masks; and 3) internal nostril masks. Full nasal masks fit at the bridge of the nose, on the upper lip and at the side of the nostrils. The soft surface can be either cushioned or flailed. The cushion of the nasal mask can be filled with air or gel. Although full nasal masks have also been used for the treatment of acute hypercapnic [1, 2] and hypoxaemic [25] respiratory failure, they are preferentially chosen for chronic patients on long-term home ventilation. In patients with chronic respiratory failure of mixed aetiology, full nasal masks are better tolerated than facial masks and nasal pillows, but less effective in ameliorating gas exchange [23].

External nostril masks are recently developed interfaces that have the advantage to minimise the bulk of the mask, to eliminate the occurrence of claustrophobia, and to allow the patient to wear glasses while the ventilator is in use. External nostril masks are applied around the outer wall of the nostrils, thereby assuring minimal facial contact and no pressure on the bridge of the nose.

Internal nostril masks, often called nasal plugs, are available from a few manufacturers and consist of soft plastic plugs inserted into the nostrils. The pressure applied during inspiration helps to seal the wall of the pillows against the inner surface of the nasal vestibule. Nasal pillows are held in place with specifically designed

Table 2. – Advantages and disadvantages of mouthpiece

Advantages	Disadvantages
Negligible dead space	Ineffective if patient cannot maintain mouth seal
Less interference with speech (patient allowed to use the ventilator intermittently)	Difficult to use overnight
	Nasal leaks
	Possible gag reflex, salivation, vomit
	Possible orthodontic deformities over time

headgears. The nasal pillows can be as effective as oro-nasal masks in improving gas exchange but less tolerated than full nasal masks [23].

Dual pressure ports are common for allowing oxygen administration and pressure check. Most masks are available with exhalation ports directly included in the shell to eliminate the exhaled air and avoid rebreathing. This apparatus represents a real anti-rebreathing system and should not be used when the circuit has separated inspiratory and expiratory limbs or when an expiratory valve or another external device for CO_2 elimination is present. In order to avoid erroneous connections between masks and circuits, some manufactures make a distinction between interfaces with and without vent holes, using different colours or connections. Advantages and disadvantages of nasal masks are listed in table 3.

Oro-nasal interfaces. Oro-nasal interfaces can be divided into: 1) facial masks, comprehensive of the surface around nose and mouth; 2) total face mask, which also include the eyes [26]; and 3) helmet, including the whole head. They are available in a variety of sizes and are often equipped with an anti-asphyxia valve, which automatically opens when airway pressure falls below a minimal pressure (2–3 cmH$_2$O), enabling the patient to breathe room air while still wearing the mask. As it may occur during power failure or machine malfunctioning, oro-nasal masks are preferred for severely dyspnoeic patients with acute respiratory failure, who breathe through both the nose and the mouth.

Facial masks fit on the nasal bridge, below the lower lip and beside the nose. Facial masks can be cushioned or flailed. The cushion is either air-filled or foam-filled. In some masks the cushion is inflatable; air is added or removed to improve mask fit [27, 28]. A transparent dome is preferred because it allows visual assessment of the presence of secretions [22]. Facial masks are also available with exhalation vents. Technical improvements, such as more-comfortable seals, improved air sealing capabilities, quick-release straps and anti-asphyxia valves have increased the acceptability of the facial masks also for long-term application [14].

The total face mask has a soft flail that seals around the perimeter of the face. The total face mask can be an alternative for patients who are unable to obtain a good seal [14]. As it covers the entire face, the total face mask does not exert pressure on the nose bridge. Its use is characterised by large air leaks, which make it compatible only with ventilators with high air leak compensation capability.

The helmet is a transparent hood secured by two armpit braces at two hooks sited on a metallic ring that joins the hood to a soft collar. It was designed to deliver a precise oxygen fraction during hyperbaric oxygen therapy, but is now used in Europe to apply CPAP and, less commonly, NIV, in the acute setting. The helmet has no indication for long term NIV.

Table 4 shows advantages and disadvantages oro-nasal interfaces.

Table 3. – Advantages and disadvantages of nasal interfaces

Advantages	Disadvantages
Less risk of aspiration	Mouth leaks
Less interference with cough	Less effective with nasal obstruction
Allow patient to eat and drink	Nasal irritation and rhinorrhea
Less claustrophobic	Mouth dryness
No risk of asphyxia in case of ventilator malfunctioning	Problematic expiratory tidal volume monitoring[¶]
Not pressure over the bridge of the nose[#]	
Allow patient to wear glasses[#]	

[#]: only for external and internal nostril masks; [¶]: only for internal nostril masks.

Table 4. – Advantages and disadvantages of face mask and total face mask

Advantages	Disadvantages
No mouth leaks	Claustrophobic
Effective in mouth breathers	Increased risk of aspiration
More stable airway pressure	Difficult communication
Lower resistance to airflow	Impossible to eat and drink
Less need for patient cooperation	Disconnection necessary to expectorate

Securing system. The use of an appropriate mask is obvious but equal attention should be also directed to the choice of the headgear. The securing system is an important determinant of air-leak control, mask stability and overall patient comfort. The headgear secures the mask by means of hooks or straps, which can be attached on either the outer edge or the centre of the body mask. Attachment of the headgear to the outer edge of the mask may result in a better distribution of the pressure and facilitate the seal. Some styles of headgear are designed as a cap to minimise movement of the interface. Oro-nasal masks should be rapidly pulled out in emergency by means of headgear quick-release systems. Table 5 lists the ideal characteristics of the securing system.

Selecting the right interface

The choice of the interface requires a careful evaluation of patient, underlying disease, type of ventilator and circuit, and ventilatory mode and settings. In the present authors' opinion, a large availability of different types and sizes of interfaces is helpful to make the right choice.

Physiological issues. Air leaks may reduce the efficiency of NIV by reducing tolerance, increasing patient–ventilator dyssynchrony, altering trigger sensitivity and promoting arousals that lead to sleep fragmentation [29, 30]. Leaks hinder the achievement of the inspiration-termination criteria during pressure support [31, 32] and are associated with daytime hypercapnia in neuromuscular patients receiving nocturnal NIV for treatment of chronic hypercapnic respiratory failure [33].

SCHETTINO *et al.* [34] studied air-leak dynamics and mask mechanics and estimated the pressure determining the adhesion of the mask on the skin (Pmask-occl) as the difference between the pressure pushing the mask upon the face (Pmask-fit), assessed as the pressure inside the cushion, and airway pressure (Paw). The air leak was

Table 5. – Ideal characteristics of the securing system

Characteristics of the ideal securing system
Stable
Easy to put on and remove
Nontraumatic
Light and soft
Made of transpiring material
Available in different sizes
Nonspecific for a single interface
Re-washable
Quick-release system

negligible and nearly constant for Pmask-occl values >2 cmH$_2$O; when Pmask-occl decreased below that threshold, however, air leaks became relevant [34]. As a consequence, increasing Pmask-occl promote air-leak containment, which can be obtained either lowering the overall pressure applied by the ventilator or tightening the headgear (*i.e.* increasing Pmask-fit). With the latter approach, however, Pmask-fit may exceed skin capillary pressure, which impairs tissue perfusion and cause skin abrasions [14, 35].

The improvement in alveolar ventilation can be limited by an increase in the dynamic dead space (VD,dyn), which is the physiologic dead space (VD,phys) plus the dead space of the apparatus (VD,app), which depends on the inner volume of the interface. Different flow patterns and pressure waveforms may also influence the dead space of the apparatus. SAATCI *et al.* [36] found that the face mask produced an increase in VD,dyn (from 32 to 42% of tidal volume) during spontaneous breathing. The addition of positive end-expiratory pressure (PEEP) lowered VD,dyn close to VD,phys [36]. Pressure support without PEEP reduced VD,dyn to a lesser extent, from 42 to 39% of tidal volume, leaving VD,dyn higher than VD,phys. In presence of PEEP, an exhalation port close to the bridge of the nose made VD,dyn lower than VD,phys. FERGUSON and GILMARTIN [37] first showed that reducing PEEP, below 4 cmH$_2$O, significantly increased rebreathing, unless a non rebreathing exhalation valve was used. In a lung-model study conducted to evaluate the effect of exhalation port location and mask design on CO$_2$ re-breathing during NIV, SCHETTINO *et al.* [38] reported a lower volume of rebreathed CO$_2$ with the exhalation port in the mask, compared with the exhalation port in the circuit. The authors concluded that masks with exhalation ports located within the mask minimised rebreathing during NIV. In a study performed on 7 COPD patients, moving the path for exhalation reduced CO$_2$ rebreathing to almost zero [39]. Masks that do not have ports sited in the optimal place, however, may still perform quite well, probably due to unintentional air leaks [40].

Clinical issues. Mouthpieces are utilised for long-term ventilation in patients affected by severe chronic respiratory failure due to neuromuscular diseases [24]. In acute patients, the mouthpiece has been shown to be as effective as the oro-nasal mask in improving gas exchange [41, 42]; compared with the mask, however, the mouthpiece was considered less comfortable by the patients [41]. A recent study, still in abstract form, demonstrated that the mouthpiece is able to reduce inspiratory effort, although to a lesser extent than facial and nasal masks [43].

During daytime, the mouthpiece can be attached to the wheelchair and mounted close to the mouth, so that the patients may use the ventilator either intermittently or breath by breath, according their own needs [14]. During sleep, some patients use strapless custom mouthpieces and others use strapped-on lip seals [24]. Although a few individuals have learned to use such mouthpieces during sleep, the majority of patients use the mouthpiece only during daytime and switch overnight to another interface [44, 45]. In a retrospective evaluation of a cohort of 257 patients, requiring continuous or quasi-continuous ventilatory support, BACH *et al.* [24] reported the use of mouthpiece alone or in association with other interfaces. The mouthpiece was the preferential interface for providing daytime ventilatory support for 228 individuals. In some cases, a narrow flexed mouthpiece was used during the day-time and a nasal mask overnight, but in 163 individuals, 61 of whom had little or no measurable vital capacity, a standard mouthpiece with lip seal retention or a custom moulded orthodontic bite was used also for nocturnal aid [24]. The authors concluded that for patients with chronic respiratory muscle insufficiency and intact bulbar function, mouthpieces may be an effective alternative to tracheostomy [24]. The use of mouthpieces has also been reported in a series of patients with respiratory failure secondary to cystic fibrosis [46].

Compared with oro-nasal masks, nasal interfaces add less static dead space, are less claustrophobic and allow communication, expectoration and oral intake without removing the mask [15]. Oro-nasal interfaces are preferable for treating severe episodes of acute respiratory failure because dyspnoeic patients breathe through the mouth, which makes nasal masks prone to increased air leakage and lower effectiveness [47, 48]. In order to reduce mouth leaks while wearing a nose mask, a chin strap has been proposed [33]; this approach is, in the present authors' opinion, often of limited benefit and always ineffective in edentulous patients. Total face mask may be advantageous in patients who are unable to tolerate a nasal mask because of nasal pathologies or clinically relevant mouth leaks persisting, despite application of chinstrap. Finally, compared with nasal masks, facial masks allow application of higher positive pressure and require less patient co-operation.

Patient tolerance is primarily improved by avoiding air leaks and skin breakdown [14]. Small amounts of air leakage may be well tolerated if the tidal volume is adequate. Air leaks, however, often profoundly affect the patient's tolerance and long-term response to NIV by causing side effects, such as eyes irritation, mouth and nose dryness, noise, impaired ventilator cycling and patient–machine dyssynchrony. Air leaks also deteriorate sleep quality, worsen gas exchange and increase inspiratory muscle effort contributing to treatment failure [49].

The site involved by bruising depends upon the type of interface: nose bridge and upper lip from the full nasal mask, nose bridge and chin from the facial mask, nasal mucosa and upper lip from the nasal pillows and pit from the helmet. Skin sensitivity to certain materials and excessive sweating may facilitate bruising. A common mistake is to fit the headgear too tight. While further tightening of the headgear does not necessarily improve the fit of the mask, it does frequently worsen the patient's comfort. With this latter approach, in fact, the pressure exerted by the mask may exceed skin capillary pressure, which impairs tissue perfusion and determines abrasions [14, 34, 35]. A good "rule of thumb" is to keep the straps loose enough to allow one or two fingers to pass between the headgear and the skin [35]. In order to improve the mask fit and avoid leaks it is also helpful to maintain the headgear straps parallel to one another. There are several helpful strategies to limit the risk of skin breakdown, such as rotational use of different types of interfaces, skin and mask hygiene and the use of forehead spacers.

Humidification

The importance of heating and humidifying the inhaled air is well recognised for patients undergoing invasive mechanical ventilation in both the acute [50] and long term [51] setting. On the contrary, few studies have, so far, evaluated this aspect during NIV. Inhaling dry cold air can effect release of inflammatory mediators [52], increase mucosal blood flow [53], and increase nasal airway resistance [54] In OSAs patients receiving nocturnal CPAP, the lack of humidification increases nasal resistance and causes nasal symptoms [16]. These side-effects, which have been primarily attributed to mouth leaks causing unidirectional inspiratory nasal airflow and progressive drying of the nasal mucosa, are attenuated by heated humidification, while the use of cold pass-over humidifier is no beneficial [16]. Dryness of inhaled air during CPAP is attenuated by heated humidification, even with mouth leaks, and further reduced by using a face mask in place of a nasal mask [55]. Although heated humidification of nasal CPAP has been repeatedly demonstrated to reduce upper airway symptoms [56, 57], its use has produced controversial results with respect to patient's compliance to treatment, which resulted in significant improvement in one study [58], slightly and only initially ameliorated in a second study [56] and unchanged in a third [57].

Most patients on long-term domiciliary NIV use nasal masks and are, therefore, subject to air leaking through the mouth [18]. Recently, a daytime study performed on healthy individuals showed that a short period of mouth leak during nasal NIV increases nasal resistance, which negatively affects the delivered tidal volume [18]. These effects were reduced using heated humidification, which improved comfort, both in the absence of leaks and following a period of increased leak [18]. These data indicate that heated humidification may improve the comfort by attenuating the adverse effects of mouth leak in patients on domiciliary NIV.

In acute patients, heated humidification and heat-and-moisture exchanger (HME) have been compared in two recent studies [59, 60]. Compared with heated humidification, HME reduced NIV efficiency, resulting in higher Pa,CO_2, respiratory rate and minute ventilation [59], and increased the work of breathing [60]. In principle, HME should be avoided with nasal NIV because the air leaked through the mouth makes it less effective or ineffective at all. Furthermore, the additional resistance imposed by HME [60] may interfere with ventilator triggering. Very recently, NAVA et al. [61] performed a pilot randomised cross-over 12-month study on 16 patients with stable chronic hypercapnic respiratory failure who underwent NIV with either heated humidification or HME. Although a higher number of patients decided to continue NIV with heated humidification, no significant difference was found with respect to NIV compliance, airway symptoms, rate of hospitalisation consequent to acute exacerbation [61].

In conclusion, data from physiological studies suggest a beneficial effect of heated humidification for patients on long term noninvasive ventilation and, in particular, for those using a nasal mask who have nasal symptoms. Further randomised controlled trials are needed to evaluate the long-term effects of heated humidification and the efficacy of the different humidification devices.

Summary

The choice of the interface is crucial for the success of noninvasive ventilation (NIV) in both the acute and chronic setting. Type (oral, nasal, oro-nasal), size, design, material and securing system of the interface may affect the patient's comfort with respect to many aspects, such as air-leaks, claustrophobia, skin erythema, eye irritation and skin breakdown. Although the continuous development of new products has increased the availability of interfaces and the chance to meet different requirements, in patients necessitating several daily hours of NIV, the rotational use of different interfaces remains an excellent strategy to decrease the risk of skin breakdown.

While the importance of heating and humidification for long-term invasive mechanical ventilation is well known, it is less recognised for the patient receiving long term NIV. Recent work, however, suggests that, in the presence of airleaks, cold dry air increases nasal resistance, causes nasal symptoms and reduces the patient's compliance to NIV, and that heated humidification has the potential to reduce these adverse effects.

Keywords: Air heating and humidification, long-term mechanical ventilation, mechanical ventilation, noninvasive ventilation, noninvasive ventilation interfaces.

References

1. Bott J, Carroll MP, Conway JH, *et al.* Randomised controlled trial of nasal ventilation in acute ventilatory failure due to chronic obstructive airways disease. *Lancet* 1993; 341: 1555–1557.
2. Kramer N, Meyer TJ, Meharg J, Cece RD, Hill NS. Randomized, prospective trial of noninvasive positive pressure ventilation in acute respiratory failure. *Am J Respir Crit Care Med* 1995; 151: 1799–1806.
3. Brochard L, Mancebo J, Wysocki M, *et al.* Noninvasive ventilation for acute exacerbations of chronic obstructive pulmonary disease. *N Engl J Med* 1995; 333: 817–822.
4. Meduri GU, Turner RE, Abou-Shala N, Wunderink R, Tolley E. Noninvasive positive pressure ventilation *via* face mask. First-line intervention in patients with acute hypercapnic and hypoxemic respiratory failure. *Chest* 1996; 109: 179–193.
5. Plant PK, Owen JL, Elliott MW. Early use of non-invasive ventilation for acute exacerbations of chronic obstructive pulmonary disease on general respiratory wards: a multicentre randomised controlled trial. *Lancet* 2000; 355: 1931–1935.
6. Antonelli M, Conti G, Rocco M, *et al.* A comparison of noninvasive positive-pressure ventilation and conventional mechanical ventilation in patients with acute respiratory failure. *N Engl J Med* 1998; 339: 429–435.
7. Hilbert G, Gruson D, Vargas F, *et al.* Noninvasive ventilation in immunosuppressed patients with pulmonary infiltrates, fever, and acute respiratory failure. *N Engl J Med* 2001; 344: 481–487.
8. Meyer TJ, Hill NS. Noninvasive positive pressure ventilation to treat respiratory failure. *Ann Intern Med* 1994; 120: 760–770.
9. Shneerson JM, Simonds AK. Noninvasive ventilation for chest wall and neuromuscular disorders. *Eur Respir J* 2002; 20: 480–487.
10. Simonds AK. Home ventilation. *Eur Respir J* 2003; 22: Suppl. 47, 38S–46S.

11. Antonelli M, Conti G, Moro ML, *et al.* Predictors of failure of noninvasive positive pressure ventilation in patients with acute hypoxemic respiratory failure: a multi-center study. *Intensive Care Med* 2001; 27: 1718–1728.

12. Squadrone E, Frigerio P, Fogliati C, *et al.* Noninvasive *vs* invasive ventilation in COPD patients with severe acute respiratory failure deemed to require ventilatory assistance. *Intensive Care Med* 2004; 30: 1303–1310.

13. Criner GJ, Brennan K, Travaline JM, Kreimer D. Efficacy and compliance with noninvasive positive pressure ventilation in patients with chronic respiratory failure. *Chest* 1999; 116: 667–675.

14. Mehta S, Hill NS. Noninvasive ventilation. *Am J Respir Crit Care Med* 2001; 163: 540–577.

15. Schönhofer B, Sortor-Leger S. Equipment needs for noninvasive mechanical ventilation. *Eur Respir J* 2002; 20: 1029–1036.

16. Richards GN, Cistulli PA, Ungar RG, Berthon-Jones M, Sullivan CE. Mouth leak with nasal continuous positive airway pressure increases nasal airway resistance. *Am J Respir Crit Care Med* 1996; 154: 182–186.

17. Bachour A, Maasilta P. Mouth breathing compromises adherence to nasal continuous positive airway pressure therapy. *Chest* 2004; 126: 1248–1254.

18. Tuggey JM, Delmastro M, Elliott MW. The effect of mouth leak and humidification during nasal non-invasive ventilation. *Respir Med* 2007; 101: 1874–1879.

19. Navalesi P, Frigerio P, Gregoretti C. Interfaces for noninvasive ventilation. *ERJ Buyers' Guide* 2001: 40–41.

20. McDermott I, Bach JR, Parker C, Sortor S. Custom-fabricated interfaces for intermittent positive pressure ventilation. *Int J Prosthodont* 1989; 2: 224–233.

21. Cornette A MD. Ventilatory assistance via the nasal route: mask and fitting. *Eur Respir Rev* 1993; 3: 250–253.

22. Meduri G, Spencer S. Noninvasive mechanical ventilation in the acute setting. Technical aspects, monitoring and choice of interface. *In*: Muir JF, Ambrosino N, Simonds AK, eds. Noninvasive Mechanical Ventilation. *Eur Respir Mon* 2001; 16: 106–124.

23. Navalesi P, Fanfulla F, Frigerio P, Gregoretti C, Nava S. Physiologic evaluation of noninvasive mechanical ventilation delivered with three types of masks in patients with chronic hypercapnic respiratory failure. *Crit Care Med* 2000; 28: 1785–1790.

24. Bach JR, Alba AS, Saporito LR. Intermittent positive pressure ventilation *via* the mouth as an alternative to tracheostomy for 257 ventilator users. *Chest* 1993; 103: 174–182.

25. Pennock BE, Crawshaw L, Kaplan PD. Noninvasive nasal mask ventilation for acute respiratory failure. Institution of a new therapeutic technology for routine use. *Chest* 1994; 105: 441–444.

26. Criner GJ, Travaline JM, Brennan KJ, Kreimer DT. Efficacy of a new full face mask for noninvasive positive pressure ventilation. *Chest* 1994; 106: 1109–1115.

27. Gregoretti C, Confalonieri M, Navalesi P, *et al.* Evaluation of patient skin breakdown and comfort with a new face mask for non-invasive ventilation: a multi-center study. *Intensive Care Med* 2002; 28: 278–284.

28. Munckton K, Ho KM, Dobb GJ, Das-Gupta M, Webb SA. The pressure effects of facemasks during noninvasive ventilation: a volunteer study. *Anaesthesia* 2007; 62: 1126–1131.

29. Bach JR, Robert D, Leger P, Langevin B. Sleep fragmentation in kyphoscoliotic individuals with alveolar hypoventilation treated by NIPPV. *Chest* 1995; 107: 1552–1558.

30. Meyer TJ, Pressman MR, Benditt J, *et al.* Air leaking through the mouth during nocturnal nasal ventilation: effect on sleep quality. *Sleep* 1997; 20: 561–569.

31. Calderini E, Confalonieri M, Puccio PG, Francavilla N, Stella L, Gregoretti C. Patient–ventilator asynchrony during noninvasive ventilation: the role of expiratory trigger. *Intensive Care Med* 1999; 25: 662–667.

32. Mehta S, McCool FD, Hill NS. Leak compensation in positive pressure ventilators: a lung model study. *Eur Respir J* 2001; 17: 259–267.

33. Gonzalez J, Sharshar T, Hart N, Chadda K, Raphaël JC, Lofaso F. Air leaks during mechanical ventilation as a cause of persistent hypercapnia in neuromuscular disorders. *Intensive Care Med* 2003; 29: 596–602.

34. Schettino GP, Tucci MR, Sousa R, Valente Barbas CS, Passos Amato MB, Carvalho CR. Mask mechanics and leak dynamics during noninvasive pressure support ventilation: a bench study. *Intensive Care Med* 2001; 27: 1887–1891.

35. Meduri GU. Noninvasive positive-pressure ventilation in patients with acute respiratory failure. *Clin Chest Med* 1996; 17: 513–553.

36. Saatci E, Miller DM, Stell IM, Lee KC, Moxham J. Dynamic dead space in face masks used with noninvasive ventilators: a lung model study. *Eur Respir J* 2004; 23: 129–135.

37. Ferguson GT, Gilmartin M. CO_2 rebreathing during BiPAP ventilatory assistance. *Am J Respir Crit Care Med* 1995; 151: 1126–1135.

38. Schettino GP, Chatmongkolchart S, Hess DR, Kacmarek RM. Position of exhalation port and mask design affect CO_2 rebreathing during noninvasive positive pressure ventilation. *Crit Care Med* 2003; 31: 2178–2182.

39. Chen R, Zhang X, He G. [Modification of facial mask on the dead space effect in non-invasive mask ventilation]. *Zhonghua Jie He He Hu Xi Za Zhi* 2000; 23: 734–736.

40. Hill NS, Carlisle C, Kramer NR. Effect of a nonrebreathing exhalation valve on long-term nasal ventilation using a bilevel device. *Chest* 2002; 122: 84–91.

41. Schneider E, Dualé C, Vaille JL, *et al.* Comparison of tolerance of facemask *vs.* mouthpiece for non-invasive ventilation. *Anaesthesia* 2006; 61: 20–23.

42. Glerant JC, Rose D, Oltean V, Dayen C, Mayeux I, Jounieaux V. Noninvasive ventilation using a mouthpiece in patients with chronic obstructive pulmonary disease and acute respiratory failure. *Respiration* 2007; 74: 632–639.

43. Lellouche F FA, Taillé S, Deye N, *et al.* Physiological evaluation of five interfaces during non-invasive ventilation in healthy subjects. Abstract. *Intensive Care Med* 2002.

44. Toussaint M, Chatwin M, Soudon P. Mechanical ventilation in Duchenne patients with chronic respiratory insufficiency: clinical implications of 20 years published experience. *Chron Respir Dis* 2007; 4: 167–177.

45. Toussaint M, Soudon P, Kinnear W. Effect of non-invasive ventilation on respiratory muscle loading and endurance in patients with Duchenne muscular dystrophy. *Thorax* 2008; 63: 430–434.

46. Madden BP, Kariyawasam H, Siddiqi AJ, Machin A, Pryor JA, Hodson ME. Noninvasive ventilation in cystic fibrosis patients with acute or chronic respiratory failure. *Eur Respir J* 2002; 19: 310–313.

47. Carrey Z, Gottfried SB, Levy RD. Ventilatory muscle support in respiratory failure with nasal positive pressure ventilation. *Chest* 1990; 97: 150–158.

48. Soo Hoo GW, Santiago S, Williams AJ. Nasal mechanical ventilation for hypercapnic respiratory failure in chronic obstructive pulmonary disease: determinants of success and failure. *Crit Care Med* 1994; 22: 1253–1261.

49. Hess DR. Noninvasive ventilation in neuromuscular disease: equipment and application. *Respir Care* 2006; 51: 896–911.

50. Ricard JD, Cook D, Griffith L, Brochard L, Dreyfuss D. Physicians' attitude to use heat and moisture exchangers or heated humidifiers: a Franco-Canadian survey. *Intensive Care Med* 2002; 28: 719–725.

51. Heffner JE. Management of the chronically ventilated patient with a tracheostomy. *Chron Respir Dis* 2005; 2: 151–161.

52. Togias AG, Naclerio RM, Proud D, *et al.* Nasal challenge with cold, dry air results in release of inflammatory mediators. Possible mast cell involvement. *J Clin Invest* 1985; 76: 1375–1381.

53. Hayes MJ, McGregor FB, Roberts DN, Schroter RC, Pride NB. Continuous nasal positive airway pressure with a mouth leak: effect on nasal mucosal blood flux and nasal geometry. *Thorax* 1995; 50: 1179–1182.

54. Takagi Y, Proctor DF, Salman S, Evering S. Effects of cold air and carbon dioxide on nasal air flow resistance. *Ann Otol Rhinol Laryngol* 1969; 78: 40–48.

55. Martins De Araújo MT, Vieira SB, Vasquez EC, Fleury B. Heated humidification or face mask to prevent upper airway dryness during continuous positive airway pressure therapy. *Chest* 2000; 117: 142–147.

56. Neill AM, Wai HS, Bannan SP, Beasley CR, Weatherall M, Campbell AJ. Humidified nasal continuous positive airway pressure in obstructive sleep apnoea. *Eur Respir J* 2003; 22: 258–262.

57. Mador MJ, Krauza M, Pervez A, Pierce D, Braun M. Effect of heated humidification on compliance and quality of life in patients with sleep apnea using nasal continuous positive airway pressure. *Chest* 2005; 128: 2151–2158.

58. Massie CA, Hart RW, Peralez K, Richards GN. Effects of humidification on nasal symptoms and compliance in sleep apnea patients using continuous positive airway pressure. *Chest* 1999; 116: 403–408.

59. Jaber S, Chanques G, Matecki S, *et al.* Comparison of the effects of heat and moisture exchangers and heated humidifiers on ventilation and gas exchange during non-invasive ventilation. *Intensive Care Med* 2002; 28: 1590–1594.

60. Lellouche F, Maggiore SM, Deye N, *et al.* Effect of the humidification device on the work of breathing during noninvasive ventilation. *Intensive Care Med* 2002; 28: 1582–1589.

61. Nava S, Cirio S, Fanfulla F, *et al.* Comparison of two humidification systems for long-term noninvasive mechanical ventilation. *Eur Respir J* 2008; 32: 460–464.

CHAPTER 24

Sleep and NIV: monitoring of the patient under home ventilation

J-L. Pépin*,#, J.C. Borel*,#, J-P. Janssens¶, R. Tamisier*,#, P. Lévy*,#

*Pulmonary Function Test and Sleep Laboratory, Dept of Rehabilitation and Physiology, and #HP2 Laboratory, INSERM-ERI 17, University Hospital, Grenoble, France, and ¶Division of Pulmonary Diseases, Geneva University Hospitals, Geneva, Switzerland.

Correspondence: J-L. Pépin, Pôle Rééducation et Physiologie, CHU de Grenoble, BP 217 X, 38043, Grenoble, France. Fax: 33 476765586; E-mail: JPepin@chu-grenoble.fr

Introduction

Sleep is a unique physiological state associated with deep changes in upper airway (UA) resistance, respiratory control and lung mechanics. In patients with chronic respiratory diseases, this specific situation induces different categories of consequences. First, as minute ventilation decreases particularly in rapid eye movement (REM) sleep, sleep-related hypoventilation is the first sign of respiratory failure, systemically preceding the development of daytime chronic hypercapnic failure. Secondly, as abnormal respiratory events occur specifically during sleep, noninvasive ventilation (NIV) settings which are appropriate for ventilating awake patients may not work appropriately during the night. Alternatively, sleep itself increases nonintentional leaks, patient–ventilator asynchrony and periodic breathing or glottic closures, thus justifying a specific monitoring of NIV efficacy during the night.

In the present chapter, the overall mechanisms for ventilatory changes occurring during sleep, the ability of NIV to suppress respiratory events during night and improve sleep quality, and the tools that can be proposed for monitoring NIV efficacy during sleep, will be successively reviewed. These topics will be covered for patients suffering from chronic respiratory failure, in stable state and home-ventilated by NIV.

During sleep changes in ventilation

There are several mechanisms explaining that, even in normal subjects, ventilation is slightly reduced during sleep. Modifications occur in muscle activity, respiratory drive and lung mechanics. Depending upon the underlying respiratory disease, these different mechanisms isolated or in association may aggravate or reveal respiratory failure during sleep.

Reduction of activity of respiratory muscles

During sleep, the loss of the wakefulness stimulus is associated with a decreased activity of the medullary respiratory neurons [1] leading to a reduction of respiratory muscles tonic activity. There is a concomitant fall in ventilation [2]. In normal individuals, arterial carbon dioxide tension (Pa,CO$_2$) rises by 2–8 mmHg, arterial oxygen

Eur Respir Mon, 2008, 41, 350–366. Printed in UK - all rights reserved. Copyright ERS Journals Ltd 2008; European Respiratory Monograph; ISSN 1025-448x.

tension (P_a,O_2) decreases by 3–10 mmHg and oxygen saturation drops by <2% [3–5]. These changes occur despite the reduction in oxygen consumption and carbon dioxide production during sleep [4]. The decrease in ventilation occurs during all stages of sleep and worsens during REM, particularly during phasic REM sleep [1, 6, 7]. Phasic REM sleep is associated with a dramatic reduction in intercostal muscle phasic and tonic activity and a reduction in diaphragm tonic activity, whereas diaphragmatic phasic inspiratory activity is preserved [8, 9]. During this period, breathing is more irregular, rapid and shallow (fig. 1) [10].

Diaphragmatic functioning is absolutely critical in REM sleep because the other respiratory muscles alone cannot maintain normal alveolar ventilation. Subjects with diaphragmatic weakness, as in neuromuscular disorders or breathing with a diaphragm in unfavourable mechanic conditions, as in morbid obesity or chronic obstructive pulmonary disease (COPD) with hyperinflated lungs, are highly prone to hypoventilate during REM sleep.

Changes in ventilatory control

Ventilatory control is physiologically altered during sleep, resulting in a diminished responsiveness to chemical, mechanical and cortical inputs. During REM sleep [8, 9], there is virtually no metabolic control in ventilation. The respiratory muscles also exhibit a diminished response to ventilatory drive during sleep [8]. This reduction in ventilatory response is particularly deleterious in patients who already have an abnormal chemosensitivity during wakefulness, such as patients with myotonic dystrophy or obesity hypoventilation syndrome (OHS). In OHS, daytime ventilatory responses to carbon dioxide are highly related to percentage of REM sleep spent in hypoventilation [11].

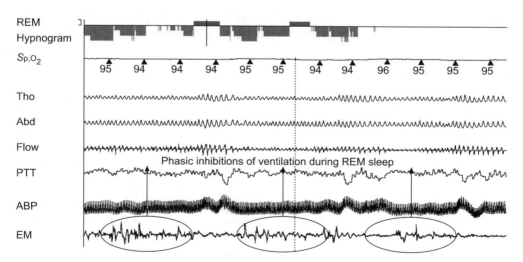

Fig. 1. – Irregular, rapid and shallow breathing during phasic rapid eye movement (REM) sleep. Decrease in ventilation during phasic REM sleep episodes: a sustained reduction in flow and thoracic and abdominal movements occurs concurrently with rapid eye movements. This occurs to various degrees in normal subjects and is aggravated or revealing in patients with respiratory failure. S_p,O_2: arterial oxygen saturation measured by pulse oximetry; Tho: thoracic movements; Abd: abdominal movements; Flow: flow signal; PTT: pulse transit time; ABP: arterial blood pressure; EM: eye movements.

Changes in functional residual capacity

In normal subjects, functional residual capacity (FRC) decreases during REM sleep as a result of supine position and atonia of the intercostals muscles [12–14]. This reduction in FRC is particularly marked in morbidly obese subjects and in patients using their accessory muscles to compensate for either a diaphragm weakness or a diaphragm working in an unfavourable geometrical position.

Change in ventilation/perfusion mismatch

Breathing irregularity and rapid shallow breathing during REM sleep [15] also increase the physiological dead space in COPD patients and, thus, impair gas exchange [14, 16–18].

Associated sleep-disordered breathing

The UA resistance is increased, secondary to a reduction in tonic and phasic activity of the UA muscles. These UA muscles are responsible for both preventing pharyngeal collapse during the contraction of the diaphragm (phasic activity) and maintaining the UA tone during sleep (tonic activity) [1, 6, 7]. Obstructive sleep apnoea is a common condition and thus its association with another frequent disease, such as COPD, is expected. However, sleep apnoea is not more prevalent in COPD than in the general population. Conversely, prevalence of sleep apnoea seems to be increased in kyphoscoliosis and in neuromuscular disorders. Finally, severe sleep apnoea is almost always present in OHS and is a key factor in the pathophysiology of chronic respiratory failure in these patients.

NIV can suppress or reduce sleep-related hypoventilation and episodes of upper airway collapse and improve sleep quality

In order to limit its impact on quality of life and to compensate for the physiological decreases in nocturnal ventilation which may be critical in chronic respiratory failure, NIV is mainly applied during night. Efficacy of NIV is mainly assessed by daytime outcome measures, such as blood gases, health-related quality-of-life scores and number of hospitalisations. Surprisingly, there is a limited number of studies specifically addressing the question of NIV efficacy during the night in terms or improving nocturnal hypoventilation and sleep quality.

In restrictive chronic respiratory failure patients, SCHONHOFER et al. [19] showed that nocturnal hypoventilation improved and both slow wave sleep and REM sleep increased after 1 yr of home NIV. Interestingly, after 6 months of treatment, a one-night withdrawal of NIV was associated with a significant but lesser degree of sleep hypoventilation compared with baseline. This suggests that long-term NIV improved respiratory drive and limited immediate recurrence of severe REM sleep hypoventilation. A recent meta-analysis [20], in neuromuscular and chest wall disorders, found only eight trials (144 participants) eligible. In these studies, alleviation of sleep hypoventilation or correction of sleep-disordered breathing was measured by nocturnal pulse-oximetry only. Arterial oxygen saturation (Sa,O_2) is, however, a surrogate marker which cannot clearly discriminate between apnoeas or hypopnoeas and episodes of REM sleep hypoventilation. Using NIV, the average increase in mean nocturnal Sa,O_2

was 5.45% (95% confidence interval (CI) 1.47–9.44) [20]. In a similar population of neuromuscular and chest wall disorders, WARD et al. [21] noted that patients with nocturnal hypoventilation (nocturnal transcutaneous carbon dioxide tension (Ptc,CO_2) >6.5 kPa) but with normal daytime Pa,CO_2 at baseline are likely to deteriorate with the development of daytime hypercapnia and/or progressive symptoms within 2 yrs. Early introduction of nocturnal NIV, before occurrence of daytime hypercapnia, reduced levels of nocturnal Ptc,CO_2.

O'DONOGHUE et al. [22] documented sleep hypoventilation in >43% of a group of hypercapnic COPD. Sleep hypoventilation was associated with significant increases in night-to-morning Pa,CO_2 and proposed as contributing to long-term elevations in Pa,CO_2. Accordingly, in a randomised controlled trial, MEECHAM-JONES et al. [23] showed using Ptc,CO_2 measurements that degree of improvement in daytime Pa,CO_2 was correlated with the improvement in mean overnight Ptc,CO_2 by using NIV. A meta-analysis, addressing the issue of efficacy of NIV in COPD patients with chronic respiratory failure, suggested a detrimental (although nonsignificant) effect of the device in terms of sleep efficiency [24]. However, the small sample size precludes a definitive statement regarding the clinical implications of such a result. In another systematic review of NIV in COPD, sleep-related difficulties were reported in four out of the 15 included studies [25].

In OHS patients, NIV treats associated sleep apnoea syndrome, improves ventilatory responses and sleep quality, and suppresses REM sleep hypoventilation [11]. Conversely, in a percentage of extremely obese subjects, continuous positive airway pressure (CPAP) treatment alone corrected upper airway collapse but severe oxygen desaturation persisted and NIV was required [26] in this situation in order to treat sleep-related hypoventilation.

Thus, in different diseases associated with chronic respiratory failure, NIV is capable of counteracting the different mechanisms associated with sleep-related hypoventilation. Even though robust data are lacking, it is generally accepted that sleep quality is improved. However, in the real life of home-ventilated patients, the situation appears more problematic and sleep hypoventilation or sleep fragmentation is far from being perfectly corrected [27–29].

Potential undesirable respiratory events and sleep fragmentation induced by NIV

Nonintentional leaks, around the mask or through the mouth are common during sleep [27–30] and remain one of the main events which impair effectiveness of ventilatory support. Leaks can either alter the functioning of the NIV apparatus (i.e. triggering, pressurisation delay) [31, 32] or directly decrease level of ventilation [33] inducing recurrent episodes of hypoventilation and oxygen desaturations. GONZALEZ et al. [34] demonstrated a significant relationship between air leaks and persistent hypercapnia. Moreover, by increasing microarousals related to leaks, sleep efficiency can be significantly altered [27, 29, 30].

Although nonintentional leaks may lead to inappropriate ventilatory support, other patterns of sleep-disordered breathing (i.e. periodic breathing, closure of the glottis and patient–ventilator asynchrony) may be induced by the ventilatory support itself [35–37], independently of leaks.

NIV has the potential to induce periodic breathing during sleep. In a recent polysomnography study, 40% of obese patients using NIV showed a high index of periodic breathing, mostly occurring in light sleep and associated with severe nocturnal hypoxaemia [36]. A Pa,CO_2 apnoeic threshold exists during sleep at 1.5–5.8 Torr below eupnoeic Pa,CO_2 [38]. If NIV settings lead to hyperventilation, bursts of central apnoeas or hypopnoeas can occur, particularly during transitions between sleep onset and wakefulness. The susceptibility to periodic breathing varies considerably among subjects; its occurrence under NIV is thus difficult to predict and needs to be specifically monitored (fig. 2). High levels of pressure support are more frequently associated with this abnormality.

Hyperventilation, associated with NIV use, can also lead to glottis narrowing and closures [37, 39]. Glottis narrowing seems more related to a controlled mode (both in volumetric and barometric support). In spontaneous cycles, initiation of inspiration by the patient may allow an activation of the inspiratory glottis abductors inducing vocal-cord abduction [40]. High levels of ventilation and hypocapnia are more frequently associated with these adverse events. During NIV, ventilatory responses to hypoxia are highly dependent on carbon dioxide levels and can be definitely abolished by severe hypocapnia (Pa,CO_2 <27 mmHg) [41]. This means that glottis closures can be associated with severe desaturations before reopening of the glottis and resumption of effective ventilation.

Profound modifications in the recruitment of the respiratory muscles may occur during the various stages of sleep, potentially leading to inappropriate triggering. Patient–ventilator dyssynchrony may be a cause of suboptimal ventilation and sleep fragmentation (fig. 3) [42]. In a systematic polysomnographic study in OHS, 55% of the patients exhibited desynchronisation, occurring mostly in slow-wave sleep and REM sleep and associated with arousals [36]. Auto-triggering was more sporadic and usually limited to one or two breaths [36]. Similarly, FANFULLA et al. [43], including 48 patients enrolled in a long term home NIV programme, found a mean of 48 ± 37 ineffective efforts per hour during sleep compared with none during wakefulness.

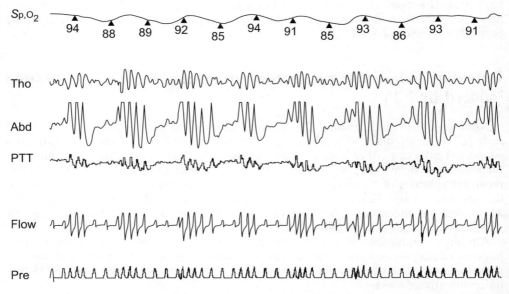

Fig. 2. – 5-min epoch of polysomnography with central events induced by noninvasive ventilation. Arterial oxygen saturation measured by pulse oximetry (Sp,O_2) oscillations related to central events occurring in stage-1 sleep. Note the decrease in respiratory effort during events, identified by pulse transit time (PTT). Tho: thoracic movements; Abd: abdominal movements; Flow: flow signal measured using a pneumotachograph; Pre: pressure.

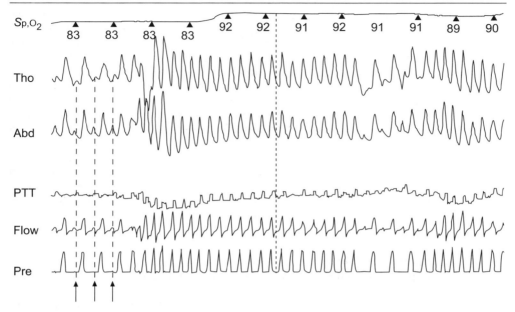

Fig. 3. – 5-min epoch of polysomnography with patient–ventilator asynchrony. Ineffective efforts (arrows) and arterial oxygen saturation oscillations related to patient–ventilator asynchrony. Sp,O_2: arterial oxygen saturation measured by pulse oximetry; Tho: thoracic movements; Abd: abdominal movements; PTT: pulse transit time; Flow: flow signal; Pre: pressure.

How should NIV be monitored during sleep?

During sleep, specific respiratory events result from both physiological changes and the use of NIV. An appropriate strategy for monitoring these respiratory events should be proposed. Monitoring tools can be limited to the recognition of consequences such as oxygen desaturation or increases in Ptc,CO_2. More complex and complete evaluations can be performed by polygraphic or polysomnographic recordings. These assessments provide more insights as to the mechanisms involved but are more costly and less available. Finally, manufacturers have developed software, using signals included in NIV devices, that provide interesting information. The following chapter aims to describe the different techniques and their respective contribution for assessing home ventilated patients during sleep.

Nocturnal pulse-oximetry

The amount of nocturnal oxygen desaturation is considered as one of the major determinants of adverse neurocognitive and cardiovascular consequences occurring during chronic respiratory failure and sleep apnoea syndrome [44, 45]. It is obviously an important item to monitor in home-ventilated patients. It has been suggested that the morphological pattern of Sa,O_2 desaturation could be specific to the different mechanisms explaining their occurrence [46]. When Sa,O_2 measurements are performed in spontaneous breathing, repetitive episodes of brief desaturation/reoxygenation sequences with simultaneous acceleration/deceleration of heart frequency (fig. 4a) are generally accepted as being associated with obstructive or central apnoeas. However, overnight nocturnal pulse-oximetry cannot distinguish between central and obstructive events [47]. In patients using NIV at night, repetitive oscillations in Sa,O_2 should be interpreted more cautiously, as they may reflect central events (fig. 2), residual obstructive events (fig. 5), patient–ventilator asynchrony (fig. 3) or repetitive leaks interrupted by microarousals. Another characteristic pattern of Sa,O_2 recordings in spontaneous breathing is a prolonged desaturation (10–30 min) with concurrent acceleration of heart frequency, occurring approximately every 90–120 min, during the night. This is a typical pattern of REM sleep hypoventilation (fig. 4b). In ventilated patients, however, the same aspect can result not only from persistent REM sleep hypoventilation (fig. 6), but also from prolonged leaks or insufficient pressure support irrespective of sleep stage.

In summary, the occurrence of desaturations is highly sensitive to detect breathing abnormalities in NIV users but the different patterns are difficult to interpret. When abnormalities are present, polygraphy or polysomnography is required for understanding the relevant mechanisms and adjusting ventilator settings and/or interfaces.

P_{tc},CO_2 monitoring

Assessing Pa,CO_2 overnight is essential for evaluating efficacy of NIV during sleep. The simplest approach is to measure Pa,CO_2 by arterial puncture at the end of the night to document night-to-morning increases in Pa,CO_2 [22]. However, blood is most often sampled after arousal and thus after a short period of appropriate ventilation. In this condition a normal morning Pa,CO_2 actually does not reflect the abnormal time course of

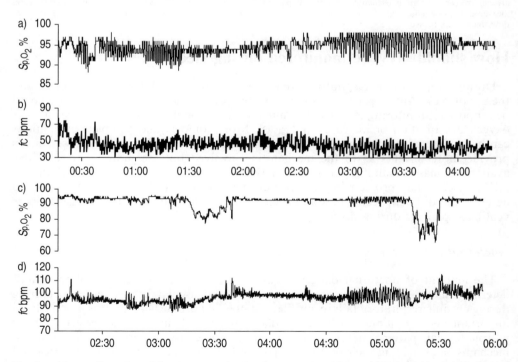

Fig. 4. – 4-h recordings of arterial oxygen saturation in spontaneous breathing. a and b) Repetitive episodes of brief desaturation/reoxygenation sequences with simultaneous acceleration/deceleration of cardiac frequency (*f*C) generally accepted as associated with obstructive or central apnoeas. c and d) Persistent desaturation (10–30 min) with concurrent acceleration of the *f*C and occurring approximately every 90–120 min during the night. This corresponds to a typical of pattern of rapid eye movement sleep hypoventilation. Sp,O_2: arterial oxygen saturation measured by pulse oximetry.

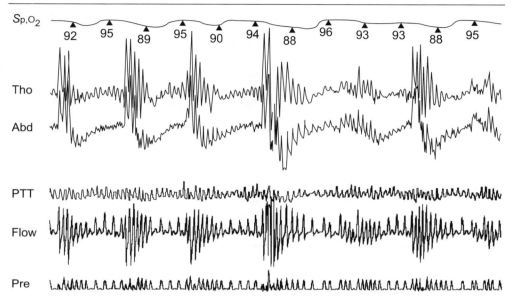

Fig. 5. – 5-min epoch of polysomnography with residual obstructive events. S_{p,O_2}: arterial oxygen saturation measured by pulse oximetry; Tho: thoracic movements; Abd: abdominal movements; PTT: pulse transit time; Flow: flow signal measured using a pneumotachograph; Pre: pressure.

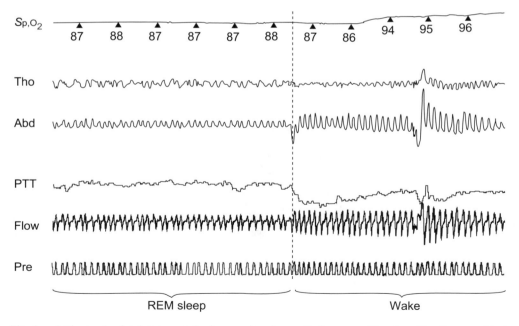

Fig. 6. – 5-min epoch of polysomnography in a noninvasive ventilation user with a transition from persistent hypoventilation during rapid eye movement (REM) sleep and awakening. See flow reduction during REM sleep with sustained desaturation. S_{p,O_2}: arterial oxygen saturation measured by pulse oximetry; Tho: thoracic movements; Abd: abdominal movements; PTT: Pulse transit time; Flow: Flow signal measured using a pneumotachograph; Pre: pressure.

Pa,CO_2 during the night. Repeated sampling of arterial blood from a catheter in the radial artery remains the "gold standard" for estimating Pa,CO_2 changes but is not conceivable for routine assessment in stable state patients. End-tidal carbon dioxide is unreliable in patients with chronic respiratory failure, particularly in COPD and is technically difficult to measure with the continuous flow related to bi-level pressure support. Continuous Ptc,CO_2 recordings (fig. 7) show good agreement with arterial measurements [48–50] even if high levels of Pa,CO_2 may increase $Pa,CO_2/Ptc,CO_2$ bias [48]. Importantly, further studies [48–53] have reported that the good agreement between Ptc,CO_2 and Pa,CO_2 is preserved when patients are treated by CPAP or pressure support. A limitation of the technique is the requirement for periodic calibration and changes of membrane in order to ensure sufficient precision of transcutaneous measurements. Despite these precautions, Ptc,CO_2 sensor drift has been reported during overnight recordings [22]. Compensation of this drift has been proposed by using linear interpolation but this actually requires two arterial measures of Pa,CO_2 (at the beginning and at the end of Ptc,CO_2 recording) [22]. One study, however, showed that, in 28 subjects under NIV, Ptc,CO_2 recordings could be performed continuously for 8 h at a probe temperature of 43°C, without any local discomfort or significant signal drift [51].

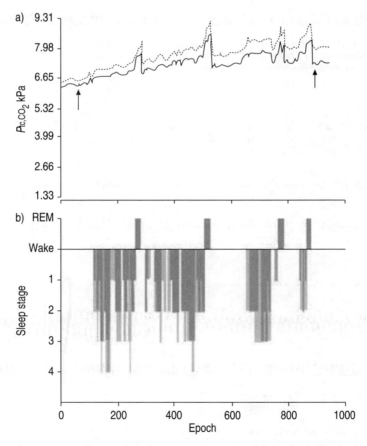

Fig. 7. – During night evolution of transcutaneous carbon dioxide tension (Ptc,CO_2). Note the systematic increase in Ptc,CO_2 (a) concurrently with rapid eye movement (REM) sleep (b). Arrows depict significant increase in arterial carbon dioxide tension night-to-morning. Modified from [22].

More-recent devices, combining Ptc,CO_2 and arterial oxygen tension measured by pulse oximetry (Sp,O_2) earlobe sensors, have been validated in acute care and chronic clinical settings, are designed for continuous recording over 8-h periods without requiring recalibration and are feasible for routine use [53–55]. All Ptc,CO_2 sensors have a lag-time (~2 min) which precludes monitoring of rapid changes of Pa,CO_2 such as those which could be associated with recurrent apnoeas, hypopnoeas or brief leaks [49].

In summary, nocturnal Ptc,CO_2 should be considered as a reliable noninvasive tool to monitor nocturnal Pa,CO_2 for patients treated with NIV on a long-term basis. Limitations of the technique are the cost of the devices, the increase in bias between arterial and transcutaneous values at high Pa,CO_2 values [48], and the occasional occurrence of unexplained errant values. Recent devices, however, are easy to use, have user-friendly software and can be connected to polysomnography software. Finally, nocturnal Ptc,CO_2 reveals the occurrence of episodes of hypoventilation but provides no information as to their cause (inappropriate settings, leaks, *etc.*).

Data available from NIV machines

The majority of industrial companies have designed NIV devices to include flow and pressure sensors and to store raw data of these parameters on a long-term basis. Specific software allows home-care providers or clinicians to download these data onto a personal computer.

Downloaded data can be separated in three categories. The first is a "synthesis report" (*i.e.* a trend of each parameter recorded during a given period; fig. 8). Depending on the manufacturers and the machines (table 1), compliance, settings, mean

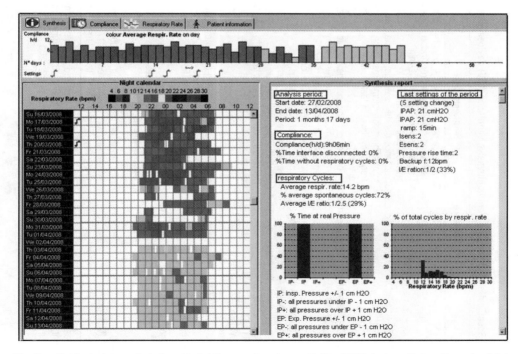

Fig. 8. – Synthesis data analysis downloaded from noninvasive ventilation (NIV) device software. Example of data downloaded from GK 425 Tyco Healthcare^{TM} using Silverlining 3.0 software. Compliance data, mean respiratory rate and percentage of spontaneous cycles are available.

Table 1. – Specifications of software from noninvasive ventilation (NIV) devices allowing the download of data

Device	Software	Synthesis data	Detailed data	Polygraphic data
VPAP3-ST (A) ResMed™	ReScan 3.5	Compliance per day, settings, minute ventilation, tidal volume, respiratory frequency, level of leaks# L·min-1, residual AHI n·h-1	Minute ventilation, respiratory frequency, level of leaks# L·min-1, residual AHI n·h-1	Simultaneous recording of S_{p,O_2} and heart rate (available with additional module: RESLINK)
HARMONY SYNCHRONY Respironics™	Encore pro 1.8	Compliance per day, settings, minute ventilation, tidal volume, respiratory frequency, level of leaks¶, flow, alarms	Minute ventilation, tidal volume, respiratory frequency, level of leaks¶, flow (cycle to cycle acquisition is available with additional module STARDUST)	Simultaneous recording of S_{p,O_2}, heart rate and respiratory effort (available with additional module STARDUST)
VENTIMOTION Weinman™ (Hamburg, Germany)	Ventisupport™	Compliance per day, settings, minute ventilation, tidal volume, respiratory frequency, level of leaks#, flow, inspiratory time/total time, alarms	Pressure, flow, level of leaks	Pressure, flow, level of leaks could be transferred to any polygraph with the "analog box-Weinmann"
GK 425 Tycohealthcare™ (Pleasanton, CA, USA)	Silverlining 3™	Compliance per day, settings, respiratory frequency, pressure		
SMARTAIR, SMARTAIR+ LEGENDAIR SUPPORTAIR Airox-Covidien™ (Pau, France)	Airox com 3.5.1	Compliance per day, settings, technical alarms and ventilation alarm	Tidal volume, respiratory frequency, inspiratory time/total time, leaks#, pressure/ time curve, flow/time curve (acquisition requires a connection to a computer when the patient is under NIV)	Simultaneous recording of S_{p,O_2} available with SUPPORTAIR monitoring of S_{p,O_2}
VS ULTRA, VS INTEGRA SAIME™ (Savigng le Temple, France)	Easydiag1.1.3	Compliance per day, settings, minute ventilation, tidal volume, respiratory frequency, level of leaks, flow, inspiratory time/total time	Tidal volume, respiratory frequency, level of leaks#(+), flow (direct acquisition is possible when the patient is under NIV)	
ELYSEE 150 SAIME™	Easyview 150 (2.11)	Compliance per day, settings, minute ventilation, tidal volume, respiratory frequency, level of leaks	Minute ventilation, tidal volume, respiratory frequency, level of leaks (direct acquisition is possible when the patient is under NIV)	
VIVO 30-40 Breas™ (Mölngcke, Sweden)	Vivo PS software 2.5	Compliance per day, settings, minute ventilation, tidal volume, respiratory frequency, level of leaks¶, flow, alarms	Pressure, flow, tidal volume, level of leaks (acquisition cycle to cycle directly on the patient is under NIV) or differed)	

AHI: apnoea/hypopnoea index; S_{p,O_2}: arterial oxygen tension measured by pulse oximetry. #: level of nonintentional leaks (mask must be recognised to ensure a valid assessment of leaks) expressed in L·min-1 (or L·s-1); ¶: level of total leaks (including intentional leaks of masks and nonintentional leaks) expressed in L·min-1 (or L·s-1); +: when using double way tubing, the level of leaks is expressed as the ratio (insufflated tidal volume/expired tidal volume).

level of leaks, tidal volume, respiratory frequency and/or minute ventilation could be provided. The second category is "detailed data analysis". Raw data of a given parameter could be analysed cycle by cycle (fig. 9). The third category provides "polygraphic data analysis". In this situation, by adding an external module connected to the machine (Reslink; Resmed™, North Ryde, Australia, or Stardust; Respironics™, Murrysville, PA, USA), physiological parameters such as oxygen saturation, heart rate and respiratory effort can be recorded and displayed, in addition to the signals already stored by the device (fig. 10).

There are large discrepancies in parameters provided by the different software. This reflects the fact that relevant parameters for monitoring NIV have not been yet clearly defined by clinicians and that recommendations in this field should be proposed by scientific societies. Additionally, the validity of several parameters estimated by the NIV devices (minute ventilation, tidal volume, apnoea hyponoea index) is questionable and must be validated by independent clinical and/or bench test studies. For pulse-oximetry, these data should be used as screening tools for identifying, in a large population of home ventilated patients, those requiring further investigations.

Polygraphy and polysomnography

As illustrated by figures 1–7, polysomnography is the most integrative assessment of NIV during sleep, allowing in most circumstances a precise description of the different mechanisms involved in desaturations, episodes of hypoventilation, or disrupted sleep structure. Identifying the mechanisms involved in these respiratory events is crucial for

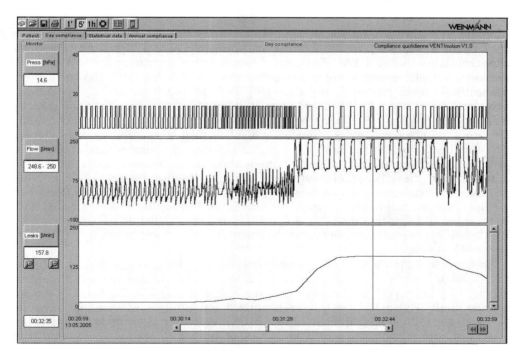

Fig. 9. – Detailed data analysis downloaded from noninvasive ventilation device softwares (5-min epoch). Pressure (press), flow and leaks monitored respiratory cycle by respiratory cycle (download from Ventimotion Weinmann™ using Ventisupport 1.01 software) are shown. Owing to the increase of leaks, pressure support move to back-up frequency (spontaneous cycles are replaced by controlled cycles; widening of inspiratory pressure delay).

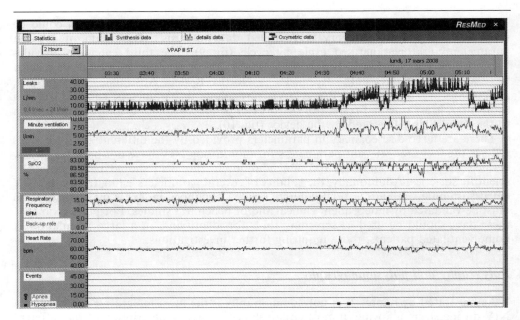

Fig. 10. – Polygraphic data by using the noninvasive ventilation (NIV) device associated with an external module (2-h epoch). Combination of data usually provided by the NIV machine and physiological data (arterial oxygen saturation measured by pulse oximetry (SpO2) and heart rate); download from VPAP 3 ST Resmed^{TM} using Rescan 5.3 software). Note oxygen desaturation explained by a huge increase in leaks levels.

adapting NIV settings or interfaces. Thus, documenting residual obstructive events in an obese patient will lead to an increase in positive expiratory pressure. Persistent hypoventilation during REM sleep may warrant either increasing level of pressure support or implementing a volume-targeting mode which has been shown to more efficiently decrease Ptc,CO_2 during sleep [56]. Periodic breathing and glottis closure, frequently associated with hypocapnia and hyperventilation, might be diminished by reducing the levels of ventilation and increasing inspiratory trigger sensitivity than favouring spontaneous cycles. Finally, patient–ventilator asynchrony may require adjusting inspiratory and expiratory triggers and reducing nonintentional leaks, when present. Leaks increase the probability of most abnormal respiratory events under NIV, thus reducing the efficacy of ventilatory support. It must be kept in mind that relationships between these events and quality of sleep are extremely complex. For example, volume targeting may improve ventilation but seems to be associated with increased sleep fragmentation [57]. Moreover, increasing ventilation to correct residual REM sleep hypoventilation can favour the emergence of periodic breathing particularly in non-REM sleep.

An important contribution of polysomnography is to document sleep fragmentation and to relate microarousals to their cause. Microarousals related to leaks should be managed by improving the interface or using a mouth strip [28, 29, 58]. Conversely, microarousals related to other above-mentioned respiratory events require adapting NIV settings. Guo et al. [36] reported that patient ventilator asynchrony is usually not associated with significant changes in Ptc,CO_2 or oxygen saturation (Sp,O_2) and thus polysomnography was necessary in order to identify these respiratory events and improve NIV settings.

For all these reasons, periodic polysomnography is recommended by experts in the follow-up of home ventilated patients [58, 59]. However, in the field of sleep medicine, interpreting polysomnography under NIV is probably one of the most difficult tasks. Resulting flow and pressure signals are influenced by not only the patients' ventilation but also the technical specifications of the device and the ventilatory mode. Specific recommendations regarding the channels that need to be recorded and consensus criteria for scoring are highly desirable.

Polygraphy is easier to perform in an outpatient setting and clearly useful for identifying events such as patient–ventilator asynchrony, periodic breathing, auto-triggering, and their impact on Sp,O_2. Obviously, impact on sleep structure of these events will not be detected, although integration of signs of "autonomic arousals" in portable polygraphy recordings may be useful in the near future.

Conclusions

Overall sleep and breathing during NIV are far from ideal. Screening studies using ventilator software and/or nocturnal pulse-oximetry are useful for identifying patients with significant problems but these tools may not suffice. Polysomnography (or polygraphy) under NIV, interpreted by trained specialists, may allow for improved ventilator settings, respiration during sleep and hopefully sleep quality. Future studies are needed to establish whether recognition and correction of these abnormalities, during sleep, positively impact either on long-term efficacy of NIV, compliance or quality of life.

Summary

The present chapter first reiterates the different mechanisms underlying ventilatory changes occurring during sleep and the capability of noninvasive ventilation (NIV) in correcting abnormal respiratory events and improving sleep quality in different diseases. In order to ensure long-term NIV efficiency, appropriate strategies for monitoring ventilation and sleep, during NIV treatment, are proposed. Different tools, allowing monitoring of chronic respiratory failure patients treated using long-term home NIV, and their respective interests and limitations are successively reviewed. Tools only aiming to recognise the consequences of residual events, such as oxygen desaturations or increases in nocturnal transcutaneous carbon dioxide tension are distinguished compared with more complex strategies, such as respiratory polygraphy and polysomnography. Finally, specific software, designed by ventilator manufacturers for at-home monitoring, and the use of flow signals included in NIV devices, are remarked upon. These data may provide useful information for clinicians.

Keywords: Chronic respiratory failure, long-term respiratory care, noninvasive ventilation, sleep-disordered breathing.

References

1.   Hudgel DW, Martin RJ, Johnson B, Hill P. Mechanics of the respiratory system and breathing pattern during sleep in normal humans. *J Appl Physiol* 1984; 56: 133–137.
2.   White DP, Weil JV, Zwillich CW. Metabolic rate and breathing during sleep. *J Appl Physiol* 1985; 59: 384–391.

3. Bulow K. Respiration and wakefulness in man. *Acta Physiol Scand Suppl* 1963; 209: 1–110.
4. Douglas NJ, White DP, Weil JV, Pickett CK, Zwillich CW. Hypercapnic ventilatory response in sleeping adults. *Am Rev Respir Dis* 1982; 126: 758–762.
5. Robin ED, Whaley RD, Crump CH, Travis DM. Alveolar gas tensions, pulmonary ventilation and blood pH during physiologic sleep in normal subjects. *J Clin Invest* 1958; 37: 981–989.
6. Lopes JM, Tabachnik E, Muller NL, Levison H, Bryan AC. Total airway resistance and respiratory muscle activity during sleep. *J Appl Physiol* 1983; 54: 773–777.
7. Skatrud JB, Dempsey JA. Airway resistance and respiratory muscle function in snorers during NREM sleep. *J Appl Physiol* 1985; 59: 328–335.
8. Gothe B, Altose MD, Goldman MD, Cherniack NS. Effect of quiet sleep on resting and CO_2-stimulated breathing in humans. *J Appl Physiol* 1981; 50: 724–730.
9. Phillipson EA. Respiratory adaptations in sleep. *Annu Rev Physiol* 1978; 40: 133–156.
10. Bourke SC, Gibson GJ. Sleep and breathing in neuromuscular disease. *Eur Respir J* 2002; 19: 1194–1201.
11. Chouri-Pontarollo N, Borel JC, Tamisier R, Wuyam B, Levy P, Pepin JL. Impaired objective daytime vigilance in obesity-hypoventilation syndrome: impact of noninvasive ventilation. *Chest* 2007; 131: 148–155.
12. Hudgel DW, Devadatta P. Decrease in functional residual capacity during sleep in normal humans. *J Appl Physiol* 1984; 57: 1319–1322.
13. Hudgel DW, Martin RJ, Capehart M, Johnson B, Hill P. Contribution of hypoventilation to sleep oxygen desaturation in chronic obstructive pulmonary disease. *J Appl Physiol* 1983; 55: 669–677.
14. Tusiewicz K, Moldofsky H, Bryan AC, Bryan MH. Mechanics of the rib cage and diaphragm during sleep. *J Appl Physiol* 1977; 43: 600–602.
15. Gould GA, Gugger M, Molloy J, Tsara V, Shapiro CM, Douglas NJ. Breathing pattern and eye movement density during REM sleep in humans. *Am Rev Respir Dis* 1988; 138: 874–877.
16. Gothe B, Goldman MD, Cherniack NS, Mantey P. Effect of progressive hypoxia on breathing during sleep. *Am Rev Respir Dis* 1982; 126: 97–102.
17. Krieger J, Turlot JC, Mangin P, Kurtz D. Breathing during sleep in normal young and elderly subjects: hypopneas, apneas, and correlated factors. *Sleep* 1983; 6: 108–120.
18. Stradling JR, Chadwick GA, Frew AJ. Changes in ventilation and its components in normal subjects during sleep. *Thorax* 1985; 40: 364–370.
19. Schonhofer B, Kohler D. Effect of non-invasive mechanical ventilation on sleep and nocturnal ventilation in patients with chronic respiratory failure. *Thorax* 2000; 55: 308–313.
20. Annane D, Orlikowski D, Chevret S, Chevrolet JC, Raphael JC. Nocturnal mechanical ventilation for chronic hypoventilation in patients with neuromuscular and chest wall disorders. *Cochrane Database Syst Rev* 2007; CD001941.
21. Ward S, Chatwin M, Heather S, Simonds AK. Randomised controlled trial of non-invasive ventilation (NIV) for nocturnal hypoventilation in neuromuscular and chest wall disease patients with daytime normocapnia. *Thorax* 2005; 60: 1019–1024.
22. O'Donoghue FJ, Catcheside PG, Ellis EE, *et al.* Sleep hypoventilation in hypercapnic chronic obstructive pulmonary disease: prevalence and associated factors. *Eur Respir J* 2003; 21: 977–984.
23. Meecham-Jones DJ, Paul EA, Jones PW, Wedzicha JA. Nasal pressure support ventilation plus oxygen compared with oxygen therapy alone in hypercapnic COPD. *Am J Respir Crit Care Med* 1995; 152: 538–544.
24. Wijkstra PJ, Lacasse Y, Guyatt GH, *et al.* A meta-analysis of nocturnal noninvasive positive pressure ventilation in patients with stable COPD. *Chest* 2003; 124: 337–343.
25. Kolodziej MA, Jensen L, Rowe B, Sin D. Systematic review of noninvasive positive pressure ventilation in severe stable COPD. *Eur Respir J* 2007; 30: 293–306.
26. Banerjee D, Yee BJ, Piper AJ, Zwillich CW, Grunstein RR. Obesity hypoventilation syndrome: hypoxemia during continuous positive airway pressure. *Chest* 2007; 131: 1678–1684.
27. Bach JR, Robert D, Leger P, Langevin B. Sleep fragmentation in kyphoscoliotic individuals with alveolar hypoventilation treated by NIPPV. *Chest* 1995; 107: 1552–1558.

28. Rabec CA, Reybet-Degat O, Bonniaud P, Fanton A, Camus P. Leak monitoring in noninvasive ventilation. *Arch Bronconeumol* 2004; 40: 508–517.

29. Teschler H, Stampa J, Ragette R, Konietzko N, Berthon-Jones M. Effect of mouth leak on effectiveness of nasal bilevel ventilatory assistance and sleep architecture. *Eur Respir J* 1999; 14: 1251–1257.

30. Meyer TJ, Pressman MR, Benditt J, *et al.* Air leaking through the mouth during nocturnal nasal ventilation: effect on sleep quality. *Sleep* 1997; 20: 561–569.

31. Calderini E, Confalonieri M, Puccio PG, Francavilla N, Stella L, Gregoretti C. Patient-ventilator asynchrony during noninvasive ventilation: the role of expiratory trigger. *Intensive Care Med* 1999; 25: 662–667.

32. Highcock MP, Shneerson JM, Smith IE. Functional differences in bi-level pressure preset ventilators. *Eur Respir J* 2001; 17: 268–273.

33. Tuggey JM, Delmastro M, Elliott MW. The effect of mouth leak and humidification during nasal non-invasive ventilation. *Respir Med* 2007; 101: 1874–1879.

34. Gonzalez J, Sharshar T, Hart N, Chadda K, Raphael JC, Lofaso F. Air leaks during mechanical ventilation as a cause of persistent hypercapnia in neuromuscular disorders. *Intensive Care Med* 2003; 29: 596–602.

35. Delguste P, Aubert-Tulkens G, Rodenstein DO. Upper airway obstruction during nasal intermittent positive-pressure hyperventilation in sleep. *Lancet* 1991; 338: 1295–1297.

36. Guo YF, Sforza E, Janssens JP. Respiratory patterns during sleep in obesity-hypoventilation patients treated with nocturnal pressure support: a preliminary report. *Chest* 2007; 131: 1090–1099.

37. Jounieaux V, Aubert G, Dury M, Delguste P, Rodenstein DO. Effects of nasal positive-pressure hyperventilation on the glottis in normal awake subjects. *J Appl Physiol* 1995; 79: 176–185.

38. Meza S, Mendez M, Ostrowski M, Younes M. Susceptibility to periodic breathing with assisted ventilation during sleep in normal subjects. *J Appl Physiol* 1998; 85: 1929–1940.

39. Parreira VF, Jounieaux V, Aubert G, Dury M, Delguste PE, Rodenstein DO. Nasal two-level positive-pressure ventilation in normal subjects. Effects of the glottis and ventilation. *Am J Respir Crit Care Med* 1996; 153: 1616–1623.

40. Parreira VF, Delguste P, Jounieaux V, Aubert G, Dury M, Rodenstein DO. Glottic aperture and effective minute ventilation during nasal two-level positive pressure ventilation in spontaneous mode. *Am J Respir Crit Care Med* 1996; 154: 1857–1863.

41. Jounieaux V, Parreira VF, Aubert G, Dury M, Delguste P, Rodenstein DO. Effects of hypocapnic hyperventilation on the response to hypoxia in normal subjects receiving intermittent positive-pressure ventilation. *Chest* 2002; 121: 1141–1148.

42. Fanfulla F, Delmastro M, Berardinelli A, Lupo ND, Nava S. Effects of different ventilator settings on sleep and inspiratory effort in patients with neuromuscular disease. *Am J Respir Crit Care Med* 2005; 172: 619–624.

43. Fanfulla F, Taurino AE, Lupo ND, Trentin R, D'Ambrosio C, Nava S. Effect of sleep on patient/ventilator asynchrony in patients undergoing chronic non-invasive mechanical ventilation. *Respir Med* 2007; 101: 1702–1707.

44. Carroll N, Bain RJ, Smith PE, Saltissi S, Edwards RH, Calverley PM. Domiciliary investigation of sleep-related hypoxaemia in Duchenne muscular dystrophy. *Eur Respir J* 1991; 4: 434–440.

45. Santos C, Braghiroli A, Mazzini L, Pratesi R, Oliveira LV, Mora G. Sleep-related breathing disorders in amyotrophic lateral sclerosis. *Monaldi Arch Chest Dis* 2003; 59: 160–165.

46. Pepin JL, Levy P, Lepaulle B, Brambilla C, Guilleminault C. Does oximetry contribute to the detection of apneic events? Mathematical processing of the SaO_2 signal. *Chest* 1991; 99: 1151–1157.

47. Series F, Kimoff RJ, Morrison D, *et al.* Prospective evaluation of nocturnal oximetry for detection of sleep-related breathing disturbances in patients with chronic heart failure. *Chest* 2005; 127: 1507–1514.

48. Cuvelier A, Grigoriu B, Molano LC, Muir JF. Limitations of transcutaneous carbon dioxide measurements for assessing long-term mechanical ventilation. *Chest* 2005; 127: 1744–1748.

49. Janssens JP, Howarth-Frey C, Chevrolet JC, Abajo B, Rochat T. Transcutaneous P_{CO_2} to monitor noninvasive mechanical ventilation in adults: assessment of a new transcutaneous P_{CO_2} device. *Chest* 1998; 113: 768–773.

50. Storre JH, Steurer B, Kabitz HJ, Dreher M, Windisch W. Transcutaneous P_{CO_2} monitoring during initiation of noninvasive ventilation. *Chest* 2007; 132: 1810–1816.

51. Janssens JP, Perrin E, Bennani I, de Muralt B, Titelion V, Picaud C. Is continuous transcutaneous monitoring of P_{CO_2} (TcP_{CO_2}) over 8 h reliable in adults? *Respir Med* 2001; 95: 331–335.

52. Maniscalco M, Zedda A, Faraone S, Carratu P, Sofia M. Evaluation of a transcutaneous carbon dioxide monitor in severe obesity. *Intensive Care Med* 2008; 34: 1340–1344.

53. Senn O, Clarenbach CF, Kaplan V, Maggiorini M, Bloch KE. Monitoring carbon dioxide tension and arterial oxygen saturation by a single earlobe sensor in patients with critical illness or sleep apnea. *Chest* 2005; 128: 1291–1296.

54. Bendjelid K, Schutz N, Stotz M, Gerard I, Suter PM, Romand JA. Transcutaneous P_{CO_2} monitoring in critically ill adults: clinical evaluation of a new sensor. *Crit Care Med* 2005; 33: 2203–2206.

55. Parker SM, Gibson GJ. Evaluation of a transcutaneous carbon dioxide monitor ("TOSCA") in adult patients in routine respiratory practice. *Respir Med* 2007; 101: 261–264.

56. Storre JH, Seuthe B, Fiechter R, *et al.* Average volume-assured pressure support in obesity hypoventilation: a randomized crossover trial. *Chest* 2006; 130: 815–821.

57. Janssens J-P, Metzger M, Sforza E. Impact of volume targetling on efficacy of bi-level non-invasive ventilation and sleep in obesity–hypoventilation. *Respir Med* 2008; [Epub ahead of print PMID: 18579368].

58. Rodenstein DO, Levy P. To sleep, perchance to leak. *Eur Respir J* 1999; 14: 1241–1243.

59. Lofaso F, Quera-Salva MA. Polysomnography for the management of progressive neuromuscular disorders. *Eur Respir J* 2002; 19: 989–990.

CHAPTER 25

NIV: discharging the ventilator-dependent patient

J. Escarrabill

Correspondence: *J. Escarrabill, Institut d'Estudis de la Salut, C/ Roc Boronat, 81-95 1st floor, 08005 Barcelona, Spain. Fax: 34 932607576; E-mail: jescarrabill@gencat.cat*

Introduction

The continuity of care is one of the key elements in evaluating the quality of healthcare [1]. There are many difficulties in guaranteeing the coordination of this care. In the majority of cases, multiple health providers intervene and this intervention can be unplanned (in some cases as a result of decisions made by the patient or by the health services) and, what's more, the interoperability of these information systems is not guaranteed. In addition, the coordination requires time and a consideration of the problems in terms of the bigger picture, things that are not systematically promoted in clinical practice, which focuses mainly on acute problems.

The discharge of a patient who has been admitted to hospital is not an administrative procedure. The process of discharge has a big impact on the later evolution and progress of the patient. NEALE *et al.* [2] observed that 18% of the errors made in clinical practice to patients admitted to two London hospitals take place during the process of discharge.

In patients with complex needs, such as patients with noninvasive ventilation (NIV), the coordination of the caregivers and the planning of the process of discharge are especially important. This planning must be considered in two situations: in the moment that NIV begins and following hospital admission due to an acute exacerbation. The process of discharge, having initiated the NIV, determines the future course of treatment: adaptation to the ventilation, and completion by, and security of, the patient and the caregiver. From a practical point of view, this process of discharge from the initiation of the ventilation can be divided into three main periods: 1) evaluation and adaptation, 2) critical period (moment of discharge and the first few days at home) and 3) progress beyond.

It is difficult to identify the best manner of clinical practice, especially when we refer to patients with complex needs in very different welfare and social contexts. HAYNES *et al.* [3] suggest that good practice depends on diverse factors: the scientific evidence, the preferences of the patient, the circumstances and the clinical situation and, especially, the skills of the team. The decisions can vary from one circumstance to the other, according to the support that the patient has or the accessibility to healthcare mechanisms.

In any case, the organisation of the healthcare services has to be prepared in order to respond to the needs of the patient. The care team must make sure that the patient (and the caregiver) is fully informed, that they retain control over the decisions, that they participate in the care programme and that individual values are respected in the process of care [4]. In a general way, the basic elements of the "patient-centred care" are summed up in table 1.

Eur Respir Mon, 2008, 41, 367–376. Printed in UK - all rights reserved. Copyright ERS Journals Ltd 2008; European Respiratory Monograph; ISSN 1025-448x.

Table 1. – Patient-centred care

Respect for patients' values and preferences
Coordination and integrated care
Information, communication and education
Physical comfort
Emotional support
Involvement of family and friends

Data from the Institute of Medicine (Washington, DC, USA) [4].

The six elements that define the quality of the healthcare service are: safety (an unsafe treatment cannot be a quality treatment), effect (it produces benefits in actual conditions of use), focus on the needs of the patient, time (waiting does not help to improve the quality of treatment), efficiency and equitability.

Feasibility

Feasibility has to do with whether a proposed project is practical or not. At the same time as raising the possibility that NIV is needed, we must respond to the question of viability. A decisive aspect, obviously, is the clinical criteria that hint at the use of the NIV, but next we must determine whether the circumstances make this proposal viable.

The clinical criteria refer to the characteristics of the illness, the natural history and technical aspects and to the physiological response to the ventilation support. The circumstances refer to the situation in terms of a caregiver, the preferences of the patient, the characteristics of the household and the availability, or not, of technical home support. That is to say, the viability depends on both technical and social aspects of the case. If from the beginning it is clear that the patient will not be able to receive care at home, it will be necessary to consider alternatives (*e.g.* hospices), which will affect the design of the therapeutic plan.

Evaluation and adaptation to the NIV

The indication of the NIV can raise itself in the course of an acute exacerbation (with the patient admitted to the hospital) or in the monitoring of patients with restrictive illnesses. In any case the doctor faces an important decision for the patient as, in order to obtain benefits to their wellbeing (to ensure survival and improve their general state of health), they must accept important changes to their lifestyle (becoming dependent on a ventilator).

The adaptation to the ventilation is a process that can take several days. The technical criteria of indication have been discussed in other chapters of this *European Respiratory Monograph*. The adaptation is a process which requires the collaboration of the patient and the caregiver, as the rhythm cannot be established in the same way for every patient. In general it is recommended to try first to achieve a good adaptation with the patient awake, beginning with a few minutes and then, little by little, lengthening the time on the ventilator. When the patient is well adapted during the day it is necessary to weigh up the efficacy of the ventilation with the parameters used: ventilator parameters that do not manage to improve the gaseous exchange with the patient awake will not manage it during the night.

Table 2. – Roles for the discharge plan

Role	Functions/needs
Patient	Education
	Risk management
Caregiver	Education/risk management
	Special attention to formal caregivers without direct relationship with the hospital team
Hospital	Experience
	Case manager
	Accessibility
Case manager	Integral evaluation of the patient and caregiver
	Home conditions
	Mobility
	Communication
Health service	Financial issues
Supplier	Technical competence
	Relationship with hospital team
	Service 24 h/7 days

If the patient is admitted to hospital (or if it is an outpatient adaptation), it is very important to make use of this period to educate the patient and the caregiver. Table 2 sums up the roles of those who intervene in the plan of discharge of a patient with NIV.

Outpatient NIV

The possibility of starting the ventilation without the need to admit the patient depends on the gravity of the patient's condition, the accessibility to the hospital (outpatient NIV is more difficult with patients who live very far from the hospital), the possibility of having a place adapted to running a training programme and, in some countries, on financial limitations.

According to the circumstances and to the health resources available, it will be crucial to evaluate the effort and the cost for the patient and the team who will have to carry out the outpatient treatment. When a patient is admitted, if complications do not arise, the adaptation takes 4–6 days. Trying to reduce the consumption of resources (hospital stays) has very little impact (on the whole) on the consumption of resources of the patients with chronic respiratory illnesses [5].

For patients with serious respiratory insufficiency or for those who are suffering an acute exacerbation it seems more prudent to carry out the adaptation "in-house" (at the hospital). For the rest of the patients, either option should be satisfactory: inpatient or outpatient adaptation.

The process of adaptation

Informing and educating the patient and the carer are basic elements of the process of adaptation. This whole process requires time and that time varies between patients [6]. There is a risk of overwhelming the patient and caregiver with an excess of information. It is important to provide written information and to make sure that the essential elements are properly understood. In the long term, NIV is a safe procedure, but it is crucial to make sure that the patient and the caregiver are aware that zero risk does not exist. Although fatal accidents have been registered in patients on NIV relating to electrical power failures, we must insist that these occurrences were exceptional and that it is possible to minimise the risks. Table 3 summarises the key elements with regard to risk management for the patient undergoing NIV in the safest possible way.

Table 3. – Risk management

Problem	Resolution
Ventilator	
Power supply failure	Spare ventilation parts
	Additional batteries
Apparatus problems	Regular review
	Service 24 h/7 days
Accessories	
Mask (fixing)	Basic spare parts
Circuits	Regular cleaning
	Replacement of security
Medical	
Exacerbation	Signs of alarm
	Telephone contact
	Ambulance contact
Monitoring	Telephone contact of the expert team
	Regular updates of the knowledge of patient (and caregiver)
	Self-management
	Regular review of written care plans
Compliance and consumption of resources	
Compliance	Regular access to the hours of ventilation
Consumption of resources	Repeated alarm calls, technical problems, unclear or unscheduled visits
	or emergencies

Data taken from SIMONDS [7].

In a very short space of time, a lot of information must be conveyed and, therefore, it is advisable that the welfare teams make a check-list with all the information they must give to the patient, the educational targets and the necessary equipment for the proper administering of treatment. This systematic action is especially important in the management of patients with complex needs and involving the coordination of various professionals.

Critical period: planning for discharge

The adaptation process is concluded on the day on which it is decided that the patient has adapted well and can be administered the ventilation alone at home. This is the critical period when they must put into practice everything that they have been preparing for.

The discharge plan is defined as designing a customised plan for each patient, which takes place before leaving the hospital (or before starting independent treatment at home). The discharge plan for patients with complex needs is a multidisciplinary effort with the goal that this transition between hospital and home is made efficiently and safely [8]. The discharge plan is aimed at preparing the patient and the caregiver from a technical and a psychological standpoint, in order to achieve maximum possible independence for the patient and, simultaneously, to ensure the continuity of care.

The discharge plan must include considerations of the practical aspects of daily life, which, in the end, are the ones the patient will have to resolve at home. Therefore, in addition to the respiratory needs, it is important to bear in mind all the basic needs of the patient: communication, hygiene, transfers, mobility, social activities, *etc*. In some cases the patient, before starting NIV, must make changes to the structure of their house or have a vehicle adapted. These elements, while they cannot be resolved by the welfare team, must be kept in mind to facilitate the successful outcome of the NIV. In many cases it is useful for a member of the care team to visit the home of the patient before they are discharged, so that adjustments can be suggested in order to help with the installation of the equipment that the patient will need.

From a practical perspective, the discharge plan must contemplate the simplest option that obtains the maximum benefits.

The care team must take particular care on the first day of NIV at home. A phone call or a visit after the first night of NIV at home can be especially useful. The strategy of the discharge plan is simpler than it looks. BERTOYE *et al.* [9] magnificently described how the first inpatients who required ventilatory support after long-term acute poliomyelitis accepted the challenge of returning home with the ventilator. The key elements for a successful transfer from hospital to home are: 1) agreement between the doctor, patient and caregiver; 2) clinical stability; 3) a willing and competent caregiver; 4) availability of technical elements, with the financial coverage necessary; and 5) a good plan for risk management. Ventilation at home is possible through this agreement between the patient (and the caregiver) and the doctor, assuming a certain risk and all the work that will go into the care.

Case manager

The discharge plan is a result of the work of a team, but, in the case of a patient with complex needs, it is unlikely that the team, spontaneously through the routine work, will be able to respond to all the requirements of the patient. In the most complex cases it is easy for duplications or deficiencies to arise, related more to fragmentation of care than to the knowledge of the team members.

The figure of the nurse case manager plays a vital role in implementing the plan of care for patients with NIV. It is useful for all patients, but it is imperative for those with more complex needs, such as constant need for ventilation, major limitations with autonomy (*e.g.* for a neuromuscular disease) or where there are doubts about the competency of the caregiver, or, simply, for those that live far from the expert team.

The nurse case manager is the one who sees the bigger picture of the problem and identifies the needs. The patient and the caregiver have a competent advisor, the intervening professionals have a mediator to resolve any doubts or propose changes in the treatment and the doctor can focus his energy on the clinical problems, with the reassurance that the overall treatment plan is being executed as planned.

Most of the problems associated with outpatient NIV are the result of mismanagement of the care rather than problems with technical or clinical issues.

The nurse case manager has a broad and diverse field of activity, but table 4 summarises those particular activities or skills that will facilitate the development of the discharge plan.

Table 4. – Case management competencies

1	Identify competences that health professionals need to care for specific patients:
	In the course of the diseases there are a lot of professionals that cooperate with the expert team
2	Leading complex care coordination:
	Different providers
	Social services
3	Proactive management of clinical problems
4	Managing mental well-being (of the patient and the caregiver)
5	Supporting self-management
6	Proactive risk management
7	Managing care at end of life

General needs

Having initiated the NIV, most teams deal with all the respiratory needs of the patients: ventilators, access to airways, suction cleaners for secretions, supplementary oxygen, humidification, nebulisation, complementary batteries to counter any failure in the power supply, *etc*. However, addressing the needs of the patients to perform the activities of daily life is just as important as thinking about respiratory needs [10].

The needs of daily life can be grouped into different dimensions as follows.

Communication. The discharge plan must consider the ability of the patient to communicate and the availability (and ease of operation) of alarms to call the caregiver when they are not in attendance.

Ensuring patient communication does not exclusively require the use of sophisticated technology. A poster with photographs or small book with icons may be sufficient for basic communication. Having alarms (in addition to those of the ventilator) is an important element in giving confidence to the patient.

Accessibility. The accessibility in the home is an element that can affect the activities of daily living for the patient and limit or facilitate their autonomy and social relations. Narrow stairs or the absence of a lift (elevator) facility are factors to be considered with patients who, in addition to the disability related to their illness, require a wheelchair.

Mobility. With patients who have mobility problems and must move around with the ventilator, special care must be taken to adapt the unit to the chair. Social services can be a big help in terms of facilitating travel by public transport or by identifying means to adapt private vehicles.

Adaptation of the home. The adaptation of the home can be a problem for many patients. The bathroom and the bedroom are very important because their adjustments must be mindful of the transferences that the patient will have to undergo.

Technological support. There are countless technological tools that facilitate the adaptation to the activities of daily life for patients with disabilities. In many cases it is necessary to resort to expert advice in order to find the best solution to each problem. With rapidly evolving diseases, such as amyotrophic lateral sclerosis (ALS), the technological support needs change rapidly. For the patient and the caregiver this fact is an inconvenience, both from an economic perspective and in choosing the best option. The creation of "banks of material" can facilitate a quick solution to the problems posed by the changing needs for technological support.

Relationship with community resources

There is no team or assistive device that is capable of answering all the welfare needs of complex patients in a continuous manner. The expert teams should assume the bulk of the assistance for the patient but, to a greater or lesser extent, they will have to look to and coordinate the collaboration of other professionals [11]. The health organisations are very different in each country but in a general way, the expert teams must coordinate with the welfare and social resources closest to the patient. General practitioners, the nurses and physiotherapists from the community and the social workers play a greater role, which can be assigned from the perspective of a centre of expertise. This effective coordination should be based on a level of cooperation, so that the transmission of information is made in a way that is quick and complete and there are open discussions about improved therapeutic alternatives, and accessibility should be the desired formal framework. The community resources are not there to comply with the orders of the expert team but to contribute to its skill and knowledge of the treatment plan.

The discharge plan after an exacerbation

The discharge plan is not a one-off but a plan that is developed progressively depending on the needs of the patient. The patient's needs can change, in which case the care plan must be adapted, as previously mentioned.

However, when there is an admission caused by a worsening of the symptoms (especially when the admission is unexpected), it may be necessary to reformulate an in-depth care plan. The discharge after an exacerbation may require a care plan as complex as the one designed at the time of the NIV initiation. One of the worst situations for the care of patients with complex needs is the routine repetition of care.

Follow-up

Even once the patient is stabilised and well adapted to their home, the care plan is incomplete if it does not include a long-term monitoring programme. The European study on home mechanical ventilation (HMV; Eurovent survey) [12] showed a great variability in the care plans for patients with HMV: more than half the patients with HMV did not have a home-care specialist. Access to healthcare alternatives to conventional hospitalisation was also very heterogeneous. Additionally, there are many differences between countries and within the same country when it comes to technical checks on the ventilators [13].

The monitoring of the patients with NIV must be proactive (it is not enough to facilitate access to a consultation) and plan visits according to the patient's clinical condition. The role of the nurse case manager is very important. In the first phase the patient should be monitored very closely. Most patients to be discharged from the hospital after beginning the ventilation will not yet have reached the maximum degree of improvement that can be expected. In fact, most patients do not obtain the maximum benefits of the NIV until 2 or 3 months after the initiation of treatment [14].

One very important aspect is the quality control of the ventilators. FARRÉ et al. [15] noted that the prescribed parameters did not coincide with the parameters observed during surveillance of the ventilators in the home. A larger study confirmed these discrepancies between the prescribed and observed parameters, although they did not observe any negative impact on the number of admissions [16] or the clinical condition of the patients. The control of the ventilators and complaints from patients regarding their operation is not a subject that has been studied in depth, but it is possible that in addition to the routine checks it will be necessary to pay closer attention to the patient/ventilator interrelationship.

The monitoring of the patients must be planned in accordance with the available resources. Information and communication technology could facilitate this monitoring [17], especially in the case of patients who live far from the hospital. However, in general, these technologies are there to compliment the care and they do not completely replace home visits or external consultation visits.

Care of the caregiver

The monitoring of patients with NIV must include attention to the caregiver. Caring for a patient with NIV can lead to psychological problems. Overall, 15% of caregivers for patients with long-term home ventilation develop symptoms of depression 6 months after the discharge [18]. Sometimes the role of informal caregivers is underestimated, given that sometimes this role is played by very young people [19]. Even though it may seem that the opposite is the case, and in spite of the chronicity, the patients and the caregivers do need regular information about their condition and the therapeutic recommendations [20]. This necessity for information is even more important as the patient approaches the final phases of life [21]. In patients with ALS, the burden on the caregiver can be very great, requiring between 12 and 14 h a day [22]. It has also been shown that 60% of caregivers with patients with ALS and tracheotomy must leave their jobs to care for the patient [22].

TALLEY and CREWS [23] insist that there is still little interest in caring for the caregiver, despite the recognised fact that if the caregiver falls ill, the whole fragile system of welfare can collapse. The caregiver may give up due to health problems, when they "forget" to take care of themselves, e.g. to comply with medication or visit the doctor. Therefore, when analysing the problems of patients with NIV, we should always consider the triangle of patients, health professionals and caregivers. The carers need communication and temporary discharges of obligations of care [24]. The social isolation caused by caring for a very dependent patient has an enormous impact on the satisfaction of the caregiver [25]. On other occasions the impact of care can be difficult to detect. In highly dependent patients, the biggest impact for the caregiver can manifest itself in interruptions of sleep [26]. Caregivers of patients with neuromuscular diseases must mobilise them up to 10 or 12 times every night.

Since the impact on health is sometimes imperceptible, some authors call the caregiver the "hidden client" [27].

Ultimately, the success of home treatment for patients with complex needs, such as patients with NIV, is partly based on an appropriate discharge plan and adapted to the needs of the patient [7, 28].

Summary

In patients with complex needs, such as patients with noninvasive ventilation (NIV), the coordination of the caregivers and the planning of the process of discharge are especially important. The care team must make sure that the patient (and the caregiver) is fully informed, that they retain control over the decisions, that they participate in the care programme and that individual values are respected in the process of care.

The adaptation to the ventilation is a process that can take several days and it requires the collaboration of the patient and the caregiver. The discharge plan is defined as designing a customised plan for each patient that takes place before leaving the hospital (or before starting independent treatment at home). The discharge plan must contemplate the simplest option that obtains the maximum benefits. The figure of the nurse case manager plays a vital role in implementing the plan of care for patients with NIV.

Keywords: Caregiver, case manager, home mechanical ventilation.

References

1. Bodenheimer T. Coordinating care – a perilous journey through the health care system. *N Engl J Med* 2008; 358: 1064–1071.
2. Neale G, Woloshynowych M, Vincent C. Exploring the causes of adverse events in NHS hospital practice. *J R Soc Med* 2001; 94: 322–330.
3. Haynes RB, Devereaux PJ, Guyatt GH. Physicians' and patients' choices in evidence based practice. *BMJ* 2002; 324: 1350.
4. Institute of Medicine, Crossing the Quality Chasm: A New Health System for the 21st Century. Washington, National Academy Press, 2001.
5. Luján M, Moreno A, Veigas C, Montón C, Pomares X, Domingo C. Non-invasive home mechanical ventilation: effectiveness and efficiency of an outpatient initiation protocol compared with the standard in-hospital model. *Respir Med* 2007; 101: 1177–1182.
6. Vitacca M, Guerra A, Pizzocaro P, *et al.* [Time consuming of physicians and nurses before discharge in patients with chronic respiratory failure submitted to home mechanical ventilation]. *Rassegna di Patologia dell'Apparto Respiratorio* 2005; 20: 275–283.
7. Simonds AK. Risk management of the home ventilator dependent patient. *Thorax* 2006; 61: 369–371.
8. O'Donohue WJ Jr, Giovannoni RM, Goldberg AI, *et al.* Long-term mechanical ventilation. Guidelines for management in the home and at alternate community sites. Report of the Ad Hoc Committee, Respiratory Care Section, American College of Chest Physicians. *Chest* 1986; 90: Suppl. 1, 1S–37S.
9. Bertoye A, Garin JP, Vincent P, Giroud M, Monier P, Humbert G. Le retour à domicili des insuffisants respiratoires chroniques [The return home of equipped chronic respiratory insufficiency patients]. *Lyon Med* 1965; 214: 389–410.
10. Schönhofer B, Sortor-Leger S. Equipment needs for noninvasive mechanical ventilation. *Eur Respir J* 2002; 20: 1029–1036.
11. Goldberg AI. Noninvasive mechanical ventilation at home: building upon the tradition. *Chest* 2002; 121: 321–324.
12. Lloyd-Owen SJ, Donaldson GC, Ambrosino N, *et al.* Patterns of home mechanical ventilation use in Europe: results from the Eurovent survey. *Eur Respir J* 2005; 25: 1025–1031.
13. Farré R, Lloyd-Owen SJ, Ambrosino N, *et al.* Quality control of equipment in home mechanical ventilation: a European survey. *Eur Respir J* 2005; 26: 86–94.
14. Escarrabill J, Estopà R, Robert D, Casolivé V, Manresa F. [Long-term effects of home mechanical ventilation with positive pressure using a nasal mask]. *Med Clin (Barc)* 1991; 97: 421–423.
15. Farré R, Giró E, Casolivé V, Navajas D, Escarrabill J. Quality control of mechanical ventilation at the patient's home. *Intensive Care Med* 2003; 29: 484–486.
16. Farré R, Navajas D, Prats E, *et al.* Performance of mechanical ventilators at the patient's home: a multicentre quality control study. *Thorax* 2006; 61: 400–404.
17. Vitacca M, Escarrabill J, Galavotti G, *et al.* Home mechanical ventilation patients: a retrospective survey to identify level of burden in real life. *Monaldi Arch Chest Dis* 2007; 67: 142–147.
18. Douglas SL, Daly BJ. Caregivers of long-term ventilator patients: physical and psychological outcomes. *Chest* 2003; 123: 1073–1081.
19. Doran T, Drever F, Whitehead M. Health of young and elderly informal carers: analysis of UK census data. *BMJ* 2003; 327: 1388.
20. Rossi Ferrario S, Zotti AM, Zaccaria S, Donner CF. Caregiver strain associated with tracheostomy in chronic respiratory failure. *Chest* 2001; 119: 1498–1502.
21. Gilgoff I, Prentice W, Baydur A. Patient and family participation in the management of respiratory failure in Duchenne's muscular dystrophy. *Chest* 1989; 95: 519–524.
22. Kaub-Wittemer D, Steinbüchel N, Wasner M, Laier-Groeneveld G, Borasio GD. Quality of life and psychosocial issues in ventilated patients with amyotrophic lateral sclerosis and their caregivers. *J Pain Symptom Manage* 2003; 26: 890–896.

23. Talley RC, Crews JE. Framing the public health of caregiving. *Am J Public Health* 2007; 97: 224–228.

24. Koopmanschap MA, van Exel NJ, van den Bos GA, van den Berg B, Brouwer WB. The desire for support and respite care: preferences of Dutch informal caregivers. *Health Policy* 2004; 68: 309–320.

25. Ibañez M, Aguilar JJ, Maderal MA, *et al.* Sexuality in chronic respiratory failure: coincidences and divergences between patient and primary caregiver. *Respir Med* 2001; 95: 975–979.

26. Creese J, Bédard M, Brazil K, Chambers L. Sleep disturbances in spousal caregivers of individuals with Alzheimer's disease. *Int Psychogeriatr* 2008; 20: 149–161.

27. Bergs D. "The Hidden Client" – women caring for husbands with COPD: their experience of quality of life. *J Clin Nurs* 2002; 11: 613–621.

28. Lewarski JS, Gay PC. Current issues in home mechanical ventilation. *Chest* 2007; 132: 671–676.

CHAPTER 26

Cost-effectiveness of NIV applied to chronic respiratory failure

E.M. Clini*,#, E. Crisafulli#, M. Moretti*, L.M. Fabbri*

*University of Modena, Dept of Oncology, Haematology and Pneumology and #Ospedale Villa Pineta, Dept of Rehabilitation, Pavullo, Modena, Italy.

Correspondence: E.M. Clini, Dept of Oncology, Haematology and Pneumology, University of Modena, Ospedale Villa Pineta, Via Gaiato 127, 41026, Pavullo n/F (MO), Italy. Fax: 39 053642039; E-mail: enrico.clini@unimore.it

Introduction

Home mechanical ventilation (HMV) is an established therapy for severe chronic hypercapnic respiratory failure (HRF). The 1990s saw a substantial rise in the HMV attributed to: 1) increased numbers of patients surviving the critical care; 2) increased awareness and experience with indications and technologies; and 3) improved life expectancy and reduced morbidity of treated patients, especially those with chest wall and neuromuscular disease [1]. In particular, HMV delivered noninvasively (either with positive or negative modalities) has received growing interest. The expansion of HMV in the last 15 yrs was stimulated by the introduction of noninvasive mask ventilation and the recognition that more patient groups could benefit [2].

A report in France has shown that most of the population of ventilated individuals were using tracheostomy HMV during the 1990s; this figure has changed in the last decade, showing a progressive increase of noninvasive HMV, thus paralleling the numbers of tracheostomised patients [3].

The rapidly growing number of patients on noninvasive HMV in France mirrors the development in other countries; in particular, a recent European survey has reported updates on centre characteristics, user demographics and equipment choice for 329 centres and 21,526 users [4]. In this survey, an estimated HMV prevalence of about 6 per 100,000 citizens (range 0.1–17 per 100,000 for different countries) was shown; the presence of detailed observatories or national registers might have explained the highest prevalence of HMV in countries nearer the northern borders of Europe. Moreover, the vast majority of patients were treated noninvasively; 34% of users (>7,000 people) had parenchymal lung disorders, the majority of whom probably represented chronic obstructive pulmonary disease (COPD) patients.

Impact and effectiveness of long-term noninvasive mechanical ventilation

The most recent evidence suggests that HMV delivered by mask ventilation has proven effective in terms of both physiological and clinical outcomes in several conditions [5, 6]. In other chapters of this *European Respiratory Monograph* this aspect is extensively discussed. We here briefly summarise and report the major findings in

Eur Respir Mon, 2008, 41, 377–391. Printed in UK - all rights reserved. Copyright ERS Journals Ltd 2008; European Respiratory Monograph; ISSN 1025-448x.

Table 1. – Mechanisms of action of ventilatory support in respiratory failure due to restrictive disease

Supposed mechanism of action	Positive study		Negative study	
	First author [ref.]	Outcome	First author [ref.]	Outcome
Resetting the CO_2 sensitivity of the central ventilatory controller	NICKOL [7] ANNANE [8]	Increased ventilatory response to CO_2 Decreased Pa,CO_2		
Changes in lung mechanics: increased lung volume, improved compliance, reduced dead space by recruitment of atelectatic lung	DELLBORG [9] SIMONDS [10]	Increased VC	NICKOL [7] ANNANE [8]	No improvement in lung mechanics
Increase in muscle strength	NICKOL [7] DELLBORG [9]	Increased MIP and MEP	NICKOL [7] ANNANE [8]	No improvement in muscle strength

Pa,CO_2: arterial carbon dioxide tension; VC: vital capacity; MIP: maximum inspiratory pressure; MEP: maximum expiratory pressure.

restrictive and obstructive patients treated by noninvasive HMV. Tables 1 and 2 report the mechanisms of action which have been suggested in noninvasive HMV.

Restrictive disorders

Since the 1980s, extensive experience has been gained in using all forms of home ventilatory support in chest wall and neuromuscular disorders. Nowadays, noninvasive mask ventilation is a well-established long-term treatment in patients with symptomatic HRF secondary to restrictive thoracic disease [20].

Hypercapnia develops in restrictive ventilatory disorders when the force that can be generated by the respiratory muscles is outweighed by the extra load placed on them by

Table 2. – Mechanisms of action of ventilatory support in respiratory failure due to chronic obstructive pulmonary disease

Supposed mechanism of action	Positive study		Negative study	
	First author [ref.]	Outcome	First author [ref.]	Outcome
Downward resetting of the respiratory centre sensitivity to CO_2	MEECHAM JONES [11] ELLIOTT [12]	Improved sleep quality, decreased Pa,CO_2 and increased ventilatory response to CO_2	GAY [13] LIN [14]	No reduction in daytime Pa,CO_2
Reduction in lung hyperinflation	DÍAZ [15]	Decreased FRC, RV and TLC		
Increase in muscle strength	BRAUN [16] GUTIÉRREZ [17]	Decreased Pa,CO_2 Increased VC, MIP and MEP	ZIBRAK [18] SCHÖNHOFER [19]	No improvement in daytime gas exchange or inspiratory muscle strength [18] Daytime gas improvement without increase in respiratory muscle strength [19]

Pa,CO_2: arterial carbon dioxide tension; FRC: functional residual capacity; RV: residual volume; TLC: total lung capacity; VC: vital capacity; MIP: maximum inspiratory pressure; MEP: maximum expiratory pressure.

the reduced compliance of the respiratory system. The increased work of breathing and reduced respiratory muscle activity leads to hypercapnia during sleep and, later, wakefulness [21]. Improvement in arterial blood gases in these individuals rests on three main hypotheses: 1) increased ventilatory sensitivity to carbon dioxide during spontaneous breathing; 2) resting of the fatigued respiratory muscles; and 3) improved pulmonary mechanics [22]. In particular, NICKOL et al. [7] found a relationship between hours of use and fall in arterial carbon dioxide tension (Pa,CO_2) and sleepiness score. Nonetheless, the respiratory muscle resting with noninvasive positive pressure ventilation still remains a controversial hypothesis [8–10].

The most common chest skeletal abnormalities leading to respiratory failure include scoliosis and, less frequently, kyphosis with rib deformity, sequelae of thoracoplasty and (although rarely) spinal disorders (i.e. ankylosing spondylitis). There is considerable evidence that long-term HMV improves physiological measures, survival, quality of life and psychosocial functions [23, 24] in these patients. Very interestingly, the probability of survival in patients with kyphoscoliosis using noninvasive HMV greatly exceeds that provided by the use of long-term oxygen therapy (LTOT) [25].

Several neuromuscular conditions, either nonprogressive (e.g. poliomyelitis), slowly progressive (e.g. some myopathies and muscular dystrophy variants) or rapidly progressive (e.g. amyotrophic lateral sclerosis (ALS)) may take advantage of HMV when in the stage of respiratory failure.

Recent advances in the respiratory care of neuromuscolar diseases have improved the outlook for these patients, and many caregivers have changed from a traditional noninterventional approach to a more aggressive, supportive approach. Significant improvements in nocturnal and diurnal gas exchange, mortality and quality of life are reported in patients with slowly progressive conditions, especially when HMV is delivered by mask ventilation [24].

Patients with Duchenne muscular dystrophy, who are at substantial risk for sleep-disordered breathing, may benefit from noninvasive HMV, since improvement in quality of life and reduction in morbidity and early mortality have been reported [26]. This benefit is likely to be due to a slower rate of decline in pulmonary function compared with the untreated control subjects. In patients with ALS, where even a small elevation in diurnal Pa,CO_2 indicates high risk for incumbent decompensation, noninvasive HMV should be prompted by the occurrence of early symptoms of nocturnal hypoventilation or lung function impairment, thus favouring both survival [27] and residual life quality [28].

Obstructive disorders

The possibility that noninvasive HMV might aid patients with stable hypercapnic COPD has intrigued clinicians and researchers for decades. At least theoretically, ventilation could be beneficial in these patients through the following mechanisms: 1) reduction of hyperinflation; 2) improved CO_2 response of the respiratory centre; and 3) improved respiratory muscle function. Notwithstanding, these suggested mechanisms for improvement still remain controversial [11–19].

Due to the high prevalence of associated sleep-disordered breathing (e.g. obstructive sleep apnoea or hypoventilation) in these patients [29], the use of long-term ventilatory support is likely to be successful when adopted during night. Indeed, early studies reported favourable effects in this condition [11, 30]. In addition, the beneficial effect of noninvasive HMV in stable hypercapnic COPD has proven effectiveness by reducing lung hyperinflation [15], improving the inspiratory muscle strength [18, 19] and lowering the diaphragmatic fatigue threshold [31].

From a clinical point of view, the efficacy (quality of life, survival and hospitalisation rate) of noninvasive HMV in COPD patients still remains controversial [5]. Both observational and controlled studies on small case series with short follow-up did not completely answer the question [5]. Many factors, such as sample characteristics, degree of severity and setting of ventilator used, could explain these differences. A 2-yr prospective, randomised Italian study [32] is the largest trial showing that the addition of nocturnal mask ventilation to LTOT in stable hypercapnic COPD patients may improve daytime Pa,CO_2, dyspnoea and health-related quality of life compared with oxygen alone. Although, at present, the data do not clearly demonstrate a definitive benefit (*i.e.* improved survival) due to chronic ventilatory support in these patients, this approach has become popular in several European countries [4]. This optimistic attitude could be supported by clinical evidence and experimental data showing that noninvasive HMV is associated with a reduction in hospitalisation for acute-on-chronic ventilatory failure in the most severe hypercapnic COPD [33].

Analysis of costs

In the management of healthcare resources, cost-analysis currently represents a method for evaluation of the expenditure due to the effects on health of a new (or specific) intervention and for assessing it in the economic perspective [34].

Cost-effectiveness analysis (CEA) is a systematic methodology that measures health outcomes expressed in "natural units", *i.e.* the number of cases of disease prevented, the number of lives saved or the number of life-yrs gained by a new medical act [35]. However, the costs and the benefits in CEA are considered in "noncomparable units" and their ratio provides a yardstick with which to assess the productive efficiency [36]. For example, if an intervention is both more expensive and more effective than an alternative, then the criterion for efficiency becomes the ratio of the net increase in costs to the net increase in effectiveness (the incremental cost-effectiveness ratio).

In cost-benefit analysis (CBA), it is possible to establish, first, whether an individual intervention offers an overall net welfare gain and, secondly, how the welfare gain from that intervention compares with that from alternative interventions. Increased use of interventions with the greatest net gain will increase efficiency. Therefore, by valuing all costs and benefits in the same units, CBA compares diverse interventions using the net benefit criterion.

To complete the analysis of costs in healthcare, cost-utility analysis (CUA) could also be used [37]. This is an adaptation of CEA that measures an intervention's effect on both the quantitative and qualitative aspects of health (*i.e.* morbidity and mortality). This ratio provides a yardstick based on outcomes such as quality years of life gained; the relative efficiency is here assessed using the incremental cost-utility ratio. An intervention is deemed productively efficient, relative to an alternative, if it results in higher (or equal) benefits at lower costs. Therefore, CUA can address both productive and allocative efficiency.

In general, these three types of analysis (CEA, CBA and CUA) should be performed in more than one perspective, thus comparing all the costs, effectiveness and benefits deriving from a intervention. This would allow selection of the mix that can maximise health for a given set of resources. More often the cost-analysis studies are conducted at a complex level (involving more than just a local programme) and with periods of follow-up to look at the long-term impact of interventions [38].

Application of a cost-analysis

Most cost-analysis studies pursue an incremental approach that compares the additional costs of an intervention over the current practice with additional health benefits [39, 40].

The overall philosophy is that a new strategy intervention is being compared with the existing practice ("gold standard") or any other relevant alternative (best-available, low-cost or do-nothing) in the calculation of the cost-effectiveness ratio:

$$\text{Cost-effectiveness ratio} = \frac{\text{Cost}_{\text{(with new strategy)}} - \text{Cost}_{\text{(with current practice)}}}{\text{Effect}_{\text{(with new strategy)}} - \text{Effect}_{\text{(with current practice)}}} \quad (1)$$

The first step is needed in order to compare a set of interrelated interventions with the same target (*e.g.* to reduce the risk of cardiovascular disease, improve the health of children under 5 yrs of age, *etc.*) and then to provide information, which involves comparison of costs and outcomes of all the different types of possible interventions, and is useful to the decision on how to allocate resources. This requires cost-effectiveness to be estimated using an outcome indicator that measures changes in health, taking into account fatal and nonfatal outcomes. Disability-adjusted life-yrs (DALYs), healthy-yr equivalents (HYEs) and quality-adjusted life-yrs (QALYs) are all time-based measures of health that include the impact of interventions on years of life lost due to premature mortality and years of life lived with a nonfatal health outcome, weighted by the severity of that outcome [41, 42]. A CEA is, therefore, expressed as the cost spent for a DALY, HYE or QALY unit of measurement.

GOLD *et al.* [43] argue that people take into account the impact of an intervention on their future production when providing utility weights for QALYs, so that the effects are implicitly included in the denominator of the CEA ratio.

DALYs were first used jointly by the World Bank, the World Health Organization (WHO) and Harvard School of Public Health in the Global Burden of Disease (GBD) study [44, 45]. This study began in 1988 with the objectives of quantifying the burden of disease and injury of human populations and of defining the main health challenges at the global level using a measure that could also be used for CEA. Using DALYs, the GBD calculated by 1990 was projected up to 2020. Moreover, DALYs were used in 1993 to estimate the disease burden combined with cost-effectiveness in the World Development Report [46], in order to define priorities for investments in health. This summary measure of population health was then refined and it is now used routinely by WHO as a measure of CEA and to report health status in populations [47].

Table 3. – Advantages and disadvantages of cost-analysis studies

Pros	Cons
Promotes fiscal accountability in programmes	Requires a great deal of technical skill and knowledge
Establishes priorities when resources are limited	Difficult to assign a value in money to social programme (as human lives saved) independently of any moral issue
Extremely useful to the legislators, policy makers and other funders	Market costs (what people actually pay for something) don't always reflect "real" social costs
	Sometimes there are multiple competing goals, thus need to weight or prioritise them in some way
	The best-known cost-benefit studies have looked at long-term outcomes, but most programme evaluations don't have the time or resources to conduct long-term follow-up studies

The advantages and disadvantages of cost-analysis studies in healthcare are briefly summarised in table 3.

The costs and benefits of a set of related interventions should be evaluated with respect to the counterfactual of the "null set" of the related interventions. The counterfactual scenario for estimating population effectiveness is the null set, defined as the lifetime health experience of a defined population in a situation where all related interventions directed against a disease or condition are stopped. The null set can be estimated using natural history models, using trial data or by back-adjusting using coverage rates and effectiveness of currently implemented interventions. Data on the efficacy of interventions ideally comes from systematic reviews of studies. Efficacy can be expressed as relative risks for rates and effect sizes for means. Efficacy should be adjusted to a specific population, taking into account factors like coverage, quality of care, adherence and other local factors. Figure 1 shows the integrated assessment for healthcare costs calculation.

In the calculation of costs in the cost-analysis models every aspect has to be taken into account. Indeed, direct medical costs (directly linked and incurred by medical providers, such as for hospitalisations, drugs and visits), direct nonmedical costs (imposed on nonmedical care personnel, such as for patient and family member transportation and childcare), indirect costs (*e.g.* loss of productivity due to illness, time spent in medical appointments and disability) and intangible costs (*e.g.* pain and human suffering) should be calculated. Therefore, the actual cost of a studied drug might be only a small part of the total final cost involved [37].

Cost of care in long-term noninvasive mechanical ventilation

The delivery of noninvasive mechanical ventilation (NIV) in the acute-care hospital has been depicted as a labour-intensive therapy, which indicates that some patients treated with this modality may incur substantial healthcare costs [48, 49]. In this setting, the overall cost should be balanced by the reimbursement from the local healthcare system. To date, the financial balance between costs and diagnosis-related group reimbursement for acute-care NIV has been shown to be inappropriate, needing a different payment scale [50]. Although disappointing, this evaluation mainly referred to the hospital costs, which are known to be related more to the cost of healthcare personnel (~60% of total cost) than to the use of specific supplies, drugs and technologies. This is particularly evident in those patients who are bedridden and require significant medical and nursing therapy to treat the underlying condition.

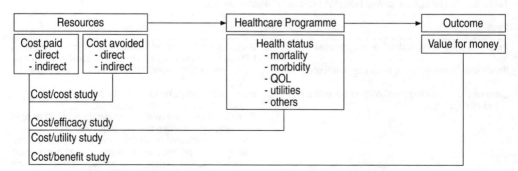

Fig. 1. – Integrated assessment for healthcare costs calculation. QOL: quality of life. Data taken from TORRANCE [37].

Different problems and perspectives can be addressed when considering the use of NIV as a long-term treatment in those candidates suffering from chronic respiratory insufficiency.

Although the effectiveness of noninvasive HMV has been addressed [20], and this treatment has been recognised in the last decades as useful in terms of individual physiological improvement and/or survival [51–54], the impact of this treatment on the overall costs has not been clearly reported or demonstrated.

So far, the cost of a formal home-care service for ventilator-dependent individuals in the USA has been estimated at ~US$6,000·month^{-1}·patient^{-1} [55]. However, it is rather difficult to compute costs related to the prolonged use of mechanical ventilation. Indeed, in contrast to the costs related to hospital care, several different factors related to the patient (including the family burden) and even to the local organisation may contribute to this calculation. In actual fact, the majority of data related to costs of noninvasive HMV in patients suffering from chronic respiratory failure relate to COPD.

A list of both direct and indirect costs related to NIV is included in table 4.

Direct costs

When chronic respiratory patients develop HRF, they report incremental use of healthcare resources. Indeed, they are more likely have increased exacerbations, access to primary care, use of medications and hospital and intensive care admissions [56], as well as a further deterioration of their health-related quality of life [57].

Most of these individuals, especially those with COPD, have been prescribed LTOT, which is known to provide better survival [58]. Notwithstanding, it is still unclear whether the addition of noninvasive HMV may be associated to further benefits in these patients [5], as already mentioned. Nevertheless, due to some recognised physiological and clinical advantages, which also include the improvement of individual physical performance [59], noninvasive HMV is currently popular among physicians [4].

Recently, a retrospective study in chronically ventilated COPD patients reported an analysis of direct costs of care [33]. The authors calculated the cost·day^{-1}·patient^{-1} of major healthcare charges (oxygen, drugs and hospitalisations) over 2 yrs in COPD patients treated by nocturnal noninvasive HMV in addition to the usual LTOT regimen compared with similar patients continuing LTOT alone. They were able to show that the addition of HMV is associated with a 20% saving of these direct costs compared with LTOT alone; in particular, they reported that the burden of costs due to the ventilatory equipment provision and management increased the whole costs up to the same limit reached by those patients using LTOT alone.

Table 4. – List and categories of main costs related to noninvasive mechanical ventilation

Direct		Indirect
Medical	Nonmedical	
Ward (capital, nursing workload, pharmacy)	Transportation	Loss of productivity and other financial issues
Intensive care (daily costs)	Childcare	Unemployment
Equipment (ventilator, humidifier, consumables, annual servicing, training)		Time spent in appointments
Drugs		Disability
Outpatient attendance (scheduled and unscheduled visits)		Professional relationships
		Housekeeping
		Social isolation

However, it seems difficult to compare this analysis of direct costs with others that have been previously published [50, 60]. Indeed, different healthcare systems and reimbursement policies in different countries might have biased the results, making comparisons rather difficult to draw.

Among the results that arose from the Italian randomised trial [33], it was interesting to note that a reduction in the use of healthcare resources in terms of hospital readmission was fairly well correlated with the use of NIV in these individuals. This research has confirmed that the overall burden of care costs is not increased when noninvasive HMV is adopted and that this regimen is associated with a 34% cost saving related to the re-hospitalisation rate, in particular. Very interestingly, this saving of costs was associated with a significant reduction in the high-cost admissions in the critical care areas.

The use of medications is another important category of direct costs in COPD. It has been calculated that costs due to drug acquisition account for ~40% of direct costs in these patients, with a proportional increase according to severity of the disease [61].

In the Italian study [33], the mean percentage cost of drugs out of the total direct costs was less than approximately 15%. This is not surprising, since this particular subgroup of patients with a very advanced disease are likely to have reached a threshold limit in their standard (evidence-based addressed) pharmacological treatment, which therefore accounts for a proportionally lower amount of the total cost that includes other advanced nonpharmacological therapies (including oxygen) or different direct costs. Additionally, the computed cost for medications in that group of COPD patients did not take into account the increased use of pharmacological resources during hospital admissions. As a matter of fact, CLINI et al. [33] did not find any difference in the current cost of medications between the two study groups, thus underlining the fact that this part of the direct cost is less likely to influence the overall burden in these patients.

These particular individuals suffering from COPD therefore represent patients for which a third part's payment decision making should not be exclusively based on a rough rather than on a precise cost-effectiveness analysis of cost [62].

Indirect costs

Direct cost gives only a partial estimate of the total costs. Indeed, this view limits the logical and more important burden of indirect costs often associated with the use of noninvasive HMV.

Among these, the indirect costs related to the family caregivers may be extremely relevant and may even further affect the efficacy of any domiciliary programme, especially in those individuals who are totally home-bound or confined to bed. Indeed, patients with COPD and neuromuscular disorders under noninvasive HMV have important burdens (e.g. high dependency, high levels of pre-morbidity score, recurrent exacerbations with following hospitalisation), which in turn may impact on the quality of their families' lives. Overall, more than 50% of ventilator-dependent patients at home suffer from two or more burdens needing specific family care [63].

In a cross-sectional survey conducted among primary family caregivers of patients who were ventilator dependent and who were living at home, it was shown that the total cost of home-care services was substantial (>US$6,000·month^{-1}·patient^{-1} in the mid-1990s) [55, 60]. Very interestingly, the monthly cost increased up to two-fold when various values of caregiver effort were incorporated into this calculation [55]. The incorporation of the caregiver's time value into cost estimates did not substantially reduce the proportion of patients for whom home care was the least expensive alternative, except when caregiver effort was valued at a registered nurse's wage rate. However, the long-term economic impact on caregivers who reduce their work hours or forego employment or educational opportunities may further increase the burden, but this has never been strictly calculated.

Therefore, home care for these patients is labour intensive and costly. Thus, although models of home-care programmes in patients with noninvasive HMV may merely prove clinical effectiveness [64, 65], the development of policies and programmes to support home placement is still lacking. Since the use of main public healthcare services for ventilator-dependent patients may be significantly affected by factors related to caregivers, the situation of caregivers should be considered when implementing the use of resources and should be included in the policy making [66].

In a recent study, the subjective and objective burdens imposed on families of 50 patients under noninvasive HMV were explored [67]. It was found that profound objective burden was reported in the field of social relations (49% of cases), household management (43%), financial issues (32%) and employment issues (29%). Interestingly, family members of these patients experienced a lower subjective burden and they were used to adopting several strategies to cope with the imposed burden, including re-orientation of life goals (92% of cases), resignation (88%), passivity (63%), hopefulness (45%), ambivalence (20%) and guilt (14%). Therefore, clinicians caring for patients with chronic respiratory failure should consider the family's needs when noninvasive HMV is prescribed. The domains causing major distress in the family (financial issues, professional relationships and housekeeping) are sectors commonly faced by the caregivers. Their impact should be taken into account by policymakers when home care is organised and/or implemented.

Additional research regarding indirect factors that may affect the global burden, as well as the ability or willingness of family members to accept the cost and to share the responsibility for caring for the patients, is now required. Indeed, it has been calculated that the use of major services and resources may be decided more by the needs of caregivers than by the care level of the applicants [66].

Another aspect, which is still far from being considered in the evaluation of indirect costs, is the estimation of those charges needed for initiating domiciliary ventilation. For example, it could be important to calculate how many patients have to try the noninvasive HMV equipment before the staff could find that the patient is likely to accept the treatment. Moreover, it could also be important to include among the indirect costs the time and effort spent by the staff to train the patient and his/her relatives during the hospital stay.

Only one observational study refers to costs related to patient training during hospital care [68], comparing periods without or with noninvasive HMV. Based on a previous economic analysis [69], the ongoing training of ward nursing staff showed similar charges in the two periods.

Similar analysis specifically related to personnel involved in training patients and relatives outside acute care and before discharging home with noninvasive HMV has not yet been reported, but it is likely that this cost may also contribute substantially to the global burden of this treatment even in the long term.

Economic analysis

To date, very few data based on true economic analysis in patients under noninvasive HMV have been published. To the best of our knowledge, the most recent and retrospective audit on the cost of noninvasive HMV in hypercapnic COPD has been conducted in a very small sample of patients in the UK [68].

The analysis performed in this study was based on the costs data (hospital admissions in a ward or in an intensive care unit, healthcare personnel charges, equipment, training and outpatient attendance) comparing 1 yr before and after initiation of noninvasive HMV in 13 COPD patients with chronic hypercapnia and recurrent admissions [68]. It was found that the year spent with noninvasive HMV resulted in significantly lower costs (~60% saving) compared with the year before, in this small sample. Therefore, it was concluded that noninvasive HMV, once its clinical efficacy is proved, may be cost-effective in a highly selected group of COPD patients with recurrent admissions, thus potentially minimising costs.

Notwithstanding, this study identified costs and placed values on these costs from the perspective of the acute hospital. Indeed, on the one hand, the acute hospital has the most to gain financially from reducing admissions and, on the other hand, it may result in a increased demand (and costs) on services in the primary care.

It has been calculated that, for the provision of home NIV to become cost neutral, the increased burden on primary care would have to be in excess of 450 consultations or 200 home visits per patient [70]. As a matter of fact, the study by JONES et al. [71] actually found a reduction in general practitioner consultations after noninvasive HMV was instituted.

Such evidence could be important in obtaining financial support for providing a service dedicated to HMV. For example, it has been shown that the cost-efficacy of prolonged mechanical ventilation provision in hospital settings varies dramatically based on factors like age and the likelihood of poor outcomes [72]. Therefore, identifying patients likely to have unfavourable prognosis due to their underlying diagnosis and reducing costly readmissions should be future priorities in improving the clinical value of prolonged mechanical ventilation especially in the domiciliary setting.

Other and more detailed analysis of costs could eventually be considered when studying chronic patients at home under prolonged mechanical ventilation. In particular, the effectiveness and the utility of this treatment would both be useful aspects to be assessed with regard to the impact of noninvasive HMV on patient survival and quality of life (or health status), respectively.

It has been shown that noninvasive HMV in hypercapnic COPD patients provides a median survival of ~29 months [68], which is comparable to that achieved by providing noninvasive ventilation during acute exacerbations or with the conventional medical treatment alone [73]. If acute ventilation per se does indeed prolong life in these patients, it is possible that noninvasive HMV postpones the costs related to the acute-care setting to a period often longer than that usually observed in the analysis of costs. Thus, the savings observed early after the institution of noninvasive HMV would be lost in the longer period. Therefore, a cost-effectiveness analysis taking survival time into account would better balance the true impact of noninvasive HMV therapy on the disease.

Similarly, long-term noninvasive HMV has shown that quality of life and health status are maintained [74] and even significantly improved [32]. This could be evaluated by a specific economic analysis of the outcome in Euros per QALY [75] (see also the foregoing discussion).

The Italian study on nocturnal noninvasive HMV in COPD patients failed to show any advantage in QALY compared with LTOT alone (Italian Association of Pneumologists, Salerno, Italy; personal communication). However, this was mainly due to the uncompleted availability of quality-of-life data in the database and the partial recordings of computed costs, with the absence of any aspect referring to the indirect costs related to this treatment. Nonetheless, it is quite interesting to note that, in a cohort from the USA in the acute-care setting, incremental costs per QALY gained by prolonged mechanical ventilation provision exceeded US$100,000 in patients aged >68 yrs (with a predicted 1-yr survival >50%) [72].

Thus, new information on stable chronic patients with noninvasive HMV is welcomed from this point of view. It is likely that this kind of analysis might further help the overall decision making and selection of candidates for noninvasive HMV.

Conclusions

The indication and use of noninvasive HMV have become popular in the last decades, since it has been proven effective on both physiological and clinical grounds in a large population of patients suffering from chronic respiratory failure.

Noninvasive mechanical ventilation has been described as a labour-intensive treatment in these patients. Notwithstanding, there is lack of accurate calculations of costs and specific analysis of costs in this population.

Direct and (partially) indirect cost calculations have been observed and reported, especially in chronic obstructive pulmonary disease patients under noninvasive home mechanical ventilation. The most recent data underline the large impact of noninvasive home mechanical ventilation on both patient outcome (reduction of recurrent admissions and increase in quality of life) and family burden (unemployment, financial and social issues), thus prompting further studies with appropriate cost-effectiveness and/or cost-utility analysis which, at present, are still lacking. This would better help in addressing the overall policy on decision making and selection of candidates.

Summary

The expansion of home mechanical ventilation (HMV) in the last 15 yrs was stimulated by the introduction of noninvasive mask ventilation and the recognition that more patient groups could benefit.

In the management of healthcare resources, cost-analysis currently represents a method for evaluation of the expenditure due to the effects on health of a new (or specific) intervention and for assessing it in the economic perspective. Disability-adjusted life-yrs, healthy-yr equivalents and quality-adjusted life-yrs are all time-based measures of health that include the impact of interventions on years of life lost due to premature mortality and years of life lived with a nonfatal health outcome, weighted by the severity of that outcome.

Although the effectiveness of noninvasive HMV has been addressed, the impact of this treatment on the overall costs has not been clearly reported or demonstrated and very few data based on a true economic analysis in patients under noninvasive HMV have been published. Direct and (partially) indirect cost calculations have been observed and reported, especially in chronic obstructive pulmonary disease patients under noninvasive HMV. The most recent data underline the large impact of noninvasive HMV on both patient outcome (reduction of recurrent admissions and increase in quality of life) and family burden (unemployment, financial and social issues), thus prompting further studies with appropriate cost-effectiveness and/or cost-utility analysis.

Keywords: Cost analysis, home care, mechanical ventilation, respiratory insufficiency.

Support Statement: E.M. Clini has received an unrestricted research grant (project no. 21 of the research programme 2005/2006) from the Italian Association of Pulmonologists (Salerno, Italy).

References

1. Chailleux E, Fauroux B, Binet F, Dautzenberg B, Polu JM. Predictors of survival in patients receiving domiciliary oxygen therapy or mechanical ventilation. A 10-year analysis of ANTADIR Observatory. *Chest* 1996; 109: 741–749.

2. Adams AB, Shapiro R, Marini JJ. Changing prevalence of chronically ventilator-assisted individuals in Minnesota: increases, characteristics, and the use of noninvasive ventilation. *Respir Care* 1998; 43: 643–649.

3. Fédération Association Nationale pour le Traitement A Domicile l'Innovation et la Recherche (ANTADIR). www.antadir.com Date last updated: December 31, 2007. Date last accessed: June 10, 2008.

4. Lloyd-Owen SJ, Donaldson GC, Ambrosino N, *et al.* Patterns of home mechanical ventilation use in Europe: results from the Eurovent survey. *Eur Respir J* 2005; 25: 1025–1031.

5. Kolodziej MA, Jensen L, Rowe B, Sin D. Systematic review of noninvasive positive pressure ventilation in severe stable COPD. *Eur Respir J* 2007; 30: 293–306.

6. Annane D, Orlikowski D, Chevret S, Chevrolet JC, Raphaël JC. Nocturnal mechanical ventilation for chronic hypoventilation in patients with neuromuscular and chest wall disorders. *Cochrane Database Syst Rev* 2007; 4: CD001941.

7. Nickol AH, Hart N, Hopkinson NS, Moxham J, Simonds A, Polkey MI. Mechanisms of improvement of respiratory failure in patients with restrictive thoracic disease treated with non-invasive ventilation. *Thorax* 2005; 60: 754–760.

8. Annane D, Quera-Salva MA, Lofaso F, *et al.* Mechanisms underlying effects of nocturnal ventilation on daytime blood gases in neuromuscular diseases. *Eur Respir J* 1999; 13: 157–162.

9. Dellborg C, Olofson J, Hamnegård CH, Skoogh BE, Bake B. Ventilatory response to CO_2 re-breathing before and after nocturnal nasal intermittent positive pressure ventilation in patients with chronic alveolar hypoventilation. *Respir Med* 2000; 94: 1154–1160.

10. Simonds AK, Parker RA, Branthwaite MA. The effect of intermittent positive-pressure hyperinflation in restrictive chest wall disease. *Respiration* 1989; 55: 136–143.

11. Meecham Jones DJ, Paul EA, Jones PW, Wedzicha JA. Nasal pressure support ventilation plus oxygen compared with oxygen therapy alone in hypercapnic COPD. *Am J Respir Crit Care Med* 1995; 152: 538–544.

12. Elliott MW, Mulvey DA, Moxham J, Green M, Branthwaite MA. Domiciliary nocturnal nasal intermittent positive pressure ventilation in COPD: mechanisms underlying changes in arterial blood gas tensions. *Eur Respir J* 1991; 4: 1044–1052.

13. Gay PC, Hubmayr RD, Stroetz RW. Efficacy of nocturnal nasal ventilation in stable, severe chronic obstructive pulmonary disease during a 3-month controlled trial. *Mayo Clin Proc* 1996; 71: 533–542.

14. Lin CC. Comparison between nocturnal nasal positive pressure ventilation combined with oxygen therapy and oxygen monotherapy in patients with severe COPD. *Am J Respir Crit Care Med* 1996; 154: 353–358.

15. Díaz O, Bégin P, Torrealba B, Jover E, Lisboa C. Effects of nonivasive ventilation on lung hyperinflation in stable hypercapnic COPD. *Eur Respir J* 2002; 20: 1490–1498.

16. Braun NM, Marino WD. Effect of daily intermittent rest of respiratory muscles in patients with severe chronic airflow limitation (CAL). *Chest* 1984; 85: 59S–60S.

17. Gutiérrez M, Beroíza T, Contreras G, *et al.* Weekly cuirass ventilation improves blood gases and inspiratory muscle strength in patients with chronic air-flow limitation and hypercarbia. *Am Rev Respir Dis* 1988; 138: 617–623.

18. Zibrak JD, Hill NS, Federman EC, Kwa SL, O'Donnell C. Evaluation of intermittent long-term negative-pressure ventilation in patients with severe chronic obstructive pulmonary disease. *Am Rev Respir Dis* 1988; 138: 1515–1518.

19. Schönhofer B, Polkey M, Suchi S, Köhler D. Effect of home mechanical ventilation on inspiratory muscle strength in COPD. *Chest* 2006; 130: 1834–1838.

20. Clinical indications for noninvasive positive pressure ventilation in chronic respiratory failure due to restrictive lung disease, COPD, and nocturnal hypoventilation – a consensus conference report. *Chest* 1999; 116: 521–534.

21. Sawicka EH, Branthwaite MA. Respiration during sleep in kyphoscoliosis. *Thorax* 1987; 42: 801–808.

22. Hill NS. Noninvasive ventilation. Does it work, for whom, and how? *Am Rev Respir Dis* 1993; 147: 1050–1055.

23. Simonds AK. Home ventilation. *Eur Respir J* 2003; 22: Suppl. 47, 38s–46s.

24. Baydur A, Layne E, Aral H, *et al.* Long term non-invasive ventilation in the community for patients with musculoskeletal disorders: 46 year experience and review. *Thorax* 2000; 55: 4–11.

25. Gustafson T, Franklin KA, Midgren B, Pehrsson K, Ranstam J, Ström K. Survival of patients with kyphoscoliosis receiving mechanical ventilation or oxygen at home. *Chest* 2006; 130: 1828–1833.

26. Simonds AK, Muntoni F, Heather S, Fielding S. Impact of nasal ventilation on survival in hypercapnic Duchenne muscular dystrophy. *Thorax* 1998; 53: 949–952.

27. Pinto AC, Evangelista T, Carvalho M, Alves MA, Sales Luís ML. Respiratory assistance with a non-invasive ventilator (Bipap) in MND/ALS patients: survival rates in a controlled trial. *J Neurol Sci* 1995; 129: Suppl. 1, 19–26.

28. Bourke SC, Bullock RE, Williams TL, Shaw PJ, Gibson GJ. Noninvasive ventilation in ALS: indications and effect on quality of life. *Neurology* 2003; 61: 171–177.

29. Fleetham J, West P, Mezon B, Conway W, Roth T, Kryger M. Sleep, arousals, and oxygen desaturation in chronic obstructive pulmonary disease. The effect of oxygen therapy. *Am Rev Respir Dis* 1982; 126: 429–433.

30. Elliott MW, Steven MH, Phillips GD, Branthwaite MA. Non-invasive mechanical ventilation for acute respiratory failure. *BMJ* 1990; 300: 358–360.

31. Nava S, Ambrosino N, Rubini F, *et al.* Effect of nasal pressure support ventilation and external PEEP on diaphragmatic activity in patients with severe stable COPD. *Chest* 1993; 103: 143–150.

32. Clini E, Sturani C, Rossi A, *et al.* The Italian multicentre study on noninvasive ventilation in chronic obstructive pulmonary disease patients. *Eur Respir J* 2002; 20: 529–538.

33. Clini EM, Magni G, Crisafulli E, Viaggi S, Ambrosino N. Home non-invasive mechanical ventilation and long-term oxygen therapy in stable hypercapnic chronic obstructive pulmonary disease patients: comparison of costs. *Respiration* 2008; [Epub ahead of print PMID: 18417954].

34. Weinstein MC, Siegel JE, Gold MR, Kamlet MS, Russell LB. Recommendations of the Panel on Cost-effectiveness in Health and Medicine. *JAMA* 1996; 276: 1253–1258.

35. Russell LB, Gold MR, Siegel JE, Daniels N, Weinstein MC. The role of cost-effectiveness analysis in health and medicine. Panel on Cost-effectiveness in Health and Medicine. *JAMA* 1996; 276: 1172–1177.

36. Phelps CE, Mushlin AI. On the (near) equivalence of cost-effectiveness and cost-benefit analyses. *Int J Technol Assess Health Care* 1991; 7: 12–21.

37. Torrance GW. Measurement of health state utilities for economic appraisal. *J Health Econ* 1986; 5: 1–30.

38. Weinstein MC, Stason WB. Foundations of cost-effectiveness analysis for health and medical practices. *N Engl J Med* 1977; 296: 716–721.

39. Drummond M, McGuire A, eds, Economic Evaluation in Health Care. Merging Theory with Practice. 1st Edn. Oxford, Oxford University Press, 2001.

40. Neumann PJ, Rosen AB, Weinstein MC. Medicare and cost-effectiveness analysis. *N Engl J Med* 2005; 353: 1516–1522.

41. Fox-Rushby JA, Hanson K. Calculating and presenting disability adjusted life years (DALYs) in cost-effectiveness analysis. *Health Policy Plan* 2001; 16: 326–331.

42. Gafni A, Birch S. QALYs and HYEs (healthy years equivalent). Spotting the differences. *J Health Econ* 1997; 16: 601–608.

43. Gold MR, Siegel JE, Russel LB, Weinstein MC, eds, Cost-effectiveness in Health and Medicine. New York, Oxford University Press, 1996.

44. Murray CJL, Lopez AD. The Global Burden of Disease: a Comprehensive Assessment of Mortality and Disability from Diseases, Injuries, and Risk Factors in 1990 and Projected to 2020. 1st Edn. Cambridge, Harvard University Press, 1996.

45. Murray CJL, Lopez AD. Global Health Statistics: a compendium of incidence, prevalence, and mortality estimates for over 200 conditions. 2nd Edn. Cambridge, Harvard University Press, 1996.

46. The World Bank, World Development Report 1993: Investing in Health. New York, Oxford University Press, 1993.

47. Fox-Rushby JA. Disability Adjusted Life Years (DALYs) for Decision-making? An Overview of the Literature. London, Office of Health Economics, 2002.

48. Chevrolet JC, Jolliet P, Abajo B, Toussi A, Louis M. Nasal positive pressure ventilation in patients with acute respiratory failure. Difficult and time-consuming procedure for nurses. *Chest* 1991; 100: 775–782.

49. Nava S, Evangelisti I, Rampulla C, Compagnoni ML, Fracchia C, Rubini F. Human and financial costs of noninvasive mechanical ventilation in patients affected by COPD and acute respiratory failure. *Chest* 1997; 111: 1631–1638.

50. Criner GJ, Kreimer DT, Tomaselli M, Pierson W, Evans D. Financial implications of noninvasive positive pressure ventilation (NPPV). *Chest* 1995; 108: 475–481.

51. Wedzicha JA, Muir JF. Noninvasive ventilation in chronic obstructive pulmonary disease, bronchiectasis and cystic fibrosis. *Eur Respir J* 2002; 20: 777–784.

52. Cuvelier A, Muir JF. Noninvasive ventilation and chronic respiratory failure: indications and obstructive lung diseases. *In*: Muir JF, Ambrosino N, Simonds AK, eds. Noninvasive Mechanical Ventilation. *Eur Respir Mon* 2001; 16: 187–203.

53. Simonds AK. Neuromuscular disease. *In*: Muir JF, Ambrosino N, Simonds AK, eds. Noninvasive Mechanical Ventilation. *Eur Respir Mon* 2001; 16: 218–226.

54. Shneerson JM. Noninvasive ventilation in chronic respiratory failure due to restrictive chest wall and parenchymal lung disease. *In*: Muir JF, Ambrosino N, Simonds AK, eds. Noninvasive Mechanical Ventilation. *Eur Respir Mon* 2001; 16: 204–217.

55. Sevick MA, Bradham DD. Economic value of caregiver effort in maintaining long-term ventilator-assisted individuals at home. *Heart Lung* 1997; 26: 148–157.

56. Vitacca M, Foglio K, Scalvini S, Marangoni S, Quadri A, Ambrosino N. Time course of pulmonary function before admission into ICU. A two-year retrospective study of COLD patients with hypercapnia. *Chest* 1992; 102: 1737–1741.

57. Seemungal TA, Donaldson GC, Paul EA, Bestall JC, Jeffries DJ, Wedzicha JA. Effect of exacerbation on quality of life in patients with chronic obstructive pulmonary disease. *Am J Respir Crit Care Med* 1998; 157: 1418–1422.

58. Croxton TL, Bailey WC. Long-term oxygen treatment in chronic obstructive pulmonary disease: recommendations for future research: an NHLBI workshop report. *Am J Respir Crit Care Med* 2006; 174: 373–378.

59. Schönhofer B, Dellweg D, Suchi S, Köhler D. Exercise endurance before and after long-term noninvasive ventilation in patients with chronic respiratory failure. *Respiration* 2008; 75: 296–303.

60. Sevick MA, Kamlet MS, Hoffman LA, Rawson I. Economic cost of home-based care for ventilator-assisted individuals: a preliminary report. *Chest* 1996; 109: 1597–1606.

61. Miravitlles M, Murio C, Guerrero T, Gisbert R. Costs of chronic bronchitis and COPD: a 1-year follow-up study. *Chest* 2003; 123: 784–791.

62. Barbieri M, Drummond M, Willke R, Chancellor J, Jolain B, Towse A. Variability of cost-effectiveness estimates for pharmaceuticals in Western Europe: lessons for inferring generalizability. *Value Health* 2005; 8: 10–23.

63. Vitacca M, Escarrabill J, Galavotti G, *et al.* Home mechanical ventilation patients: a retrospective survey to identify level of burden in real life. *Monaldi Arch Chest Dis* 2007; 67: 142–147.

64. Clini E, Vitacca M, Foglio K, Simoni P, Ambrosino N. Long-term home care programmes may rduce hospital admissions in COPD with chronic hypercapnia. *Eur Respir J* 1996; 9: 1605–1610.

65. Nauffal D, Doménech R, Martínez García MA, Compte L, Macián V, Perpiñá M. Noninvasive positive pressure home ventilation in restrictive disorders: outcome and impact on health-related quality of life. *Respir Med* 2002; 96: 777–783.

66. Tamiya N, Yamaoka K, Yano E. Use of home health services covered by new public long-term care insurance in Japan: impact of the presence and kinship of family caregivers. *Int J Qual Health Care* 2002; 14: 295–303.

67. Tsara V, Serasli E, Voutsas V, Lazarides V, Christaki P. Burden and coping strategies in families of patients under noninvasive home mechanical ventilation. *Respiration* 2006; 73: 61–67.

68. Tuggey JM, Plant PK, Elliott MW. Domiciliary non-invasive ventilation for recurrent acidotic exacerbations of COPD: an economic analysis. *Thorax* 2003; 58: 867–871.

69. Plant PK, Owen JL, Parrott S, Elliott MW. Cost effectiveness of ward based non-invasive ventilation for acute exacerbations of chronic obstructive pulmonary disease: economic analysis of randomised controlled trial. *BMJ* 2003; 326: 956–961.

70. Netton A, Curtis L. Unit costs of health and social care. Canterbury, Personal Social Services Research Unit, 2000.

71. Jones SE, Packham S, Hebden M, Smith AP. Domiciliary nocturnal intermittent positive pressure ventilation in patients with respiratory failure due to severe COPD: long-term follow up and effect on survival. *Thorax* 1998; 53: 495–498.

72. Cox CE, Carson SS, Govert JA, Chelluri L, Sanders GD. An economic evaluation of prolonged mechanical ventilation. *Crit Care Med* 2007; 35: 1918–1927.

73. Plant PK, Owen JL, Elliott MW. Non-invasive ventilation in acute exacerbations of chronic obstructive pulmonary disease: long term survival and predictors of in-hospital outcome. *Thorax* 2001; 56: 708–712.

74. Perrin C, El Far Y, Vandenbos F, *et al.* Domiciliary nasal intermittent positive pressure ventilation in severe COPD: effects on lung function and quality of life. *Eur Respir J* 1997; 10: 2835–2839.

75. Drummond MF, O'Brien BJ, Stoddart GL, Torrance G. Methods for the Economic Evaluation of Health Care Programmes. Oxford, Oxford University Press, 1997.

CHAPTER 27

Home NIV: results and lessons from a European survey

J. Goldring, J. Wedzicha

Academic Unit of Respiratory Medicine, Royal Free and University College Medical School, London, UK.

Correspondence: J.A. Wedzicha, Academic Unit of Respiratory Medicine, Royal Free and University College Medical School, Rowland Hill Street, London, NW3 2PF, UK. Fax: 44 2074726141; E-mail: j.a.wedzicha@medsch.ucl.ac.uk

Introduction

The prevalence of chronic respiratory failure in Europe continues to rise, mostly because of an aging population demographic but also because of an increase in the uptake of smoking in Russia and the former Eastern Bloc countries [1, 2]. This has been accompanied by the expansion [3–5] over the last three decades in the use of home mechanical ventilation (HMV) to treat chronic hypercapnic respiratory failure. HMV is usually delivered as noninvasive ventilation (NIV), with the majority of patients using only nocturnal or nocturnal plus part-daytime NIV, and in many cases has been shown to reduce mortality and morbidity [6, 7] and to improve quality of life [8].

The magnitude of the rise in HMV is impressive, with the numbers of patients receiving home ventilatory support increasing from 130 patients, in one survey, in 1988 to 3,120 patients in 1998 [3]. This expansion has been driven by not only the growing population of individuals with chronic respiratory failure but also the increasing recognition that NIV can be of benefit in many different causes of ventilatory failure [9]. Technological advances have meant that ventilators are easier to use and that the interfaces are more comfortable. Additionally, HMV offers the individual the advantage of retaining an independent lifestyle and it offers the state a health–economic benefit as it is less costly when compared with invasive mechanical ventilation [10]. As well as the patient, there are industrial manufacturers and distributors of the machines, who will also benefit from the increasingly widespread use of HMV. It is, of course, important that the growth of HMV in Europe is on a properly planned basis and not simply driven by market considerations. However, it will be seen from the present chapter that the use of HMV in Europe is not presently standardised, regulated or consistent.

The present chapter will describe and explore the wide variation in practises that occur within and between the countries of Europe with regards to HMV. Firstly, it will look at predominantly national surveys which took place in the 1990s before progressing to the most recent pan-European survey which took place in 2001–2002.

Surveys within Europe in the 1990s

The most comprehensive early questionnaire survey of HMV to have been undertaken in Europe took place in 1992 [11]. The European Working Group on Home Treatment for Chronic Respiratory Insufficiency looked at the organisation of HMV, continuous

Eur Respir Mon, 2008, 41, 392–399. Printed in UK - all rights reserved. Copyright ERS Journals Ltd 2008; European Respiratory Monograph; ISSN 1025-448x.

positive airway pressure (CPAP) and long-term oxygen therapy (LTOT) in 13 European countries. The group were well aware that differences existed between the countries and the stated aim was to characterise these variations and to allow the individual countries to benefit from the comparison of data. The group's efforts were hampered by information that was "incomplete, erratic in detail and characterised only by its paucity in outcome modalities". Only France, with its *Association Nationale pour le Traitement à Domicile del'Insuffisance Respiratoire Chronique* (National Association for Home Care Patients with Chronic Respiratory Insufficiency; ANTADIR), and Switzerland (Swiss Lung Association) had national registers at that time for HMV and which facilitated comprehensive data gathering. Since 1981, ANTADIR have been responsible for managing ~70% of patients receiving HMV in France and, since 1984, a subgroup of these patients have been surveyed annually [12]. The group were also able to obtain complete information on HMV from Denmark and Belgium *via* health-service data and commercial supply companies. The information gleaned from the remaining countries was much patchier and was generally easier to obtain for LTOT than for mechanical ventilation (MV) or CPAP, perhaps because, on the whole, LTOT has been established for longer in most of the countries studied.

The main findings from that survey were that HMV was being used substantively for chronic lung disease, chest wall deformities (CWD) and neuromuscular disease (NMD) in all of the countries, apart from Poland, which had a negligible number of ventilated patients being treated at home. This latter observation could probably be extrapolated to other European states that have recently joined the European Union [13]. The majority of ventilators in use were positive pressure and of those, most were volume-cycled as opposed to pressure-cycled. Italy and Belgium used volume-cycled machines exclusively. Prescriptions for HMV were being written by both respiratory physicians and nonspecialist physicians. Prescription rules existed in only a few countries with most having no regulation of prescribing whatsoever. The ventilators were supplied through commercial companies or nationalised health services and paid for, primarily, by the latter. Specific details on supervision and technical support for HMV were difficult to extract from the article because the data were combined with those for LTOT.

The authors concluded that major differences occurred between the 13 European countries and that these were probably explained by the "historical origin of home care in each country, the different impact of commercial companies and the supervision of insurance companies on doctor's prescriptions." In order to improve the uniformity and quality of HMV provision they proposed: the establishment of further national registries to improve data collection; a standardised Europe-wide set of guidelines to advise clinicians; and a system that would ensure adequate equipment performance and maintenance.

There are other notable single European country reviews of home respiratory care from the 1990s. A follow-up study between 1992 and 2000 provided longitudinal data on changes in HMV practice in Geneva [5]. JANSSENS *et al.* [5] noted that, during the course of the study, there was a marked increase in the proportion of patients with chronic obstructive pulmonary disease (COPD) and obesity hypoventilation syndrome (OHS) from 0 and 14% at the outset to 25 and 39%, respectively, by the end of the study. The advent of cheaper, smaller and arguably easier to use pressure-cycled ventilators also heralded a change from the exclusive use of volume-cycled ventilators in 1992 to predominantly pressure-cycled ventilators by the end of the study. A similar longitudinal study in Sweden [4] also highlighted the rapid growth of HMV prescription for patients with OHS.

MIDGREN *et al.* [14] reported on cross-sectional data from the Swedish register of HMV, which was established in 1996 by the Swedish Society of Chest Medicine. The salient findings were that: the prevalence of HMV use varied widely between healthcare regions from 1.2 to 20 per 100,000 inhabitants and only 3% of patients had COPD as the indication for HMV. The authors believed that the difference in prevalence of HMV between healthcare regions could be because "the indications for HMV are not well defined, which may make room for more individual decision making". Further analysis by LAUB *et al.* [4] demonstrated that the disparity between the regions could not be explained by socioeconomic or demographic differences. The under-representation of COPD patients was ascribed to a lack of "enthusiasm among Swedish physicians to offer patients with these diagnoses, HMV", perhaps because of the conflicting evidence of a long-term benefit for ventilation in this patient group [15, 16]. Another finding reported from the Swedish registry was that the age distribution was bimodal. The authors contrasted this discovery to Denmark, whose age distribution was unimodal because of a heavy bias towards young patients with muscular dystrophy. The bias was attributed in part by MIDGREN *et al.* [14] to the high profile Danish Muscular Dystrophy fund. Finally, with regards to the Swedish registry, there were some similarities with the Geneva study [5] in that prospective analysis of the registry data suggested that the choice of ventilator was changing from volume- to pressure-cycled.

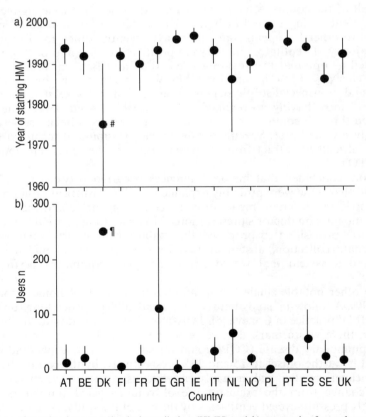

Fig. 1. – a) Year of starting home mechanical ventilation (HMV) and b) centre size for each country. Data are presented as median±interquartile range. #: median and full range shown due to only two centres being included; ¶: median only, range 250–253 for the two centres. AT: Austria; BE: Belgium; DK: Denmark; FI: Finland; FR: France; DE: Germany; GR: Greece; IE: Ireland; IT: Italy; NL: the Netherlands; NO: Norway; PL: Poland; PT: Portugal; ES: Spain; SE: Sweden. Reproduced from [17] with permission from the publisher.

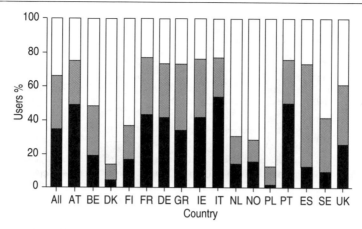

Fig. 2. – Percentage of users in each disease category by country. ■: lung/airways (chronic obstructive pulmonary disease, cystic fibrosis, bronchiectasis, pulmonary fibrosis and paediatric diseases); ▩: Chest wall deformities (kyphoscoliosis, old tuberculosis, obesity hypoventilation syndrome, surgical resection); □: neuromuscular (muscular dystrophy, motor neurone disease, post-polio kyphoscoliosis, central hypoventilation, spinal cord damage and phrenic nerve palsy). AT: Austria; BE: Belgium; DK: Denmark; FI: Finland; FR: France; DE: Germany; GR: Greece; IE: Ireland; IT: Italy; NL: the Netherlands; NO: Norway; PL: Poland; PT: Portugal; ES: Spain; SE: Sweden. Reproduced from [17] with permission from the publisher.

The "Eurovent" pan-European survey

The latest pan-European survey was undertaken in order to explore the custom and practice in 16 different countries [17] to determine if they had changed in the 10 yrs after FAROUX *et al.* [11]. The questionnaire survey, completed in 2001–2002, was more expansive and provided data on 329 centres and 21,526 HMV users, predominantly in Western Europe. More national registers were available for this study and so documentation concerning HMV from the member countries had improved over the preceding 10 yrs. However, the survey, like the previous one, continued to show wide variations in practice. For example, the prevalence of HMV per 100,000 inhabitants ranged from 0.6 in Greece to 17 in France. Overall prevalence of HMV in Europe was 6.6 per 100,000. Countries that started their HMV programme earlier (fig. 1a) had a greater prevalence and larger centre size (fig. 1b) although this could not be the only explanation for the wide variation in prevalence. The proportion in different disease categories was also wide ranging (fig. 2) with Denmark having proportionately more individuals with NMD being ventilated, whereas patients with COPD predominated in Italy and Portugal. This discrepancy also seems to be related to the date at which the HMV programme started, with the newer centres tending to focus on COPD patients. Overall, 34.4% of patients suffered from lung and airway problems, 31.2% had CWD and 34.4% had NMD.

Other findings from the Eurovent survey were that patients were most likely to have their HMV initiated and maintained by a university hospital rather than non-university hospital. The study also demonstrated that there was a bimodal distribution of users with older patients (age >66 yrs) having predominantly lung and chest wall diseases and younger patients (age <65 yrs) having predominantly NMD and neurological diseases. The latter group of patients were most likely to be ventilated for longer periods (>10 yrs), whilst the majority of those with intrinsic lung diseases had been on HMV for <1 yr. Patients with CWD ran a more intermediate course, with most of them being ventilated for 6–10 yrs. The length of time that patients had spent on HMV could be explained partly by the expected survival differences between the different diagnostic

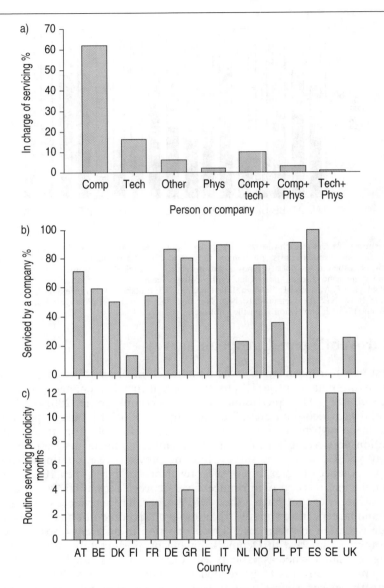

Fig. 3. – a) Answers to the question "who is in charge of the servicing and repair of ventilators in your centre?", b) centres answering that ventilator servicing was carried out by an external company, and c) answers to the question "how often is your equipment routinely serviced?" by country. Comp: ventilator company; Tech: hospital technical service; Other: other hospital department; Phys: physician in charge of the patient; AT: Austria; BE: Belgium; DK: Denmark; FI: Finland; FR: France; DE: Germany; GR: Greece; IE: Ireland; IT: Italy; NL: the Netherlands; NO: Norway; PL: Poland; PT: Portugal; ES: Spain; SE: Sweden. Reproduced from [21] with permission from the publisher.

categories [7] and partly by the fact that some centres had only recently begun recruiting COPD patients.

Pressure-cycled machines predominated in 2002 (70.6% of the total) and only a very small percentage of patients (0.005%) were using variants of negative-pressure ventilators. Ventilation was performed *via* a tracheostomy in just 13% of the overall survey population, and the patients with NMD accounted for most of these.

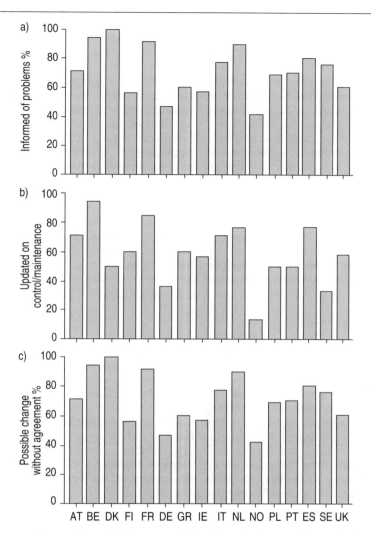

Fig. 4. – Answers to the questions: a) "Are you regularly informed of any problems with home mechanical ventilation by the person/company responsible for the maintenance of the equipment?"; b) "are you regularly updated on the specific control/maintenance of the equipment performed by the person/company responsible?"; and c) "can the person/company providing the ventilator change the model of ventilator without asking for your agreement?" by country. AT: Austria; BE: Belgium; DK: Denmark; FI: Finland; FR: France; DE: Germany; GR: Greece; IE: Ireland; IT: Italy; NL: the Netherlands; NO: Norway; PL: Poland; PT: Portugal; ES: Spain; SE: Sweden. Reproduced from [21] with permission from the publisher.

Tracheostomy ventilation was more common in France, Greece, Italy and Belgium and probably reflects local expertise in this area [18].

Quality control and servicing of HMV equipment in Europe

HMV is considered to be relatively safe [19] but a recent study demonstrated that there are sometimes considerable differences between the actual, set and prescribed values of ventilator variables and that the alarm function, when present, does not always work [20].

As an extension of the pan-European study of 2002, FARRÉ *et al.* [21] investigated the quality control procedures employed at the 329 HMV centres. Predictably, wide variations existed both within and between countries. The salient findings from the study were as follows. There was a wide variation between countries as to whether the ventilator company, a hospital technician or both took a role in servicing the machine and also in the periodicity of routine servicing (fig. 3). The timing of the servicing was unlikely to be related to technical factors so it can only be assumed that it was due to economic or administrative differences. There was also evidence for poor communication between the servicing provider and the clinician (fig. 4). An example of this is that in Sweden, it was relatively common for the ventilator to be changed without the explicit agreement of the prescriber. This might be a problem for patients whose ventilatory demands are sometimes suited to a specific ventilator model. There also appeared to be some ambivalence on the part of the prescribers to involve their patients in quality control; on average, only 56% of centres assessed whether or not the patients or their caregivers correctly maintained the equipment and only 21% gave the patients or their caregivers written information about quality control items pertaining to their particular ventilator. This is perhaps a missed opportunity, as patient self-management is now widely encouraged because of evidence of improved patient satisfaction and more importantly improved patient outcome [22].

Conclusions

The number of patients receiving HMV in Europe will continue to rise due to the combination of an aging population demographic, improved survival of patients with chronic respiratory disease and a shift towards treating more people with COPD and OHS. Indeed, in the short-to-medium term, the prevalence of COPD and OHS themselves are also expected to increase.

Other than consensus opinion on when to initiate home mechanical ventilation [23], there are as yet very few guidelines within Europe on how to practically implement it. It is probably for this reason that there is little standardisation and regulation of home mechanical ventilation between or even within European countries. This lack of uniformity extends to quality control of the equipment itself and this may impact on patient safety as well as satisfactory patient outcomes.

Summary

There has been a dramatic rise in the use of home mechanical ventilation (HMV) in Europe over the last two decades driven by the widening indications for HMV and increasing prevalence of chronic respiratory failure. The implementation of HMV differs widely among European countries and it would be desirable to standardise provision in order to provide equitable patient outcomes.

Keywords: Europe, home mechanical ventilation, prevalence surveys, quality control.

References

1. Perlman F, Bobak M, Gilmore A, McKee M. Trends in the prevalence of smoking in Russia during the transition to a market economy. *Tob Control* 2007; 16: 299–305.

2.   Helasoja VV, Lahelma E, Prättälä RS, *et al.* Determinants of daily smoking in Estonia, Latvia, Lithuania, and Finland in 1994–2002. *Scand J Public Health* 2006; 34: 353–362.

3.   Association Nationale pour le Traitement à Domicile del'Insuffisance Respiratoire Chronique. [National Association for Home Care Patients With Chronic Respiratory Insufficiency.] 1998 yearly statistics. *Observatoire*, 1998.

4.   Laub M, Berg S, Midgren B, Swedish Society of Chest Medicine. Home mechanical ventilation in Sweden – inequalities within a homogenenous health care system. *Respir Med* 2004; 98: 38–42.

5.   Janssens JP, Derivaz S, Breitenstein E, *et al.* Changing patterns in long-term noninvasive ventilation: a 7-year prospective study in the Geneva Lake area. *Chest* 2003; 123: 67–79.

6.   Leger P, Bedicam JM, Cornette A, *et al.* Nasal intermittent positive pressure: long-term follow-up in patients with severe chronic respiratory insufficiency. *Chest* 1994; 105: 100–105.

7.   Simonds AK, Elliott MW. Outcome of domiciliary nasal intermittent positive pressure in restrictive and obstructive disorders. *Thorax* 1995; 50: 604–609.

8.   Meecham Jones DJ, Paul EA, Jones PW, Wedzicha JA. Nasal pressure support ventilation plus oxygen compared with oxygen therapy alone in hypercapnic COPD. *Am J Respir Crit Care Med* 1995; 152: 538–544.

9.   Simonds AK. Home ventilation. *Eur Respir J* 2003; 22: Suppl. 47, 38s–46s.

10. Bach JR, Intintola P, Alba AS, Holland IE. The ventilator-assisted individual. Cost analysis of institutionalization *vs* rehabilitation and in-home management. *Chest* 1992; 101: 26–30.

11. Fauroux B, Howard P, Muir JF. Home treatment for chronic respiratory insufficiency: the situation in Europe in 1992. The European Working Group on Home Treatment for Chronic Respiratory Insufficiency. *Eur Respir J* 1994; 7: 1721–1726.

12. Muir JF, Voisin C, Ludot A. Organization of home respiratory care: the experience in France with ANTADIR. *Monaldi Arch Chest Dis* 1993; 48: 462–467.

13. Lloyd-Owen SJ. Organisation of home mechanical ventilation in Europe. *In*: Simonds AK ed. Noninvasive Respiratory Support: A Practical Handbook. 3rd Edn. London, Edward Arnold, 2007; pp. 375–380.

14. Midgren B, Olofson J, Harlid R, Dellborg C, Jacobsen E, Nørregaard O. Home mechanical ventilation in Sweden with reference to Danish experiences. *Respir Med* 2000; 94: 135–138.

15. Casanova C, Celli B, Tost L, *et al.* Long-term controlled trial of nocturnal nasal positive pressure ventilation in patients with severe COPD. *Chest* 2000; 118: 1582–1590.

16. Clini E, Sturani C, Rossi A, *et al.* The Italian multicentre study on noninvasive ventilation in chronic obstructive pulmonary disease patients. *Eur Respir J* 2002; 20: 529–538.

17. Lloyd-Owen SJ, Donaldson GC, Ambrosino N, *et al.* Patterns of home mechanical ventilation use in Europe: results from the Eurovent survey. *Eur Respir J* 2005; 25: 1025–1031.

18. Muir JF, Girault C, Cardinaud JP, Polu JM. Survival and long-term follow-up of tracheostomized patients with COPD treated by home mechanical ventilation. A multicenter French study in 259 patients. French Cooperative Study Group. *Chest* 1994; 106: 201–209.

19. Srinivasan S, Doty SM, White TR, *et al.* Frequency, causes, and outcome of home ventilator failure. *Chest* 1998; 114: 1363–1367.

20. Farré R, Navajas D, Prats E, *et al.* Performance of mechanical ventilators at the patient's home: a multicentre quality control study. *Thorax* 2006; 61: 400–404.

21. Farré R, Lloyd-Owen SJ, Ambrosino N, *et al.* Quality control of equipment in home mechanical ventilation: a European survey. *Eur Respir J* 2005; 26: 86–94.

22. Holman H, Lorig K. Patient self-management: a key to effectiveness and efficiency in care of chronic disease. *Public Health Rep* 2004; 119: 239–243.

23. Clinical indications for noninvasive positive pressure ventilation in chronic respiratory failure due to restrictive lung disease, COPD, and nocturnal hypoventilation – a consensus conference report. *Chest* 1999; 116: 521–534.

CHAPTER 28

Future trends in noninvasive mechanical ventilation in adults

D. Robert, L. Argaud

Medical Intensive Care Dept, Université Claude Bernard, Hôpital Edouard Herriot, 5 Place d'Arsonval 69003 Lyon, France. Fax: 33 472110042; E-mail: dominique.robert@wanadoo.fr

The modern form of noninvasive positive pressure ventilation (NPPV) using a facial interface as opposed to negative pressure ventilation, which appeared in the 1980s as an advantageous mode of ventilatory support for some patients needing long-term assistance; either with continuous positive airway pressure (CPAP) for obstructive sleep apnoea [1] or with intermittent positive pressure ventilation (NIPPV) for chronic respiratory insufficiency related to neuromuscular or parietal disorders [2–6].

Since this pioneering time, the evolution of the medical knowledge and of the technical aspects concerning NIPPV are continuously growing, with many studies opening new areas for the application of NIPPV or bringing clinical evidence of its efficacy [7–12].

Indications of NIPPV may be considered according to their clinical usefulness as "clearly validated", as "probably interesting but needing additional studies" or as "new possible fields of interest". Besides clinical considerations, NIPPV, compared with invasive ventilation, has the risk of becoming less efficient in relation to the difficulty in continuously mechanically ventilating for long periods and to inevitable nonintentional leaks, between the mask and the skin [13, 14]. So, the final results are a balance between negative and positive effects; the way to progress is to decrease the negatives and to improve the positives.

NIPPV was first used at home and in the intensive care unit (ICU) but as evidence of its efficacy emerged, NIPPV was progressively used in other places, such as emergency department, intermediary unit, medical ward and step-down unit [15–18].

The present chapter will review many points which might progress in an attempt to anticipate the future.

Clinical application of NIPPV

Acute respiratory failure

The results concerning acute failure on chronic respiratory insufficiency clearly contrast with those without previous respiratory insufficiency. According to the literature, NIPPV must be employed as the first line mode of ventilatory assistance in cases of acute failure on chronic respiratory disease [10, 16, 19–21], while several studies report conflicting results in acute failure without previous respiratory disease [22–27]. This is relatively easy to understand if it is considered that, in case of previous respiratory insufficiency, any minor additional factors, potentially easily reversible, may

Eur Respir Mon, 2008, 41, 400–414. Printed in UK - all rights reserved. Copyright ERS Journals Ltd 2008; European Respiratory Monograph; ISSN 1025-448x.

precipitate the patient in a threatening failure. NIPPV, even of imperfect efficiency in term of assistance, may allow the rapid regaining of the previous respiratory state.

Conversely, *de novo* respiratory failures, due to severe disease like infectious pneumonia or acute respiratory distress syndrome (ARDS), are not prone to rapid recovery and need the most efficient and continuous ventilatory assistance. The only way would be to be able to select the cases with a rapid potential for reversibility and/or to improve the NIPPV technique in order to deliver more continuous and more efficient ventilatory assistance. It seems probable that subgroups considered as good candidate for NPPV would be individualised among these patients. Probably chest trauma would become a recommended indication [28].

In immunocompromised patients it seems to be important to avoid infectious risk by using NIPPV as often as possible. Nevertheless, even if studies in short series favor such approach, other larger trials seem necessary in order to confirm these data [29–31]. As the number of patients living longer with chronic immunosuppressive treatment increases rapidly, new data on this field are necessary [32]. For example, the specific use of NPPV to perform early and securely bronchoalveolar lavage in such patients must be promoted in the future [33].

In asthma, some authors have speculated that the positive pressure may have a salutary effect on airway dilatation [34, 35]; one study in asthma without respiratory failure actually showed beneficial effects [36]. Nevertheless, routine use of NIPPV in severe acute asthma can not, at present, be recommended. Probably, in the future, cautious trials in severe asthma crisis not responding to the first hour of conventional therapy would be performed in order to clarify such indication [37].

In the context of extubation, NIPPV has certainly a place but the results presently available in the literature remain unclear. Several randomised controlled trials have shown that the use of NIPPV in order to advance extubation in COPD difficult to wean (assessed by the T-tube trial failure) resulted in reduced periods of endotracheal intubation, complication rates and increased survival [38, 39]. Obviously, NIPPV may avert most of the pathophysiological mechanisms associated with weaning failure in these patients. Similarly, *a priori* NIPPV applied immediately after extubation is effective in avoiding failure in patients at risk, particularly those with chronic respiratory disorders and hypercapnic respiratory failure [40]. Conversely, the use of NIPPV in the management of respiratory failure, actually occurring after extubation, did not show clinical benefits [41]. Even if the clear understanding in this context is not totally established, it seems probable that future studies will indicate that NIPPV is useful in case of previous chronic respiratory insufficiency or when nonsevere factors would explain the inability to completely manage the whole spontaneous breathing. It is likely that the efficacy to prevent respiratory complications of early NIPPV application during the post-operative period in patients at risk would be confirmed in the future with the same concept [42–44].

Cardiac pulmonary oedema is a very frequent event. Many studies have shown the efficacy of continuous positive airway pressure (CPAP) or NIPPV to get rapid improvement and to improve the survival rate. Meta-analyses have not demonstrated the superiority of either [45–54]. Additionally, the potential risk of NIPPV in unstable coronary diseases remains possible by decreasing the cardiac output and would prompt a preference for CPAP [55, 56]. Consequently, CPAP, which is simpler must be preferred and will be more early and widely used in the future, particularly during the pre-hospital emergency treatment.

NIPPV may be proposed when intubation is contraindicated. It is important to consider, as reported by different studies, that NIPPV performed in substitute of intubation may bring favorable issues. NIPPV must be considered as the possibility of offering a chance without taking the risks of intubation, which are: the necessity to be in an ICU, the invasiveness, the potential weaning difficulties and the difficulty in extubating a patient as a process to die. In spite of respiratory failure theoretically indicating intubation, its achievement may be contraindicated in three main situations, coming either from patient willingness or from the medical situation. In the first situation, the patient could have expressed an advanced "do not intubate" directive or could express refusal to be intubated [57]. Potential difficulties may occur when the physician in charge of the patient is convinced that the use of intubation is the only technique which may cure the patient. A typical example could be observed in a suicide attempt; the issue would depend on the national regulations, habits, religions and philosophical points of view. In North America, the advanced directives must be followed, while in Southern Europe, the decision of the physician and his personal conviction may be predominant at least when the patient has lost the ability to confirm possible advance directives.

In the second situation, the physician may estimate that invasive ventilation is not indicated but NIPPV may afford reasonable chances without the risks of an intubation [58]. The role of the physician is to explain to the patient and his relatives why NIPPV is the right choice.

In the third situation, the use of NIPPV has the only objective of palliation, comfort and relief of dyspnoea for patients with a very short-term poor prognosis, independent of an efficient ventilatory assistance. NIPPV may be considered either as an acceptable end point or as an inacceptable way to prolong the dying process [59, 60]. We may anticipate, in the future, new studies and recommendations, aimed to clarify the different clinical situations in which NIPPV may be applied as a ceiling treatment taking in account cultural and religious habits.

Chronic failure needing long-term domiciliary NIPPV

During the past 15 yrs, the use of long-term ventilation at home has drastically increased [61]. This is mainly explained by the facility to use NIPPV as opposed to tracheostomy, since the positive effects of long-term ventilation were already demonstrated in the 1980s [62]. Conceptually, it is important to consider five different situations: 1) cases which need full-time mechanical ventilation related to total respiratory paralysis and a relatively normal lung (neuromuscular); 2) cases which need only part-time mechanical ventilation nightly or diurnally, typically performed in diseases with thoracic cage deformities and a remaining lung, decreased in volume but relatively functional (idiopathic kyphoscoliosis, mutilating tuberculosis *etc.*); 3) cases which need part-time mechanical ventilation performed nightly in lung diseases (COPD, cystic fibrosis, bronchiectasis *etc.*); 4) sleep apnoea, which may receive NIPPV specifically during sleep, either obstructive, in cases of upper airway abnormalities or central, in cases of severe chronic left cardiac insufficiency (periodic breathing); and 5) obesity hypoventilation syndrome, which seems relatively close to the second group. Since the techniques are the same, there is a temptation to think that the results must be identical, which may lead to serious mistakes. The future trends may be anticipated according to each group.

In the neuromuscular group, the number of patients treated would continue to increase if the positive results in term of extension of the life and improvement of the quality of life are considered, even in amyotrophic lateral sclerosis (ALS), provided they have no or only modest swallowing disorders [63–68].

Even if only seldom used, at present, the long-term technique will include special approaches for secretion clearance in order to avoid and treat chest infections and atelectasis, which are the major complication and reason to die in late-stage neuromuscular disorders. In those patients, the inability to generate an effective cough can be due to low vital capacity, impaired bulbar function and expiratory muscle weakness. The goal is to reproduce cough by inflating the lung up to its maximal inspiratory capacity in order to increase the expiratory peak flow to values up to 300–400 L·min^{-1}. Different devices and methods have been proven to promote this effect: glossopharyngeal breathing (frog breathing), volume targeted ventilators, intermittent positive pressure breathing (IPPB) devices and the in-exsufflator (cough assist). The systematic use of such techniques, twice daily, has been proposed when the spontaneous expiratory peak flow is lower than 160 L·min^{-1}, and more frequently in cases of clinical mucus retention and when the arterial oxygen saturation measured by pulse oximetry (Sp,O$_2$) is <95% [69–74]. These approaches are not new but they are not routinely practiced; so they may become most popular and new indications and recommendations about the techniques will appear in the future. These techniques will continue to allow less possibility for long-term tracheostomy, at least in the adult population [75].

In thoracic cage disorders, NIPPV will remain the uncontested method but a continual decrease in the number of cases due to the spine surgery performed during childhood may be anticipated [76–81]. Nevertheless, future physiological studies will probably confirm the specific complex mechanisms of efficacy in such patients, combining the resetting of the respiratory centres, muscle rest, better oxygenation and lung recruitment [80, 82].

In COPD, the results of NIPPV are still disappointing even if, over time, COPD with concomitant chronic hypercapnic respiratory failure has become a major indication for domiciliary NIPPV [61]. Positive effects have been reported in blood gas levels; particularly a reduction of hypercapnia but the role in long-term survival is still a topic of controversy [79, 83–85]. A meta-analysis of clinical trials does not support this form of therapy [86]. Due to these uncertainties and the important and growing number of COPD prospective trials will probably bring new information in the future. Nevertheless, considering the patho-physiology of COPD, which gradually and continuously destroys the lung with a chronic inflammatory state and a general disease, it seems unlikely that NIPPV may significantly alter the natural evolution of this devasting disease.

NIPPV during exercise in COPD has been investigated and could be a future development, with the main aim being to improve exercise capabilities in daily life [87–89]. The development of a smaller portable ventilator would facilitate use during walking. Arterial oxygen tension decreases during walking in these patients when only supplemental oxygen is given but increases when NIPPV is added to the oxygen. There is also significantly less dyspnoea and a longer walking distance. Therefore, NIPPV during walking may be developed in order to provide an additional role for palliative treatment of COPD patients with hypercapnic chronic respiratory failure. Following this, forthcoming studies may be anticipated which determine the role of NIPPV during exertion and walking in addition or not of nocturnal NIPPV.

In symptomatic obstructive sleep apnea (OSA), the use of CPAP during sleep is now strongly validated with many positive effects on cardiac, vascular, cognitive, metabolic disorders and finally on survival [90]. The use of a true NIPPV, which provides inspiratory assistance, is controversial and has been advocated in case of CPAP failure. NPPV using a bilevel device has been proposed as an optional therapy in some cases where high pressure is needed and the patient experiences difficulty exhaling against a fixed pressure [91]. It may be anticipated that, in cases of OSA not combined with other abnormalities, new clinical data will have few chances to report a better efficacy of NIPPV. In cases of OSA associated with other causes of respiratory impairment featured by hypercapnia, such as obesity hypoventilation syndrome [92–95], neuromuscular diseases (myotonic dystrophy, muscular dystrophy, *etc.*) or COPD, the use of NIPPV is usually recommended even if CPAP alone could also be beneficial [91]. New clinical data will probably be reported bringing new insights for these complex cases.

In the most severe form of chronic cardiac insufficiency, periodic breathing or Cheyne–Stokes breathing is present in ~50% of cases and has been shown to be an indicator of a worsening prognosis. The main therapeutic approaches, besides the treatment of cardiac insufficiency, are nocturnal oxygen therapy, CPAP or NIPPV [96–98]. Small studies usually report equal efficacy of CPAP or NIPPV on cardiac function, exercise tolerance and quality of life. Unfortunately, a recently published trial showed no difference in survival between CPAP and medical treatment alone [99], so there are few chances to admit indication of NIPPV in this context. Nevertheless, according to the strong rationale for using CPAP or NIPPV, it is certain that new trials will be performed. Additionally, new modes combining CPAP and NIPPV have been proposed and will also be specifically studied [100–104]. Nevertheless, whatever the results of future clinical trials, it seems unlikely that important improvements of the prognosis will be observed, if we consider the extreme severity of the underlying cardiac insufficiency in such patients. The possibility of using NIPPV in the most severe cases as a bridge to heart transplantation in selected patients is also a potential issue.

Obesity is considered to be an increasingly epidemic disease with relatively modest respiratory symptoms, except in a minority of patients who present the so called obesity hypoventilation syndrome. Long-term domiciliary NIPPV normalises hypercapnia and markedly improves hypoxaemia as well as polycythaemia [105]. Additionally, NIPPV leads to a significant reduction in restrictive ventilatory disturbances, predominantly by increasing the expiratory reserve volume [106]. Nevertheless, the necessity to definitely continue NIPPV is not clearly established and would necessitate long-term comparative studies [94].

Locations where NIPPV is applied

The application of NIPPV requires a good understanding of the method but does not need sophisticated technical means besides ventilator and mask. The fact that NIPPV used at home is very successful with only the daily supervision of the patients, or their families in totally dependent patients, clearly prove its good feasibility. In addition the development of portable ventilators for the home allows its use in conventional medical wards without any particular equipment. Therefore, it is more the actual severity of the clinical situation rather than the technique itself which determines the locations where NIPPV is used.

This explains the large and rapid spread of NIPPV outside the two original locations, which were the ICU and the home. Nowadays, NIPPV is performed in many different locations such as emergency rooms, intermediary units, weaning centers, medical wards (pneumology, neurology, cardiology, *etc.*) and rehabilitation centres [14–16, 107–112]. To be safely applied, the actual and potential severity must be determined in order to choose the correct place in which dedicated professionals are trained to practice NIPPV. In addition, in case of the condition worsening, the immediate availability of a back up unit and technique must be anticipated. So NIPPV, as a technique, offers a great versatility. A recently published study showed a small series of patients already treated at home for chronic respiratory failure who were maintained at home in the context of acute threatening failure with the reinforcement of the daily duration under NPPV and medical and nurse supervision [113]. This may open the door to early home treatment of acute crises at the cost of a specific home service.

The spread of NIPPV in different locations and the involvement of numerous professionals (medical doctors, respiratory therapists and nurses) are clear advantages allowing the delivery of NIPPV at earlier stages with minor utilisation of resources other than in the ICU. Nevertheless, it may be anticipated that recommendations for good practice will be regularly proposed and that specific training for personell will be necessary, in particular to apply NIPPV outside of the ICU [114, 115]. Dedicated mobile teams would probably be proposed in order to secure the use of NIPPV across hospitals.

Technical trends

The application of NIPPV to treat acute and chronic respiratory failure is increasing tremendously in many different settings from the hospital ward and units to home. The choice of the ventilator, setting and interface is crucial for NIPPV success because poor tolerance and excessive air leaks are significantly correlated with NIPPV failure [14, 116–120]. So, in addition to the progress afforded by the manufacturers, the clinician must understand and apply all the finer points to optimise patient–ventilator synchrony to adequately set NIPPV to respond to the patient's ventilatory demand. Many advances have been recently made and will continue to appear in the forthcoming years.

Ventilators

In order to anticipate the possible evolution of the ventilators in the future the best way is to consider the progress made since the introduction of NIPPV and to continue the trail [121].

In 1990, the available ventilators were ICU ventilators and home ventilators. ICU ventilators were big, powered by high pressure air and oxygen sources and offered volume preset modes (control, assist, intermittent mandatory ventilation (IMV) and pressure preset modes (control, assist, spontaneous or pressure support, IMV) [122]. Home ventilators were portable, powered by inside electrical motor (some with an internal battery) and offered volume preset modes.

The main progresses come from conceptual and technical advances for home ventilators able to deliver enough tidal volume in spite of inevitable and jolting leaks observed during NIPPV [123–125]. Home ventilators have progressively taken the place of ICU ventilators and allow mechanical ventilation anywhere in hospital, not just the ICU [126, 127]. At the present time, the main features concern the mode, the pressure source, the alarms and the monitoring. The available modes were enriched with bi-level positive airway pressure (BiPAP) in 1990 [123]. BiPAP is a pressure targeted mode with an expiratory positive airway pressure (EPAP) and a higher inspiratory positive airway pressure (IPAP) alternatively established in a leaking one limb circuit with a risk for CO_2 rebreathing [128, 129]. Specific algorithms, aimed at correctly detecting the start and end of inspiration, in order to improve the patient–ventilator synchrony, have been proposed allowing the use of spontaneous mode *i.e.* pressure support [130]. Very small high-speed turbines, used as pressure sources, are able to produce enough flow to face the leaks observed during NIPPV. The use of microprocessors and screens allows the setting of minimal or maximal functions concerning alarms and monitoring displays reaching the level of sophistication used in the ICU.

It may, therefore, be anticipated that, in the future, most NIPPV would be delivered by these small and portable ventilators able to deliver high quality ventilation in any place leading to fewer places using the conventional ICU ventilators [121].

Modes and settings of NIPPV

Improved knowledge and major changes have occurred in recent years with regards to choice of the settings according to the objectives of NIPPV in the various clinical situations, such as acute or chronic failure, normal or obstructive or restrictive diseases and asleep or awake patient. It is anticipated that concepts will continue to progress to better improve such approaches.

The pressure targeted mode is definitely preferred to volume targeted mode in NIPPV, since they are able to compensate for air leaks provided that the flow capability is high enough [61, 131–134]. Many efforts have tried to improve triggering and cycling in pressure support mode and recent studies report that this is frequently successful but not in every case with every ventilator [135, 136]. Additionally, it appears that algorithms could work differently in normal, obstructive or restrictive diseases or even become counterproductive [130]. On the ICU ventilators and in the more-advanced bi-level ventilators, the rise time of the pressure can be set in order to try to synchronise the patient effort and the spontaneous demand of the patient [137, 138]. Such findings open the place for specific research and proposition according to the disease submitted to NIPPV. Trials using proportional assisted ventilation, which theoretically improves synchrony and adapts the level of assistance to the spontaneous pattern of breathing, have been performed. Nevertheless, at least in the original functioning in which the compliance and resistance are needed, the variable air leakages (equivalent to variable resistance), which characterise NIPPV are poorly compatible with the use of such a mode [139]. Clinical trials did not report clear superiority of this mode [140, 141]. Pressure support ventilation brings variable tidal volumes according to complex interactions between inspiratory effort, leaks, respiratory mechanics, sleep (which may produce rapid changes from hypoventilation to normoventilation) or to hyperventilation for the same patients [142]. Hypoventilation may be avoided by using dual modes, which may ensure target tidal volumes considered either as minimal, letting the possibility to ventilate more or the unique fixed objective, letting no possibility to improve the ventilation [143, 144]. More research is necessary to determine the place of such sophisticated modes. Hyperventilation, which may particularly occur during sleep, may induce central apnoea in response to low arterial carbon dioxide tension (Pa,CO_2) and arousals before the resuming of breathing. In order to avoid such a risk setting of a back up rate is more-frequently recommended and would become the rule [145]. In addition, the back up rate may be useful when a cautious sedation is administered [146].

In summary, the present knowledge on the complex interactions between more- or less-preserved physiological regulation and the ventilator clearly shows that much progress is necessary in order to optimise NIPPV to improve its efficacy and avoid invasive ventilation.

Interfaces

The quality of the different interfaces has continuously increased in order to combine minimum leaks, to improve the ventilation, and comfort, to improve the tolerance and the continuity of NIPPV when necessary. In acute situation naso-facial masks are recommended as the first-line interface and full-face as the second line [7, 9, 147–149]. Nevertheless the place of "full-head" interface as the helmet is not yet clearly known [150, 151]. Additional physiological and clinical studies are necessary. In chronic failure and long-term ventilation nasal mask is considered as better tolerated [152]. In case of inadequate ventilation, the place of other interfaces like naso-facial, oral or nasal pillow is not clearly established [153]. Numerous studies combining comfort and efficacy criteria will be published in the future.

Conclusion

It is now evident that NPPV has a place as a major tool in treating chronic and acute respiratory failure. Its application is still in progression and new important studies and knowledge appear every year concerning clinical indications, the way to use NIPPV and the quality of the ventilators and the interfaces. A main development concerning the ventilators used in the intensive care unit will probably occur by using the progresses made on the portable ventilators designed for home, which are smaller and cheaper. Another development will further the possibility of applying NIPPV outside the conventional ICU and thus save ICU resources and allow the use of NIPPV early in respiratory failure. Nevertheless, NIPPV will always demand well-trained teams and dedicated organisations in order to avoid accident and offer the whole efficacy of this relatively new therapeutic approach.

Summary

Noninvasive ventilation using intermittent positive pressure (NIPPV) which appeared in the 1980s for long-term home ventilation is now routinely used both at home and in hospital for chronic and acute respiratory failure. New indications for NIPPV have been validated but many remain to be better known with forthcoming studies. In the long term, the role in chronic obstructive pulmonary disease, in obesity-hypoventilation syndrome and in periodic breathing due to severe cardiac insufficiency, will be clarified. In acute situations, the place to apply NIPPV according to the severity is an important issue for hospital organisations. Clinical indications will be established and/or clarified, such as pneumonia occurring on normal lung, severe asthma, immune compromised patients, weaning from invasive ventilation and NIPPV as the ceiling to offer ventilatory assistance. Technical progress will also continue to appear concerning the ventilators both for chronic and acute using. New ventilators will provide a better synchronisation between patient and ventilator and would confirm the predominant use of high speed turbine as the pressure and flow generator.

Keywords: Chronic obstructive pulmonary disease, noninvasive ventilation using intermittent positive pressure trends, obesity-hypoventilation syndrome, periodic breathing, ventilator.

References

1. Sullivan CE, Issa FG, Berthon-Jones M, Eves L. Reversal of obstructive sleep apnea by continuous positive airway pressure applied the nares. *Lancet* 1981; 1: 862–865.
2. Bach JR, Alba A, Mosher R, Delaubier A. Intermittent positive pressure ventilation *via* nasal access in the management of respiratory insufficiency. *Chest* 1987; 92: 168–170.
3. Ellis ER, Bye PTP, Bruderer JW, Sullivan CE. Treatment of respiratory failure during sleep in patients with neuromuscular disease. Positive-pressure ventilation through a nose mask. *Am Rev Respir Dis* 1987; 135: 148–152.
4. Carroll N, Branthwaite M. Control of nocturnal hypoventilation by nasal intermittent positive ventilation. *Thorax* 1988; 43: 349–353.

5. Ellis ER, Grunstein RR, Chan S, Bye PT, Sullivan CE. Noninvasive ventilatory support during sleep improves respiratory failure in kyphoscoliosis. *Chest* 1988; 94: 811–815.

6. Leger P, Jennequin J, Gerard M, Gaussorgues P, Robert D. Nocturnal mechanical ventilation in intermittent positive pressure at home by nasal route in chronic restrictive respiratory insufficiency. An effective substitute for tracheotomy. *Presse Med* 1988; 17: 874.

7. International Consensus Conferences in Intensive Care Medicine: noninvasive positive pressure ventilation in acute respiratory failure. *Am J Respir Crit Care Med* 2001; 163: 283–291.

8. Hess DR. The evidence for noninvasive positive-pressure ventilation in the care of patients in acute respiratory failure: a systematic review of the literature. *Respir Care* 2004; 49: 810–829.

9. Mehta S, Hill NS. Noninvasive ventilation. *Am J Respir Crit Care Med* 2001; 163: 540–577.

10. Ram FS, Picot J, Lightowler J, Wedzicha JA. Non-invasive positive pressure ventilation for treatment of respiratory failure due to exacerbations of chronic obstructive pulmonary disease. *Cochrane Database Syst Rev* 2004; 3: CD004104.

11. Garpestad E, Brennan J, Hill NS. Noninvasive ventilation for critical care. *Chest* 2007; 132: 711–720.

12. Schettino G, Altobelli N, Kacmarek RM. Noninvasive positive-pressure ventilation in acute respiratory failure outside clinical trials: experience at the Massachusetts General Hospital. *Crit Care Med* 2008; 36: 441–447.

13. Bach JR, Robert D, Leger P, Langevin B. Sleep fragmentation in kyphoscoliotic individuals with alveolar hypoventilation treated by NIPPV. *Chest* 1995; 107: 1552–1558.

14. Carlucci A, Richard JC, Wysocki M, Lepage E, Brochard L. Noninvasive versus conventional mechanical ventilation. An epidemiologic survey. *Am J Respir Crit Care Med* 2001; 163: 874–880.

15. Paus-Jenssen ES, Reid JK, Cockcroft DW, Laframboise K, Ward HA. The use of noninvasive ventilation in acute respiratory failure at a tertiary care center. *Chest* 2004; 126: 165–172.

16. Plant PK, Owen JL, Elliott MW. Early use of non-invasive ventilation for acute exacerbations of chronic obstructive pulmonary disease on general respiratory wards: a multicentre randomised controlled trial. *Lancet* 2000; 355: 1931–1935.

17. Sinuff T, Cook D, Randall J, Allen C. Noninvasive positive-pressure ventilation: a utilization review of use in a teaching hospital. *Cmaj* 2000; 163: 969–973.

18. Vanpee D. The use of non-invasive ventilation in the emergency department. *Eur J Emerg Med* 2003; 10: 77–78.

19. Brochard L. Non-invasive ventilation for acute exacerbations of COPD: a new standard of care. *Thorax* 2000; 55: 817–818.

20. Dikensoy O, Ikidag B, Filiz A, Bayram N. Comparison of non-invasive ventilation and standard medical therapy in acute hypercapnic respiratory failure: a randomised controlled study at a tertiary health centre in SE Turkey. *Int J Clin Pract* 2002; 56: 85–88.

21. Keenan SP, Sinuff T, Cook DJ, Hill NS. Does noninvasive positive pressure ventilation improve outcome in acute hypoxemic respiratory failure? A systematic review. *Crit Care Med* 2004; 32: 2516–2523.

22. Antonelli M, Conti G, Moro ML, *et al.* Predictors of failure of noninvasive positive pressure ventilation in patients with acute hypoxemic respiratory failure: a multi-center study. *Intensive Care Med* 2001; 27: 1718–1728.

23. Ferrer M, Esquinas A, Leon M, Gonzalez G, Alarcon A, Torres A. Noninvasive ventilation in severe hypoxemic respiratory failure: a randomized clinical trial. *Am J Respir Crit Care Med* 2003; 168: 1438–1444.

24. Honrubia T, Garcia Lopez FJ, Franco N, *et al.* Noninvasive vs conventional mechanical ventilation in acute respiratory failure: a multicenter, randomized controlled trial. *Chest* 2005; 128: 3916–3924.

25. Jolliet P, Abajo B, Pasquina P, Chevrolet JC. Non-invasive pressure support ventilation in severe community-acquired pneumonia. *Intensive Care Med* 2001; 27: 812–821.

26. Wysocki M, Antonelli M. Noninvasive mechanical ventilation in acute hypoxaemic respiratory failure. *Eur Respir J* 2001; 18: 209–220.

27. Agarwal R, Reddy C, Aggarwal AN, Gupta D. Is there a role for noninvasive ventilation in acute respiratory distress syndrome? A meta-analysis. *Respir Med* 2006; 100: 2235–2238.

28. Gregoretti C, Beltrame F, Lucangelo U, *et al.* Physiologic evaluation of non-invasive pressure support ventilation in trauma patients with acute respiratory failure. *Intensive Care Med* 1998; 24: 785–790.

29. Antonelli M, Conti G, Bufi M, *et al.* Noninvasive ventilation for treatment of acute respiratory failure in patients undergoing solid organ transplantation: a randomized trial. *JAMA* 2000; 283: 235–241.

30. Hilbert G, Gruson D, Vargas F, *et al.* Noninvasive ventilation in immunosuppressed patients with pulmonary infiltrates, fever, and acute respiratory failure. *N Engl J Med* 2001; 344: 481–487.

31. Confalonieri M, Calderini E, Terraciano S, *et al.* Noninvasive ventilation for treating acute respiratory failure in AIDS patients with Pneumocystis carinii pneumonia. *Intensive Care Med* 2002; 28: 1233–1238.

32. Pancera CF, Hayashi M, Fregnani JH, Negri EM, Deheinzelin D, de Camargo B. Noninvasive ventilation in immunocompromised pediatric patients: eight years of experience in a pediatric oncology intensive care unit. *J Pediatr Hematol Oncol* 2008; 30: 533–538.

33. Antonelli M, Conti G, Rocco M, *et al.* Noninvasive positive-pressure ventilation vs. conventional oxygen supplementation in hypoxemic patients undergoing diagnostic bronchoscopy. *Chest* 2002; 121: 1149–1154.

34. Fernandez MM, Villagra A, Blanch L, Fernandez R. Non-invasive mechanical ventilation in status asthmaticus. *Intensive Care Med* 2001; 27: 486–492.

35. Meduri GU, Cook TR, Turner RE, Cohen M, Leeper KV. Noninvasive positive pressure ventilation in status asthmaticus. *Chest* 1996; 110: 767–774.

36. Soroksky A, Stav D, Shpirer I. A pilot prospective, randomized, placebo-controlled trial of bilevel positive airway pressure in acute asthmatic attack. *Chest* 2003; 123: 1018–1025.

37. Medoff BD. : Invasive and noninvasive ventilation in patients with asthma. *Respir Care* 2008; 53: 740–748.

38. Girault C, Daudenthun I, Chevron V, Tamion F, Leroy J, Bonmarchand G. Noninvasive ventilation as a systematic extubation and weaning technique in acute-on-chronic respiratory failure: a prospective, randomized controlled study. *Am J Respir Crit Care Med* 1999; 160: 86–92.

39. Nava S, Gregoretti C, Fanfulla F, *et al.* Noninvasive ventilation to prevent respiratory failure after extubation in high-risk patients. *Crit Care Med* 2005; 33: 2465–2470.

40. Ferrer M, Esquinas A, Arancibia F, *et al.* Noninvasive ventilation during persistent weaning failure: a randomized controlled trial. *Am J Respir Crit Care Med* 2003; 168: 70–76.

41. Esteban A, Frutos-Vivar F, Ferguson ND, *et al.* Noninvasive positive-pressure ventilation for respiratory failure after extubation. *N Engl J Med* 2004; 350: 2452–2460.

42. Auriant I, Jallot A, Herve P, *et al.* Noninvasive ventilation reduces mortality in acute respiratory failure following lung resection. *Am J Respir Crit Care Med* 2001; 164: 1231–1235.

43. Squadrone V, Coha M, Cerutti E, *et al.* Continuous positive airway pressure for treatment of postoperative hypoxemia: a randomized controlled trial. *JAMA* 2005; 293: 589–595.

44. Jensen C, Tejirian T, Lewis C, Yadegar J, Dutson E, Mehran A. Postoperative CPAP and BiPAP use can be safely omitted after laparoscopic Roux-en-Y gastric bypass. *Surg Obes Relat Dis* 2008; 4: 512–514.

45. Crane SD, Elliott MW, Gilligan P, Richards K, Gray AJ. Randomised controlled comparison of continuous positive airways pressure, bilevel non-invasive ventilation, and standard treatment in emergency department patients with acute cardiogenic pulmonary oedema. *Emerg Med J* 2004; 21: 155–161.

46. Lin M, Chiang HT. The efficacy of early continuous positive airway pressure therapy in patients with acute cardiogenic pulmonary edema. *J Formos Med Assoc* 1991; 90: 736–743.

47. Masip J. Noninvasive ventilation in acute cardiogenic pulmonary edema. *Curr Opin Crit Care* 2008; 14: 531–535.

48. Masip J, Betbese AJ, Paez J, *et al.* Non-invasive pressure support ventilation versus conventional oxygen therapy in acute cardiogenic pulmonary oedema: a randomised trial. *Lancet* 2000; 356: 2126–2132.

49. Masip J, Paez J, Betbese AJ, Vecilla F. Noninvasive ventilation for pulmonary edema in the emergency room. *Am J Respir Crit Care Med* 2004; 169: 1072.

50. Nava S, Carbone G, DiBattista N, *et al.* Noninvasive ventilation in cardiogenic pulmonary edema: a multicenter randomized trial. *Am J Respir Crit Care Med* 2003; 168: 1432–1437.

51. Park M, Sangean MC, Volpe Mde S, *et al.* Randomized, prospective trial of oxygen, continuous positive airway pressure, and bilevel positive airway pressure by face mask in acute cardiogenic pulmonary edema. *Crit Care Med* 2004; 32: 2407–2415.

52. Rasanen J, Heikkila J, Downs J, Nikki P, Vaisanen I, Viitanen A. Continuous positive airway pressure by face mask in acute cardiogenic pulmonary edema. *Am J Cardiol* 1985; 55: 296–300.

53. Vital FM, Saconato H, Ladeira MT, *et al.* Non-invasive positive pressure ventilation (CPAP or bilevel NPPV) for cardiogenic pulmonary edema. *Cochrane Database Syst Rev* 2008; 3: CD005351.

54. Gray A, Goodacre S, Newby DE, Masson M, Sampson F, Nicholl J. Noninvasive ventilation in acute cardiogenic pulmonary edema. *N Engl J Med* 2008; 359: 142–151.

55. Mehta S. Continuous versus bilevel positive airway pressure in acute cardiogenic pulmonary edema? A good question!. *Crit Care Med* 2004; 32: 2546–2548.

56. Mehta S, Jay GD, Woolard RH, *et al.* Randomized, prospective trial of bilevel *versus* continuous positive airway pressure in acute pulmonary edema. *Crit Care Med* 1997; 25: 620–628.

57. Levy M, Tanios MA, Nelson D, *et al.* Outcomes of patients with do-not-intubate orders treated with noninvasive ventilation. *Crit Care Med* 2004; 32: 2002–2007.

58. Schettino G, Altobelli N, Kacmarek RM. Noninvasive positive pressure ventilation reverses acute respiratory failure in select "do-not-intubate" patients. *Crit Care Med* 2005; 33: 1976–1982.

59. Curtis JR, Cook DJ, Sinuff T, *et al.* Noninvasive positive pressure ventilation in critical and palliative care settings: understanding the goals of therapy. *Crit Care Med* 2007; 35: 932–939.

60. Sinuff T, Cook DJ, Keenan SP, *et al.* Noninvasive ventilation for acute respiratory failure near the end of life. *Crit Care Med* 2008; 36: 789–794.

61. Lloyd-Owen SJ, Donaldson GC, Ambrosino N, *et al.* Patterns of home mechanical ventilation use in Europe: results from the Eurovent survey. *Eur Respir J* 2005; 25: 1025–1031.

62. Robert D, Gerard M, Leger P, *et al.* Permanent mechanical ventilation at home via a tracheotomy in chronic respiratory insufficiency. *Rev Fr Mal Respir* 1983; 11: 923–936.

63. Bach JR. Continuous noninvasive ventilation for patients with neuromuscular disease and spinal cord injury. *Semin Respir Crit Care Med* 2002; 23: 283–292.

64. Bourke SC, Tomlinson M, Williams TL, Bullock RE, Shaw PJ, Gibson GJ. Effects of non-invasive ventilation on survival and quality of life in patients with amyotrophic lateral sclerosis: a randomised controlled trial. *Lancet Neurol* 2006; 5: 140–147.

65. Robert D, Willig TN, Paulus J, Leger P. Long-term nasal ventilation in neuromuscular disorders: report of a consensus conference. *Eur Respir J* 1993; 6: 599–606.

66. Simonds AK, Elliott MW. Outcome of domiciliary nasal intermittent positive pressure ventilation in restrictive and obstructive disorders. *Thorax* 1995; 50: 604–609.

67. Simonds AK, Ward S, Heather S, Bush A, Muntoni F. Outcome of paediatric domiciliary mask ventilation in neuromuscular and skeletal disease. *Eur Respir J* 2000; 16: 476–481.

68. Peysson S, Vandenberghe N, Philit F, *et al.* Factors predicting survival following noninvasive ventilation in amyotrophic lateral sclerosis. *Eur Neurol* 2008; 59: 164–171.

69. Bach JR. Update and perspective on noninvasive respiratory muscle aids; Part 2 : the expiratory aids. *Chest* 1994; 105: 1538–1544.

70. Bach JR. Mechanical insufflation/exsufflation: has it come of age? A commentary. *Eur Respir J* 2003; 21: 385–386.

71. Bach JR, Smith WH, Michaels J, *et al.* Airway secretion clearance by mechanical exsufflation for post-poliomyelitis ventilator-assisted individuals. *Arch Phys Med Rehabil* 1993; 74: 170–177.

72. Dohna-Schwake C, Ragette R, Teschler H, Voit T, Mellies U. Predictors of severe chest infections in pediatric neuromuscular disorders. *Neuromuscul Disord* 2006; 16: 325–328.

73. Servera E, Sancho J, Zafra MJ, Marin J. Secretion management must be considered when reporting success or failure of noninvasive ventilation. *Chest* 2003; 123: 1773.

74. Winck JC, Goncalves MR, Lourenco C, Viana P, Almeida J, Bach JR. Effects of mechanical insufflation-exsufflation on respiratory parameters for patients with chronic airway secretion encumbrance. *Chest* 2004; 126: 774–780.

75. Soudon P, Steens M, Toussaint M. A comparison of invasive versus noninvasive full-time mechanical ventilation in Duchenne muscular dystrophy. *Chron Respir Dis* 2008; 5: 87–93.

76. Hill NS, Eveloff SE, Carlisle C, Goff SG. Efficacy of nocturnal nasal ventilation in patients with restrictive thoracic disease. *Am Rev Respir Dis* 1992; 145: 365–371.

77. Leger P. Long-term noninvasive ventilation for patients with thoracic cage abnormalities. *Respir Care Clin N Am* 1996; 2: 241–252.

78. Leger P, Bedicam JM, Cornette A, *et al.* Nasal intermittent positive pressure ventilation. Long-term follow-up in patients with severe chronic respiratory insufficiency. *Chest* 1994; 105: 100–105.

79. Masa JF, Celli BR, Riesco JA, Sanchez de Cos J, Disdier C, Sojo A. Noninvasive positive pressure ventilation and not oxygen may prevent overt ventilatory failure in patients with chest wall diseases. *Chest* 1997; 112: 207–213.

80. Petitjean T, Philit F, Germain-Pastenne M, Langevin B, Guerin C. Sleep and respiratory function after withdrawal of noninvasive ventilation in patients with chronic respiratory failure. *Respir Care* 2008; 53: 1316–1323.

81. Annane D, Chevrolet JC, Chevret S, Raphael JC. Nocturnal mechanical ventilation for chronic hypoventilation in patients with neuromuscular and chest wall disorders. *Cochrane Database Syst Rev* 2000; 2: CD001941.

82. Annane D, Quera-Salva MA, Lofaso F, *et al.* Mechanisms underlying effects of nocturnal ventilation on daytime blood gases in neuromuscular diseases. *Eur Respir J* 1999; 13: 157–162.

83. Clini E, Sturani C, Rossi A, *et al.* The Italian multicentre study on noninvasive ventilation in chronic obstructive pulmonary disease patients. *Eur Respir J* 2002; 20: 529–538.

84. Clini EM, Magni G, Crisafulli E, Viaggi S, Ambrosino N. Home non-invasive mechanical ventilation and long-term oxygen therapy in stable hypercapnic chronic obstructive pulmonary disease patients: comparison of costs. *Respiration* 2008; Epub ahead of print.

85. Windisch W, Kostic S, Dreher M, Virchow JC Jr, Sorichter S. Outcome of patients with stable COPD receiving controlled noninvasive positive pressure ventilation aimed at a maximal reduction of Pa(CO2). *Chest* 2005; 128: 657–662.

86. Wijkstra PJ, Lacasse Y, Guyatt GH, *et al.* A meta-analysis of nocturnal noninvasive positive pressure ventilation in patients with stable COPD. *Chest* 2003; 124: 337–343.

87. Ambrosino N. Exercise and noninvasive ventilatory support. *Monaldi Arch Chest Dis* 2000; 55: 242–246.

88. Dreher M, Storre JH, Windisch W. Noninvasive ventilation during walking in patients with severe COPD: a randomised cross-over trial. *Eur Respir J* 2007; 29: 930–936.

89. Schonhofer B, Dellweg D, Suchi S, Kohler D. Exercise endurance before and after long-term noninvasive ventilation in patients with chronic respiratory failure. *Respiration* 2008; 75: 296–303.

90. Giles TL, Lasserson TJ, Smith BH, White J, Wright J, Cates CJ. Continuous positive airways pressure for obstructive sleep apnoea in adults. *Cochrane Database Syst Rev* 2006; 3: CD001106.

91. Kushida CA, Littner MR, Hirshkowitz M, *et al.* Practice parameters for the use of continuous and bilevel positive airway pressure devices to treat adult patients with sleep-related breathing disorders. *Sleep* 2006; 29: 375–380.

92. Banerjee D, Yee BJ, Piper AJ, Zwillich CW, Grunstein RR. Obesity hypoventilation syndrome: hypoxemia during continuous positive airway pressure. *Chest* 2007; 131: 1678–1684.

93. Mokhlesi B, Kryger MH, Grunstein RR. Assessment and management of patients with obesity hypoventilation syndrome. *Proc Am Thorac Soc* 2008; 5: 218–225.

94. Perez de Llano LA, Golpe R, Ortiz Piquer M, *et al.* Short-term and long-term effects of nasal intermittent positive pressure ventilation in patients with obesity-hypoventilation syndrome. *Chest* 2005; 128: 587–594.

95. Piper AJ, Wang D, Yee BJ, Barnes DJ, Grunstein RR. Randomised trial of CPAP vs bilevel support in the treatment of obesity hypoventilation syndrome without severe nocturnal desaturation. *Thorax* 2008; 63: 395–401.

96. Bradley TD, Floras JS. Sleep apnea and heart failure: Part II: central sleep apnea. *Circulation* 2003; 107: 1822–1826.

97. Bradley TD, Logan AG, Kimoff RJ, *et al.* Continuous positive airway pressure for central sleep apnea and heart failure. *N Engl J Med* 2005; 353: 2025–2033.

98. Dohi T, Kasai T, Narui K, *et al.* Bi-level positive airway pressure ventilation for treating heart failure with central sleep apnea that is unresponsive to continuous positive airway pressure. *Circ J* 2008; 72: 1100–1105.

99. Arzt M, Floras JS, Logan AG, *et al.* Suppression of central sleep apnea by continuous positive airway pressure and transplant-free survival in heart failure: a *post hoc* analysis of the Canadian Continuous Positive Airway Pressure for Patients with Central Sleep Apnea and Heart Failure Trial (CANPAP). *Circulation* 2007; 115: 3173–3180.

100. Arzt M, Wensel R, Montalvan S, *et al.* Effects of dynamic bilevel positive airway pressure support on central sleep apnea in men with heart failure. *Chest* 2008; 134: 61–66.

101. Pepperell JC, Maskell NA, Jones DR, *et al.* A randomized controlled trial of adaptive ventilation for Cheyne-Stokes breathing in heart failure. *Am J Respir Crit Care Med* 2003; 168: 1109–1114.

102. Philippe C, Stoica-Herman M, Drouot X, *et al.* Compliance with and effectiveness of adaptive servoventilation versus continuous positive airway pressure in the treatment of Cheyne-Stokes respiration in heart failure over a six month period. *Heart* 2006; 92: 337–342.

103. Teschler H, Dohring J, Wang YM, Berthon-Jones M. Adaptive pressure support servo-ventilation: a novel treatment for Cheyne-Stokes respiration in heart failure. *Am J Respir Crit Care Med* 2001; 164: 614–619.

104. Fietze I, Blau A, Glos M, Theres H, Baumann G, Penzel T. Bi-level positive pressure ventilation and adaptive servo ventilation in patients with heart failure and Cheyne-Stokes respiration. *Sleep Med* 2008; 9: 652–659.

105. Janssens JP, Metzger M, Sforza E. Impact of volume targeting on efficacy of bi-level non-invasive ventilation and sleep in obesity-hypoventilation. *Respir Med* 2008; Epub ahead of print.

106. Heinemann F, Budweiser S, Dobroschke J, Pfeifer M. Non-invasive positive pressure ventilation improves lung volumes in the obesity hypoventilation syndrome. *Respir Med* 2007; 101: 1229–1235.

107. Corrado A, De Palma M. Respiratory intermediate intensive care units in Europe. *Monaldi Arch Chest Dis* 1999; 54: 379–380.

108. Sinuff T. Review: noninvasive ventilation reduces mortality in acute respiratory failure. *ACP J Club* 2002; 137: 50.

109. Vanpee D, Delaunois L, Lheureux P, *et al.* Survey of non-invasive ventilation for acute exacerbation of chronic obstructive pulmonary disease patients in emergency departments in Belgium. *Eur J Emerg Med* 2002; 9: 217–224.

110. Taylor DM, Bernard SA, Masci K, MacBean CE, Kennedy MP. Prehospital noninvasive ventilation: a viable treatment option in the urban setting. *Prehosp Emerg Care* 2008; 12: 42–45.

111. Tomii K, Seo R, Tachikawa R, *et al.* Impact of noninvasive ventilation (NIV) trial for various types of acute respiratory failure in the emergency department; decreased mortality and use of the ICU. *Respir Med* 2008; Epub ahead of print.

112. Yeow ME, Santanilla JI. Noninvasive positive pressure ventilation in the emergency department. *Emerg Med Clin North Am* 2008; 26: 835–847.

113. Banfi P, Redolfi S, Robert D. Home treatment of infection-related acute respiratory failure in kyphoscoliotic patients on long-term mechanical ventilation. *Respir Care* 2007; 52: 713–719.

114. Sweet DD, Naismith A, Keenan SP, Sinuff T, Dodek PM. Missed opportunities for noninvasive positive pressure ventilation: a utilization review. *J Crit Care* 2008; 23: 111–117.

115. Kacmarek RM. NPPV in acute respiratory failure: is it time to reconsider where it may be applied? *Respir Care* 2006; 51: 1226–1227.

116. Criner GJ, Tzouanakis A, Kreimer DT. Overview of improving tolerance of long-term mechanical ventilation. *Crit Care Clin* 1994; 10: 845–866.

117. Soo Hoo GW, Santiago S, Williams AJ. Nasal mechanical ventilation for hypercapnic respiratory failure in chronic obstructive pulmonary disease: determinants of success and failure. *Crit Care Med* 1994; 22: 1253–1261.

118. Kacmarek RM. NIPPV: patient-ventilator synchrony, the difference between success and failure? *Intensive Care Med* 1999; 25: 645–647.

119. Kacmarek RM. Noninvasive positive-pressure ventilation:the little things do make the difference!. *Respir Care* 2003; 48: 919–921.

120. Vitacca M, Rubini F, Foglio K, Scalvini S, Nava S, Ambrosino N. Non-invasive modalities of positive pressure ventilation improve the outcome of acute exacerbations in COLD patients. *Intensive Care Med* 1993; 19: 450–455.

121. Scala R, Naldi M. Ventilators for noninvasive ventilation to treat acute respiratory failure. *Respir Care* 2008; 53: 1054–1080.

122. Branson RD, Chatburn RL. Technical description and classification of modes of ventilator operation. *Respir Care* 1992; 37: 1026–1044.

123. Sanders M, Kern N. Obstructive sleep apnea treated by indepently adjusted inspiratory and expiratory positive airway pressures *via* nasal mask. Physiologic and clinical implications. *Chest* 1990; 98: 317–324.

124. Mehta S, McCool FD, Hill NS. Leak compensation in positive pressure ventilators: a lung model study. *Eur Respir J* 2001; 17: 259–267.

125. Vitacca M, Barbano L, D'Anna S, Porta R, Bianchi L, Ambrosino N. Comparison of five bilevel pressure ventilators in patients with chronic ventilatory failure: a physiologic study. *Chest* 2002; 122: 2105–2114.

126. Lofaso F, Brochard L, Hang T, Lorino H, Harf A, Isabey D. Home versus intensive care pressure support devices. Experimental and clinical comparison. *Am J Respir Crit Care Med* 1996; 153: 1591–1599.

127. Tassaux D, Strasser S, Fonseca S, Dalmas E, Jolliet P. Comparative bench study of triggering, pressurization, and cycling between the home ventilator VPAP II and three ICU ventilators. *Intensive Care Med* 2002; 28: 1254–1261.

128. Ferguson GT, Gilmartin M. CO_2 rebreathing during BiPAP ventilatory assistance. *Am J Respir Crit Care Med* 1995; 151: 1126–1135.

129. Lofaso F, Brochard L, Touchard D, Hang T, Harf A, Isabey D. Evaluation of carbon dioxyde rebreathing during pressure support ventilationwith airway management system (BiPAP) devices. *Chest* 1995; 108: 772–778.

130. Vignaux L, Tassaux D, Jolliet P. Performance of noninvasive ventilation modes on ICU ventilators during pressure support: a bench model study. *Intensive Care Med* 2007; 33: 1444–1451.

131. Carlucci A, Delmastro M, Rubini F, Fracchia C, Nava S. Changes in the practice of non-invasive ventilation in treating COPD patients over 8 years. *Intensive Care Med* 2003; 29: 419–425.

132. Demoule A, Girou E, Richard JC, Taille S, Brochard L. Increased use of noninvasive ventilation in French intensive care units. *Intensive Care Med* 2006; 32: 1747–1755.

133. Windisch W, Dreher M, Storre JH, Sorichter S. Nocturnal non-invasive positive pressure ventilation: physiological effects on spontaneous breathing. *Respir Physiol Neurobiol* 2006; 150: 251–260.

134. Ambrosino N, Vagheggini G. Noninvasive positive pressure ventilation in the acute care setting: where are we? *Eur Respir J* 2008; 31: 874–886.

135. Bunburaphong T, Imanaka H, Nishimura M, Hess D, Kacmarek RM. Performance characteristics of bilevel pressure ventilators: a lung model study. *Chest* 1997; 111: 1050–1060.

136. Richard JC, Carlucci A, Breton L, *et al.* Bench testing of pressure support ventilation with three different generations of ventilators. *Intensive Care Med* 2002; 28: 1049–1057.

137. Chatmongkolchart S, Williams P, Hess DR, Kacmarek RM. Evaluation of inspiratory rise time and inspiration termination criteria in new-generation mechanical ventilators: a lung model study. *Respir Care* 2001; 46: 666–677.

138. Prinianakis G, Delmastro M, Carlucci A, Ceriana P, Nava S. Effect of varying the pressurisation rate during noninvasive pressure support ventilation. *Eur Respir J* 2004; 23: 314–320.

139. Younes M, Kun J, Masiowski B, Webster K, Roberts D. A method for noninvasive determination of inspiratory resistance during proportional assist ventilation. *Am J Respir Crit Care Med* 2001; 163: 829–839.

140. Gay PC, Hess DR, Hill NS. Noninvasive proportional assist ventilation for acute respiratory insufficiency. Comparison with pressure support ventilation. *Am J Respir Crit Care Med* 2001; 164: 1606–1611.

141. Wysocki M, Richard JC, Meshaka P. Noninvasive proportional assist ventilation compared with noninvasive pressure support ventilation in hypercapnic acute respiratory failure. *Crit Care Med* 2002; 30: 323–329.

142. Hotchkiss JR, Adams AB, Dries DJ, Marini JJ, Crooke PS. Dynamic behavior during noninvasive ventilation: chaotic support? *Am J Respir Crit Care Med* 2001; 163: 374–378.

143. Branson RD. Dual control modes, closed loop ventilation, handguns, and tequila. *Respir Care* 2001; 46: 232–233.

144. Jaber S, Delay JM, Matecki S, Sebbane M, Eledjam JJ, Brochard L. Volume-guaranteed pressure-support ventilation facing acute changes in ventilatory demand. *Intensive Care Med* 2005; 31: 1181–1188.

145. Parthasarathy S, Tobin MJ. Effect of ventilator mode on sleep quality in critically ill patients. *Am J Respir Crit Care Med* 2002; 166: 1423–1429.

146. Devlin JW, Nava S, Fong JJ, Bahhady I, Hill NS. Survey of sedation practices during noninvasive positive-pressure ventilation to treat acute respiratory failure. *Crit Care Med* 2007; 35: 2298–2302.

147. Criner GJ, Travaline JM, Brennan KJ, Kreimer DT. Efficacy of a new full face mask for noninvasive positive pressure ventilation. *Chest* 1994; 106: 1109–1115.

148. Kwok H, McCormack J, Cece R, Houtchens J, Hill NS. Controlled trial of oronasal versus nasal mask ventilation in the treatment of acute respiratory failure. *Crit Care Med* 2003; 31: 468–473.

149. Hess DR. The mask for noninvasive ventilation: principles of design and effects on aerosol delivery. *J Aerosol Med* 2007; 20: Suppl. 1, S85–98.

150. Antonelli M, Conti G, Pelosi P, *et al.* New treatment of acute hypoxemic respiratory failure: noninvasive pressure support ventilation delivered by helmet--a pilot controlled trial. *Crit Care Med* 2002; 30: 602–608.

151. Navalesi P, Costa R, Ceriana P, *et al.* Non-invasive ventilation in chronic obstructive pulmonary disease patients: helmet versus facial mask. *Intensive Care Med* 2007; 33: 74–81.

152. Schonhofer B, Sortor-Leger S. Equipment needs for noninvasive mechanical ventilation. *Eur Respir J* 2002; 20: 1029–1036.

153. Schneider E, Duale C, Vaille JL, *et al.* Comparison of tolerance of facemask vs. mouthpiece for non-invasive ventilation. *Anaesthesia* 2006; 61: 20–23.

Statements of interest

N. Ambrosino received reimbursement, fee and/or funds from: AstraZeneca; GSK, Boehringer-Ingelheim; Novartis; Pfizer; Menarini; Vivisol. *(Author of Introduction, and Chapters 2 and 18)*

N. Amiot. None declared. *(Author of Chapter 4)*

L. Arguad. None declared. *(Author of Chapter 28)*

G. Aubertin. None declared. *(Author of Chapter 19)*

J.C. Borel has received a research grant from Covidien for NIV in obesity hypoventilation syndrome. In addition, J.C. Borel has also received a research grant from AIROX, a subsidiary of Covidien, for NIV and exercise. *(Author of Chapter 24)*

L. Brochard has received research grants from: Drägen for studies on SmartCare®; from Respironics for studies on NIV; from Genereal Electrics Healthcare Systems and from MAQUET for clinical trials. *(Author of Chapter 11)*

N. Carpenè. None declared. *(Author of Chapter 18)*

E. Clini has received an unrestricted research grant (Project N° 21 of the Research Program 2005/2006) from the Italian Association of Pulmonologist (AIPO). *(Author of Chapter 26)*

A. Corrado received a bursary from Vivisol in 2007 and 2008. *(Author of Chapter 3)*

E. Crisafulli. None declared. *(Author of Chapter 26)*

A. Cuvelier. None declared. *(Author of Chapters 4 and 14)*

N. Delvau received a fund from Brussels City for study physiotherapy in NIV application during 2005–2006. *(Author of Chapter 9)*

M. Dreher has received speaking fees from: Drager Medical (Germany); Weinmann Medical (Germany); Vital Aire Medical (Germany); and Boehringer Ingelheim (Germany). M. Dreher has been reimbursed from local provider of home ventilators Werner an Muller Medizintechnik (Germany) for attending the annual German conferences on home mechanical ventilation in 2003, 2005, 2006 and 2007. M. Dreher states that none of the discussed issues in the submitted work was dependent on or influenced by support funding. *(Author of Chapter 16)*

M.W. Elliott. None declared. *(Author of Chapters 6 and 13)*

J. Escarrabill. None declared. *(Author of Chapter 25)*

L.M. Fabbri. None declared. *(Author of Chapter 26)*

B. Fauroux. None declared. *(Author of Chapter 19)*

M. Ferrer. None declared. *(Author of Chapter 5)*

P. Frigerio. None declared. *(Author of Chapter 23)*

D. Georgopoulos. None declared. *(Author of Chapter 2)*

M. Gherardi. None declared. *(Author of Chapter 18)*

C. Girault received a reimbursement for attending a symposium, received fees for a workshop and logistics support for clinical research from Respironics (France). *(Author of Chapter 10)*

J. Goldring. None declared. *(Author of Chapter 27)*

M. Gonçalves. None declared. *(Author of Chapter 4)*

A. Gray. None declared. *(Author of Chapter 6)*

C. Gregoretti has received a consultant fee from Koo Company and travel reimbursment to the ERS congress was funded by Vivisol. *(Author of Chapter 23)*

Y.F. Guo. None declared. *(Author of Chapter 17)*

G. Hilbert. None declared. *(Author of Chapter 7)*

J-P. Janssens. None declared. *(Author of Chapters 17, 21 and 24)*

P. Jolliet has received funding for research projects in the form of unrestricted grants over the past three years from ResMed and Draeger. *(Author of Chapter 21)*

M. Klimathianaki. None declared. *(Author of Chapter 1)*

B. Lamia. None declared. *(Author of Chapter 4)*

M. Latham. None declared. *(Author of Chapter 13)*

P. Lévy has received consulting fees from Covidien for obesity hypoventilation syndrome. In addition, travel expenses have been reimbursed by Weinmann, ResMed, Respironics and Covidien. *(Author of Chapter 24)*

F. Lofaso. None declared. *(Author of Chapter 19)*

A. Lyazidi. None declared. *(Author of Chapter 11)*

S. Maggiore. None declared. *(Author of Chapter 12)*

G. Mercurio. None declared. *(Author of Chapter 12)*

S.D.W. Miller. None declared. *(Author of Chapter 13)*

L.C. Molano. None declared. *(Author of Chapters 4 and 14)*

M. Moretti. None declared. *(Author of Chapter 26)*

J-F Muir. None declared *(Author of Introduction, and Chapters 4 and 14)*

S. Nava has received reimbursement for symposiums from: Draefer-Fiscker; Paykel; Respironics; BREAS; and ResSMed. He has received speaking fees from: ReSMed and Respironics. He also received funds for research from Fyscrer, Payrel, ReSMed and Respironics and received funds for a member of staff from Actelion. *(Author of Chapter 20)*

P. Navalesi has received a fee for lectures from Airliquide and ResMED, and a travel grant for an ERS Congress from Vivisol. In addition, the author has received: one ICU ventilator, PC, data acquisition software for research purposes from Maquet Critical Care; one ICU ventilator for research purposes from General Electrics; other equipment from Vivisol; one PhD student financed by Covidien and a second PhD student funded by General Electrics. *(Author of Chapter 23)*

O. Nørregaard. None declared. *(Author of Chapter 8)*

J-L. Pépin received research grants from Respironics for NIV for COPD patients, and from ResMed for NIV in obesity hypoventilation syndrome. J-L. Pépin
has also received a consulting fee from COVIDEN for obesity hypoventilation syndrome. In addition, the author has received speaking fees from Respironics for NIV in COPD patients. Travel expenses have also been reimbursed by ResMed, Respironics and COVIDIEN. *(Author of Chapter 17 and 24)*

G. Prinianakis. None declared. *(Author of Chapter 1)*

D. Robert. None declared. *(Author of Chapter 28)*

J. Roeseler. None declared. *(Author of Chapter 9)*

R. Scala. None declared. *(Author of Chapter 20)*

D. Schlosshan. None declared. *(Author of Chapter 6)*

B. Schonhofer. None declared. *(Author of Chapter 22)*

A.K. Simonds has received research grants from ResMed Co. and Breas Medical. *(Author of Introduction and Chapter 15)*

S. Spencer. None declared. *(Author of Chapter 9)*

J.H. Storre has received speaking fees by Werner Müller Medizintechnik. Travel funding for international research congresses was supplied from Respironics International, Respironics (Germany) and Werner und Muller Medizintechnik. The author states that none of the discussed issues in the submitted manuscript were dependent on or influenced by support and funding. *(Author of Chapter 22)*

R. Tamisier. None declared. *(Author of Chapter 24)*

F. Templier. None declared. *(Author of Chapter 9)*

A. Thille. None declared. *(Author of Chapter 11)*

F. Thys. None declared. *(Author of Chapter 9)*

A. Torres. None declared. *(Author of Chapter 5)*

F. Vargas. None declared. *(Author of Chapter 11)*

F. Verschuren. None declared. *(Author of Chapter 9)*

L. Vignaux. None declared. *(Author of Chapter 21)*

C. Volpe. None declared. *(Author of Chapter 12)*

W. Wedzicha. None declared. *(Author of Chapter 27)*

J.C. Winck has received: a reimbursment for attending a sleep congress, a fee for speaking at an NIV meeting, and a fee for organising a postgraduate course on NIV, all from Respironics. *(Author of Chapter 3)*

W. Windisch was reimbursed by BREAS Medical AB (Sweden) for attending the annual ERS conferences between 2003 and 2005. W. Windisch has also been reimbursed from the local provider of home ventilators Werner and Muller Medizintechnik (Germany) for attending the annual German conferences on home mechanical ventilation between 2003 and 2007. W. Windisch received speaking fees from Dräger Medical (Germany); Heinen und Lowenstein (Germany); Werner und Müller Modizintechnik (Germany); VitalAire (Germany) Respironics Inc., (US); and Weinmann (Germany). W. Windisch is the leader of a research group, which has received open research grants from Respironics Inc. (US), Heinen and Lowenstein (Germany), SenTec AG (Switzerland), Werner und Müller Medizintechnik (Germany), and BREAS medical AB (Sweden). *(Author of Chapter 16)*

Previously published in the European Respiratory Monograph Series:

Monographs may be purchased from:

Publications Sales Department, Maney Publishing, Suite 1C, Joseph's Well, Hanover Walk, Leeds, LS3 1AB, UK.

Tel: 44 (0)113 2432800; Fax: 44 (0)113 3868178; E-mail: books@maney.co.uk; www.maney.co.uk

Customers in the Americas should contact: Old City Publishing Inc., 628 North 2nd Street, Philadelphia PA 19123, USA. Tel: 1 215 925 4390; Fax: 1 215 925 4371; E-mail: info@oldcitypublishing.com